Dosage Calculations

A Multi-Method Approach

Second Edition

Anthony Patrick Giangrasso, PhD
Professor of Mathematics
LaGuardia Community College
Long Island City, NY

Dolores Donahue Shrimpton, MA, RN
Professor Emerita of Nursing
Department of Nursing
Kingsborough Community College
Brooklyn, NY

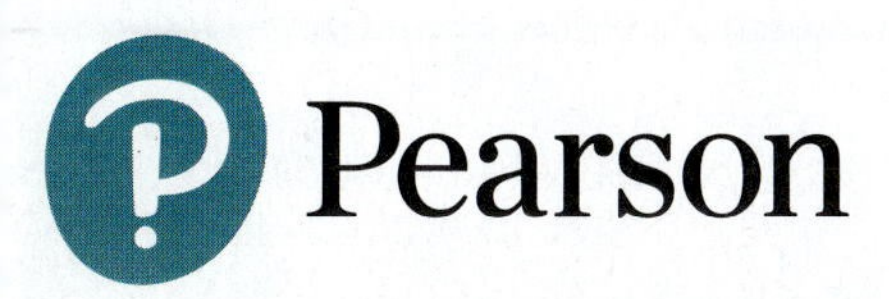
Pearson

Vice President, Health Science: Julie Levin Alexander
Nursing Director: Katrin Beacom
Executive Portfolio Manager: Lisa Rahn
Content Producer: Michael Giacobbe
Portfolio Management Assistant: Taylor Scuglik
Director of Marketing: David Gesell
Executive Product Marketing Manager: Christopher Barry
Senior Field Marketing Manager: Brittany Hammond
Vice President, Production: Paul DeLuca
Project Manager: Prathiba Rajagopal, SPi Global
Manufacturing Manager: Maura Zaldivar-Garcia

Library of Congress Cataloging-in-Publication Data

Names: Giangrasso, Anthony Patrick, author. | Shrimpton, Dolores M., author.
Title: Dosage calculations : a multi-method approach / Anthony Patrick Giangrasso, Dolores Donahue Shrimpton.
Description: Second edition. | New York, NY : Pearson, 2017. | Includes index.
Identifiers: LCCN 2017026617 | ISBN 9780134624679 | ISBN 013462467X
Subjects: | MESH: Drug Dosage Calculations | Pharmaceutical Preparations–administration & dosage | Nurses' Instruction | Problems and Exercises
Classification: LCC RS57 | NLM QV 18.2 | DDC 615.1/9–dc23 LC record available at https://lccn.loc.gov/2017026617

1 17

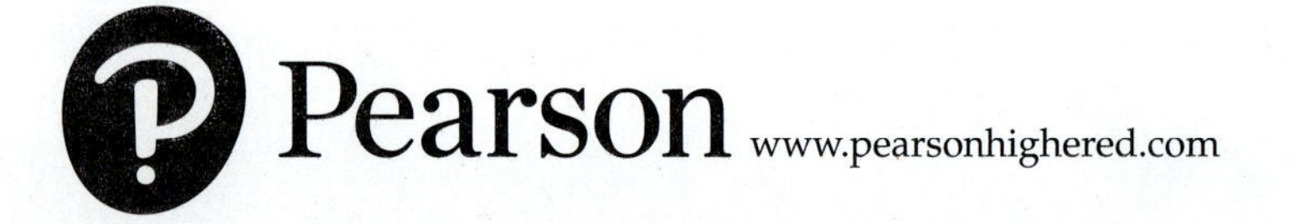

ISBN 10: 0-13-462467-X
ISBN 13: 978-0-13-462467-9

About the Authors

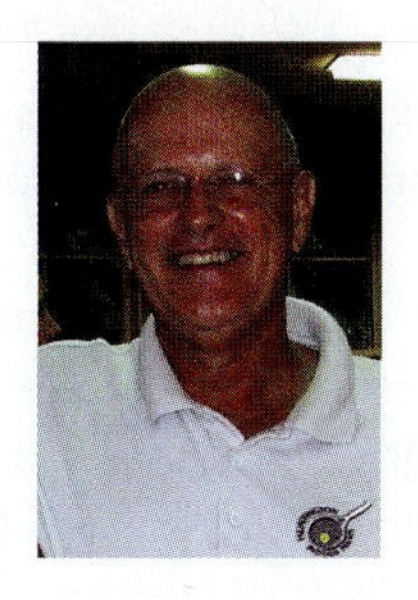

Anthony Giangrasso was born and raised in Maspeth, New York. He attended Rice High School on a scholarship and in his senior year was named in an annual citywide contest by the *New York Journal-American* newspaper as New York City's most outstanding high school scholar-athlete. He was also awarded a full-tuition scholarship to Iona College, from which he obtained a BA in mathematics, magna cum laude, ranking sixth in his graduating class of approximately 600 students.

Anthony began his teaching career as a fifth-grade teacher in Manhattan, as a member of the Christian Brothers of Ireland, and taught high school mathematics and physics in Harlem and Newark, New Jersey. He holds an MS and PhD from New York University and has taught at all levels from elementary through graduate school. He is currently teaching at Adelphi University and LaGuardia Community College, where he was chairman of the mathematics department. He has authored nine college textbooks through twenty-six editions.

Anthony's community service has included membership on the boards of directors of the *Polish-American Museum Foundation, Catholic Adoptive Parents Association,* and *Family Focus Adoptive Services.* He was the *founding Chairman of the Board* of the *Italian-American Legal Defense and Higher Education Fund, Inc.*, and the *president of the Italian-American Faculty Association of the City University of New York*—in the latter capacity he signed the first discrimination complaint filed with the *United States Department of Labor* in which Italian-Americans were recognized as a "class." This class-action complaint eventually resulted in the threat of twenty separate lawsuits by the U.S. Department of Labor individually against each of the branches of CUNY. The complaint was later dropped as part of a settlement of a separate suit in which CUNY was forced to defend itself in federal court before Judge Constance Baker Motley where Anthony was the first witness. As part of the ensuing settlement of that case, CUNY was ordered to pay all legal fees and correct some past injustices.

He and his wife, Susan, are proud parents of Anthony, Michael, and Jennifer—and grandparents of Calvin, Jackson, Isabel, and Emilia. He enjoys tennis and twice has been ranked #1 for his age group in the Eastern Section by the *United States Tennis Association*.

Dedication

For my lovely wife, Susan. Thanks for your love and support for over four decades.

—Anthony Giangrasso

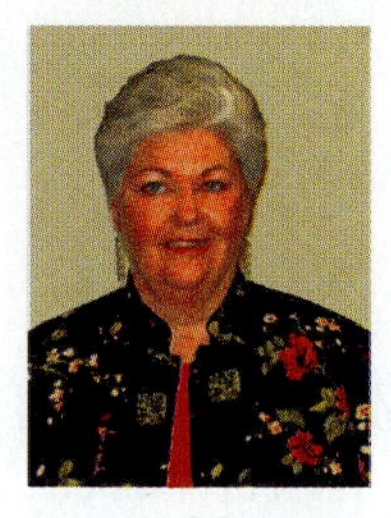

Dolores Donahue Shrimpton is Professor emerita of Nursing at Kingsborough Community College (CUNY), where she was Chairperson of the department for thirteen years. She received a diploma in nursing from Kings Country Hospital Center School of Nursing, a BS from C.W. Post College, an MA in nursing administration from New York University, and a post-Master's certificate in nursing education from Adelphi University. She is a member of the Upsilon and Mu Upilson Chapters of Sigma Theta Tau. She has taught a wide variety of courses in practical nursing, diploma, and associate degree nursing programs. She has authored three college nursing books through eight editions.

Dolores has held many leadership positions in nursing, including Board Member, Vice-President, and President of the NYS Associate Degree Nursing Council. She was the Co-Chair of the CUNY Nursing Discipline Council, and Member of the Board of Directors and Co-President of the Brooklyn Nursing Partnership. She has served on a number of Advisory Boards of LPN, associate degree, and baccalaureate degree nursing programs. She is a recipient of the Presidential Award in Nursing Leadership from the Nurses Association of Long Island (NACLI) as well as of the Mu Upsilon award for Excellence in Nursing Education and Excellence in Nursing Leadership. She has also been recognized for her commitment to nursing by the Brooklyn Nursing Partnership.

Dolores lives in Rockville Centre, New York, and enjoys cooking and spending time with her grandchildren, Brooke Elizabeth, Paige Dolores, Jack Paul, and their parents, Kim and Shawn. She also enjoys traveling and spending time with friends and family in Harwich Port, Cape Cod, Massachusetts.

Dedication

To my four amazing brothers: Frank, Al, Don, and Den. No one could find a more loving, dependable, generous, caring or considerate group as the "Donahue Boys." The Donahue's have always been happy for one another when things go well, and are there for each other when things don't. I love you all and am so fortunate that we are family. Love also to my "sister by marriage" Martina.

—Dolores Donahue Shrimpton

Preface

Safe administration of medication starts with equipping nursing students with the requisite math skills. Recent studies show that medical errors result in close to 400,000 patient deaths per year (MacDonald, 2013), 35% of which are due to medication errors (James, 2013). Worryingly, approximately 75% of novices commit medication errors (Smith & Crawford, 2003). Calculating dosages is a crucial skill, as the aforementioned statistics attest.

Many nursing students dread math. Teaching dosage calculations to an audience with a fear of the subject is daunting. Similarly, an audience with a preconceived notion that "math is difficult" inhibits learning. Students need accessible resources that provide easy-to-understand instructions and explanations, problem examples, and practice opportunities to progress their learning. The second edition of *Dosage Calculation: A Multi-Method Approach coupled with MyLab Nursing for Dosage Calculations* helps students develop dosage calculation skills and transfer those skills to administer medications safely in a clinical environment.

Dosage Calculations explains the standard methods—dimensional analysis, formula, ratio and proportion—and includes illustrated examples with worked-out solutions. Examples of solved problems appear side-by-side, which allows readers to compare methods easily. Instructors can teach their preferred method or multiple methods while allowing students to select the option that suits their learning style.

Dosage Calculation does not merely cover math skills; it provides a crucial introduction to the professional context of safe drug administration. Not only does this resource emphasize calculation skills and their rationales, but its focus on safety, accuracy, and professionalism communicate the nurses' and health professionals' role in administering medication safely.

Organization of Content

Divided into four units, *Dosage Calculation* progresses from simple math topics to more complex ones. Based on the text's organization, *MyLab Nursing for Dosage Calculations* features practice activities and assessment opportunities to support and reinforce content.

Unit	Content
1: Basic Calculation Skills and Introduction to Medication Administration	Chapter 1 reviews basic math skills. Chapter 2 presents the medication administration process. Chapter 3 introduces the dimensional analysis and ratio & proportion methods in small increments, step-by-step.
2: Systems of Measurement	Chapters 4 and 5 feature metric and household measurement systems needed to interpret medication orders and calculate dosages, with students learning to convert between and within measurement systems.
3: Oral and Parenteral Medications	Chapter 6 introduces oral drug dosage calculations using the formula method and includes dosages based on patient size. Chapter 7 discusses syringes and insulin. Chapter 8 covers solutions. Chapter 9 educates about parenteral medications and heparin.
Unit 4: Infusions and Pediatric Dosages	Chapters 10 and 11 teach how to calculate intravenous and enteral dosage rates and flow rates, including titrating IV medications. Chapter 12 explains pediatric dosages and daily fluid needs.

New Features

- *MyLab Nursing for Dosage Calculations* provides diagnostic testing and practice opportunities with hundreds of questions. (Please speak to your Pearson Health Sciences Specialist about package options.)
- Highlights safety in medication administration per the Joint Commission National Patient Safety Goals, the Institute for Safe Medical Practice, and the CDC One and Only Campaign.
- Updates drug labels and examples for both trade and generic drug names.
- Expands coverage of titration tables and IV push.
- Provides latest information on insulin administration and calculations.
- Enhances coverage of heparin administration and calculations.
- Features schematic diagrams for computations concerning solutions and IV calculations.
- Showcases new illustrated examples.

Hallmark Features

- Enhances all illustrated examples with worked-out solutions, showing each step in the process.
- Solves many examples using two different methods, side-by-side, allowing students to compare easily.
- Reinforces skills through frequent practice opportunities, offering more than 1,000 problems for students to solve.
- Presents actual drug labels, syringes, drug package inserts, prescriptions, and medication administration records (MARs).
- Provides Keystroke Sequences in Chapter 1, enabling students to check their calculations.
- Includes answers in Appendix A to Try These for Practice, Exercises, and Cumulative Review questions, making it easy for students to double check their work. (Note: the Instructor's Resource Manual provides answers to Additional Exercises.)

Student Resources

MyLab Nursing for Dosage Calculations

MyLab Nursing for Dosage Calculations enhances learning by providing diagnostic quizzing, practice exercises, and chapter assessments. Ask your Pearson Health Science Specialist for a demonstration, and to learn about packaging this powerful resource with the printed text.

- Mirrors *Dosage Calculation: A Multi-Method Approach's* organization.
- Helps students identify gaps in their knowledge by providing over 200 pre- and post-test diagnostic questions.
- Features 425 topic specific multiple choice practice exercises.
- Illustrates select questions with drug labels, package inserts, and syringe images.
- Offers automatic feedback with explanations to support learning.
- Includes access to eText of *Dosage Calculation: A Multi-Method Approach.*

Instructor Resources

Locate text-specific Instructor Resources in the *MyLab Nursing for Dosage Calculations* resource that can accompany *Dosage Calculation: A Multi-Method Approach* (see Instructor Tools section), and Pearson's Instructor Resource Center. Login credentials are required to access these ancillaries. Speak to your Pearson Health Sciences Specialist for assistance.

Instructor's Resource Manual provides an overview, instructor notes, answers to Additional Exercises in the book, exam questions and answers for every chapter.

Lecture Note PowerPoint features slides with instructions and worked examples to assist with classroom and online learning.

Classroom Response System PowerPoint offers questions with multiple choice answers to be employed with clickers.

Image Bank showcases all art and images, including examples, drug labels, prescriptions, and more.

Test Item File contains close to 400 questions that instructors can use to create tests. (Note: these questions are the same ones in the Computerized Test Bank.)

Computerized Test Bank facilitates test and exam creation easily, and includes close to 400 questions. (Note: these questions are the same ones in the Test Item File.)

Acknowledgments

Our special thanks to the nursing and mathematics faculty and the students at LaGuardia Community College and Kingsborough Community College. Also, a special thank you to our portfolio manager, Lisa Rahn, and content producer, Michael Giacobbe, and to the marketing teams at Pearson.

Thank you also to the following manufacturers for supplying labels and art for this resource:

Courtesy of Abbott Laboratories

Courtesy of AbbVie

Actavis Pharma, Inc.

B. Braun Medical Inc.

Eisai Inc.

Endo Pharmaceuticals Inc.

Meda Pharmaceuticals

Courtesy of Novartis AG

Courtesy of Pfizer, Inc.

Teva North America

Reviewers

Paul Ache, III
Kutztown University of PA

Michele Bach, MS, MS
Professor
Kansas City Kansas Community College
Kansas City, Kansas

Eileen Costello
Dean, School of Health Professions, Public Service Programs and Social Services
Mount Wachusett Community College

Jennifer Ellis, DNP, CNE
University of Cincinnati, Blue Ash College

Dr. James E. Hodge, EdD.
University of Charleston, WV

Carol A Penrosa MS, RN
Instructor
Associate Degree Nursing
Southeast Community College
Lincoln, NE

Sonia Rudolph, MSN, APRN, FNP-BC
Jefferson Community & Technical College

Jason Shea
Director of Mathematics
Goodwin College

Gladdi Tomlinson, RN, MSN
Professor of Nursing
Harrisburg Area Community College

Linda Walter
Northwestern Michigan College

Technical Reviewers

Katherine Poser, RN BScN MNEd
Professor of Nursing
St Lawrence College School of Baccalaureate Nursing
Kingston, ON

Jeffrey N. McCulloch
Consultant
Retired Mathematics Instructor
Wilmington, NC

Learn to Calculate Dosages Safely and Accurately!

The Ease of Learning Dosage Calculations

Dosage Calculations provides the ease of learning the dimensional analysis, ratio & proportion, and formula methods of calculation with a building-block approach of the basics.

The Diagnostic Test of Arithmetic helps students rediscover their understanding of basic math concepts and guides them in identifying areas for review.

Name: ______________________ Date: ______________

Diagnostic Test of Arithmetic

The following Diagnostic Test illustrates *all* the arithmetic skills needed to do the computations in this textbook. Take the test and compare your answers with the answers found in Appendix A. If you discover areas of weakness, carefully review the relevant review materials in this chapter so that you will be mathematically prepared for the rest of the textbook.

1. Write 0.375 as a fraction in lowest terms. ________
2. Write $\frac{28{,}500}{100{,}000}$ as a decimal number. ________
3. Round off 6.492 to the nearest tenth. ________
4. Write $\frac{5}{6}$ as a decimal number rounded off to the nearest hundredth. ________
5. Simplify $\frac{0.63}{0.2}$ to a decimal number rounded off to the nearest tenth. ________
6. $0.038 \times 100 =$ ________
7. $4.26 \times 0.015 =$ ________
8. $55 \div 0.11 =$ ________
9. $90 \times \frac{1}{300} \times \frac{20}{3} =$ ________
10. Write $5\frac{3}{4} \div 23$ as a fraction and as a decimal number. ________
11. Write $\frac{7}{100} \div \frac{3}{100}$ as a mixed number. ________
12. Write $\frac{\frac{4}{5}}{20}$ as a simple fraction in lowest terms. ________

Example 10.16

Order: ***For every 100 mL of urine output, replace with 40 mL of water via PEG tube q4h.*** **The client's urine output is 300 *mL*. What is the replacement volume?**

DIMENSIONAL ANALYSIS

Think of the problem as:

Output: 300 *mL* (out) [single unit of measurement]

Replacement: 100 *mL* (out)/ 40 *mL* (in) [equivalence]

Input: ? *mL* (in) [single unit of measurement]

In this example, you want to change the single unit of measurement [300 *mL(out)*] to another single unit of measurement [*mL(in)*].

$$300 \, mL(out) = ? \, mL(in)$$

The flow rate provides the equivalence [*100 mL(out)/40 mL(in)*] for the unit fraction.

$$300 \, \cancel{mL(out)} \times \frac{40 \, mL(in)}{100 \, \cancel{mL(out)}} = 120 \, mL(in)$$

RATIO & PROPORTION

Think of the problem as:

100 *mL* (*output*) = 40 *mL* (*input*) [*order*]

300 *mL* (*output*) = *x mL* (*input*) [*client*]

The proportion could be set up as

$$\frac{Out}{In} = \frac{Out'}{In'}$$

Substituting, you get

$$\frac{100 \, mL}{40 \, mL} = \frac{300 \, mL}{x \, mL}$$

$$12{,}000 = 100x$$

$$120 = x$$

So, the replacement volume is 120 *mL*.

So, the replacement volume is *120 mL*.

Learn by Example. Each chapter unfolds basic concepts and skills through completely worked-out questions with solutions.

Example 6.12

The order is *Tikosyn (dofetilide) 0.5 mg PO b.i.d.* Read the label shown in Figure 6.14. Calculate how many capsules of this antiarrythmic drug should be given to the client. Although there are two strengths on the label (*mcg* and *mg*), calculate the problem using microgram strength.

Figure 6.14 Drug label for Tikosyn.

(Reg. trademark of Pfizer Inc. Reproduced with permission.)

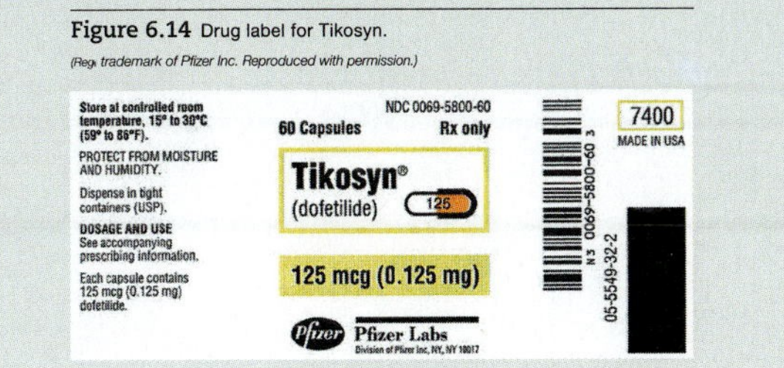

Safe and Accurate Dosage Calculation

Safe and accurate dosage calculation comes from practice and critical thinking.

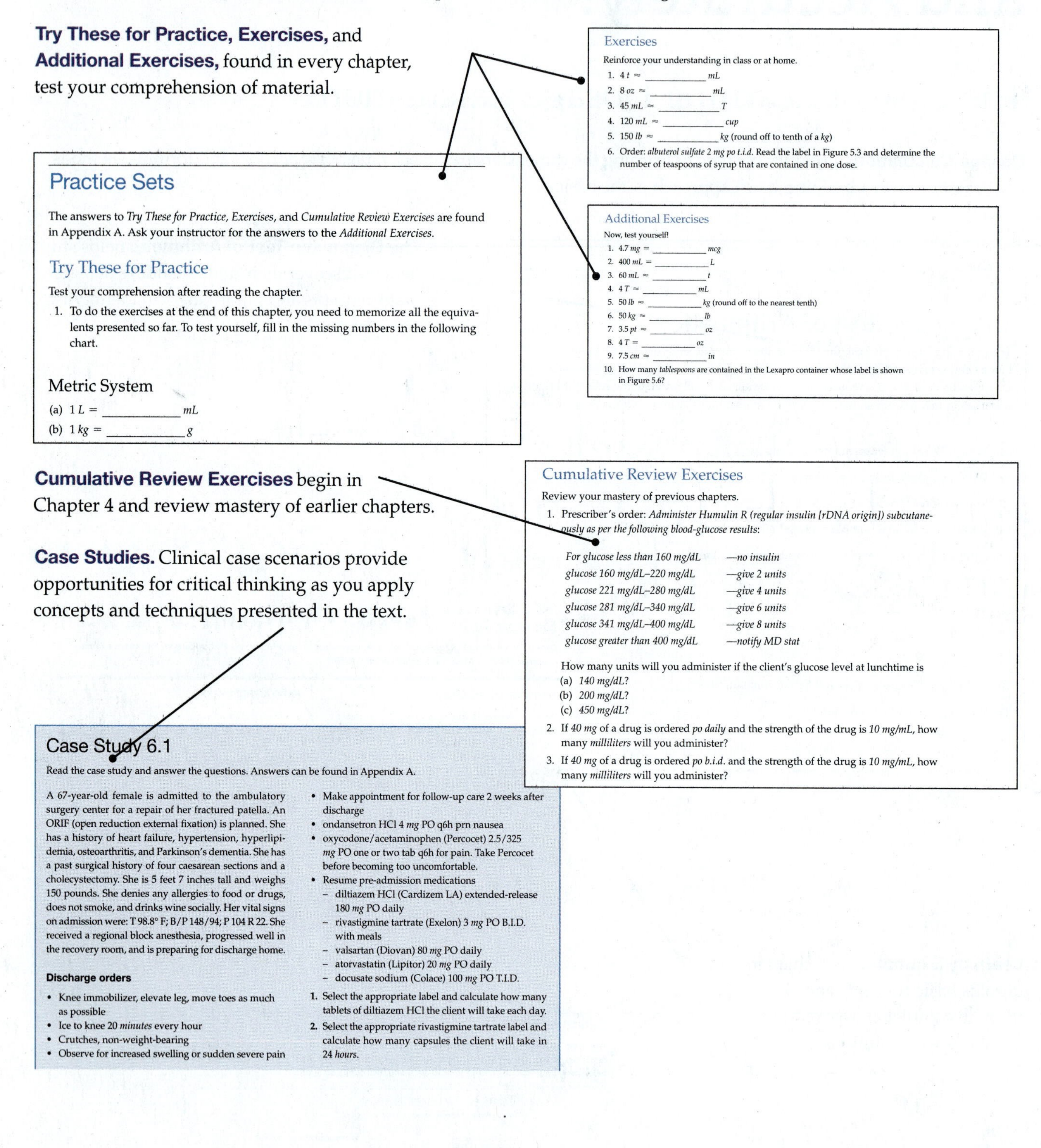

Try These for Practice, Exercises, and **Additional Exercises,** found in every chapter, test your comprehension of material.

Practice Sets

The answers to *Try These for Practice, Exercises,* and *Cumulative Review Exercises* are found in Appendix A. Ask your instructor for the answers to the *Additional Exercises*.

Try These for Practice

Test your comprehension after reading the chapter.

1. To do the exercises at the end of this chapter, you need to memorize all the equivalents presented so far. To test yourself, fill in the missing numbers in the following chart.

Metric System

(a) 1 *L* = ___________ *mL*

(b) 1 *kg* = ___________ *g*

Exercises

Reinforce your understanding in class or at home.

1. 4 *t* ≈ __________ *mL*
2. 8 *oz* ≈ __________ *mL*
3. 45 *mL* ≈ __________ *T*
4. 120 *mL* ≈ __________ *cup*
5. 150 *lb* ≈ __________ *kg* (round off to tenth of a *kg*)
6. Order: *albuterol sulfate 2 mg po t.i.d.* Read the label in Figure 5.3 and determine the number of teaspoons of syrup that are contained in one dose.

Additional Exercises

Now, test yourself!

1. 4.7 *mg* = __________ *mcg*
2. 400 *mL* = __________ *L*
3. 60 *mL* ≈ __________ *t*
4. 4 *T* ≈ __________ *mL*
5. 50 *lb* ≈ __________ *kg* (round off to the nearest tenth)
6. 50 *kg* ≈ __________ *lb*
7. 3.5 *pt* ≈ __________ *oz*
8. 4 *T* = __________ *oz*
9. 7.5 *cm* ≈ __________ *in*
10. How many *tablespoons* are contained in the Lexapro container whose label is shown in Figure 5.6?

Cumulative Review Exercises begin in Chapter 4 and review mastery of earlier chapters.

Cumulative Review Exercises

Review your mastery of previous chapters.

1. Prescriber's order: *Administer Humulin R (regular insulin [rDNA origin]) subcutaneously as per the following blood-glucose results:*

For glucose less than 160 mg/dL	*—no insulin*
glucose 160 mg/dL–220 mg/dL	*—give 2 units*
glucose 221 mg/dL–280 mg/dL	*—give 4 units*
glucose 281 mg/dL–340 mg/dL	*—give 6 units*
glucose 341 mg/dL–400 mg/dL	*—give 8 units*
glucose greater than 400 mg/dL	*—notify MD stat*

   How many units will you administer if the client's glucose level at lunchtime is
   (a) *140 mg/dL?*
   (b) *200 mg/dL?*
   (c) *450 mg/dL?*

2. If *40 mg* of a drug is ordered *po daily* and the strength of the drug is *10 mg/mL*, how many *milliliters* will you administer?
3. If *40 mg* of a drug is ordered *po b.i.d.* and the strength of the drug is *10 mg/mL*, how many *milliliters* will you administer?

Case Studies. Clinical case scenarios provide opportunities for critical thinking as you apply concepts and techniques presented in the text.

Case Study 6.1

Read the case study and answer the questions. Answers can be found in Appendix A.

A 67-year-old female is admitted to the ambulatory surgery center for a repair of her fractured patella. An ORIF (open reduction external fixation) is planned. She has a history of heart failure, hypertension, hyperlipidemia, osteoarthritis, and Parkinson's dementia. She has a past surgical history of four caesarean sections and a cholecystectomy. She is 5 feet 7 inches tall and weighs 150 pounds. She denies any allergies to food or drugs, does not smoke, and drinks wine socially. Her vital signs on admission were: T 98.8° F; B/P 148/94; P 104 R 22. She received a regional block anesthesia, progressed well in the recovery room, and is preparing for discharge home.

Discharge orders

- Knee immobilizer, elevate leg, move toes as much as possible
- Ice to knee 20 *minutes* every hour
- Crutches, non-weight-bearing
- Observe for increased swelling or sudden severe pain
- Make appointment for follow-up care 2 weeks after discharge
- ondansetron HCl 4 *mg* PO q6h prn nausea
- oxycodone/acetaminophen (Percocet) 2.5/325 *mg* PO one or two tab q6h for pain. Take Percocet before becoming too uncomfortable.
- Resume pre-admission medications
  - diltiazem HCl (Cardizem LA) extended-release 180 *mg* PO daily
  - rivastigmine tartrate (Exelon) 3 *mg* PO B.I.D. with meals
  - valsartan (Diovan) 80 *mg* PO daily
  - atorvastatin (Lipitor) 20 *mg* PO daily
  - docusate sodium (Colace) 100 *mg* PO T.I.D.

1. Select the appropriate label and calculate how many tablets of diltiazem HCl the client will take each day.
2. Select the appropriate rivastigmine tartrate label and calculate how many capsules the client will take in 24 *hours*.

ALERT

The calibrations on the 1 *mL* syringe are very small and close together. Use caution when drawing up medication in this syringe.

Notes and **Alerts** highlight concepts and principles for safe medication calculation and administration.

NOTE

The two rings on the stopper are called “top” ring and “bottom” ring because when the syringe is held with the needle facing upward, the “top” ring is above the “bottom” ring.

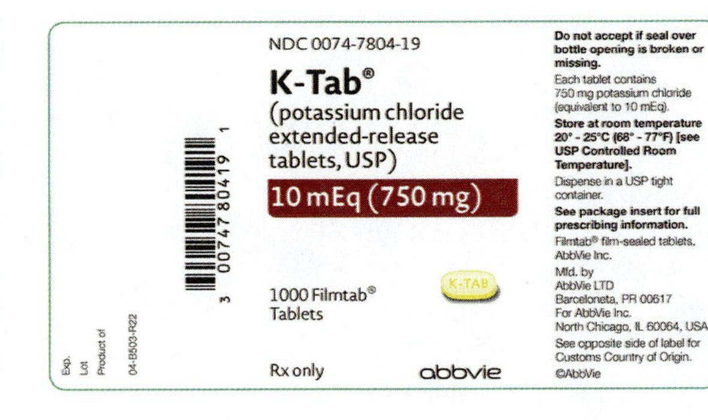

Realistic Illustrations. Real drug labels and realistic syringes aid in identifying and practicing with what you will encounter in actual clinical settings.

Figure 7.3 A sample of commonly used hypodermic syringes (35 *mL*, 12 *mL*, 5 *mL*, 3 *mL*, 1 *mL*, and 0.5 *mL*).

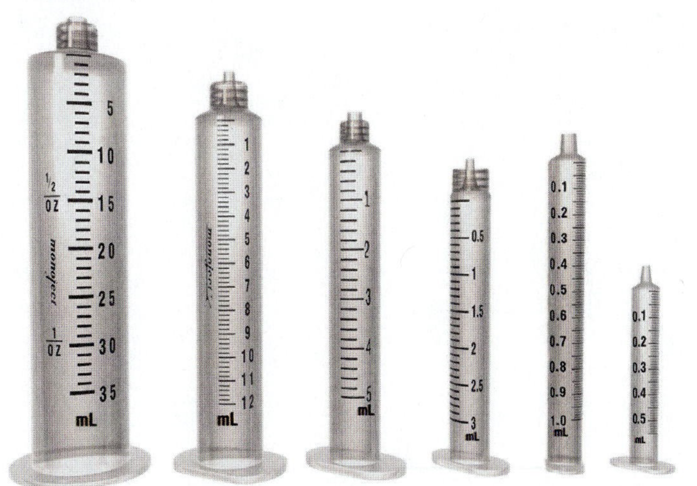

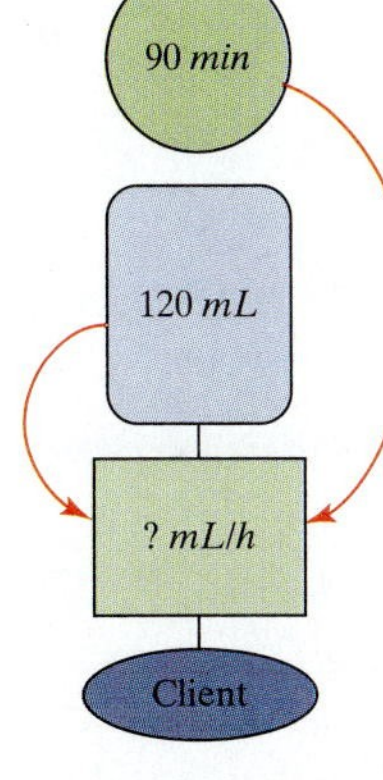

Schematic Diagrams To help students visualize some of the more difficult mathematical concepts involved in solutions and IVs.

Contents

Unit 1

Basic Calculation Skills and Introduction to Medication Administration

Chapter 1

Review of Arithmetic for Dosage Calculations

Learning Outcomes

After completing this chapter, you will be able to

1.1 Reduce and build fractions into equivalent forms.

1.2 Add, subtract, multiply, and divide fractions.

1.3 Simplify complex fractions.

1.4 Convert between decimal numbers and fractions.

1.5 Add, subtract, multiply, and divide decimal numbers.

1.6 Round decimal numbers to a desired number of decimal places.

1.7 Write percentages as decimal numbers and fractions.

1.8 Find the percent of a number and the percent of change.

1.9 Estimate answers.

1.10 Use a calculator to verify answers.

Medical dosage calculations can involve whole numbers, fractions, decimal numbers, and percentages. Your results on the *Diagnostic Test of Arithmetic*, found on the next page, will identify your areas of strength and weakness. You can use this chapter to improve your math skills or simply to review the kinds of calculations you will encounter in this text.

Name: ______________________________ Date: ____________________

Diagnostic Test of Arithmetic

The following Diagnostic Test illustrates *all* the arithmetic skills needed to do the computations in this textbook. Take the test and compare your answers with the answers found in Appendix A. If you discover areas of weakness, carefully review the relevant review materials in this chapter so that you will be mathematically prepared for the rest of the textbook.

1. Write 0.375 as a fraction in lowest terms. ________

2. Write $\frac{28,500}{100,000}$ as a decimal number. ________

3. Round off 6.492 to the nearest tenth. ________

4. Write $\frac{5}{6}$ as a decimal number rounded off to the nearest hundredth. ________

5. Simplify $\frac{0.63}{0.2}$ to a decimal number rounded off to the nearest tenth. ________

6. $0.038 \times 100 =$ ________

7. $4.26 \times 0.015 =$ ________

8. $55 \div 0.11 =$ ________

9. $90 \times \frac{1}{300} \times \frac{20}{3} =$ ________

10. Write $5\frac{3}{4} \div 23$ as a fraction and as a decimal number. ________

11. Write $\frac{7}{100} \div \frac{3}{100}$ as a mixed number. ________

12. Write $\frac{\frac{4}{5}}{20}$ as a simple fraction in lowest terms. ________

13. Write 45% as a fraction in lowest terms. ________

14. Write $2\frac{1}{2}\%$ as a decimal number. ________

15. Write $2\frac{4}{7}$ as an improper fraction. ________

16. 30% of 40 = ________

17. $4.1 + 0.5 + 3 =$ ________

18. $\frac{3}{4} = \frac{?}{8}$ ________

19. Which is larger, 0.4 or 0.21? ________

20. Express the ratio *15 to 20* as a fraction in lowest terms. ________

Decimal Numbers and Fractions

Changing Decimal Numbers to Fractional Form

A decimal number represents a fraction with a denominator of 10; 100; 1,000; and so on. Each decimal number has three parts: the whole-number part, the decimal point, and the fraction part. Table 1.1 shows the names of the decimal positions (places values).

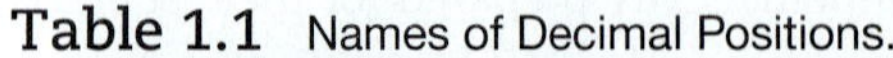

Table 1.1 Names of Decimal Positions.

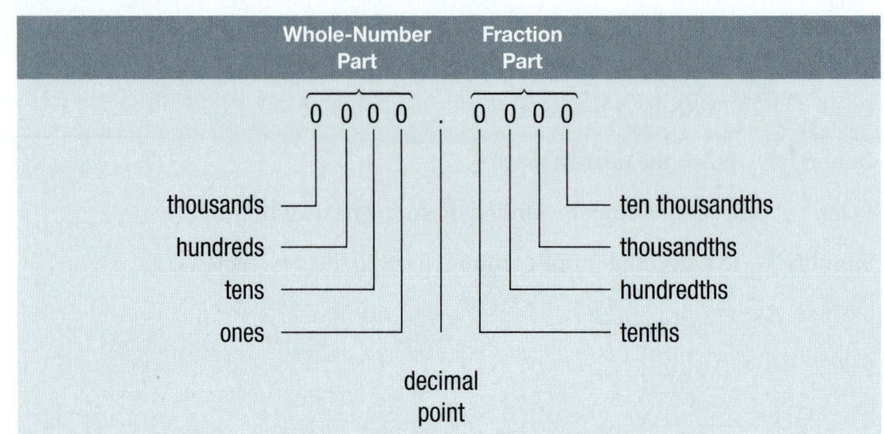

Reading a decimal number will help you write it as a fraction.

Decimal Number	⟶	Read	⟶	Fraction
4.1	⟶	four and one tenth	⟶	$4\frac{1}{10}$
0.3	⟶	three tenths	⟶	$\frac{3}{10}$
6.07	⟶	six and seven hundredths	⟶	$6\frac{7}{100}$
0.231	⟶	two hundred thirty-one thousandths	⟶	$\frac{231}{1,000}$
0.0025	⟶	twenty-five ten thousandths	⟶	$\frac{25}{10,000}$

NOTE

A decimal number that is less than 1 is written with a leading zero—for example, 0.3 and 0.0025.

A number can be written in different forms. A decimal number *less than 1*, such as 0.9, is read as *nine tenths* and also can be written as the *proper fraction* $\frac{9}{10}$. In a **proper fraction,** the **numerator** (the number on the top) of the fraction is smaller than its **denominator** (the number on the bottom).

Mixed Numbers and Improper Fractions

A decimal number *greater than 1*, such as 3.5, is read as *three and five tenths* and can also be written as the *mixed number* $3\frac{5}{10}$ or reduced to lowest terms as $3\frac{1}{2}$. A **mixed number** combines a whole number and a proper fraction. The *mixed number* $3\frac{1}{2}$ can be changed to an *improper fraction* as follows:

$$3\frac{1}{2} = \frac{3 \times 2 + 1}{2} = \frac{7}{2}$$

The numerator of an **improper fraction** is larger than or equal to its denominator.

Any number can be written as a fraction by writing it over 1. For example, 9 can be written as the improper fraction $\frac{9}{1}$.

Calculator

To help avoid medication errors, many healthcare agencies have policies requiring that calculations done by hand be verified with a calculator. "Drop-down" calculators are available on the computer screen to candidates who are taking the National Council Licensure Examination for Registered Nurses (NCLEX-RN) or the National Council Licensure Examination for Practical Nurses (NCLEX-PN). Therefore, it is important to know how to use a calculator.

A basic four-function (addition, subtraction, multiplication, and division), handheld calculator with a square-root key [√] is sufficient to perform most medical dosage calculations. See Figure 1.1.

Figure 1.1 Basic handheld calculator.

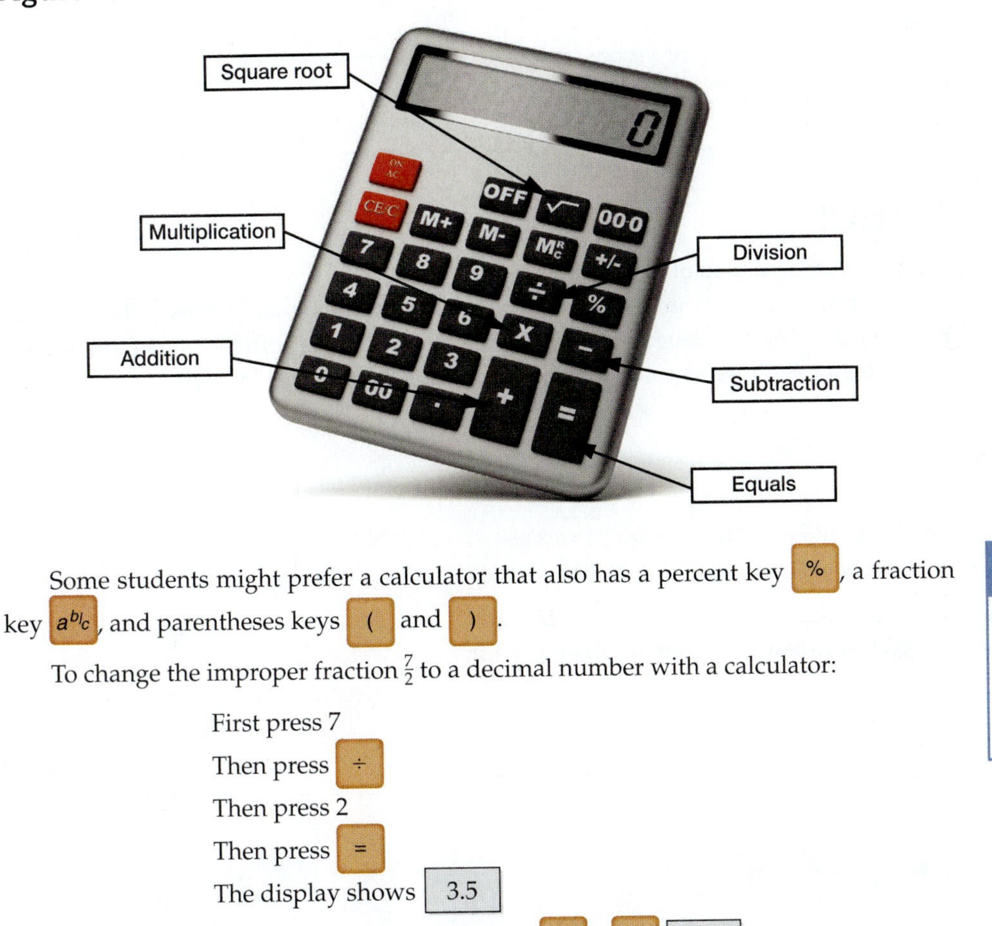

Some students might prefer a calculator that also has a percent key [%], a fraction key [a b/c], and parentheses keys [(] and [)].

To change the improper fraction $\frac{7}{2}$ to a decimal number with a calculator:

First press 7
Then press [÷]
Then press 2
Then press [=]
The display shows [3.5]

This keystroke sequence will be abbreviated as 7 [÷] 2 [=] [3.5]

If the calculator has a fraction key, the mixed-number form of $\frac{7}{2}$ will be obtained by the following keystroke sequence:

7 [a b/c] 2 [=] [$3\frac{1}{2}$]

Throughout this chapter, keystroke sequences are shown for selected examples. The calculator icon, 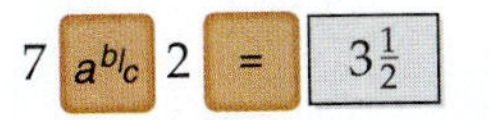, indicates where this occurs.

NOTE

Some calculators use the [Enter] key rather than the [=] key.

NOTE

The keystroke sequences presented in this chapter apply to many calculators. But not all calculators work the same way. If you have a problem, consult the user's manual for your calculator.

Example 1.1

Write 2.25 as a mixed number and as an improper fraction.

The number 2.25 is read *two and twenty-five hundredths* and is written $2\frac{25}{100}$. You can simplify:

$$2\frac{25}{100} = 2\frac{\overset{1}{\cancel{25}}}{\underset{4}{\cancel{100}}} = 2\frac{1}{4} = \frac{2 \times 4 + 1}{4} = \frac{9}{4}$$

So, 2.25 can be written as the mixed number $2\frac{1}{4}$ or as the improper fraction $\frac{9}{4}$

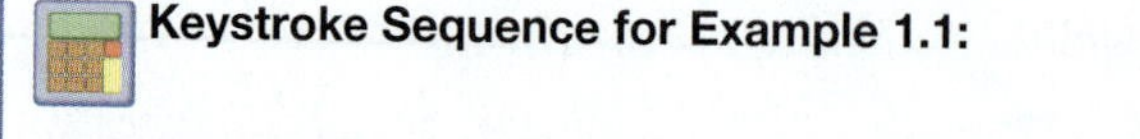

Keystroke Sequence for Example 1.1:

To obtain the simplified mixed number, enter the following keystroke sequence.

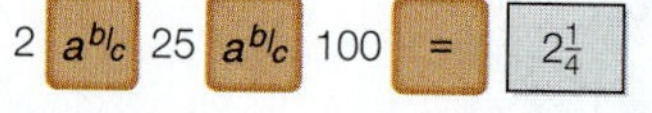

2 $a^{b}/_{c}$ 25 $a^{b}/_{c}$ 100 = $2\frac{1}{4}$

Ratios

A **ratio** is a comparison of two numbers.

The ratio of *5 to 10* can also be written as *5:10* or in fractional form as $\frac{5}{10}$. This fraction may be *reduced by cancelling* by a number that evenly divides both the numerator and the denominator. Because 5 evenly divides both 5 and 10, divide as follows:

$$\frac{5}{10} = \frac{5 \div 5}{10 \div 5} = \frac{1}{2}$$

The fraction $\frac{5}{10}$ is *reduced to lowest terms* as $\frac{1}{2}$.

So, the ratio of *5 to 10* can also be written as the ratio of *1 to 2* or *1:2*

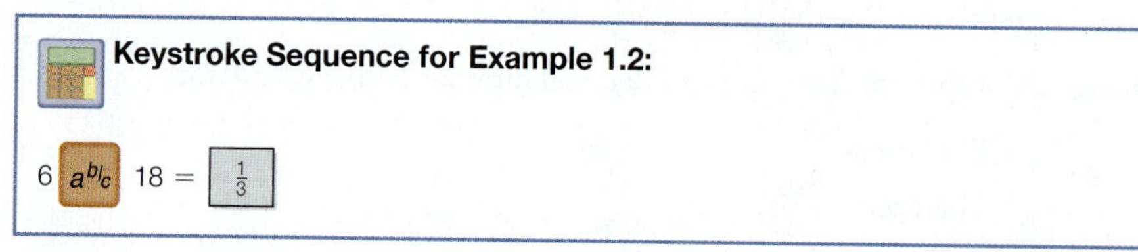

Keystroke Sequence for Example 1.2:

6 $a^{b}/_{c}$ 18 = $\frac{1}{3}$

Example 1.2

Express 6:18 as an equivalent fraction and ratio in lowest terms.

The ratio *6:18*, also written as *6 to 18*, can be written in fractional form as $\frac{6}{18}$. This fraction may be *reduced by cancelling* by a number that evenly divides both the numerator and the denominator. Because 6 divides both 6 and 18, divide as follows:

$$\frac{6}{18} = \frac{6 \div 6}{18 \div 6} = \frac{1}{3}$$

So, the ratio 6 to 18 equals the fraction $\frac{1}{3}$ and the ratio 1:3

Keystroke Sequence for Example 1.3:

To check the answer, use

12 $a^{b}/_{c}$ 120 = $\frac{1}{10}$

Example 1.3

Write the ratio 1:10 as an equivalent fraction with 120 in the denominator.

Because 1:10 as a fraction is $\frac{1}{10}$, you need to write this fraction with the larger denominator of 120. Such processes are called **building fractions.**

$$\frac{1}{10} = \frac{?}{120}$$

$\frac{1}{10}$ may be built up by *multiplying the numerator and denominator of the fraction by the same number* (12 in this case) as follows:

$$\frac{1}{10} = \frac{1 \times 12}{10 \times 12} = \frac{12}{120}$$

So, 1:10 is equivalent to $\frac{12}{120}$

NOTE

When *reducing* a fraction, you *divide* both numerator and denominator by the same number. This process is called *cancelling*.

When *building* a fraction, you *multiply* both numerator and denominator by the same number.

Changing Fractions to Decimal Numbers

To change a fraction to a decimal number, think of the fraction as a division problem. For example:

$$\frac{2}{5} \text{ means } 2 \div 5 \text{ or } 5\overline{)2}$$

Here are the steps for this division.

Step 1 Replace 2 with 2.0, and then place a decimal point directly above the decimal point in 2.0.

$$\begin{array}{r} . \\ 5\overline{)2.0} \end{array}$$

Step 2 Perform the division *twenty divided by five = four*.

$$\begin{array}{r} 0.4 \\ 5\overline{)2.0} \\ \underline{2\,0} \\ 0 \end{array}$$

So, $\frac{2}{5} = 0.4$

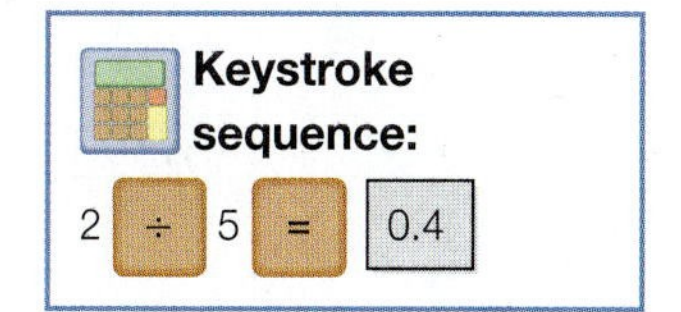

Example 1.4

Write $\frac{5}{2}$ as a decimal number.

$$\frac{5}{2} \text{ means } 5 \div 2 \text{ or } 2\overline{)5}$$

Step 1 $\begin{array}{r} . \\ 2\overline{)5.0} \end{array}$

Step 2 $\begin{array}{r} 2.5 \\ 2\overline{)5.0} \\ \underline{4} \\ 10 \\ \underline{10} \\ 0 \end{array}$

So, $\frac{5}{2} = 2.5$

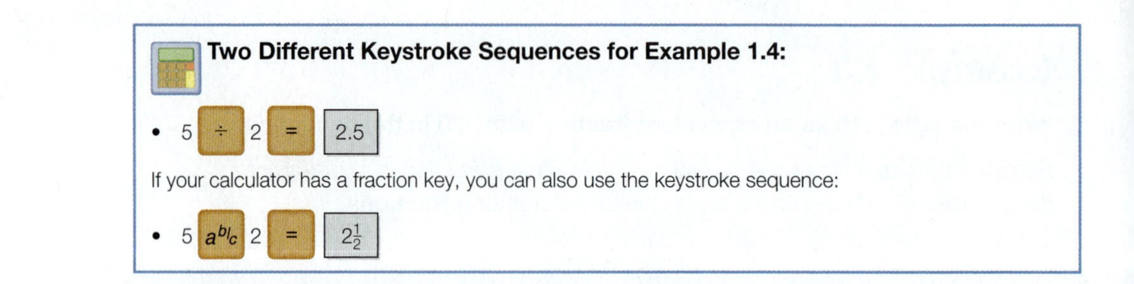

Example 1.5

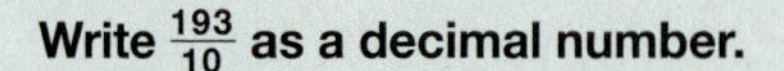

Write $\frac{193}{10}$ as a decimal number.

$$\frac{193}{10} \quad \text{means} \quad 193 \div 10 \quad \text{or} \quad 10\overline{)193}$$

Step 1 $10\overline{)193.0}$ (decimal point placed above the quotient)

Step 2

$$\begin{array}{r} 19.3 \\ 10\overline{)193.0} \\ \underline{10} \\ 93 \\ \underline{90} \\ 30 \\ \underline{30} \\ 0 \end{array}$$

So, $\frac{193}{10} = 19.3$

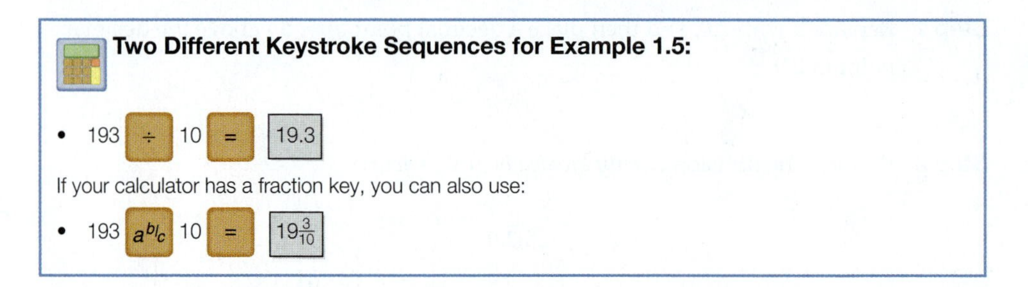

There is a quicker way to do Example 1.5. To divide a *decimal number by 10, move* the decimal point in the number *one place to the left*. Notice that there is one zero in 10.

$$\frac{193}{10} = \frac{193.}{10} = 19\underset{\smile}{3}. = 19.3$$

To *divide a number by 100, move* the decimal point in the number *two places to the left* because there are two zeros in 100. So, the quick way to divide by 10; 100; 1,000; and so on is to count the zeros and then move the decimal point to the left the same number of places; the answer should always be a *smaller* number than the original number. Check your answer to be sure.

Example 1.6

Write $\frac{9.25}{100}$ as a decimal number.

This fraction means 9.25 ÷ 100. There are two zeros in 100, so move the decimal point in 9.25 two places to the left, and fill the empty position with a zero.

$$\frac{9.25}{100} = \underset{\smile\smile}{}9.25 = 0.0925$$

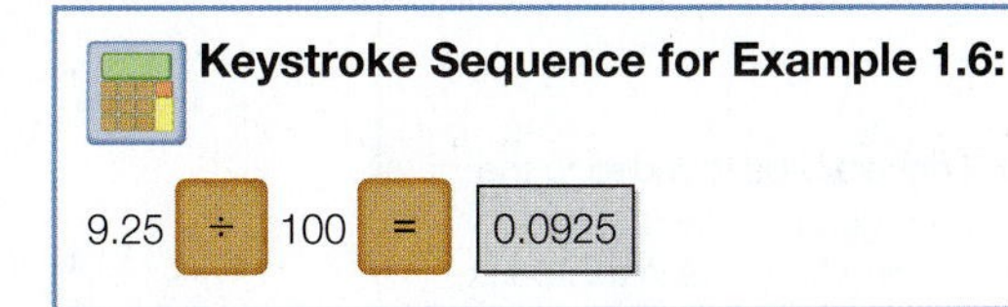

Rounding Decimal Numbers

Sometimes it is convenient to round an answer—that is, to use an approximate answer rather than an exact one.

Rounding Off

To round off 1.267 to the *nearest tenth*—that is, to round off the number to one decimal place—do the following:

> *Look at the digit after the tenths place (the hundredths-place digit). Because this digit (6) is 5 or more, round off 1.267 by adding 1 to the tenths-place digit. Finally, drop all the digits after the tenths place.*
>
> *So, 1.267 is approximated by 1.3 when rounded off to the nearest tenth.*

To round off 0.8345 to the *nearest hundredth*—that is, to round off the number to two decimal places—do the following:

> *Look at the digit after the hundredths place (the thousandths-place digit). Because this digit (4) is less than 5, round off 0.8345 by leaving the hundredths digit alone. Finally, drop all the digits after the hundredths place.*
>
> *So, 0.8345 is approximated by 0.83 when rounded off to the nearest hundredth.*

Example 1.7

Round off 4.8075 to the nearest hundredth, tenth, and whole number.

4.8075 rounded off to the nearest: hundredth $\rightarrow$ 4.81

tenth $\rightarrow$ 4.8

whole number $\rightarrow$ 5

Rounding Down and Rounding Up

In the *rounding off* process, either 0 or 1 is added to the appropriate digit of a given number; therefore, the rounded result can be either smaller or larger than the given number. In healthcare, two other types of rounding are also used. **Rounding down** and **rounding up** are similar to rounding **off**. The only difference is that in *rounding down, 0 is always added* to the appropriate digit, whereas in *rounding up, 1 is always added* to the appropriate digit.

When rounding down both 2.34 and 2.36 to the tenths place, *add 0* to the tenths-place digit and delete the remaining digits. Thus, both 2.34 and 2.36 round down to 2.3.

When rounding up 2.34 and 2.36 to the tenths place, *add 1* to the tenths-place digit and delete the remaining digits. Thus, both 2.34 and 2.36 round up to 2.4.

Generally speaking, rounding down results in a smaller quantity, whereas rounding up results in a larger quantity. So, *rounding down* a dosage helps to avoid an overdose, and *rounding up* a dosage helps to avoid an underdose. When rounding a dosage calculation, most of the time rounding off is used. However, sometimes rounding down is used, whereas rounding up is very rarely used.

NOTE

Rounding down is also referred to as *truncating*, which means "cutting off" digits.

NOTE

Unless otherwise specified, quantities *less than 1* will generally be rounded to the *nearest hundredth*, whereas quantities *greater than 1* will generally be rounded to the *nearest tenth*. For the sake of uniformity, when rounding numbers in this book, rounding *off* is used rather than rounding *down*. However, in Chapter 12, *all pediatric dosages are rounded down*.

Example 1.8

Fill in the table with the indicated rounded numbers.

Number	Round to	Rounded Off	Rounded Down	Rounded Up
0.123	hundredths			
0.129	hundredths			
3.87	tenths			
3.84	tenths			

You should have gotten the following answers:

Number	Round to	Rounded Off	Rounded Down	Rounded Up
0.123	hundredths	0.12	0.12	0.13
0.129	hundredths	0.13	0.12	0.13
3.87	tenths	3.9	3.8	3.9
3.84	tenths	3.8	3.8	3.9

ALERT

The danger of an overdose must always be guarded against. Therefore, the amount of medication to be administered is often rounded *down* instead of rounded *off*. This rounding down is sometimes done in pediatrics and when administering high-alert drugs to adults.

Adding and Subtracting Decimal Numbers

When adding or subtracting decimal numbers, write the numbers in a column with the *decimal points lined up under each other*.

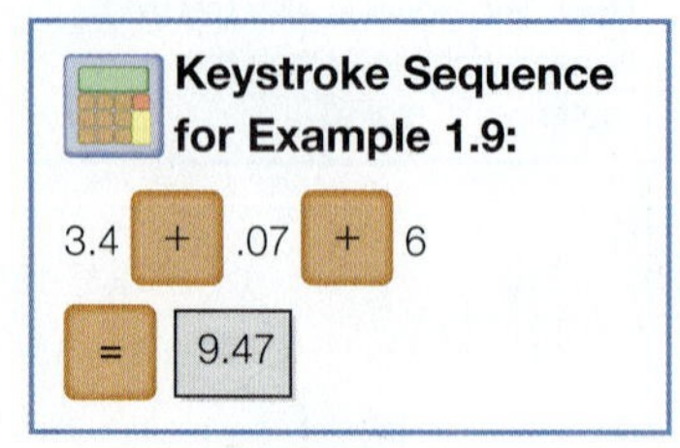

Example 1.9

3.4 + 0.07 + 6 = ?

Write the numbers in a column with the decimal points lined up. *Trailing zeros* may be included to give each number the same amount of decimal places. Therefore, write 6 as 6.00 [Think: $6 is equivalent to $6.00].

$$\begin{array}{r} 3.40 \\ 0.07 \\ +\ \underline{6.00} \\ 9.47 \end{array}$$

So, the sum of 3.4, 0.07, and 6 is 9.47

Example 1.10

5 − 0.45 = ?

Write the numbers in a column with the decimal points lined up. Include *trailing zeros* to give each number the same amount of decimal places.

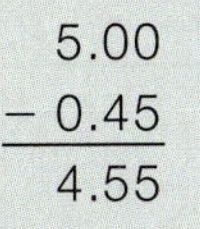

$$\begin{array}{r} 5.00 \\ -\ 0.45 \\ \hline 4.55 \end{array}$$

So, the difference between 5 and 0.45 is 4.55

Keystroke Sequence for Example 1.10:

5 [−] .45 [=] 4.55

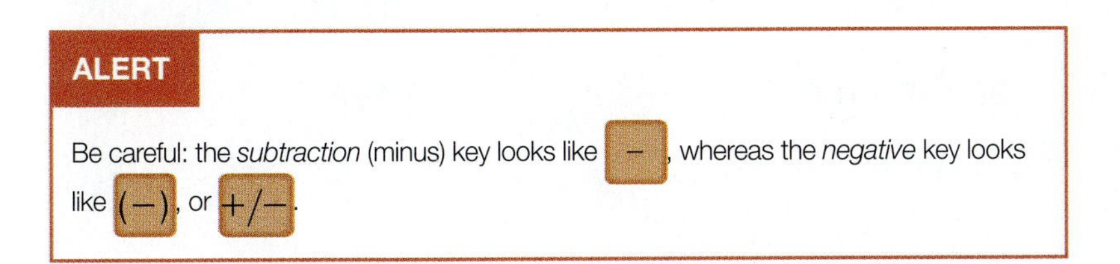

Multiplying Decimal Numbers

To multiply two decimal numbers, first multiply ignoring the decimal points. Then count the total number of decimal places (digits to the right of the decimal point) in the original two numbers. That sum equals the number of decimal places in the answer.

Example 1.11

304.2 × 0.16 = ?

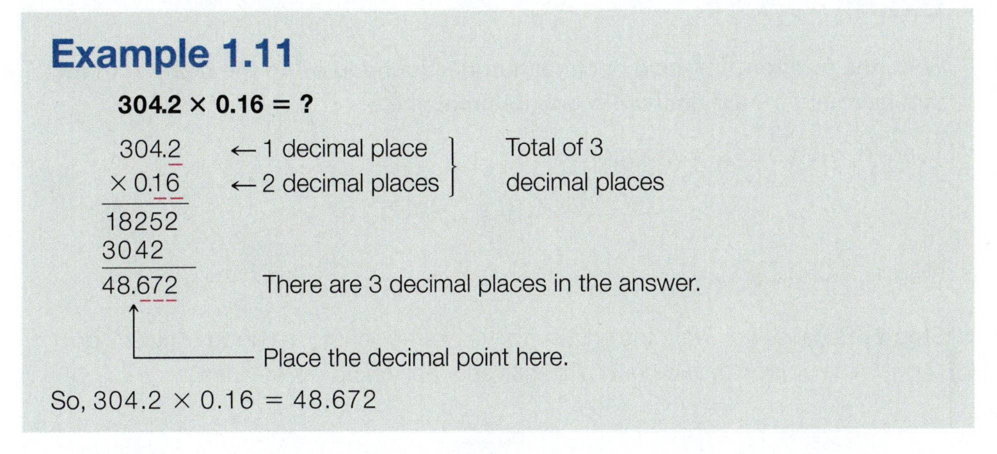

So, 304.2 × 0.16 = 48.672

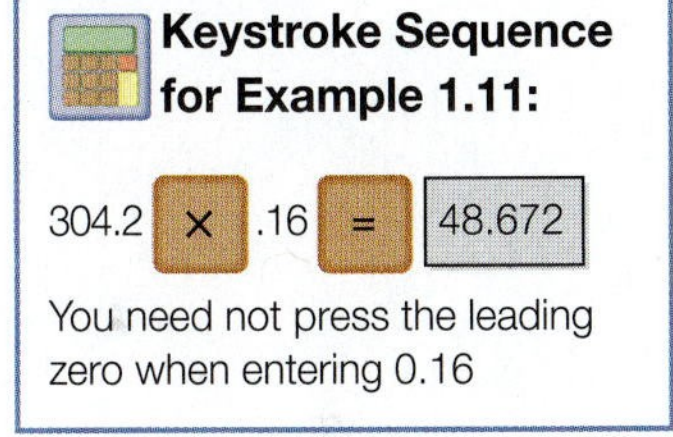

Example 1.12

304.25 × 10 = ?

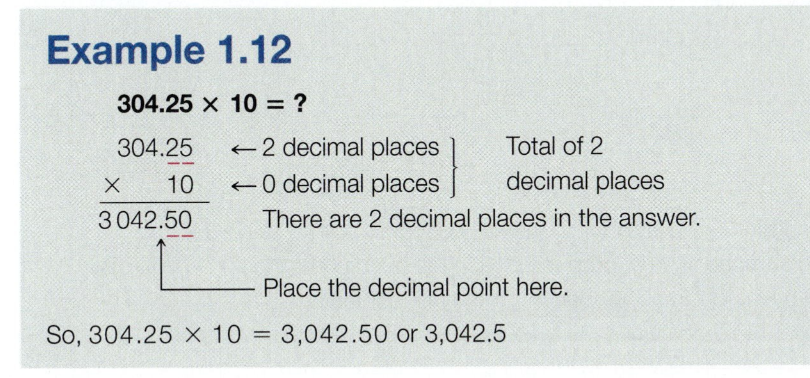

So, 304.25 × 10 = 3,042.50 or 3,042.5

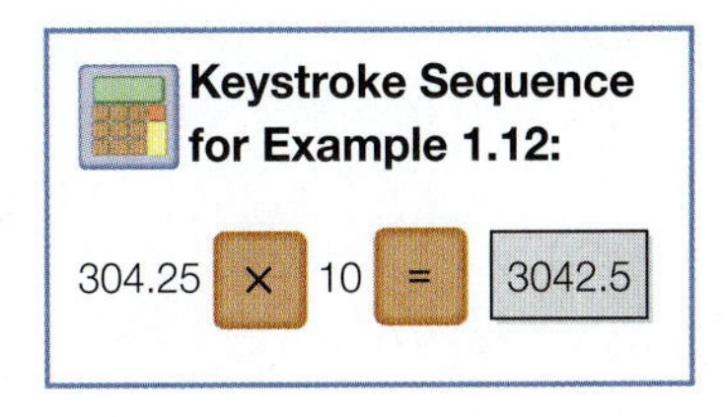

There is a quicker way to do Example 1.12. To *multiply any decimal number by 10, move* the decimal point in the number being multiplied *one place to the right*. Notice that there is one zero in 10.

304.25 × 10 = 304.25 or 3,042.5

To *multiply a number by 100, move* the decimal point in the number *two places to the right* because there are two zeros in 100. So, the quick way to multiply by 10; 100; 1,000; and so on is to count the zeros and then move the decimal point to the right the same number of places. The answer should always be a *larger* number than the original. Check your answer to be sure.

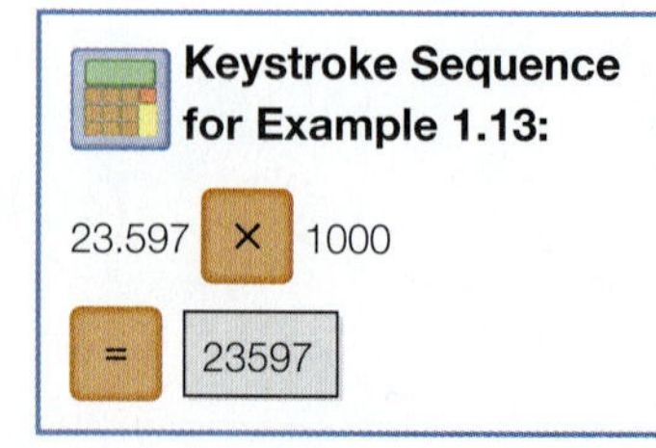

Example 1.13

23.597 × 1,000 = ?

There are three zeros in 1,000, so move the decimal point in 23.597 three places to the right.

23.597 × 1,000 = 2 3 .5 9 7 or 23,597

So, 23.597 × 1,000 = 23,597

Dividing Decimal Numbers

When dividing with decimal numbers, be sure that you are careful where you place the decimal point in the answer.

Example 1.14

Write the fraction $\frac{106.8}{15}$ as a decimal number rounded off to the nearest tenth; that is, round off the answer to one decimal place.

Treat this fraction as a division problem.

$\frac{106.8}{15}$ means $15\overline{)106.8}$

Step 1 $15\overline{)106.8}$

Step 2 Because you want the answer to the nearest tenth (one decimal place), do the division to two decimal places and then round off the answer.

$$\begin{array}{r} 7.12 \\ 15\overline{)106.80} \\ \underline{105} \\ 1\,8 \\ \underline{1\,5} \\ 30 \\ \underline{30} \\ 0 \end{array}$$

Because the hundredths-place digit in the answer is *less than 5*, leave the tenths-place digit alone. Finally, drop the digit in the hundredths place. So, $\frac{106.8}{15}$ is approximated by the decimal number 7.1 to the nearest tenth.

Keystroke Sequence for Example 1.14:

106.8 ÷ 15 = 7.12 ≈7.1 after rounding off. The symbol ≈ means "is approximately equal to."

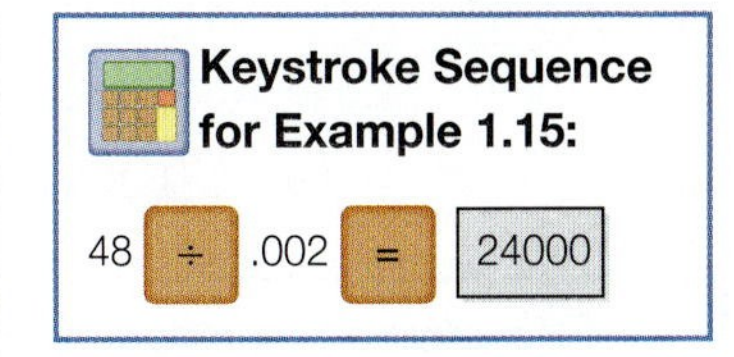

Example 1.15

Simplify $\frac{48}{0.002}$

Think of this fraction as a division problem. Because there are three decimal places in 0.002, move the decimal points in both numbers three places to the right.

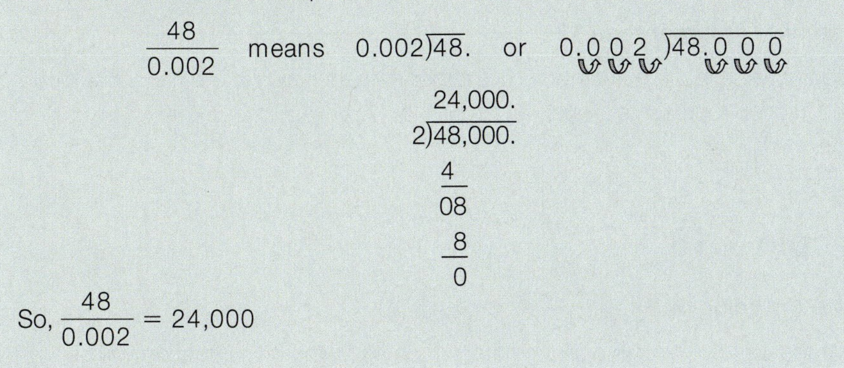

So, $\frac{48}{0.002} = 24{,}000$

Example 1.15 could also have been done by eliminating the decimal point from the given fraction by multiplying by $\frac{1000}{1000}$ as follows:

$$\frac{48}{0.002} \times \frac{1000}{1000} = \frac{48000}{2} = 24{,}000$$

Estimating Answers

When you use a calculator, errors in the keystroke sequence may lead to dangerously high or dangerously low dosages. To help avoid such mistakes:

1. *Carefully* enter the keystroke sequence. A calculator that simultaneously shows both your entries and the answer in the display is desirable.
2. Think: *Is the answer reasonable*? For example, an oral dosage of 50 tablets is not reasonable!
3. Use rounding to *estimate* the size of the answer. The product of 498 and 49 can be estimated by rounding the numbers off to 500 and 50, respectively: $500 \times 50 = 25{,}000$. Because each factor was made larger, the product of 498 and 49 is a little less than 25,000. Sometimes it is useful to know whether an answer will be larger or smaller than a given number.

Example 1.16

Which is larger, 0.4 or 0.23?

Write the numbers in a column with the decimal points lined up, and include trailing zeros to give each number the same amount of decimal places.

0.40
0.23

Because 40 hundredths is larger than 23 hundredths, 0.4 is larger than 0.23.

Keystroke Sequence for Example 1.16:

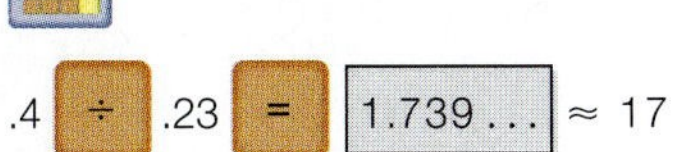

Because 1.7 is larger than 1, the first number entered (0.4) is larger than the second (0.23).

For positive numbers, when one number is divided by a second number, if the answer is larger than 1, the first number is larger. If the answer is less than 1, the second number is larger.

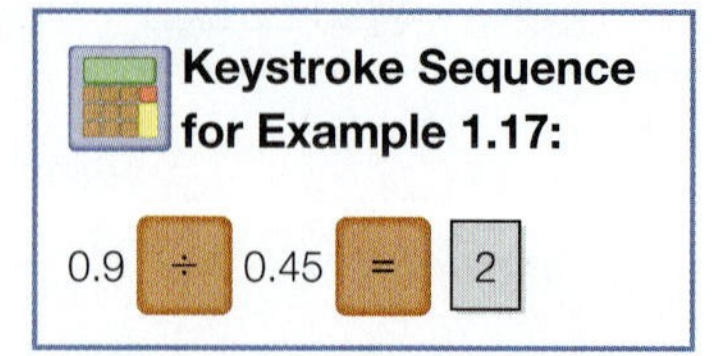

Example 1.17

Is $\frac{0.9}{0.45}$ smaller or larger than 1?

Because the value in the numerator 0.9 is larger than the value in the denominator 0.45, the fraction represents a quantity larger than 1.

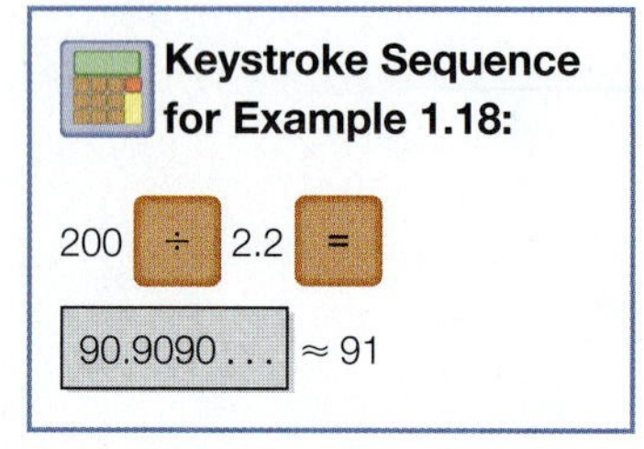

Example 1.18

Estimate the value of $\frac{200}{2.2}$

Because the denominator is approximately equal to 2, the given fraction will be close in value to $\frac{200}{2}$ or 100. In this case, by making the denominator smaller (2 instead of 2.2), you made the value of the entire fraction larger. Therefore, 100 is an overestimate. So, the actual value of $\frac{200}{2.2}$ is a number somewhat less than 100.

Multiplying Fractions

To *multiply fractions,* multiply the numerators to get the new numerator and multiply the denominators to get the new denominator.

Example 1.19

$$\frac{3}{5} \times 6 \times \frac{1}{5} = ?$$

A whole number can be written as a fraction with 1 in the denominator. So, in this example, write 6 as to make all the numbers fractions.

$$\frac{3}{5} \times \frac{6}{1} \times \frac{1}{5} = \frac{3 \times 6 \times 1}{5 \times 1 \times 5} = \frac{18}{25}$$

It is often convenient to cancel before you multiply.

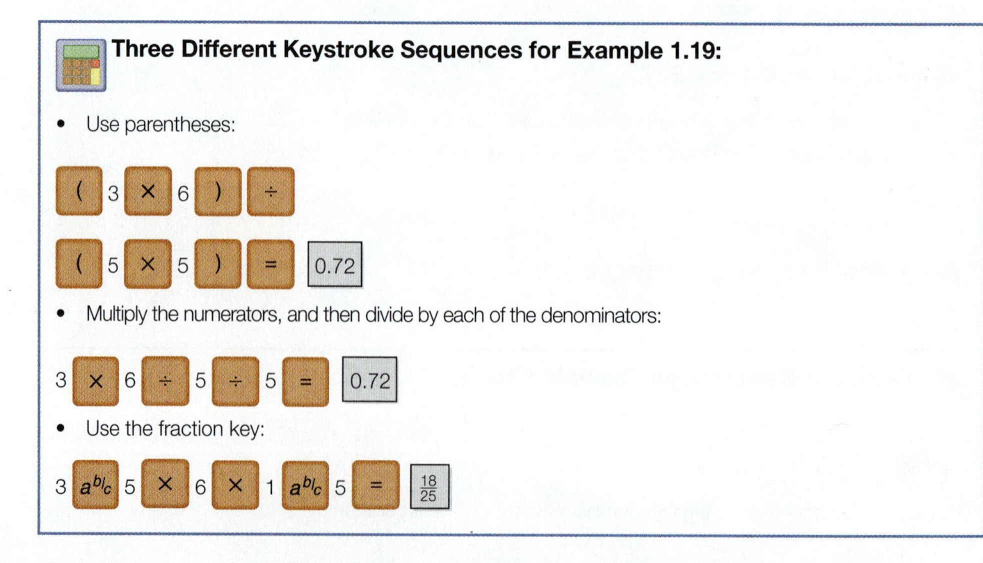

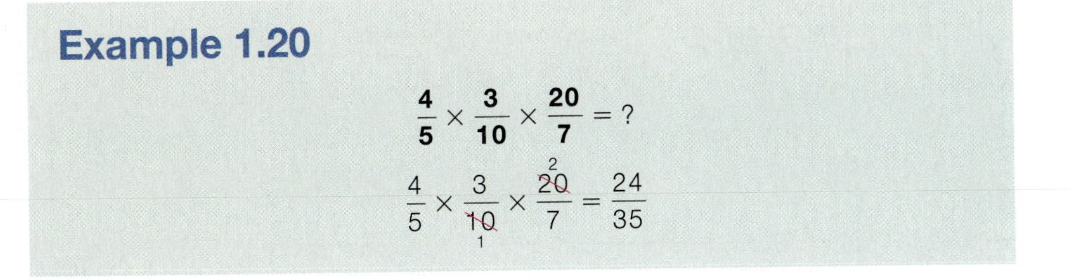

Example 1.20

$$\frac{4}{5} \times \frac{3}{10} \times \frac{20}{7} = ?$$

$$\frac{4}{5} \times \frac{3}{\cancel{10}_{1}} \times \frac{\cancel{20}^{2}}{7} = \frac{24}{35}$$

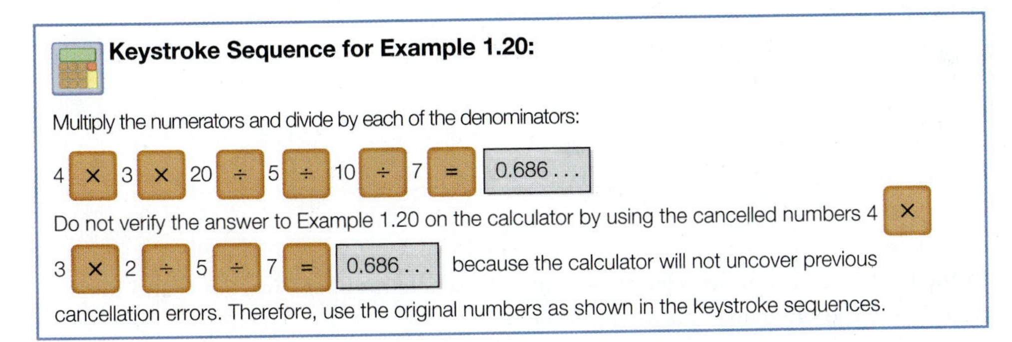

Keystroke Sequence for Example 1.20:

Multiply the numerators and divide by each of the denominators:

4 [×] 3 [×] 20 [÷] 5 [÷] 10 [÷] 7 [=] 0.686 . . .

Do not verify the answer to Example 1.20 on the calculator by using the cancelled numbers 4 [×] 3 [×] 2 [÷] 5 [÷] 7 [=] 0.686 . . . because the calculator will not uncover previous cancellation errors. Therefore, use the original numbers as shown in the keystroke sequences.

Example 1.21

Simplify $\frac{21 \times 15}{7}$

Method 1: Multiply the numbers in the numerator, which yields $\frac{315}{7}$, and then divide 315 by 7, which yields 45

Method 2: First cancel by 7, and then multiply

$$\frac{\cancel{21}^{3} \times 15}{\cancel{7}_{1}} = \frac{3 \times 15}{1} = \frac{45}{1} = 45$$

So, $\frac{21 \times 15}{7} = 45$

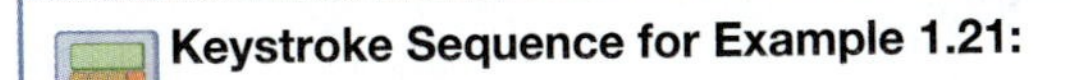

Keystroke Sequence for Example 1.21:

21 [×] 15 [÷] 7 [=] 45

Dividing Fractions

To *divide fractions*, change the division problem to an equivalent multiplication problem by inverting the second fraction.

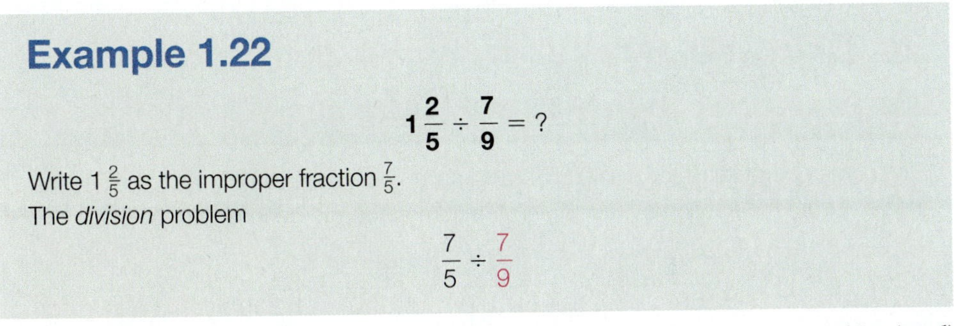

Example 1.22

$$1\frac{2}{5} \div \frac{7}{9} = ?$$

Write $1\frac{2}{5}$ as the improper fraction $\frac{7}{5}$.

The *division* problem

$$\frac{7}{5} \div \frac{7}{9}$$

(Continued)

becomes the *multiplication* problem by inverting the second fraction.

$$\frac{7}{5} \times \frac{9}{7}$$

$$\frac{\overset{1}{\cancel{7}}}{5} \times \frac{9}{\underset{1}{\cancel{7}}} = \frac{9}{5} = 1\frac{4}{5}$$

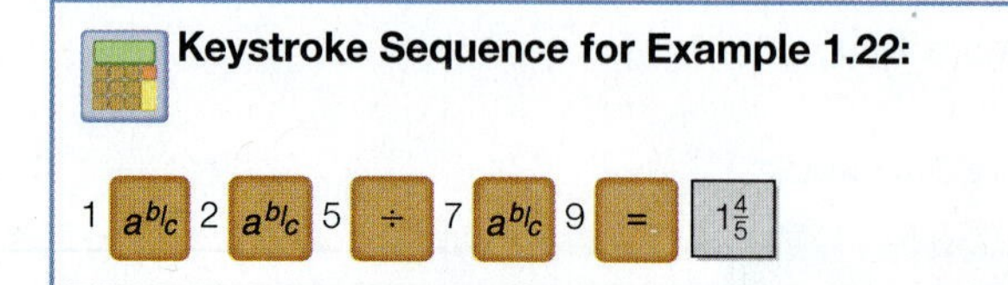

Keystroke Sequence for Example 1.22:

1 $a^b/_c$ 2 $a^b/_c$ 5 ÷ 7 $a^b/_c$ 9 = $1\frac{4}{5}$

NOTE

Avoid cancelling decimal numbers. It is a possible source of error.

In the next three examples you must deal with whole numbers, fractions, and decimal numbers in the same multiplication problem.

Example 1.23

Give the answer to the following problem in simplified fractional form.

$$\frac{1}{300} \times 60 \times \frac{1}{0.4} = ?$$

Write 60 as a fraction and cancel.

$$\frac{1}{\underset{5}{\cancel{300}}} \times \frac{\overset{1}{\cancel{60}}}{1} \times \frac{1}{0.4} = \frac{1}{5 \times 0.4} = \frac{1}{2}$$

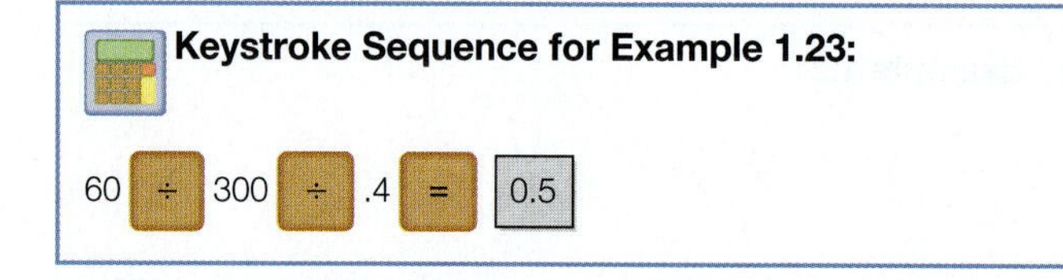

Keystroke Sequence for Example 1.23:

60 ÷ 300 ÷ .4 = 0.5

Example 1.24

Give the answer to the following problem in simplified fractional form.

$$0.35 \times \frac{1}{60} = ?$$

Write 0.35 as the fraction $\frac{0.35}{1}$.

$$\frac{0.35}{1} \times \frac{1}{60} = \frac{0.35}{60}$$

The numerator of this fraction is 0.35, a decimal number. You can eliminate the decimal number from the fraction by multiplying the numerator and denominator by 100.

$$\frac{0.35}{60} \times \frac{100}{100} = \frac{0.35}{60.00} = \frac{35}{6{,}000} = \frac{7}{1{,}200}$$

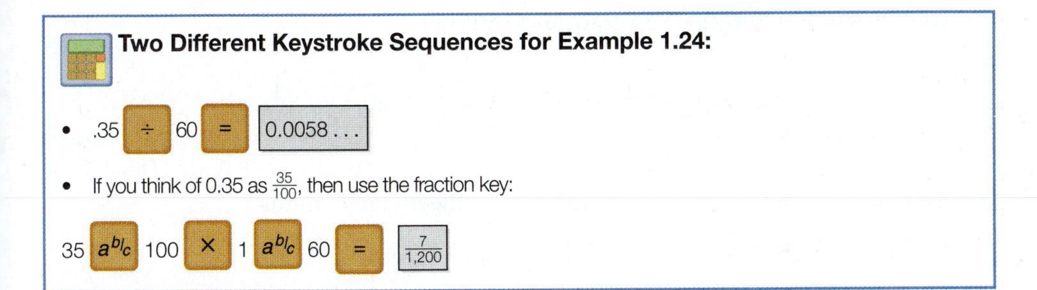

Example 1.25

Give the answer to the following problem in simplified fractional form.

$$0.88 \times \frac{1}{2.2} = ?$$

$$\frac{0.88}{1} \times \frac{1}{2.2} = \frac{0.88}{2.2}$$

Method 1: Multiply the numerator and the denominator of this fraction by 100 to eliminate both decimal numbers.

$$\frac{0.88}{2.2} \times \frac{100}{100} = \frac{0.88}{2.2} = \frac{88}{220} = \frac{2}{5}$$

Method 2: You can simplify $\frac{0.88}{2.2}$ a different way by dividing 0.88 by 2.2

$$2.2\overline{)0.88} = 0.4 \quad \text{and} \quad 0.4 = \frac{4}{10} \quad \text{or} \quad \frac{2}{5}$$

Keystroke Sequence for Example 1.25:

.88 ÷ 2.2 = 0.4

To change 0.4 to a fraction in lowest terms:

4 a b/c 10 = 2/5

Complex Fractions

Fractions that have numerators or denominators that are themselves fractions are called **complex fractions**.

The longest line in the complex fraction separates the numerator from the denominator of the complex fraction. As with any fraction, you can write the complex fraction as a division problem: *Top ÷ Bottom.*

In the complex fraction $\frac{1}{\frac{2}{5}}$, the numerator is 1 and the denominator is $\frac{2}{5}$.

You can simplify this complex fraction as follows:

$$\frac{1}{\frac{2}{5}} \quad \text{means} \quad 1 \div \frac{2}{5} \quad \text{or} \quad 1 \times \frac{5}{2}, \quad \text{which is} \quad \frac{5}{2}$$

In the complex fraction $\frac{\frac{1}{2}}{5}$, the numerator is $\frac{1}{2}$ and the denominator is 5.

You can simplify this complex fraction as follows:

$$\frac{\frac{1}{2}}{5} \text{ means } \frac{1}{2} \div 5 \text{ or } \frac{1}{2} \times \frac{1}{5}, \text{ which is } \frac{1}{10}$$

In the complex fraction $\frac{\frac{3}{5}}{\frac{2}{5}}$, the numerator is $\frac{3}{5}$ and the denominator is $\frac{2}{5}$.

You can simplify this complex fraction as follows:

$$\frac{\frac{3}{5}}{\frac{2}{5}} \text{ means } \frac{3}{5} \div \frac{2}{5} \text{ or } \frac{3}{\cancel{5}_1} \times \frac{\cancel{5}^1}{2}, \text{ which is } \frac{3}{2}$$

Example 1.26

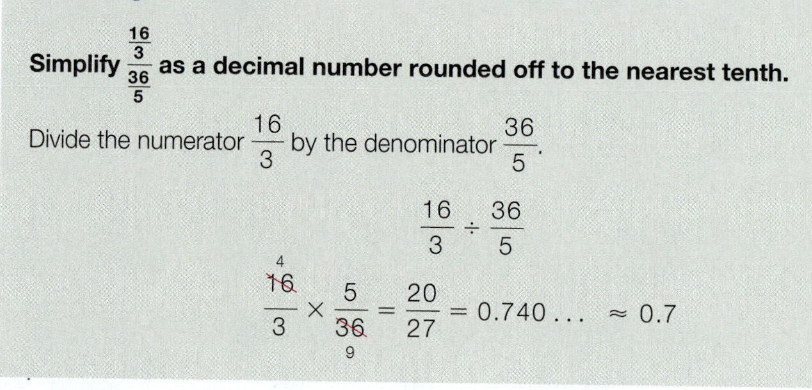

Simplify $\frac{\frac{16}{3}}{\frac{36}{5}}$ as a decimal number rounded off to the nearest tenth.

Divide the numerator $\frac{16}{3}$ by the denominator $\frac{36}{5}$.

$$\frac{16}{3} \div \frac{36}{5}$$

$$\frac{\cancel{16}^4}{3} \times \frac{5}{\cancel{36}_9} = \frac{20}{27} = 0.740\ldots \approx 0.7$$

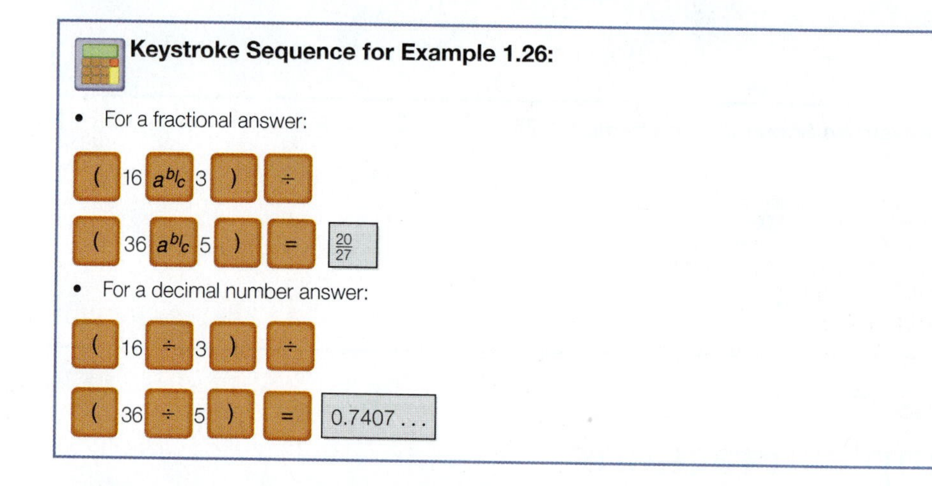

Example 1.27

$$\frac{2}{3} \times \frac{1}{\frac{3}{4}} = ?$$

Method 1: You can multiply the numerators to get the new numerator and multiply the denominators to get the new denominator, as follows:

$$\frac{2}{3} \times \frac{1}{\frac{3}{4}} = \frac{2 \times 1}{3 \times \frac{3}{4}} = \frac{2}{\frac{9}{4}}$$

Now, the numerator is 2 and the denominator is $\frac{9}{4}$, so you get

$$\frac{2}{1} \div \frac{9}{4}$$

which becomes

$$\frac{2}{1} \times \frac{4}{9} = \frac{8}{9}$$

Method 2: This problem could have been done another way by simplifying $\frac{1}{\frac{3}{4}}$ first.

You can write $\frac{1}{\frac{3}{4}}$ as $1 \div \frac{3}{4}$ as $1 \times \frac{4}{3}$ or $\frac{4}{3}$

Then

$$\frac{2}{3} \times \frac{4}{3} = \frac{8}{9}$$

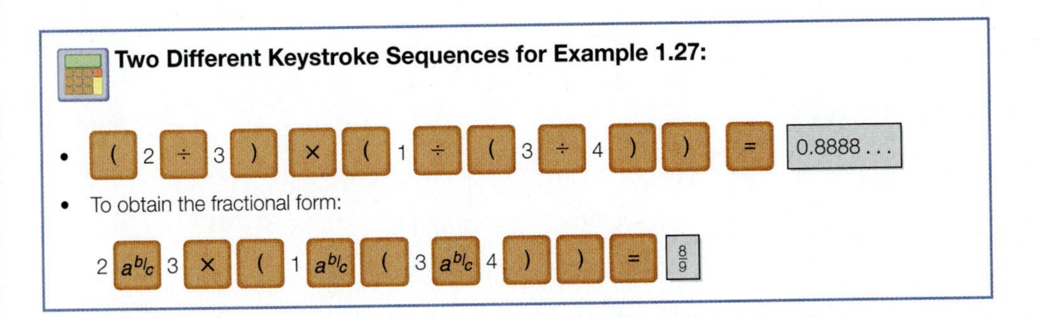

Addition and Subtraction of Fractions

Addition and subtraction of fractions in this textbook generally involves fractions with denominators of 2, 4, or 8.

Same Denominators

When adding or subtracting fractions that have the *same denominators, add or subtract the numerators and keep the common denominator.*

Add $\frac{1}{2}$ and $\frac{1}{2}$:

$$\frac{1}{2} + \frac{1}{2} = \frac{1+1}{2} = \frac{2}{2}, \text{ which equals } 1$$

From $\frac{11}{4}$ subtract $\frac{5}{4}$:

$$\frac{11}{4} - \frac{5}{4} = \frac{11-5}{4} = \frac{6}{4}, \text{ which can be reduced to } \frac{3}{2} \text{ or } 1\frac{1}{2}$$

For *mixed numbers*, add (or subtract) the whole number and fraction parts separately.

Add $3\frac{1}{4}$ and $2\frac{1}{4}$:

$$\begin{array}{rl} 3 & \frac{1}{4} \\ +\,2 & \frac{1}{4} \\ \hline 5 & \frac{1+1}{4} = 5\frac{2}{4}, \text{ which equals } 5\frac{1}{2} \end{array}$$

From $10\frac{3}{4}$ *subtract* $6\frac{1}{4}$:

$$\begin{array}{rr} 10 & \frac{3}{4} \\ -\ 6 & \frac{1}{4} \\ \hline 4 & \frac{3-1}{4} = 4\frac{2}{4}, \text{ which equals } 4\frac{1}{2} \end{array}$$

Different Denominators

When adding or subtracting fractions that have *different denominators*, build the fraction(s) so that the denominators are the same (have a common denominator), and proceed as before.

Add $\frac{1}{2}$ and $\frac{1}{4}$

This problem has fractions with different denominators. Recall that $\frac{1}{2} = \frac{2}{4}$. Then the problem becomes

$$\frac{2}{4} + \frac{1}{4} = \frac{2+1}{4} = \frac{3}{4}$$

From $\frac{3}{4}$ subtract $\frac{1}{2}$

Recall that $\frac{1}{2} = \frac{2}{4}$. Then the problem becomes

$$\frac{3}{4} - \frac{2}{4} = \frac{3-2}{4} = \frac{1}{4}$$

For *mixed numbers*, add (or subtract) the whole number and fraction parts separately.

Add $9\frac{3}{4}$ and $6\frac{1}{2}$

To make the denominators the same, use $\frac{1}{2} = \frac{2}{4}$

$$\begin{array}{rrcrr} 9 & \frac{3}{4} & = & 9 & \frac{3}{4} \\ +\,6 & \frac{1}{2} & = & 6 & \frac{2}{4} \\ \hline & & & 15 & \frac{3+2}{4} = 15\frac{5}{4}, \text{ which equals } 16\frac{1}{4} \end{array}$$

From $9\frac{3}{4}$ subtract $6\frac{3}{8}$

To make the denominators the same, use $\frac{3}{4} = \frac{6}{8}$

$$\begin{array}{rrcrr} 9 & \frac{3}{4} & = & 9 & \frac{6}{8} \\ -\,6 & \frac{3}{8} & = & 6 & \frac{3}{8} \\ \hline & & & 3 & \frac{6-3}{8} = 3\frac{3}{8} \end{array}$$

From $6\frac{1}{4}$ subtract $4\frac{3}{4}$

Method 1: Use borrowing (renaming).

Because $\frac{3}{4}$ is larger than $\frac{1}{4}$, subtraction of the fractions is not possible. Therefore, you may rename $6\frac{1}{4}$ as follows: Borrow 1 from the whole number part (6), and add the 1 to the fractional part ($\frac{1}{4}$). This results in $6\frac{1}{4} = (6 - 1) + (1 + \frac{1}{4})$ or $5\frac{5}{4}$.

$$
\begin{array}{rcl}
6\frac{1}{4} & = & 5\frac{5}{4} \\
-4\frac{3}{4} & = & 4\frac{3}{4} \\
\hline
 & & 1\,\frac{5-3}{4} = 1\frac{2}{4} \text{ or } 1\frac{1}{2}
\end{array}
$$

Method 2: Change the mixed numbers to improper fractions.

$$
\begin{array}{rcl}
6\frac{1}{4} & = & \frac{25}{4} \\
-4\frac{3}{4} & = & \frac{19}{4} \\
\hline
 & & \frac{25-19}{4} = \frac{6}{4} \text{ which also equals } 1\frac{1}{2}
\end{array}
$$

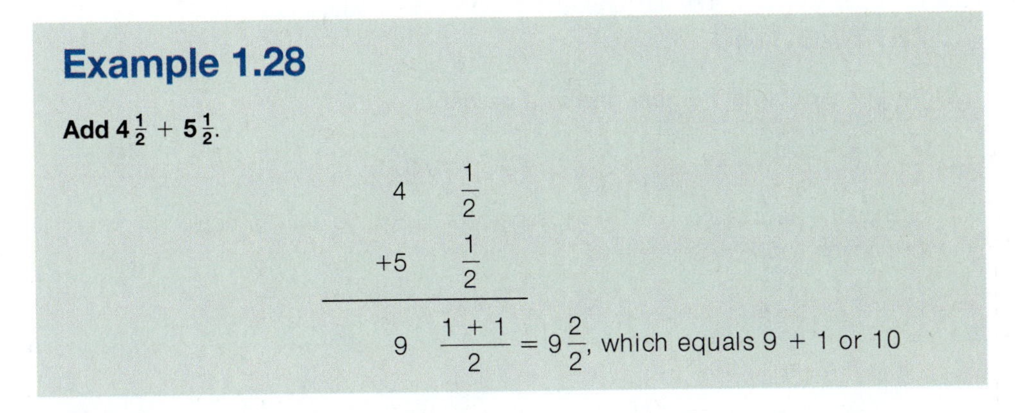

Example 1.28

Add $4\frac{1}{2} + 5\frac{1}{2}$.

$$
\begin{array}{rl}
4 & \frac{1}{2} \\
+5 & \frac{1}{2} \\
\hline
9 & \frac{1+1}{2} = 9\frac{2}{2}, \text{ which equals } 9 + 1 \text{ or } 10
\end{array}
$$

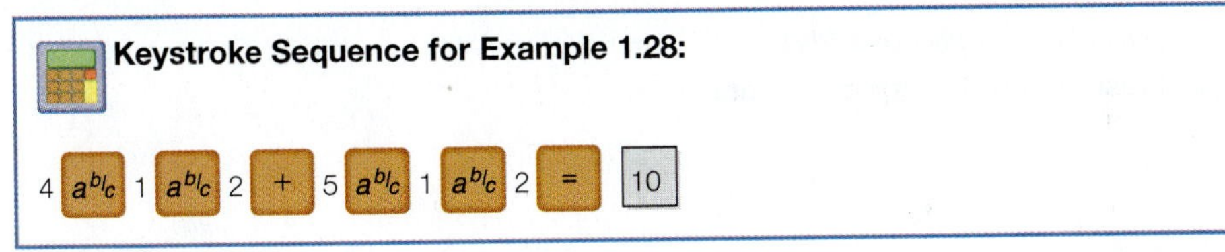

Keystroke Sequence for Example 1.28:

4 [a b/c] 1 [a b/c] 2 [+] 5 [a b/c] 1 [a b/c] 2 [=] [10]

Percentages

Percent (%) means *parts per 100* or *divided by 100*. Thus 50% means 50 *parts per hundred* or 50 *divided by 100*, which can also be written as the fraction $\frac{50}{100}$. The fraction $\frac{50}{100}$ can be changed to the decimal numbers 0.50 and 0.5 or reduced to the fraction $\frac{1}{2}$.

13% means $\frac{13}{100}$ or 0.13

100% means $\frac{100}{100}$ or 1

12.3% means $\frac{12.3}{100}$ or 0.123

$6\frac{1}{2}$% means 6.5% or $\frac{6.5}{100}$ or 0.065

ALERT

Calculating with numbers in percent form can be difficult, so percentages should be converted to either fractional or decimal form before performing any calculations.

Example 1.29

Write 0.5% as a fraction in lowest terms and as a decimal number.

$$0.5\% = \frac{0.5}{100} = \frac{5}{1{,}000} = \frac{1}{200}$$

There is another way to get the answer. Because you understand that $0.5 = \frac{1}{2}$, then

$$0.5\% = \frac{1}{2}\% = \frac{1}{2} \div 100 = \frac{1}{2} \div \frac{100}{1} = \frac{1}{2} \times \frac{1}{100} = \frac{1}{200}$$

To obtain a decimal number, write

$$0.5\% = \frac{0.5}{100} = 0.5 = 0.005$$

Example 1.30

Write $\frac{3}{4}$ as a decimal number and as a percent.

$$\frac{3}{4} = 3 \div 4 = 0.75$$

To change the decimal number 0.75 to a percent, move the decimal point two places to the right and add the percent sign.

$$0.75 = 75\%$$

To find a *percent of a number* or a *fraction of a number*, translate the word "of" as "multiplication," as illustrated in Examples 1.31 and 1.32.

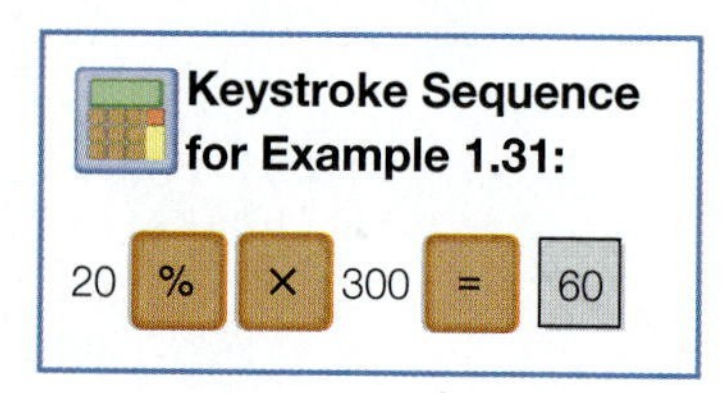

Example 1.31

What is 20% of 300?

To find a percent of a number, translate the "of" as multiplication.

$$20\% \text{ of } 300 \quad \text{means} \quad 20\% \times 300 \text{ or}$$

$$0.20 \times 300 = 60$$

So, 20% of 300 is 60.

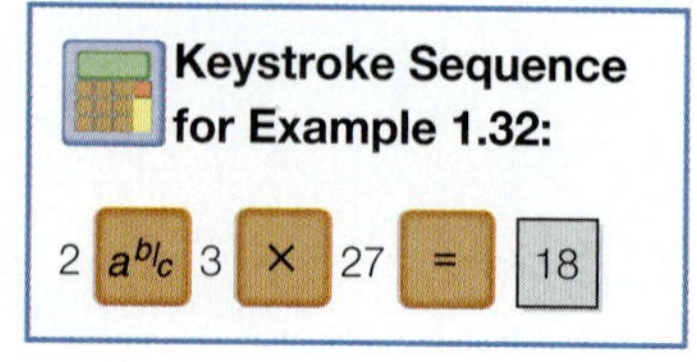

Example 1.32

What is two-thirds of 27?

To find a fraction of a number, translate the "of" as multiplication.

$$\frac{2}{3} \text{ of } 27 \quad \text{means} \quad \frac{2}{3} \times 27 = 18$$

So, two-thirds of 27 is 18.

Percent of Change

It is often useful to determine a *percent of change* (increase or decrease). For example, you might want to know if a 20-pound weight loss for a client is significant. For an adult client who was 200 pounds, a 20-pound loss would be a decrease in weight of 10%. However, for a child who was 50 pounds, a 20-pound loss would be a decrease in weight of 40%, which is far more significant than a 10% loss.

To obtain the fraction of change, you may use the formula:

$$\text{Fraction of Change} = \frac{\textit{Change}}{\textit{Original}}$$

Change the above fraction to a percent to obtain the *percent of change.*

Example 1.33

A daily dosage increases from 4 tablets to 5 tablets. What is the fraction of change and percent of change in daily dosage?

$$\text{Fraction of Change} = \frac{\textit{Change}}{\textit{Original}}$$

Because the original (old) dosage is 4 tablets and the new dosage is 5 tablets, then the change in dosage is

$$\text{Change} = 5 \text{ tablets} - 4 \text{ tablets} = 1 \text{ tablet}$$

$$\text{Fraction of Change} = \frac{\textit{Change}}{\textit{Original}} = \frac{1}{4} \text{ or } 25\%$$

So, the dosage has increased by $\frac{1}{4}$ or 25%.

Example 1.34

A person was drinking 40 ounces of fluid per day, but this was reduced to 10 ounces of fluid per day. What is the percent of change in fluid intake?

$$\text{Fraction of Change} = \frac{\textit{Change}}{\textit{Original}}$$

Because the original (old) amount is 40 ounces and the new amount is 10 ounces, the change is

$$\text{Change} = 40 - 10 = 30 \text{ ounces}$$

$$\text{Fraction of Change} = \frac{\textit{Change}}{\textit{Original}} = \frac{30}{40} = \frac{3}{4} \text{ or } 75\%$$

So, this is a 75% decrease in fluid intake.

Summary

In this chapter, all the essential mathematical skills that are needed for dosage calculation were reviewed.

When working with fractions:

- Proper fractions have smaller numbers in the numerator than in the denominator.
- Improper fractions have numerators that are larger than or equal to their denominators.
- Improper fractions can be changed to mixed numbers, and vice versa.
- Any number can be changed into a fraction by writing the number over 1.

- Cancel first when you multiply fractions.
- Change a fraction to a decimal number by dividing the numerator by the denominator.
- A ratio may be written as a fraction.
- Simplify complex fractions by dividing the numerator by the denominator.

When working with decimals:

- Line up the decimal points when adding or subtracting.
- Move the decimal point three places to the right when multiplying a decimal number by 1,000.
- Move the decimal point three places to the left when dividing a decimal number by 1,000.
- Count the total number of places in the numbers you are multiplying to determine the number of decimal places in the answer.
- Avoid cancelling with decimal numbers.

When working with percentages:

- Change to fractions or decimal numbers before doing any calculations.
- "Of" means multiply when calculating a percent of a number.
- Fraction of Change $= \frac{Change}{Original}$

Practice Sets

The answers to *Try These for Practice* and *Exercises* are found in Appendix A. Ask your instructor for the answers to the *Additional Exercises.*

Try These for Practice

Test your comprehension after reading the chapter.

1. Write $\frac{7}{16}$ as a decimal number rounded off to the hundredths place. ______________________________
2. Find 23% of 59 and round down the answer to the tenths place. ______________________________
3. Fill in the missing numbers in this chart.

Fraction	Decimal	Percent
$^1/_2$	0.5	50%
$^3/_5$		
	0.45	
		3%

4. Write the value of this expression as a fraction: $\frac{14}{33} \times \frac{55}{8} \times \frac{12}{35}$
5. Write this expression as an ordinary fraction in lowest terms: $\frac{\frac{5}{4}}{10}$

Exercises

Reinforce your understanding in class or at home.

Convert to whole numbers, proper fractions, or mixed numbers (Questions 1–7).

1. $0.55 =$ ________
2. $4\frac{1}{4} + 3\frac{3}{4} =$ ________
3. $15 \times \frac{3}{5} \times \frac{4}{27} =$ ________
4. $2\frac{3}{4} \div 7 =$ ________
5. $36 \div \frac{9}{10} =$ ________
6. $0.72 \div \frac{9}{20} =$ ________

7. $20{,}000 \times \frac{7}{15{,}000} \times \frac{1}{56} =$ ________

Convert to decimal numbers (Questions 8–19).

8. $\frac{3}{8} =$ ________ (round down to the hundredths place)

9. $\frac{16}{25} =$ ________

10. $6\frac{7}{10} =$ ________

11. $\frac{3}{200} =$ ________

12. $\frac{5}{24} =$ ________ (round off to the hundredths place)

13. $\frac{457}{1{,}000} =$ ________

14. $\frac{6.55}{500}$

15. $\frac{11}{13}$ (round down to the hundredths place)

16. $\frac{0.48}{0.8}$

17. $\frac{0.054}{0.06}$

18. $16\frac{2}{3}\%$ (round off to two decimal places)

19. 0.9%

Simplify and write the answer in decimal form (Questions 20–24).

20. 5.437×0.05 (round off to the nearest hundredth)

21. $0.0657 \times 1{,}000$

22. $4.7 \div 100$

23. $9 \div 0.17$ (round off to the hundredths place)

24. 0.45×0.03 (round up to two decimal places)

Simplify and write the answer in fractional and in decimal form rounded off to the nearest tenth (Questions 25–30).

25. $\frac{6}{35} \times \frac{55}{18} \times 14$

26. $\frac{\frac{3}{4}}{\frac{3}{7}}$

27. $\frac{(7\%)\left(\frac{2}{3}\right)}{6\%}$

28. What is half of $\frac{1}{4}$? ________

29. 7.5% = ________

30. 125% = ________

31. Express the ratio 35:40 as a fraction in lowest terms. ________

32. Mentally approximate to the nearest whole number: $\frac{603}{198}$ ________

33. Find the numerator of the equivalent fraction with the given denominator. $\frac{3}{4} = \frac{?}{12}$ ________

34. Find the denominator of the equivalent fraction with the given numerator. $\frac{3}{4} = \frac{120}{?}$ ________

35. Simplify $0.04 + 21 + 3.7$ ________

36. Simplify $2 - 0.002$ ________

37. Which is larger, 0.9 or 0.22? ________

38. What is 20% of 30? ________

39. A dose was increased from 250 milligrams to 500 milligrams. What is the percent of increase? ________

40. A dose was decreased from 500 milligrams to 250 milligrams. What is the percent of decrease? ________

Additional Exercises

Now, test yourself!

Convert to proper fractions or mixed numbers (Questions 1–7).

1. $0.65 =$ ________
2. $3\frac{1}{4} + 4\frac{1}{4} =$ ________
3. $50 \times \frac{3}{5} \times \frac{1}{30} =$ ________
4. $6\frac{3}{5} \div 11 =$ ________
5. $60 \div \frac{13}{5} =$ ________
6. $6.3 \div \frac{3}{4} =$ ________
7. $52 \times \frac{5}{8{,}400} \times \frac{21}{0.13} =$ ________

Convert to decimal numbers (Questions 8–19).

8. $\frac{1}{8} =$ ________ (round down to the hundredths place)
9. $\frac{14}{25} =$ ________
10. $5\frac{3}{10} =$ ________
11. $\frac{1}{200} =$ ________
12. $\frac{1}{75} =$ ________ (round off to the nearest hundredth)
13. $\frac{870}{1{,}000} =$ ________
14. $\frac{4.56}{200} =$ ________
15. $\frac{20}{7} =$ ________ (round down to the tenths place)
16. $\frac{0.72}{0.9} =$ ________

17. $\frac{0.072}{0.08} =$ __________

18. $6\frac{1}{4}\% =$ __________

19. $0.9\% =$ __________

Simplify and write the answer in decimal form (Questions 20–24).

20. $0.24 \times 6.23 =$ __________ (round off to the nearest hundredth)

21. $0.0047 \times 100 =$ __________

22. $0.0047 \times 1{,}000 =$ __________

23. $0.77 \div 0.3$ __________ (round off to the nearest tenth)

24. $7 \div 0.13$ __________ (round down to the hundredths place)

Simplify and write the answer in fractional form and in decimal form rounded off to the nearest tenth (Questions 25–30).

25. $0.56 \div \frac{1}{0.9} =$ __________

26. $\frac{13}{\frac{3}{4}} =$ __________

27. $\frac{\frac{5}{7}}{100} \times \frac{200}{7} =$ __________

28. $\frac{15 \times \frac{3}{8}}{\frac{7}{8}} =$ __________

29. $12.5\% =$ __________

30. $37\frac{1}{2}\% =$ __________

31. Express the ratio 25:50 as a fraction in lowest terms.

____

32. Express the ratio 24 to 36 as a fraction in lowest terms.

____

33. Find the numerator of the equivalent fraction with the given denominator. $\frac{3}{5} = \frac{?}{100}$

____

34. Find the numerator of the equivalent fraction with the given denominator.

$\frac{3}{4} = \frac{?}{8}$ __________

35. Simplify $0.4 + 7 + 2.55$ __________

36. Simplify $2.06 - 1.222$ __________

37. Which is larger, 0.7 or 0.24? __________

38. What is 20% of 80? __________

39. The number of patients in the hospital has increased from 160 to 200. What is the percent of change? __________

40. A patient weighed 400 pounds before a diet program. After the program she weighed 280 pounds. What was the percent of change in the patient's weight? __________

Chapter 2
Safe and Accurate Medication Administration

Learning Outcomes

After completing this chapter, you will be able to

2.1 Describe the six "rights" of safe medication administration.

2.2 Explain the legal implications of medication administration.

2.3 Describe the routes of medication administration.

2.4 Identify common abbreviations used in medication administration.

2.5 Compare the trade name and generic name of drugs.

2.6 Describe the forms in which medications are supplied.

2.7 Identify and interpret the components of a Drug Prescription, Physician's Order, and Medication Administration Record.

2.8 Interpret information found on drug labels and in prescribing information.

This chapter introduces the process of safe and accurate medication administration. Client safety is an ongoing critical issue and a primary goal for all healthcare providers. Safety in medication administration involves more than merely calculating accurate dosages. Client rights, knowledge of potential sources of error, critical thinking, and attention to detail are all important in ensuring client safety. The responsibilities of the people involved in the administration of medication are described.

The various forms and routes of drugs are presented, as well as abbreviations used in prescribing and documenting the administration of medications. You will learn how to interpret information found in drug labels, website "prescribing information," the *Physician's Desk Reference (PDR)*, package inserts, and drug guide books.

The Medication Administration Process

Medication administration is a process involving a chain of healthcare professionals. It includes five stages: (1) ordering/prescribing, (2) transcribing and verifying, (3) dispensing and delivering, (4) administering, and (5) monitoring and reporting.

Physicians, medical doctors (MD), osteopathic doctors (DO), podiatrists (DPM), and *dentists (DDS)* can legally prescribe medications. In many states, *physician's assistants, certified nurse midwives,* and *nurse practitioners* can also prescribe a range of medications related to their areas of practice.

Nurses and pharmacists are involved in transcribing, verifying, dispensing, and delivering medications.

The **prescriber writes** the order, the **pharmacist fills** the order, and the **nurse administers** the medication to the client; each is responsible for the accuracy of the order.

Although prescribers may administer drugs to clients, the *registered professional nurse (RN), licensed practical nurse (LPN), licensed vocational nurse (LVN),* and in some states, the *medication technician* may be responsible for administering drugs ordered by the prescriber.

To ensure client safety, all healthcare professionals must understand how a client's medications act and interact. Drugs can be life-saving or life-threatening. Every year, thousands of deaths occur because of medication errors. Errors can occur at any point in the medication process.

NOTE

The National Coordinating Council for Medication Error Reporting and Prevention is operated by the ISMP. The Council defines a medication error as "any preventable event that may cause or lead to inappropriate medication use or client harm while the medication is in the control of the health care professional, client, or consumer. Such events may be related to professional practice, health care products, procedures, and systems, including prescribing; order communication; product labeling, packaging, and nomenclature; compounding; dispensing; distribution; administration; education; monitoring; and use."* When a medication error is identified, the National Alert Network (NAN) issues alerts.

Preventing Medication Errors

Medication errors may occur anywhere in the medication administration process. When an error occurs it may be caused by failure to comply with the required policies or procedures, errors in calculating dosages, failure to follow the "six rights of medication administration," and miscommunication of orders. Miscommunication of orders can include illegible handwriting, incorrect use of zeros and decimal points, confusion of metric and other dosing units, as well as inappropriate abbreviations.

Other causes of medication errors include confusing drug names (look-alike or sound-alike); unclear or absent drug labels and packages; and lack of information about the drug or the client (e.g., allergies, other medications the client is taking). *High-alert* medications are those that have the highest risk of causing injury when misused. The top high-alert medications are insulin, heparin, injectable potassium chloride, opiates and narcotics, neuromuscular drugs, and chemotherapy drugs.

The **Institute for Safe Medication Practices (ISMP)**, the **United States Pharmacopeia (USP)**, and **The Joint Commission (TJC)** are organizations that are actively involved in preventing medication errors and monitoring medication error reports. The ***Quality and Safety Education for Nurses (QSEN)*** project has a goal to prepare student nurses with the knowledge, skills, and attitudes (KSAs) that are necessary to improve the quality and safety of client care. Safety, one of QSEN's "six competencies," is vital to medication administration; for further information, go to *qsen.org*. Personnel who administer medications must be familiar with and follow applicable laws, policies, and procedures relative to the administration of medications, and they have a legal and ethical responsibility to report medication errors. When an error occurs, it must be reported immediately, the client assessed for any ***adverse drug events (ADEs)***, and an incident report prepared. The reason for the error must be determined, and corrective policies or procedures must be instituted. Best practices for preventing ADEs begin with a review of the client's current drug regimen, allergies, and diagnosis. The healthcare professional must be knowledgeable of the drug's expected benefits, actions, adverse reactions, interactions, and appropriateness for the client's diagnosis.

*From National Coordinating Council for Medication Error Reporting and Prevention. Used by permission of National Coordinating Council for Medication Error Reporting and Prevention.

TJC requires healthcare facilities to "maintain and communicate accurate patient medication information" (National Patient Safety Goal 03.06.01, 2013). ***Medication Reconciliation*** is a process that includes developing a list of all current medications that a client is taking, making a list of medications to be prescribed, comparing the lists, making clinical decisions based on the comparison, and communicating the new list to appropriate caregivers and to the client. This procedure must be performed at every transition of care, including changes in setting, service, practitioner, and level of care. Medication Reconciliation helps to prevent medication errors such as omissions, duplications, dosing errors, or drug interactions.

NOTE

For additional information about preventing medication errors and about Medication Reconciliation, refer to The Joint Commission's National Patient Safety Goals (www.jointcommission.org), the Institute for Healthcare Improvement (www.ihi.org), and the Institute for Safe Medication Practices (www.ismp.org).

ALERT

The person who administers the drug has the last opportunity to identify an error before a client might be injured.

Six Rights of Medication Administration

To prepare and administer drugs safely, it is imperative that you understand and follow the **Six Rights of Medication Administration**:

- Right drug
- Right dose
- Right route and form
- Right time
- Right client
- Right documentation

These six "rights" should be checked before administering any medications. Failure to achieve any of these rights constitutes a medication error.

Some institutions recognize additional rights, such as the *right to know* and the *right to refuse*. Clients need to be educated about their medications, and if a client refuses a medication, the reason must be documented and reported. The IOM report "Preventing Medication Errors" emphasizes the need for open communication between nurses and clients. This includes talking as well as active listening to clients. TJC began a "Speak Up" campaign that urges clients to take an active role in preventing errors by becoming more active in their own care. Clients are encouraged to ask questions about their medications and receive satisfactory answers. Printed information and videos of the Speak Up campaign are found online at www.jointcommission.org/speakup.

NOTE

A generic drug may be manufactured by different companies under different trade names. For example, the generic drug ibuprofen is manufactured by McNeil PPC under the trade name Motrin, and by Pfizer Consumer Healthcare under the trade name Advil. The active ingredients in Motrin and Advil are the same, but the size, shape, color, or fillers may be different. Be aware that clients may become confused and worried about receiving a medication that has a different name or appears to be dissimilar from their usual medication. State and federal governments now permit, encourage, and, in some states, mandate that the consumer be given the generic form when buying prescription drugs.

The Right Drug

A drug is a chemical substance that acts on the physiological processes in the human body. For example, the drug insulin is given to clients whose bodies do not manufacture sufficient insulin. Some drugs have more than one action. Aspirin, for example, is an antipyretic (fever-reducing), analgesic (pain-relieving), and anti-inflammatory drug that also has anticoagulant properties (keeps the blood from clotting). A drug may be taken for one, some, or all its therapeutic properties.

The **generic** name is the official accepted name of a drug, as listed in the United States Pharmacopeia (USP). The designation of USP after a drug name indicates that the drug meets government standards. A drug has only one generic name, but can have many trade names. By law, generic names must be identified on all drug labels.

Many companies may manufacture the same drug using different **trade** (patented, brand, or proprietary) names. The drug's trade name is prominently displayed and followed by the trademark symbol (™) or the registration symbol (®). For example, Nitrostat is the trade name and nitroglycerin is the generic name for the drug shown in Figure 2.1.

> **NOTE**
>
> At the time of administration, the name, purpose, and effects of the medication should be discussed with the client and/or caregiver, especially upon first-time administration, and reviewed upon subsequent administrations.

Figure 2.1 Drug label for Nitrostat.

SOURCE: Courtesy of Pfizer, Inc.

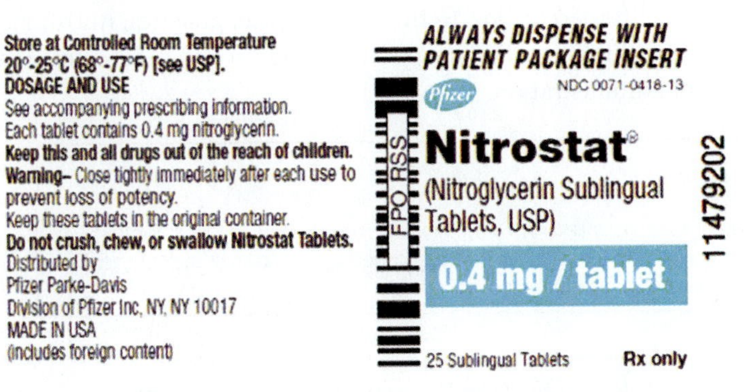

Dosage strength indicates the amount of drug in a specific unit of measurement. The dosage strength of Nitrostat is 0.4 *mg* per tablet.

Each drug has a unique identification number. This number is called the **National Drug Code (NDC) number**. The NDC number for Nitrostat is 0071-0418-13. It is printed on the label and is also encoded in the bar code. Bar codes are used with a bar code-scanning system and computerized database. The healthcare facility's bar code scanners are linked to their electronic medical records. When a medication is scanned, the medication information is compared to the client's database, and the system alerts the healthcare provider to potential problems. The *Food and Drug Administration (FDA)* regulates the manufacturing, sale, and effectiveness of all medications sold in the United States. The FDA is responsible for the "black box" warnings on certain medications, alerting the healthcare provider to serious risks associated with the medication. Legislatures and other governmental agencies also regulate the administration of medications. The FDA estimates that the bar coding of prescription drugs reduces medication errors by as much as 50 *percent*.

To help avoid errors, drugs should be prescribed with only the generic name or with both generic and trade names. Many drugs have names that sound alike, or have names or packaging that look alike. To avoid medication errors, the *FDA, Institute for Safe Medication Practice (ISMP), Joint Commission,* and *National Board of Pharmacy* recommend the use of TALL MAN Lettering in drug names. TALL MAN letters are uppercase letters used in a drug name to highlight the primary dissimilarities with look-alike drug names (ISMP Nov, 2010).

To meet the National Patient Safety Goals of The Joint Commission, a healthcare organization must develop its own list of look-alike/sound-alike drugs that it stores, dispenses, or administers. Table 2.1 includes a sample list of drugs whose names may be confused. See Appendix B for more complete FDA and ISMP Lists of Look-Alike Drug Names with Recommended Tall Man letters. See www.ismp.org for the ISMP's List of *Confused Drug Names.*

ALERT

Giving the wrong drug is a common medication error. To avoid errors, carefully read drug labels at the following times, even if the dose is prepackaged, labeled, and ready to be administered:

- When reaching for or preparing the medication.
- Immediately before administering the medication.
- When discarding the container or replacing it in its storage location.

These are referred to as the *three checks.* To minimize interuptions in the preparation of medications, some facilities have instituted "no interuption zones" that help prevent distractions to those preparing medications. *Always question the client concerning any allergies to medications!* Make sure the drug is not expired, and never give a drug from a container that is unlabeled or has an unreadable label.

The Right Dose

A person prescribing or administering medications has the *legal responsibility* of knowing the correct dose. Calculations may be necessary, and appropriate equipment must be used to measure the dose. Because no two people are exactly alike, and no drug affects every human body in exactly the same way, drug doses must be individualized. Responses to drug actions may differ according to the gender, race, genetics, nutritional and health status, age, and weight of the client (especially children and older adults), as well as the route and time of administration.

ALERT

The calibrated dropper *supplied with a medication* should be used ONLY for that medication. For example, the dropper that is supplied with digoxin (Lanoxin) cannot be used to measure furosemide (Lasix).

Table 2.1 Look-Alike/Sound-Alike Drugs with Tall Man Lettering.

Drug Name	Confused with
aceta**ZOLAMIDE**	aceto**HEXAMIDE**
bu**PROP**ion	bus**PIR**one
chloropro**MAZINE**	chloropro**PAMIDE**
DAUNOrubicin	**DOXO**rubicin
DOBUTamine	**DOP**amine
EPINEPHrine	e**PHED**rine
fenta**NYL**	**SUF**entanil
glipi**ZIDE**	gly**BURIDE**
hydr**ALAZINE**	hydr**OXY**zine
Huma**LOG**	Humu**LIN**
ni**CAR**dipine	**NIFE**dipine
predniso**LONE**	prednisone
TOLAZamide	**TOLBUT**amide
vin**BLAS**tine	vin**CRIS**tine

The **standard adult dosage** for each drug is determined by its manufacturer. A standard adult dosage is recommended based on the requirements of an average-weight adult and may be stated either as a *set dose* (20 *mg*) or as a *range* (150–300 *mg*). In the latter case, the minimum and maximum recommended dosages given are referred to as the **safe dosage range**. Recommended dosage may be found in many sources, including the package insert, the Hospital Formulary, and the prescribing information on the manufacturer's website.

Body surface area (BSA) is an estimate of the total skin area of a person measured in meters squared (m^2). BSA is determined by formulas based on height and weight (see Chapter 6). Many drug doses administered to children or used for cancer therapy are calculated based on BSA.

Carefully read the drug label to determine the *dosage strength.* Perform and *check calculations*, and pay special attention to decimal points. When giving an intravenous drug to a pediatric client or giving a high-alert drug, always *double-check the dosage and pump settings*, and confirm these with a colleague. Be sure to check for the recommended *safe dosage range* based on the client's age, BSA, or weight. After you have calculated the dose, be certain to use a standard measuring device such as a calibrated medicine dropper, syringe, or cup to administer the drug.

Medications may be prepared by the pharmacist or drug manufacturer in unit-dose packaging or multiple-dose packaging. **Unit-dose** medications may be in the form of single tablets, capsules, or a liquid dosage sealed in an individual package. Unit-dose medications may be packaged in vials, bottles, prefilled syringes, or ampules, each of which contains only one dosage of a medication. When more than one dose is contained in a package, this is referred to as **multidose** packaging. See Figures 2.2 and 2.3.

ALERT

Be very attentive when reading the drug label. For example, you might mistake the total amount in a multidose container for a unit dose. Giving the wrong dose is a medication error.

Figure 2.2 Unit-dose packages.

SOURCE: Chaloemphan/Fotolia

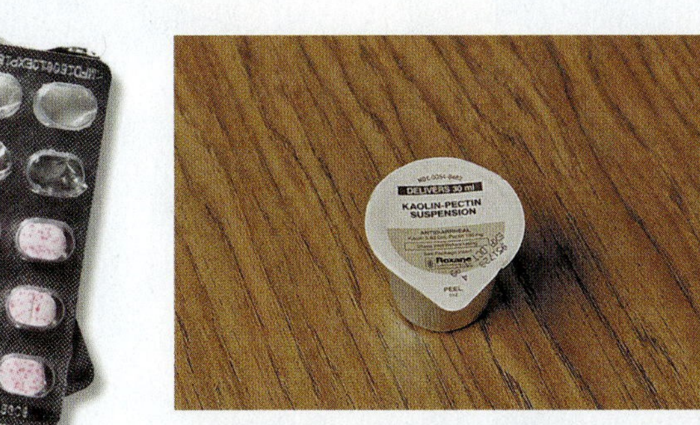

SOURCE: George Draper/Pearson Education, Inc.

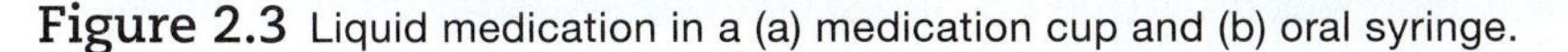

Figure 2.3 Liquid medication in a (a) medication cup and (b) oral syringe.

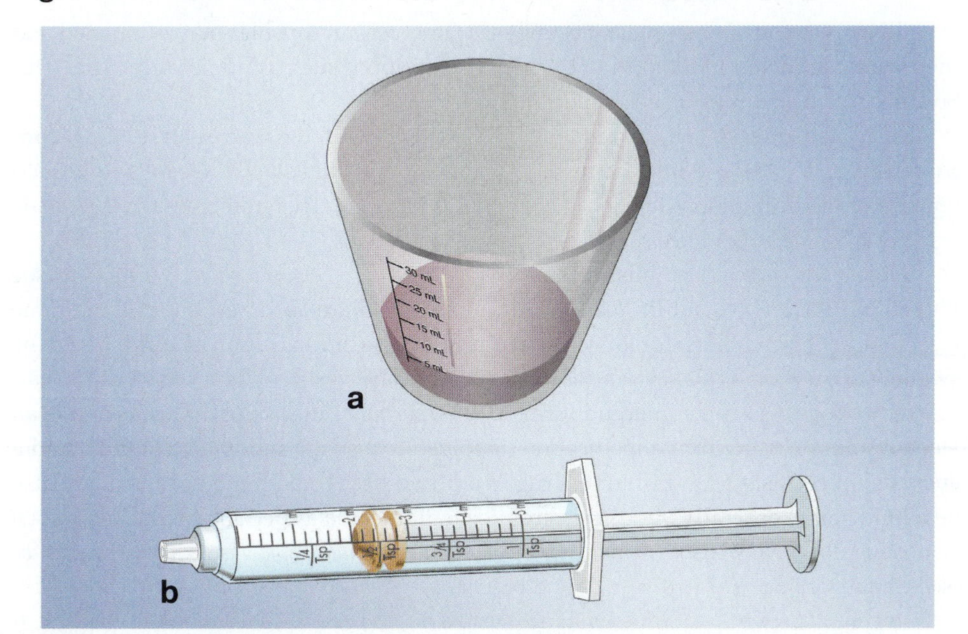

The Right Route and Form

Medications must be administered *in the form* and *via the route specified by the prescriber.* Medications are manufactured in the **form** of tablets, capsules, liquids, suppositories, creams, patches, inhalants, and injectable medications (which are supplied in solution or in a powdered form to be reconstituted). The form (preparation) of a drug affects its speed of onset, intensity of action, and route of administration. The **route** indicates the site of the body and method of drug delivery.

ORAL MEDICATIONS Oral medications are administered **by mouth** (PO) and are supplied in both solid and liquid form. The most common solid forms are *tablets* (tab), *capsules* (cap), and *caplets* (Figure 2.4).

Scored tablets have a groove down the center so that the tablet can be easily broken in half and some are also scored twice so that they can be broken into quarters. To avoid an incorrect dose, unscored tablets should never be broken.

Enteric-coated tablets are meant to dissolve in the intestine rather than in the stomach. Therefore, they should be swallowed whole and neither chewed nor crushed. A **capsule** is a gelatin case containing a powder, a liquid, or granules (pulverized fragments

Figure 2.4 Forms of oral medications.

SOURCE: Pearson Education, Inc.

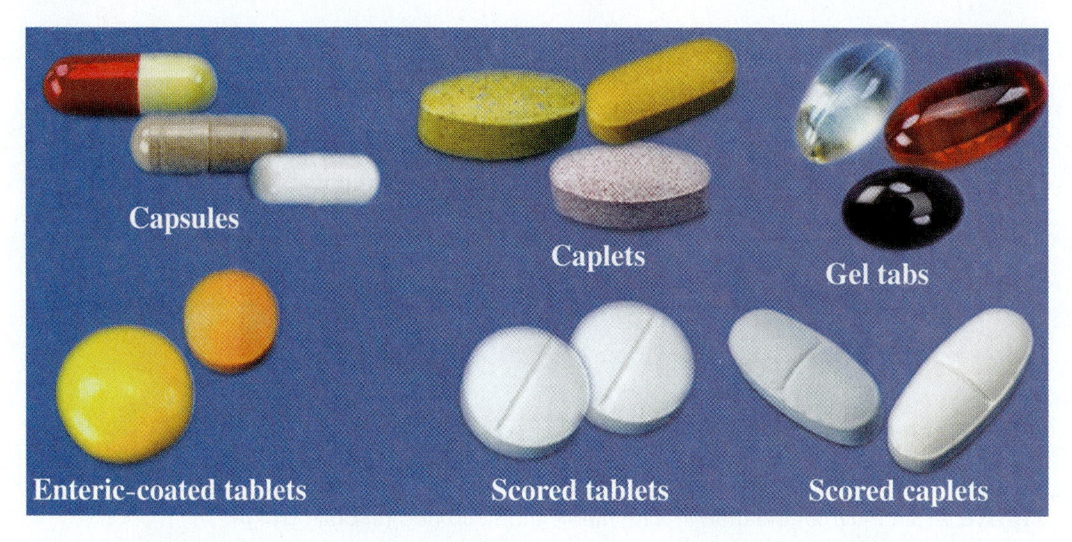

of solid medication). When a client cannot swallow, certain capsules may be opened and their contents mixed in a liquid or sprinkled on a food, such as applesauce. Theo-dur Sprinkles is an example of such a medication.

Sustained-release (SR), extended-release (ER or **XL), delayed-release (DR), controlled-release (CR),** and **long-acting (LA)** tablets or capsules slowly release a controlled amount of medication into the body over a period of time. Therefore, these drugs *should not be opened, chewed, or crushed.*

Tablets for **buccal** administration are absorbed by the mucosa of the mouth (see Figure 2.5). Tablets for **sublingual (SL)** administration are absorbed under the tongue (see Figure 2.6). Tablets for buccal or sublingual administration should never be swallowed.

Oral drugs also come in liquid forms: *elixirs, syrups,* and *suspensions.* An **elixir** is an alcohol solution, a **syrup** is a medication dissolved in a sugar-and-water solution, and a **suspension** consists of an insoluble drug in a liquid base. Liquid medications may also be administered **enterally** into the gastrointestinal tract via a specially placed tube, such as a *nasogastric (NG), gastrostomy (GT),* or *percutaneous endoscopic gastrostomy (PEG) tube* (see Chapter 10).

Figure 2.5 Buccal route: Tablet between cheek and teeth.

SOURCE: Pearson Education, Inc.

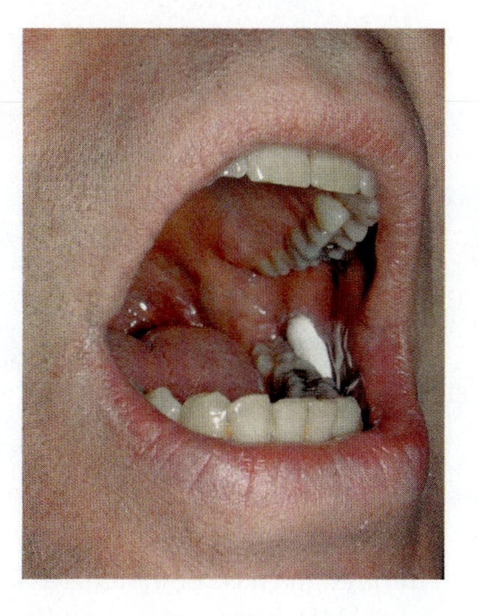

Figure 2.6 Sublingual route: Tablet under tongue.

SOURCE: Pearson Education, Inc.

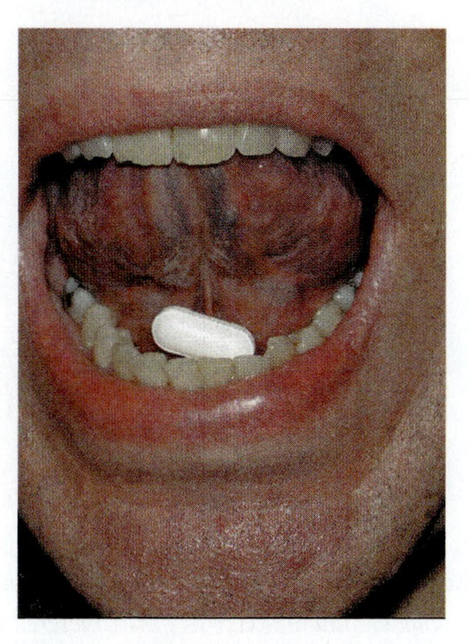

ALERT

DO NOT substitute a different route for the prescribed route because a serious overdose or underdose may occur. Giving medication by the wrong route is a medication error.

Parenteral Medications. Parenteral medications are those that are injected (via needle) into the body by various routes. They are absorbed faster and more completely than drugs given by other routes. Drug forms for parenteral use are sterile and must be administered using aseptic technique. See Chapters 7 and 9.

The most common parenteral sites are:

- **Epidural:** into the epidural space (in the lumbar region of the spine)
- **Intramuscular (IM):** into the muscle
- **Subcutaneous (subcut):** into the subcutaneous tissue
- **Intravenous (IV):** into the vein
- **Intradermal (ID):** beneath the skin
- **Intracardiac (IC):** into the cardiac muscle
- **Intrathecal:** into the spinal column or in the space under the arachnoid membrane of the brain or spinal cord
- **Intra-articular:** into a joint

Cutaneous Medications. Cutaneous medications are those that are administered through the skin or mucous membrane. Cutaneous routes include:

- **Topical:** administered *on the skin surface* and may provide either a *local* or a *systemic* effect. Those drugs applied for a **local** effect are absorbed slowly, and amounts reaching the general circulation are minimal. Those administered for a **systemic** effect provide a slow release and absorption in the general circulation.
- **Transdermal:** contained *in a patch or disk and applied to the skin.* These are administered for their *systemic* effect. Patches allow constant, controlled amounts of drug to be released over 24 *hours* or more. Examples include nitroglycerin for angina or chest pain, nicotine to control the urge to smoke, and fentanyl for chronic pain. See Figure 2.7.

Figure 2.7 Transdermal patch: (a) protective coating removed; (b) patch immediately applied to clean, dry, hairless skin and labeled with date, time, and initials.

SOURCE: Pearson Education, Inc.

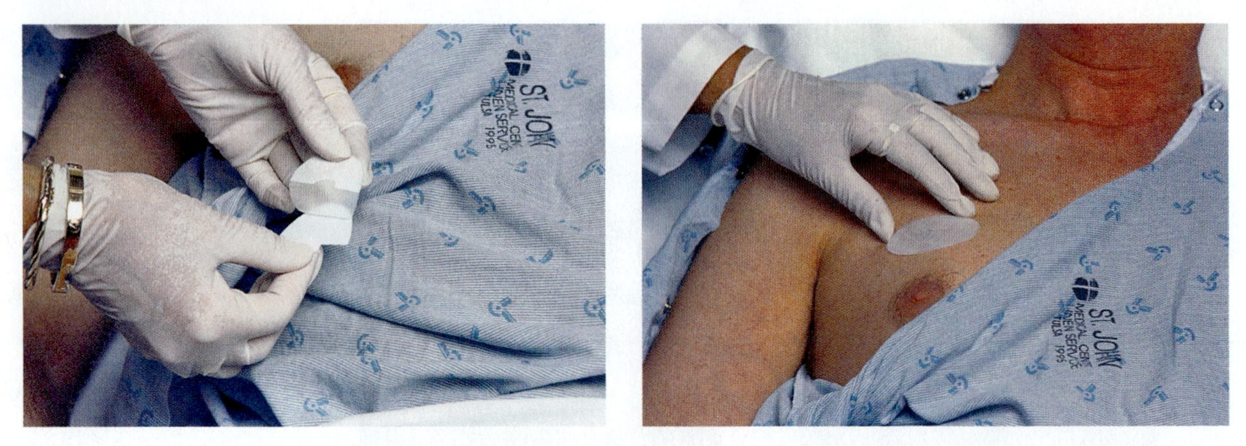

- **Inhalation:** breathed into the respiratory tract through the nose or mouth. *Nebulizers, dry powder inhalers (DPIs),* and *metered-dose inhalers (MDIs)* are types of devices used to administer drugs via inhalation. A **nebulizer** vaporizes a liquid medication into a fine mist that can then be inhaled using a face mask or handheld device. A **DPI** is a small device used for solid drugs. The device is activated by the process of inhalation, and a fine powder is inhaled. An **MDI** uses a propellant to deliver a measured dose of medication with each inhalation. See Figure 2.8.

Figure 2.8 Inhalation devices: (a) nebulizer with face mask; (b) dry powder inhaler; (c) metered dose inhaler.

SOURCE: Pearson Education, Inc.

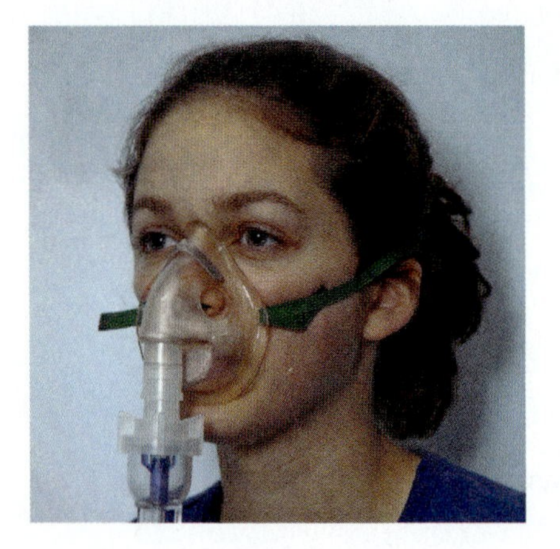

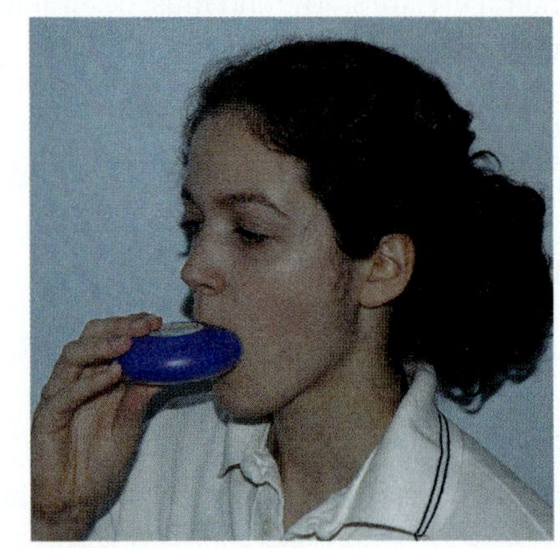

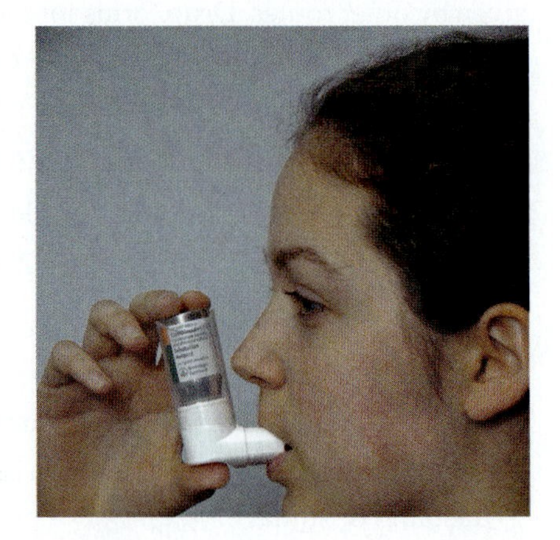

- **Solutions and ointments:** applied to the mucosa of the eyes (optic), nose (nasal), ears (otic), or mouth
- **Suppositories:** are shaped for insertion into a body cavity (vagina, rectum, or urethra) and dissolve at body temperature

Some drugs are supplied in multiple forms and therefore can be administered by a variety of routes. For example, Tigan (trimethobenzamide HCl) is supplied as a capsule, suppository, or solution for injection.

The Right Time

The prescriber will indicate when and how often a medication should be administered. Oral medications can be given either before or after meals, depending on the action of the drug. Factors such as the purpose of the drug, drug interactions, absorption of the drug, and side effects must be considered when medication times are scheduled. Medications can be ordered *once a day* (daily), *twice a day* (b.i.d.), *three times a day* (t.i.d.), and *four times a day* (q.i.d). Most healthcare facilities designate specific times for these administrations. To maintain a more stable level of the drug in the client, the period between administrations of the drug should be prescribed at regular intervals, such as q4h (every four hours), q6h, q8h, or q12h.

Incorrect interpretation of abbreviations related to medication administration times could result in drug errors. For example, *30 mg B.I.D.* (twice a day) is not necessarily the same as *30 mg q12h* (every twelve hours). Depending on the institution's drug delivery time schedule, *30 mg B.I.D.* may mean to administer 30 *mg* at 10:00 A.M. and 30 *mg* at 6:00 P.M., whereas *30 mg q12h* may mean to administer 30 *mg* at 10:00 A.M. and 30 *mg* at 10:00 P.M.

B.I.D. should also not be confused with "daily in two divided doses." For example, *30 mg B.I.D.* requires administering two doses of 30 *mg* each for a total daily dose of 60 *mg*. In contrast, *30 mg daily in two divided doses* requires administering two doses of 15 *mg* each for a total daily dose of 30 *mg*.

In 2011, the **Centers for Medicare and Medicaid Services (CMS)** revised the so-called "30-minute rule" on the administration of medication, which had established a uniform 30-minute window before or after the scheduled time for all medication administration. Hospitals now must establish policies and procedures for the timing of medication administration that take into account the nature of the prescribed medication, specific clinical applications, and client needs.

NOTE

Because regulations are evolving, healthcare providers should refer to the CMS website (www.cms.gov) for current regulations.

"Hospitals are expected to identify those medications which require exact or precise timing of administration, and which are not, therefore, eligible for scheduled dosing times." Some examples are stat doses, loading doses, one-time doses (doses specifically timed for procedures), and time-sequenced doses (doses timed for serum drug levels).

ALERT

The timing of medication administration can be critical for maintaining a stable concentration of the drug in the blood and avoiding interactions with other drugs. Know the agency policy, and always administer the dose immediately after it is prepared.

"For medications that are eligible for scheduled dosing times, hospitals are expected to distinguish between those that are time-critical and those that are not, and to establish policies governing timing of medication administration accordingly. **Time-critical** scheduled medications are those for which an early or late administration of greater than thirty minutes might cause harm." Some examples are antibiotics, insulin, anticoagulants, anticonvulsants, and pain medication.

"**Non-time-critical** scheduled medications are those for which a longer or shorter interval of time since the prior dose does not significantly change the medication's therapeutic effect or otherwise cause harm." Therefore, the hospital may establish, as appropriate, either a 1- or 2-hour window for administration.

The Right Client

Before administering any medication, it is essential to determine the identity of the recipient. Administering a medication to a client other than the one for whom it was ordered is one example of a medication error. The Joint Commission continues to include proper client identification in its National Patient Safety Goals, and it requires the use of at least two forms of client identification. Suggested identifiers include the client identification bracelet information, verbalization of the client's name and birth date by the client, family member, legal guardian, or parent, the client's home telephone number, and the client's hospital number.

ALERT

The client's bed number or room number is *not* to be used for client identification. Know and use the identifiers recognized and required by your agency. Administering a medication to the wrong client is one of the most common medication errors.

After identifying the client, match the drug order, client's name, and age to the Medication Administration Record (MAR). To help reduce errors, many agencies now use computers at the bedside or use handheld devices (scanners) to read the bar code on a client's identification bracelet and on the medication packages. See Figure 2.9.

Figure 2.9 Bar codes: (a) unit-dose drug; (b) scanner reading a client's identification band.

SOURCE: Shirlee Snyder/Pearson Education, Inc.

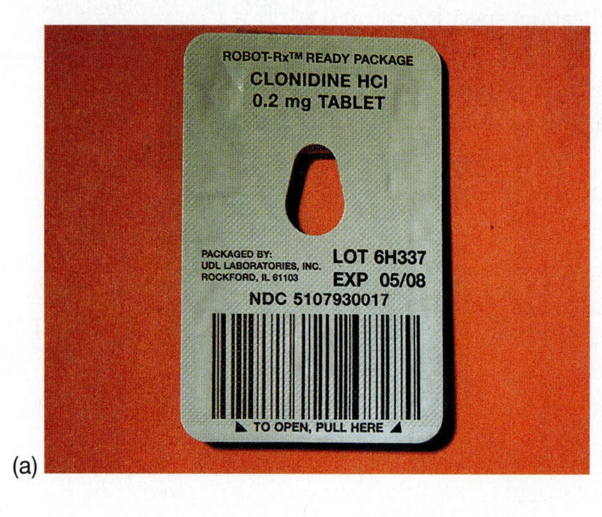

(a)

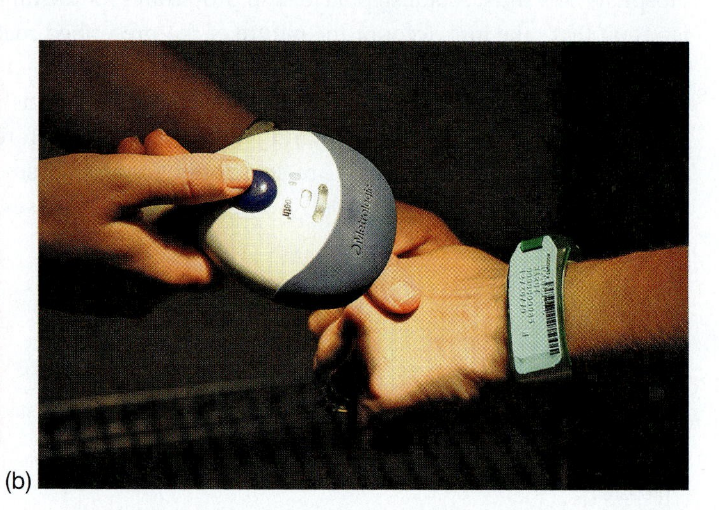

(b)

The Right Documentation

Always document the name and dosage of the drug, as well as the route and time of administration on the MAR. Sign your initials *immediately after, but never before*, the dose is given. It is important to include any relevant information. For example, document client allergies to medications, client pain level, heart rate (when giving digoxin), and blood pressure (when giving antihypertensive drugs). All documentation must be legible. Remember the axiom "If it's not documented, it's not done."

Anticipate side effects! A **side effect** is an undesired physiologic response to a drug. For example, codeine relieves pain, but its side effects include constipation, nausea, drowsiness, and itching. Be sure to record any observed side effects and discuss them with the prescriber.

Safe drug administration requires a knowledge of common abbreviations. For instance, when the prescriber writes "*Demerol 75 mg IM q4h prn pain*," the person administering the drug reads this as "Administer the drug Demerol; the dose is seventy-five milligrams, the route is intramuscular, the time is every four hours, and it is to be given when the client has pain." Be cautious with abbreviations because they can be a source of medication error. Only approved abbreviations should be used (Table 2.2).

Table 2.2 Common Abbreviations Used for Medication Administration.

Abbreviation	Meaning
Route:	
GT	gastrostomy tube
ID	intradermal
IM	intramuscular
IV	intravenous
IVP	intravenous push
IVPB	intravenous piggyback
NGT	nasogastric tube
PEG	percutaneous endoscopic gastrostomy
PO	by mouth
PR	by rectum
SL	sublingual
subcut	subcutaneously
Supp	suppository
Frequency:	
ac	before meals
ad lib	as desired
B.I.D. or b.i.d.	two times a day
h, hr	hour
hs	at bedtime
pc	after meals
prn	whenever needed or necessary
q	every
q2h	every two hours
q4h	every four hours
q6h	every six hours
q8h	every eight hours
q12h	every twelve hours
Q.I.D. or q.i.d.	four times per day
Stat	immediately
T.I.D. or t.i.d.	three times per day
General:	
c	with
CR	controlled release
cap	capsule
d.a.w.	dispense as written
DR	delayed release
ER	extended release
g	gram
gtt	drop
kg	kilogram
L	liter
LA	long acting
mcg	microgram
mg	milligram
mL	milliliter
NKDA	no known drug allergies
NPO	nothing by mouth

Table 2.2 *(Continued)*

Abbreviation	Meaning
s	without
Sig	directions to client
Susp	suspension
SR	sustained release
t or tsp	teaspoon
T or tbs	tablespoon
tab	tablet
XL or XR	extended release

The Joint Commission requires healthcare organizations to follow its official *"Do Not Use List"* that applies to all medication orders and all medication documentation. See Table 2.3.

Table 2.3 JCAHO Official "Do Not Use List"[1]

SOURCE: © The Joint Commission, 2017. Reprinted with permission.

Do Not Use	Potential Problem	Use Instead
U (for unit)	Mistaken for "0" (zero), the number "4" (four), or "cc"	Write "unit"
IU (International Unit)	Mistaken for IV (intravenous) or the number 10 (ten)	Write "International Unit"
Q.D., QD, q.d., qd (daily)	Mistaken for each other	Write "daily"
Q.O.D., QOD, q.o.d, qod (every other day)	Period after the Q mistaken for "I" and the "O" mistaken for "I"	Write "every other day"
Trailing zero (X.0 *mg*)[2]	Decimal point is missed	Write X *mg*
Lack of leading zero (.X *mg*)		Write 0.X *mg*
MS	Can mean morphine sulfate or magnesium sulfate	Write "morphine sulfate" Write "magnesium sulfate"
MSO_4 and $MgSO_4$	Confused for one another	

[1]Applies to all orders and all medication-related documentation that is handwritten (including free-text computer entry) or on preprinted forms.

[2]**Exception:** A "trailing zero" may be used only where required to demonstrate the level of precision of the value being reported, such as for laboratory results, imaging studies that report size of lesions, or catheter/tube sizes. It may not be used in medication orders or other medication-related documentation.

Additional Abbreviations, Acronyms, and Symbols
(For *possible* future inclusion in the Official "Do Not Use" List)

Do Not Use	Potential Problem	Use Instead
> (greater than)	Misinterpreted as the number	Write "greater than"
< (less than)	"7" (seven) or the letter "L"; Confused for one another	Write "less than"
Abbreviations for drug names	Misinterpreted due to similar abbreviations for multiple drugs	Write drug names in full
Apothecary units	Unfamiliar to many practitioners; Confused with metric units	Use metric units
@	Mistaken for the number "2" (two)	Write "at"
cc	Mistaken for U (units) when poorly written	Write "mL" or "milliliters"
µg	Mistaken for *mg* (milligrams) resulting in one thousand-fold overdose	Write "*mcg*" or "micrograms"

Drug Prescriptions

Before a healthcare provider can administer any medication, there must be a legal order or prescription for the medication.

A **drug prescription** is a directive to the pharmacist for a drug to be given to a client who is being seen in a medical office or clinic or is being discharged from a healthcare facility. A prescription may be written, or it can be faxed, phoned, or emailed from a secure, encrypted computer system to a pharmacist. All prescriptions should contain the following:

- Prescriber's full name, address, telephone number, and (when the prescription is given for a controlled substance) the Drug Enforcement Administration (DEA) number
- Date the prescription is written
- Client's full name, address, and age or date of birth
- Drug name (generic name should be included), dosage, route, frequency, and amount to be dispensed
- Indication whether it is acceptable to substitute a generic form (when only the trade name is given)
- Directions to the client that must appear on the drug container
- Number of refills permitted

If any of this information is missing or unclear, the prescription is considered incomplete and is therefore *not* a legal order. Every state has a drug substitution law that either mandates or may permit a less-expensive generic drug substitution by the pharmacist. If the prescriber has an objection to a generic drug substitute, the prescriber will write "do not substitute," "dispense as written," "no generic substitution," or "medically necessary" (Figure 2.10). Some states require bar codes on prescription forms.

Figure 2.10 Drug prescription for Zocor.

Adam Smith, M.D.
100 Main Street
Utopia, New York 10000
Phone (212) 345-6789

DEA # 56777 **License # 123456**

Name: *Joan Soto* **Date:** *November 24, 2020*

Address: *4205 Main Street*
Utopia, NY 10000 **Age/DOB:** *04/20/48*

℞ *Zocor 10 mg tablets*

Sig: *1 tablet PO, daily in the evening*

Dispense: *90*
Refills: *0*

THIS PRESCRIPTION WILL BE FILLED GENERICALLY UNLESS THE PRESCRIBER WRITES "d a w" IN THE BOX BELOW.

d a w

Adam Smith MD

Handwritten prescriptions are becoming a thing of the past. Health systems, hospitals, physicians, and pharmacies are increasingly using electronic prescriptions. Electronic prescribing is meant to improve client safety and quality of care. Illegibility of handwritten prescriptions is eliminated, decreasing the risk of medication errors. The system can alert prescribers to contraindications, adverse reactions, and duplicate therapies.

This prescription is interpreted as follows:

- **Prescriber:** Adam Smith, M.D.
- **Prescriber address:** 100 Main Street, Utopia, NY 10000
- **Prescriber phone number:** (212) 345-6789
- **Date prescription written:** November 24, 2020
- **Client's full name:** Joan Soto
- **Client address:** 4205 Main Street, Utopia NY 10000
- **Client date of birth:** April 20, 1948
- **Drug name:** Zocor (trade name)
- **Dosage:** 10 *mg*
- **Route:** by mouth (PO)
- **Frequency:** once a day
- **Amount to be dispensed:** 90 *tablets*
- **Acceptable to substitute a generic form?** no, the prescriber has written "d a w"
- **Directions to the client:** take 1 *tablet* by mouth daily in evening
- **Refill instructions:** no refills permitted

Medication Orders

ALERT

If persons administering medications have difficulty understanding or interpreting the orders, it is their responsibility to clarify the orders with the prescribers.

Medication orders are directives to the pharmacist for the drugs prescribed in a hospital or other healthcare facility. The terms *medication orders, drug orders*, and *physician's orders* are used interchangeably, and the forms used will vary from agency to agency. No medication should be given without a medication order. Medication orders can be *written* or *verbal.* Each medication order should follow a specific sequence: drug name, dose, route, and frequency.

Written medication orders are documented in a special book for doctors' orders, on a physician's order sheet in the client's chart, or in a computer.

A **verbal** order must contain the same components as a written order—otherwise, it is invalid. The Joint Commission requires that an *authorized person* write the order in the client's chart and then read it back to the prescriber. The prescriber must confirm that the order is correct. Hospitals must have policies stating when the order must be signed by the prescriber—for example, within 24 *hours*. To provide for the safety of the client, generally verbal orders may be taken only in an emergency.

Types of Medication Orders

The most common type of medication order is the **routine order**, which indicates that the ordered drug is administered until a discontinuation order is written or until a specified date is reached.

A **standing order** is prescribed in anticipation of sudden changes in a client's condition. Standing orders are used frequently in critical care units, where a client's condition may change rapidly and immediate action would be required. Standing orders may also be used in long-term care facilities where a physician may not be readily available; for example, "*Tylenol (acetaminophen) 650 mg PO q4h for temperature of 101°F or higher.*" This is interpreted as "Administer the drug Tylenol (acetaminophen), a dose of six hundred fifty milligrams; the route is by mouth, the time is every four hours, and it is to be given whenever the client's temperature is one hundred one degrees Fahrenheit or more."

Example 2.1

Read the prescription in Figure 2.11 and complete the following information.

Figure 2.11 Drug prescription for Dilantin (phenytoin sodium).

OFFICIAL STATE PRESCRIPTION

Primary Care Associates

1234 Spring Street, Manhattan, Kansas 10001

(913) 999-5678

CERT#: Fxxxxxx DEA#: xxxxxx

Patient Name *Steven James*

Address *124 Winding Lane* Date *10/22/20*

City *Manhattan* State *KS* Zip *10001* Age *64* Sex ☑M ☐F

℞

Dilantin (phenytoin sodium) 100 mg

1 cap po t.i.d.

 # 90

Refills: *2* *300 mg*

Prescriber Signature *Alicia Rodriguez NP*

no substitution

Substitution is mandatory unless the words "no substitution" appear in the box above.

- Date prescription written: ______
- Client full name: ______
- Client address: ______
- Client age: ______
- Generic drug name: ______
- Dosage: ______
- Route: ______
- Frequency: ______
- Amount to be dispensed: ______
- Acceptable to substitute a generic form? ______
- Directions to the client: ______
- Refill instructions: ______

This is what you should have found:

- Date prescription written: 10/22/2020
- Client full name: Steven James

• Client address:	124 Winding Lane Manhattan, Kansas 10001
• Client age:	64
• Generic drug name:	phenytoin sodium
• Dosage:	100 *mg*
• Route:	by mouth
• Frequency:	three times a day
• Amount to be dispensed:	90 *capsules*
• Acceptable to substitute a generic form?	No
• Directions to the client:	take one capsule three times a day
• Refill instructions:	may be refilled two times

A **prn order** is written by the prescriber for a drug to be given when a client needs it; for example, "*morphine sulfate 5 mg subcut q4h prn mild-moderate pain.*" This is interpreted as "Administer the drug morphine sulfate, a dose of five milligrams; the route is subcutaneous, the time is every four hours, and it is to be given as needed when the client has mild or moderate pain."

A **stat order** is an order that is to be administered immediately. Stat orders are usually written for emergencies or when a client's condition suddenly changes; for example, "*Lasix (furosemide) 80 mg IV stat.*" This is interpreted as "Administer the drug Lasix (furosemide), a dose of eighty milligrams; the route is intravenous, and the drug is to be given immediately."

Components of a Medication Order

The essential components of a medication order are:

- **Client's full name and date of birth:** Often this information is stamped or imprinted on the medication order form. Additional information may include the client's admission number, religion, type of insurance, and physician's name.
- **Date and time the order was written:** This includes the month, day, year, and time of day. Many institutions use military time, which is based on a "24-hour clock" that does not use A.M. or P.M. (Figure 2.12). Military times are written as four-digit numbers followed by the word *hours.*

Figure 2.12 Clocks showing 10:10 A.M. (1010 h) and 10:10 P.M. (2210 h).

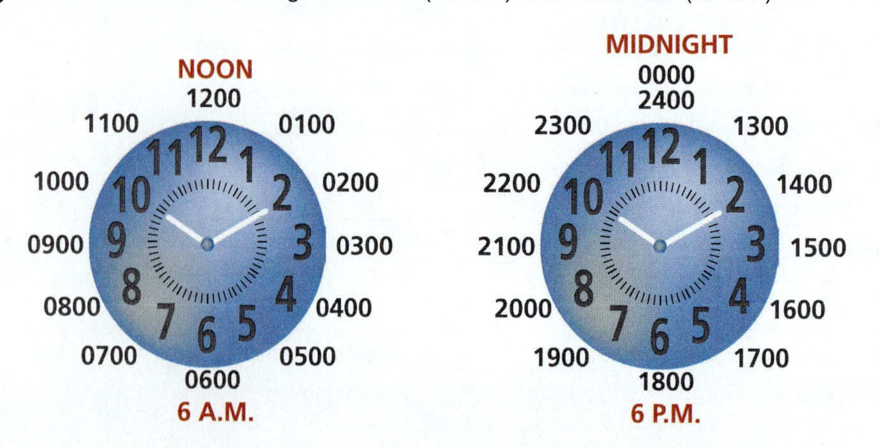

Thus, 2:00 A.M. in military time is 0200 *h* (pronounced *Oh two hundred hours*), 12 noon is 1200 *h* (pronounced *twelve hundred hours*), 2:00 P.M. is 1400 *h* (pronounced *fourteen hundred hours*), and midnight is 2400 *h*.

There is confusion between the meanings of 12:00 A.M. and 12:00 P.M. Twelve noon, for example, is literally neither A.M. (ante meridiem: before midday) nor P.M. (post meridiem: after midday). Noon *is* midday! Therefore, to avoid confusion when administering medications, for noon and midnight use *12 noon* and *12 midnight*, or use military time (*1200h* and *2400h*). The FDA recomends the use of military time.

- **Name of the medication:** The generic name is recommended. If a prescriber desires to prescribe a trade name drug, "no generic substitution" must be specified.
- **Dosage of the medication:** The amount of the drug.
- **Route of administration:** Only approved abbreviations may be used.
- **Time and frequency of administration:** When and how often the drug is to be given.
- **Signature of the prescriber:** The medication order is not legal without the signature of the prescriber.
- **Signature of the person transcribing the order:** This may be the responsibility of a nurse or others identified by agency policy.

ALERT

When the dose includes a large number involving many zeros, use *words* instead of zeros. For example, write *500 thousand units* instead of *500,000 units*, and write *10 million units* instead of *10,000,000 units*.

Figure 2.13 Physician's order for Cymbalta (duloxetine HCl).

GENERAL HOSPITAL

PRESS HARD WITH BALLPOINT PEN. WRITE DATE & TIME AND SIGN EACH ORDER.

DATE 11/20/2020 TIME 0800h

Cymbalta (duloxetine HCl) delayed release 60 mg PO daily

SIGNATURE I. Patel M.D.

IMPRINT
602412 11/20/20
John Camden 2/11/55
23 Jones Ave. RC
New York, NY 10024 BCBS
I. Patel, M.D.

ORDERS NOTED
DATE 11/20/20 TIME 0830 A.M. P.M.
NURSE'S SIG. Mary Jones, RN

FILLED BY DATE

PHYSICIAN'S ORDERS

NOTE

Drug orders follow a specific sequence: drug name, dosage, route, and frequency.

The physician's order in Figure 2.13 can be interpreted as:

Name of client: John Camden

Birth date: Feb. 11, 1955

Date of admission: Nov. 20, 2020

Admission number: 602412

Religion: Roman Catholic (RC)

Insurance: Blue Cross Blue Shield (BCBS)

Date and time the order was written: 11/20/2020 at 0800*h* or 8:00 A.M.

Name of the medication: Cymbalta (duloxetine HCl delayed release)

Dosage: 60 *mg*

Route of administration: PO (by mouth)

Frequency of administration: once a day

Signature of person writing the order: I. Patel, MD

Person who transcribed the order: Mary Jones, RN

Example 2.2

Interpret the physician's order sheet shown in Figure 2.14 and record the following information.

Figure 2.14 Physician's order for Timoptic.

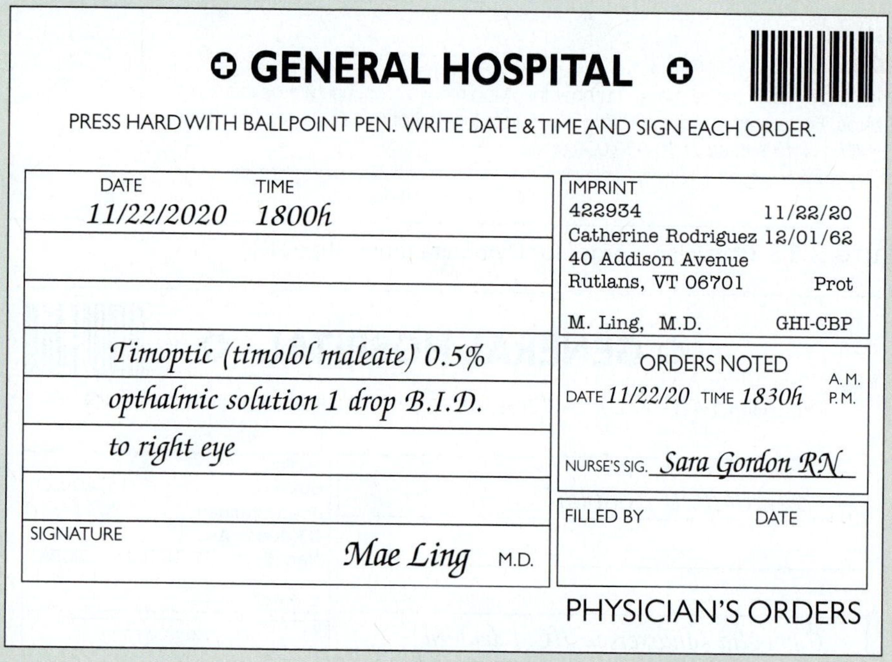

GENERAL HOSPITAL

PRESS HARD WITH BALLPOINT PEN. WRITE DATE & TIME AND SIGN EACH ORDER.

DATE 11/22/2020 TIME 1800h

Timoptic (timolol maleate) 0.5%
opthalmic solution 1 drop B.I.D.
to right eye

SIGNATURE Mae Ling M.D.

IMPRINT
422934 11/22/20
Catherine Rodriguez 12/01/62
40 Addison Avenue
Rutlans, VT 06701 Prot
M. Ling, M.D. GHI-CBP

ORDERS NOTED
DATE 11/22/20 TIME 1830h A.M. P.M.
NURSE'S SIG. Sara Gordon RN

FILLED BY DATE

PHYSICIAN'S ORDERS

Date order written: ______________________

Time order written: ______________________

Name of drug: ______________________

Dosage: ______________________

Route of administration: ______________________

Frequency of administration: ______________________

Name of prescriber: ______________________

Name of client: ______________________

Birth date: ______________________

Religion: ______________________

Type of insurance: ______________________________

Person who transcribed the order: ______________________________

This is what you should have found:

• Date order written:	11/22/2020
• Time order written:	1800 *h* or 6:00 P.M.
• Name of drug:	Timoptic (timolol maleate) 0.5% ophthalmic solution
• Dosage:	1 *drop*
• Route:	topical to right eye
• Frequency of administration:	2 times a day
• Name of prescriber:	Mae Ling, M.D.
• Name of client:	Catherine Rodriguez
• Birth date:	December 1, 1962
• Religion:	Protestant
• Type of insurance:	GHI-CBP
• Person who transcribed the order:	Sara Gordon, RN

Medication Administration Records

A **Medication Administration Record (MAR)** is a form used by healthcare facilities to document all drugs administered to a client. It is a legal document, part of the client's medical record, and the format varies from agency to agency. Client confidentiality must be maintained, and photocopying of any part of the medical record requires client permission. Every agency develops policies related to using the MAR, including how to add new medications, discontinue medications, document one-time or stat medications, the process to follow if a medication is not administered or a client refuses a medication, and correct an error on the MAR.

ALERT

Before administering any medication, always compare the label on the medication with the information on the MAR. If there is a discrepancy, you must check the prescriber's original order.

Routine, PRN, and STAT medications all may be written in separate locations on the MAR. PRN and STAT medications may also have a separate form. If a medication is to be given regularly, a complete schedule is written for all administration times. Each time a dose is administered, the healthcare worker initials the time of administration. The full name, title, and initials of the person who gave the medication must be recorded on the MAR.

After a prescriber's order has been verified, a nurse or other healthcare provider transcribes the order to the MAR. This record is used to check the medication order; prepare the correct medication dose; and record the date, time, and route of administration.

The essential components of the MAR include:

- **Client information:** a stamp or printed label with client identification (name, date of birth, medical record number).
- **Dates:** when the order was written, when to start the medication, and when to discontinue it.
- **Medication information:** full name of the drug, dose, route, and frequency of administration.
- **Time of administration:** frequency as stated in the prescriber's order—for example, t.i.d. Times for PRN and one-time doses are recorded *precisely* at the time they are administered.

- **Initials:** the initials and the signature of the person who administered the medication are recorded.
- **Special instructions:** instructions relating to the medication—for example, "Hold if systolic BP is less than 100."

Example 2.3

Study the MAR in Figure 2.15, and then complete the following chart and answer the questions.

Figure 2.15 MAR for Wendy Kim.

UNIVERSITY HOSPITAL

DAILY MEDICATION ADMINISTRATION RECORD

789652
Wendy Kim
44 Chester Avenue
New York, NY 10003

9/11/2020
12/20/60
RC
Medicaid

Dr. Juan Rodriguez, M.D.

PATIENT NAME *Wendy Kim*

ROOM # *422*

ALLERGIC TO (RECORD IN RED): *tomato, codeine*

IF ANOTHER RECORD IS IN USE ☐

DATES GIVEN

DATE DISCHARGED:

RED CHECK INITIAL	ORDER DATE	INITIAL	EXP DATE	MEDICATION, DOSAGE, FREQUENCY AND ROUTE	HOURS	12	13	14	15
	9/12	JY	9/19	**ceftriaxone** (Rocephin) 1 g	0600	/	MC	MC	
				IVPB q12h for 7 days begin at 1800h	1800	MJ	SG	SG	
	9/12	JY	9/18	**digoxin** 0.125 mg PO daily	0900	JY	JY	JY	
	9/12	JY	9/18	**enalapril maleate** (Vasotec)	0900	JY	JY	JY	
				20 mg PO q12h	2100	MJ	SG	SG	
	9/12	JY	9/18	**clopidogrel bisulfate** (Plavix)	0900	JY	JY	JY	
				75 mg PO daily					
	9/12	JY	9/18	**oxybutynin chloride** (Ditropan XL)	2100	MJ	SG	SG	
				10 mg PO HS					

INT.	NURSES' FULL SIGNATURE AND TITLE	INT.	CODES FOR INJECTION SITES	
JY	Jim Young, RN		A- left anterior thigh	H- right anterior thigh
MC	Marie Colon, RN		B- left deltoid	I- right deltoid
MJ	Mary Jones, LPN		C- left gluteus medius	J- right gluteus medius
SG	Sara Gordon, RN		D- left lateral thigh	K- right lateral thigh
			E- left ventral gluteus	L- right ventral gluteus
			F- left lower quadrant	M- right lower quadrant
			G- left upper quadrant	N- right upper quadrant

Name of Drug	Dose	Route of Administration	Time of Administration

1. Identify the drugs and their doses administered at 9:00 A.M.

 ____

2. Identify the drugs and their doses administered at 9:00 P.M.

 ____

3. Who administered the clopidogrel bisulfate on 9/14?

 ____

4. What is the route of administration for ceftriaxone?

 ____

5. What is the time of administration for enalapril maleate?

 ____

This is what you should have found:

Name of Drug	Dose	Route of Administration	Time of Administration
ceftriaxone	1 *g*	IVPB	0600 *h* (6 A.M.) &1800 *h* (6 P.M.)
digoxin	0.125 *mg*	PO	0900 *h* (9 A.M.)
enalapril maleate (Vasotec)	20 *mg*	PO	0900 *h* (9 A.M.) & 2100 *h* (9 P.M.)
clopidogrel bisulfate (Plavix)	75 *mg*	PO	0900 *h* (9 A.M.)
oxybutynin chloride (Ditropan XL)	10 *mg*	PO	2100 *h* (9 P.M.)

1. digoxin 0.125 *mg*; enalapril maleate (Vasotec) 20 *mg*; clopidogrel bisulfate (Plavix) 75 *mg*
2. enalapril maleate (Vasotec) 20 *mg* and oxybutynin chloride (Ditropan XL) 10 *mg*
3. Jim Young, RN
4. Intravenous
5. 0900 *h* (9:00 A.M.) and 2100 *h* (9:00 P.M.)

Example 2.4

Study the MAR in Figures 2.16a and 2.16b, and then fill in the following chart and answer the questions.

Figure 2.16a MAR for Mohammad Kamal.

UNIVERSITY HOSPITAL

DAILY MEDICATION ADMINISTRATION RECORD

659204 11/20/2020
Mohammad Kamal 10/2/52
4103 Ely Avenue Musl
Bronx, NY 10466 GHI-CBP

Dr. Indu Patel, M.D.

PATIENT NAME *Mohammad Kamal*

ROOM # *302*

IF ANOTHER RECORD IS IN USE ☐

ALLERGIC TO (RECORD IN RED): *sulfa, fish*

DATES GIVEN MONTH/DAY **YEAR:** *2020*

RED CHECK INITIAL	ORDER DATE	INITIAL	EXP DATE	MEDICATION, DOSAGE, FREQUENCY AND ROUTE	TIME	11/20	11/21	11/22	11/23	11/24	11/25	11/26
	11/20	MC	11/26	**pantoprazole sodium** (Protonix DR) 40 mg	10 AM	—	MC	MC	MC	MJ	MJ	JY
				PO daily								
	11/20	MC	11/26	**captopril** 25 mg	10 AM	—	MC	MC	MC	MJ	MJ	JY
				PO B.I.D.	BP	—	160/110	150/70	160/110	138/86	130/80	130/80
					6 PM	MC	MC	MC	MC	MJ	MJ	JY
					BP	160/100	150/90	160/100	140/80	130/80	128/80	128/80
	11/20	MC	11/26	**furosemide** (Lasix) 20 mg PO daily	10 AM	—	MC	MC	MC	MJ	MJ	JY
	11/20	SG	11/27	**cefotaxime**	10 AM	—	MC	MC	MC	MJ	MJ	JY
				1g IVPB q12hr for 7 days	10 PM		SG	SG	SG	SG	SG	SG
	11/21	MC	11/27	**epoetin alfa** (Procrit) 3,000 units	10 AM	—	MC	—	MC	—	MJ	—
				subcutaneous, three times per week,								
				start on 11/21								
	11/21	MC	11/27	**digoxin**, 0.125 mg PO daily	10 AM	—	MC	MC	MC	MJ	MJ	JY
					HR	—	72	70	96	76	80	80

INT.	NURSES' FULL SIGNATURE AND TITLE	INT.	NURSES' FULL SIGNATURE AND TITLE
MC	Marie Colon, RN		
SG	Sara Gordon, RN		
MJ	Mary Jones, LPN		
JY	Jim Young, RN		

Figure 2.16b MAR for Mohammad Kamal.

UNIVERSITY HOSPITAL

DAILY MEDICATION ADMINISTRATION RECORD

659204 11/20/2020
Mohammad Kamal 10/2/52
4103 Ely Avenue Musl
Bronx, NY 10466 GHI-CBP

Dr. Indu Patel, M.D.

PATIENT NAME *Mohammad Kamal*

ROOM # *302*

ALLERGIC TO (RECORD IN RED): *sulfa, fish*

IF ANOTHER RECORD IS IN USE ☐

DATES GIVEN ↓ MONTH/DAY YEAR: *2020*

PRN MEDICATION

ORDER DATE	EXPIRATION DATE/TIME	MEDICATION, DOSAGE, FREQUENCY AND ROUTE	DOSES GIVEN								
11/20	11/27	**acetaminophen** (Tylenol) 650 mg PO q6h prn mild pain	DATE	11/20	11/21	11/22					
			TIME	6 PM	10 AM	6 PM					
			INIT	MJ	MC	6 PM					
11/20	11/27	Robitussin DM 10 ml PO q12h prn	DATE	11/20	11/21						
			TIME	10 AM	10 PM						
			INIT	MJ	SG						

STAT-ONE DOSE-PRE-OPERATIVE MEDICATIONS

◯ Check here if additional sheet in use.

ORDER DATE	MEDICATION-DOSAGE ROUTE	DATE	TIME	INIT	ORDER DATE	MEDICATION-DOSAGE ROUTE	DATE	TIME	INIT
11/23	**labetalol** 20 mg IVP over 2 min stat	11/23	10 AM	MC					

INT.	NURSES' FULL SIGNATURE AND TITLE	INT.	NURSES' FULL SIGNATURE AND TITLE
MJ	Mary Jones, RN		
MC	Marie Colon, RN		
SG	Sara Gordon, RN		

Name of Routine Drug	Dose	Route of Administration	Time of Administration

1. Which drugs were administered at 10:00 A.M. on 11/23?

____

2. Which drug was given stat, and what was the route? Date and time?

____

3. Who administered the captopril at 6:00 P.M. on 11/21?

____

(Continued)

4. What is the route of administration for epoetin alfa?

____

5. How many doses of captopril did the client receive by 7:00 P.M. on 11/24?

____

Here is what you should have found:

Name of Routine Drug	Dose	Route of Administration	Time of Administration
pantoprazole sodium *(Protonix DR)*	40 *mg*	PO	10:00 A.M.
captopril	25 *mg*	PO	10:00 A.M. & 6:00 P.M.
furosemide *(Lasix)*	20 *mg*	PO	10:00 A.M.
cefotaxime	1 *g*	IVPB	10:00 A.M. & 10:00 P.M.
epoetin alfa *(Procrit)*	3,000 *units*	subcutaneously	three times a week at 10:00 A.M.
digoxin	0.125 *mg*	PO	10:00 A.M.

1. pantoprazole sodium 40 *mg*, captopril 25 *mg*; furosemide 20 *mg*; cefotaxime 1 *g*, epoetin alfa 3,000 *units*, digoxin 0.125 *mg*, labetalol 20 *mg*.

2. labetalol IV on 11/23 at 10:00 A.M.

3. Marie Colon, RN

4. subcutaneous

5. 9

Technology in the Medication Administration Process: Preventing Medication Errors

Many healthcare agencies have computerized the medication process. Those who prescribe or administer medications must use security codes and passwords to access the computer system. Prescribers input orders and all other essential client information directly into a computer terminal. This system may be referred to as **Computerized Physician Order Entry (CPOE)**. The order is received in the pharmacy, where a client's drug profile (list of drugs) is maintained. The nurse verifies the order on the computer and inputs his or her digital ID on the **eMAR (electronic Medication Administration Record)** after the medication is administered. A computer printout replaces the handwritten MAR.

One advantage of a computerized system is that handwritten orders do not need to be deciphered or transcribed. The computer program can also identify possible interactions among the client's medications and automatically alert the pharmacist and persons administering the drugs. However, though technology can reduce medication errors and enhance client safety, it also has the potential to cause new types of unintended errors.

NOTE

Healthcare facilities must provide employees with adequate training regarding medication administration devices and routinely verify that users are competent with the equipment.

Some institutions use *Automated Dispensing Cabinets (ADCs)* to dispense medications. See Figure 2.17. The healthcare provider must still be vigilant when using such technology and must be sure to follow the "Six Rights of Medication Administration"; refer to the ISMP guidelines for the safe use of ADCs.

Figure 2.18 is a portion of a *computerized MAR* for a 24-hour period stated in military time. This MAR divides the day into three shifts. Note that no medications have yet been recorded for the 3:01 P.M.–11:00 P.M. shift (1501 *h*–2300 *h*).

Figure 2.17 Automated Dispensing Cabinet (ADC).

SOURCE: Pearson Education, Inc.

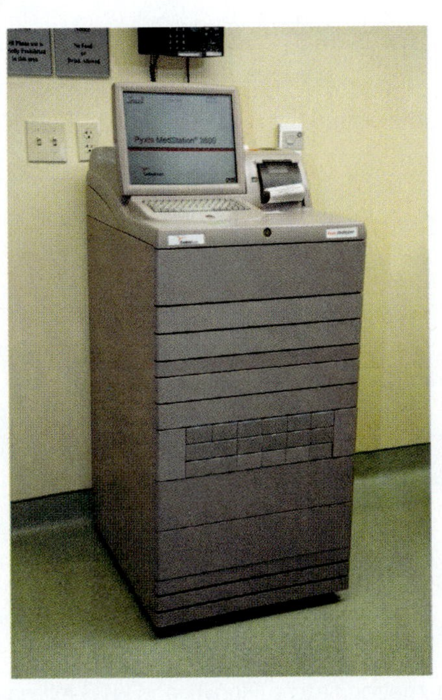

Figure 2.18 A portion of an eMAR.

SCHEDULED	12/06/20–12/07/20 2301–0700	12/07/20 0701–1500	12/07/20 1501–2300
℞ Cefepime (Maxipime)		0840 2 g IVPB MAB	2015
℞ Emoxaparin Na (Lovenox)		1026 40 mg subcutaneous MAB	
℞ Furosemide (Lasix)	0611 20 mg IVP DJS		
℞ Hetastarch (he SPAN)		0920 250 mL IVPB MAB	
℞ KCl (Potassium chloride)		1026 20 mEq ER tab PO MAB	
℞ Metoprolol XL (Toprol XL)		1000 CANCEL MAB	2200
℞ Metronidazole (Flagyl)	0611 500 mg IVPB DJS	1324 500 mg IVPB MAB	2200
℞ NTG (Nitroglycerin)	0110 15 mg oint topical DJS 061115 mg oint topical DJS	1231 15 mg oint topical MAB	1800
℞ Pantoprazole (Protonix) 40 mg IVPB		1026 40 mg IVPB MAB	
PRN	**12/06/20–12/07/20 2301–0700**	**12/07/20 0701–1500**	**12/07/20 1501–2300**
℞ Saline flush	0110 2 mL IV flush DJS	0829 2 mL IV flush MAB	1600
℞ Morphine	0115 4 mg IVP DJS 0439 4 mg IVP DJS	1306 2 mg IVP MAB	
IV	**12/06/20–12/07/20 2301–0700**	**12/07/20 0701–1500**	**12/07/20 1501–2300**
℞ NS (NaCl, 0.9%, 1 L)		0810	2130

PRN ORDERS	
Hydrocodone 5 mg and Acetaminophen 500 mg	x 1–2 tab PO q4h prn process if pain
Saline flush	2 mL IV flush q8 at 0000/0800/1600 and prn
Insulin, human regular sliding scale {Novolin R SS}	See scale prn if BS 200–249 mg/dL give 4 Units of Reg insulin subcut

Scheduled (routine), IV, and PRN orders are shown. For each order administered, the MAR indicates the time, order, and the nurse's digital identification. Currently there is a variety of computerized medication systems in use. The healthcare provider has a responsibility to be both knowledgeable of the facility's policies and proficient in using its system.

Example 2.5

Use the MAR in Figure 2.18 to answer the following questions:

1. Which drug was ordered in milliequivalents?

   ____

2. What drugs were administered at 6:11 A.M. on 12/07/2020?

   ____

3. Identify the dosage, route, and time that Flagyl was administered after noon on 12/07/2020.

   ____

4. Identify the name, dosage, route, and time of administration of the PRN drugs administered after noon on 12/07/2020.

   ____

5. What is the form and route of administration for nitroglycerin on 12/07/2020?

   ____

This is what you should have found:

1. KCl (potassium chloride)
2. furosemide (Lasix), metronidazole (Flagyl), and NTG (nitroglycerin)
3. 500 *mg*, IVPB at 1324 *h* (1:24 P.M.)
4. morphine 2 *mg* IVP was given at 1306 *h* (1:06 P.M.)
5. Ointment, topical

Drug Labels

You will need to understand the information found on drug labels to calculate drug dosages. The important features of a drug label are identified in Figure 2.19.

1. Name of drug: Trilipix is the trade name. In this case, the name begins with an uppercase letter, is in large type, and is boldly visible on the label. The generic name is fenofibric acid, written in a smaller font.
2. Form of drug: The drug is in the form of a capsule.
3. National Drug Code (NDC) number: 0074-9189-90.
4. Bar code: Has the NDC number encoded in it.
5. Dosage strength: 135 *mg* of the drug are contained in one capsule.
6. Dosage recommendations: Note that the manufacturer informs you to see the package insert for prescribing information.
7. Trilipix® is the registered trade name for the drug.
8. Storage directions: Some drugs have to be stored under controlled conditions if they are to retain their effectiveness. This drug should be stored at 25°C (77°F).

Figure 2.19 Drug label for Trilipix.

SOURCE: Courtesy of AbbVie

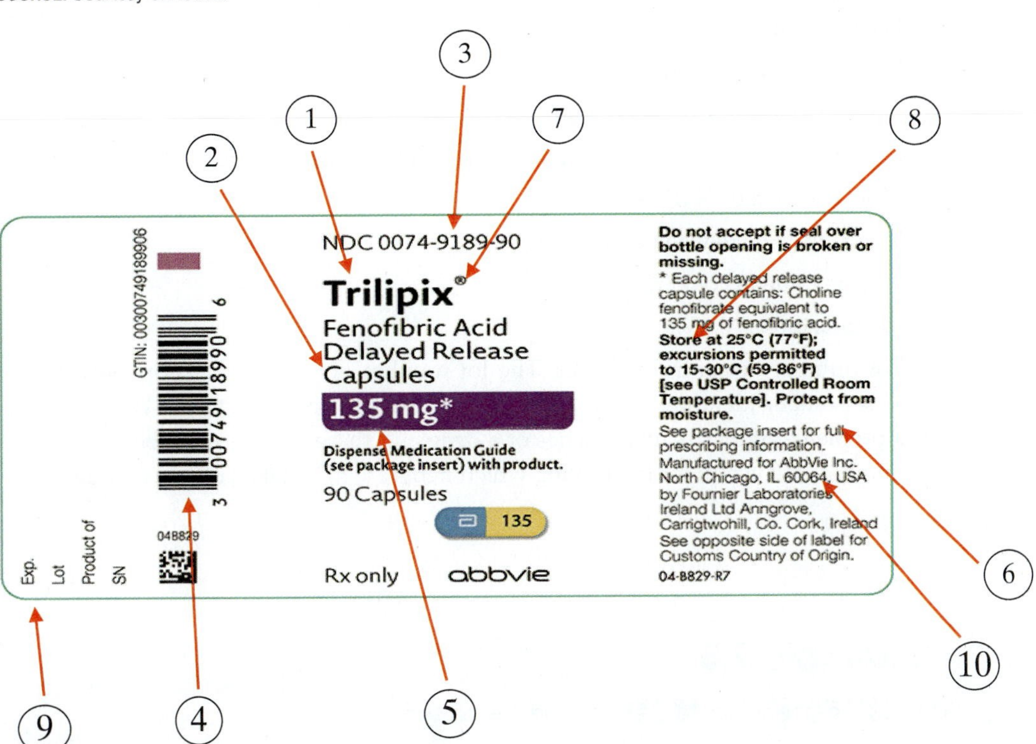

9. Expiration date: The expiration date specifies when the drug should be discarded. For the sake of simplicity, not every drug label in this textbook will have an expiration date.
10. Manufacturer: AbbVie Inc.

ALERT

Always read the expiration date! After the expiration date, the drug may lose its potency or act differently in a client's body. Follow the healthcare facility's policy regarding disposal of expired drugs. Never give expired drugs to clients!

NOTE

The label in Figure 2.20 expresses the strength as 250 *mg/5 mL*. The ISMP recommends that the slash mark (/) not be used to indicate *per* or to separate two doses because it might be mistaken for the number *1*.

Figure 2.20 Drug label for Biaxin.

SOURCE: Courtesy of AbbVie

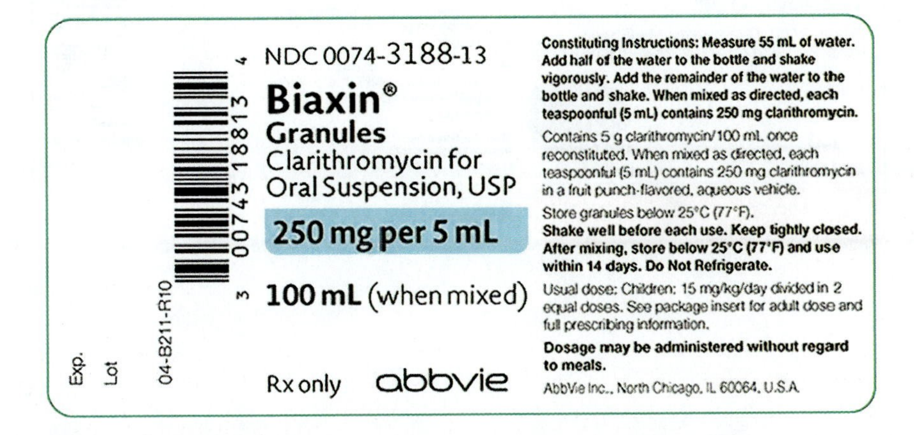

The label in Figure 2.20 indicates the following information:

1. Trade name: Biaxin
2. Generic name: clarythromycin
3. Form: oral suspension
4. Dosage strength: *250 mg per 5 mL*
5. Dosage recommendations: See package insert for full prescribing information
6. NDC number: 0074-3188-13
7. Directions: Shake well before using
8. Total volume in container: 100 mL
9. Manufacturer: AbbVie
10. Lot number or control number: The lot number of this drug is not shown here. This number identifies where and when a drug was manufactured. When there is a problem with particular batches of a drug and these batches must be recalled, lot numbers are useful for identifying which items are to be taken off the market.

Example 2.6

Read the label in Figure 2.21 and find the following:

1. Trade name: ______________________________
2. Generic name: ______________________________
3. Form: ______________________________
4. Dosage strength: ______________________________
5. NDC number: ______________________________
6. Dosage and use: ______________________________
7. Instructions for dispensing: ______________________________

Figure 2.21 Drug label for Gabapentin.

SOURCE: Copyright TEVA, Used with permission

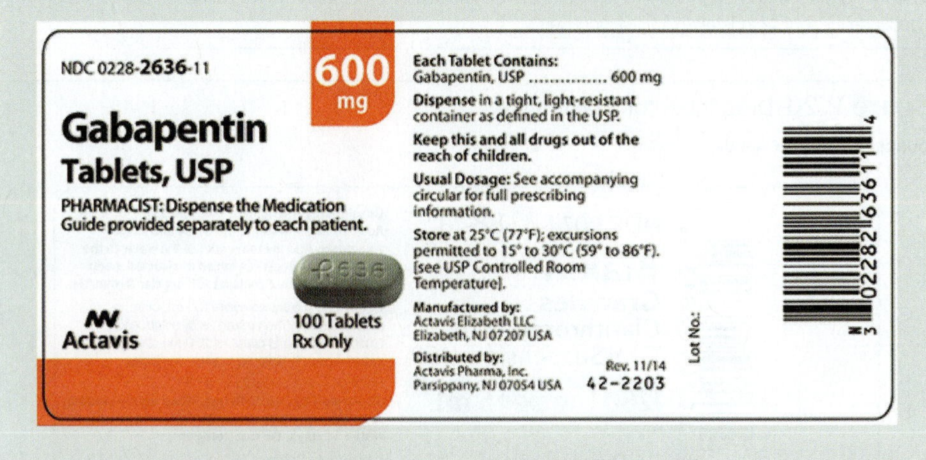

The label for the antiseizure drug gabapentin in Figure 2.21 indicates the following:

1. Trade name: None. This is a generic drug
2. Generic name: gabapentin
3. Form: tablets
4. Dosage strength: 600 *mg* per tablet
5. NDC number: 0228-2636-11
6. Dosage and use: See accompanying information
7. Instructions for dispensing: Dispense in a tight light-resistant container as defined in the USP

Example 2.7

Examine the label shown in Figure 2.22 and record the following information.

1. Trade name: ______________________
2. Generic name: ______________________
3. Form: ______________________
4. Dosage strength: ______________________
5. Amount of drug in container: ______________________
6. Storage temperature: ______________________
7. Special instructions: ______________________

This is what you should have found:

1. Trade name: Norvir
2. Generic name: Ritonavir
3. Form: Oral solution
4. Dosage strength: 80 *mg* per *mL*
5. Amount of drug in container: 240 *mL*
6. Storage temperature: Do not refrigerate
7. Special instructions: ALERT: Find out about medicines that should NOT be taken with Norvir.

Figure 2.22 Drug label for Norvir.

SOURCE: Courtesy of AbbVie

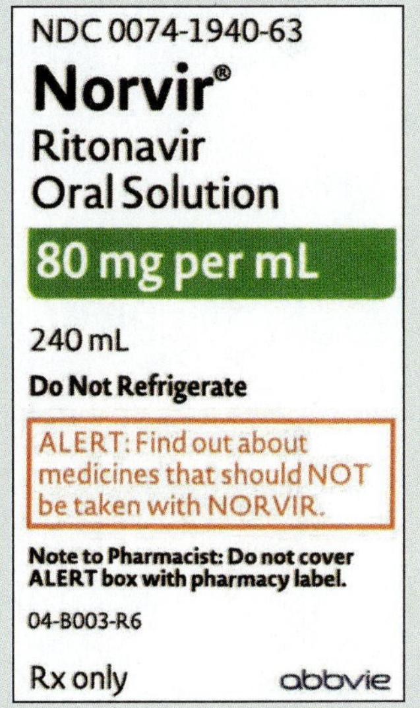

NDC 0074-1940-63
Norvir®
Ritonavir
Oral Solution
80 mg per mL
240 mL
Do Not Refrigerate
ALERT: Find out about medicines that should NOT be taken with NORVIR.
Note to Pharmacist: Do not cover ALERT box with pharmacy label.
04-B003-R6
Rx only
abbvie

Example 2.8

Examine the label shown in Figure 2.23 and record the following information.

1. Trade name: ______________________
2. Generic name: ______________________
3. Form: ______________________
4. Dosage strength: ______________________

(Continued)

Figure 2.23 Drug label for Lidoderm.

SOURCE: Endo Pharmaceuticals Inc.

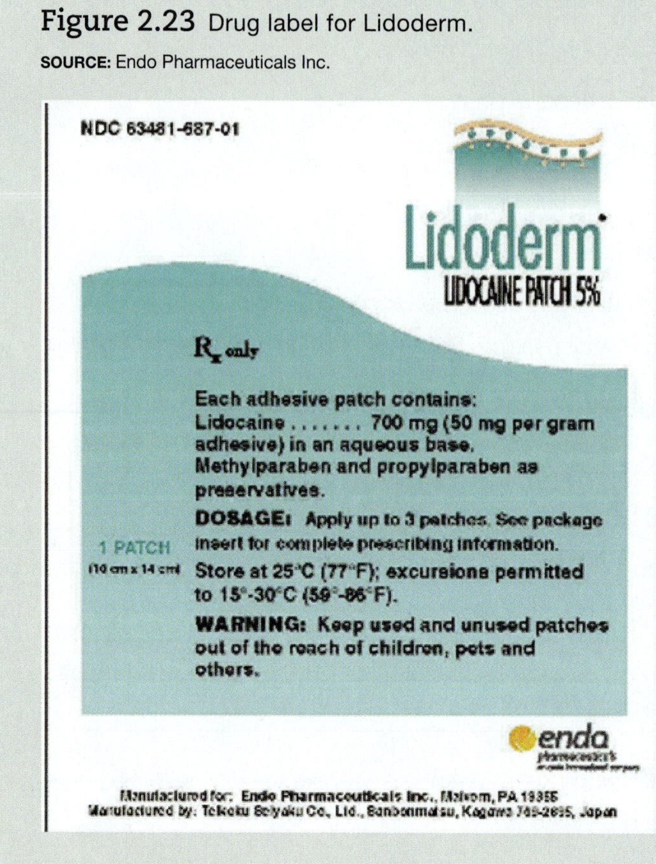

This is what you should have found:

1. Trade name: Lidoderm
2. Generic name: lidocaine 5%
3. Form: patch
4. Dosage strength: 700 *mg* per patch

Combination Drugs

Combination drugs contain two or more generic drugs in one form. Both names and strengths of each drug are on the label. Two such medication labels follow.

Examine the label shown in Figure 2.24. The label for this narcotic analgesic drug indicates that each tablet contains 2.5 *mg* of oxycodone and 325 *mg* of acetaminophen. A combination drug is sometimes prescribed indicating both the dose and the number of tablets or milliliters to be administered. For example, *Percocet (oxycodone and acetaminophen) 2.5 mg/325 mg 1 tab po q6h prn pain.*

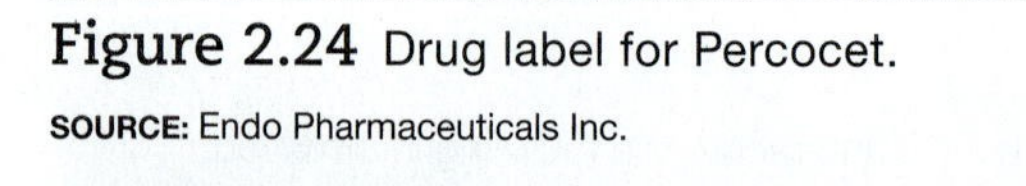

Figure 2.24 Drug label for Percocet.

SOURCE: Endo Pharmaceuticals Inc.

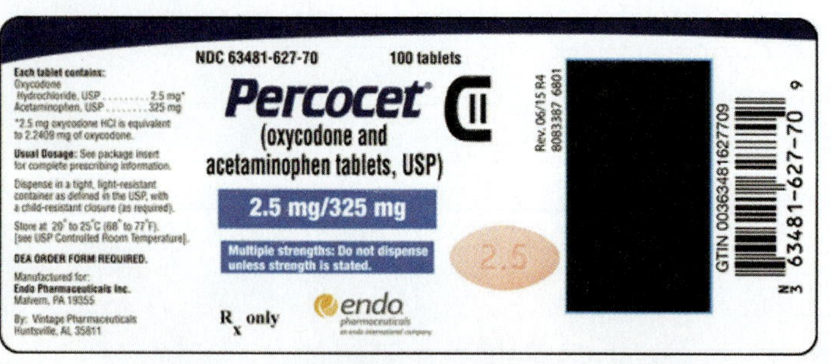

Example 2.9

Examine the label shown in Figure 2.25 and answer the following questions.

Figure 2.25 Drug label for Vicodin ES.

SOURCE: Courtesy of AbbVie

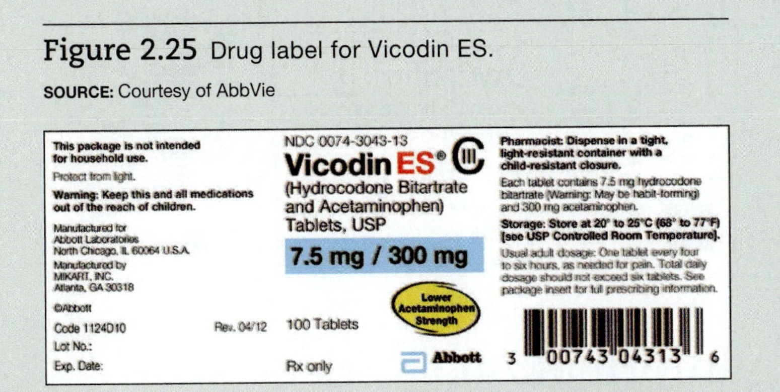

1. What is the trade name and dosage strength of the drug?

   ____

2. What is the dosage strength of acetaminophen?

   ____

3. What is the route of administration?

   ____

4. What is the amount of drug in the container?

   ____

5. What is the usual adult dose?

   ____

This is what you should have found:

1. Vicodin ES is the trade name, and the dosage strength is 7.5 *mg*/300 *mg* per tablet
2. 300 *mg* of acetaminophen per tablet
3. By mouth
4. 100 *tablets*
5. 1 *tablet* q4-6h prn pain, not to exceed 6 *tab/d*

Controlled Substances

Certain drugs that can lead to abuse or dependence are classified by law as **controlled substances**. These drugs are divided into five categories, called schedules. Schedule I drugs are those with the highest potential for abuse (e.g., heroin, marijuana). Schedule V drugs are those with the lowest potential for abuse (e.g., cough medications containing codeine). Controlled substances must be stored, handled, disposed of, and administered according to regulations established by the *U.S. Drug Enforcement Agency (DEA)*. Hospitals and pharmacies must register with the DEA and use their assigned numbers to purchase scheduled drugs. Those who prescribe medications must have a DEA number to prescribe controlled substances.

The controlled substance OxyContin (oxycodone hydrochloride) is a Schedule II drug, as indicated by the CII on the label. (See the arrow in Figure 2.26.)

Figure 2.26 Drug label for OxyContin.

SOURCE: © Purdue, used with permission.

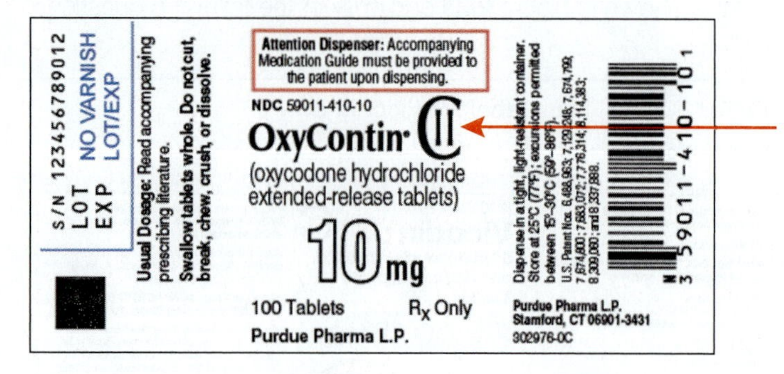

Drug Information

In an effort to manage the risks of medications and reduce medical errors and adverse drug events, the U.S. Food and Drug Administration (FDA) mandates the format in which information about drugs is provided.

Drug information can be obtained online. Prescription drug information is also found on the package insert, whereas information on over-the-counter (OTC) drugs is found on the packaging itself.

NOTE

Prescription drug information is accessible on "Daily Med," an interagency online health information clearinghouse created cooperatively by the FDA and the National Library of Medicine (NLM) at http://dailymed.nlm.nih.gov.

Prescription Drug Package Inserts

The FDA has mandated that a new format for package inserts be phased in by 2016. The new categories for the format are:

- **Highlights of Prescribing Information:** provides immediate access to the most important facts.
- **Proprietary name, dosage form, route of administration, and initial U.S. approval (year):** gives the date of initial product approvals, thereby making it easier to determine how long a product has been on the market.
- **Boxed Warning:** identifies the dangers of the medication.
- **Recent Major Changes:** notes the changes made within the past year to ensure the most up-to-date information.
- **Indications and Usage:** includes conditions for which the product is effective.
- **Dosage and Administration:** describes the recommended dose and routes of administration.
- **Dosage Forms and Strengths:** indicates how the product is supplied and its strength (e.g., 10 *mg*/*tab*).
- **Contraindications:** gives reasons for which it is inadvisable to use the product.
- **Warnings and Precautions:** provides notice of things that may cause harm.
- **Adverse Reactions:** The following statement must be included in this section: "To report SUSPECTED ADVERSE REACTIONS, contact (manufacturer) at (phone # and Web address) or FDA at 1-800-FDA-1088 or www.fda.gov/medwatch."

- **Drug Interactions:** lists other drugs that, when taken in combination, may cause concern.
- **Use in Specific Populations:** indicates target populations (e.g., pregnancy, nursing mothers, pediatric and geriatric clients).

Over-the-Counter (OTC) Labels

Over-the-counter (OTC) medicines are drugs that can be obtained without a prescription. In the United States, the FDA decides which drugs are safe enough to sell over the counter. Taking OTC drugs still has risks. Some interact with other drugs, supplements, foods, or drinks, whereas others may cause problems for people with certain medical conditions. The FDA format for OTC drug labels is much simpler than that for prescription drugs. The categories are:

- **Drug Facts:** includes the name of the drug and its purpose.
- **Uses:** indicates the conditions for which the drug is effective.
- **Warnings:** indicates the effects of the medication of which to be aware.
- **Directions:** specifies the quantity of the drug to take and how often to take it—for example, 2 *tablets* every 8 *hours* with water.
- **Other Information:** provides miscellaneous information—for example, expiration date and storage directions.
- **Inactive Ingredients:** lists other substances in the drug that are not active ingredients.
- **Questions or Comments:** provides a contact number for consumer questions.

Figure 2.27 shows an excerpt from the prescribing information for the drug Bosulif (bosutinib).

Figure 2.27 Excerpts of package insert for Bosulif.

SOURCE: From Package Insert for Bosulif. Copyright by Pfizer Inc.

HIGHLIGHTS OF PRESCRIBING INFORMATION

These highlights do not include all the information needed to use BOSULIF safely and effectively. See full prescribing information for BOSULIF.

BOSULIF® (bosutinib) tablets, for oral use Initial U.S. Approval: 2012

----------- INDICATIONS AND USAGE -----------

- BOSULIF is a kinase inhibitor indicated for the treatment of adult patients with chronic, accelerated, or blast phase Ph+ chronic myelogenous leukemia (CML) with resistance or intolerance to prior therapy.

------- DOSAGE AND ADMINISTRATION --------

- Recommended Dose: 500 *mg* orally once daily with food.
- Consider dose escalation to 600 *mg* daily in patients who do not reach complete hematologic response by week 8 or complete cytogenetic response by week 12 and do not have Grade 3 or greater adverse reactions.
- Adjust dosage for hematologic and non-hematologic toxicity.
- Hepatic impairment (at baseline): reduce BOSULIF dose to 200 *mg* daily.

------- DOSAGE FORMS AND STRENGTHS -----

Tablets: 100 *mg* and 500 *mg*.

------------- CONTRAINDICATIONS --------------

Hypersensitivity to BOSULIF.

-------- WARNINGS AND PRECAUTIONS --------

- Gastrointestinal toxicity: Monitor and manage as necessary. Withhold, dose reduce, or discontinue BOSULIF.
- Myelosuppression: Monitor blood counts and manage as necessary.
- Hepatic toxicity: Monitor liver enzymes at least monthly for the first three months and as needed. Withhold, dose reduce, or discontinue BOSULIF.
- Fluid retention: Monitor patients and manage using standard of care treatment. Withhold, dose reduce, or discontinue BOSULIF.
- Embryofetal toxicity: May cause fetal harm. Females of reproductive potential should avoid becoming pregnant while being treated with BOSULIF.

------------- ADVERSE REACTIONS --------------

Most common adverse reactions (incidence greater than 20%) are diarrhea, nausea, thrombocytopenia, vomiting, abdominal pain, rash, anemia, pyrexia, and fatigue.

To report SUSPECTED ADVERSE REACTIONS, contact Pfizer Inc. at 1-800-438-1985 or FDA at 1-800-FDA-1088 or www.fda.gov/medwatch.

------------- DRUG INTERACTIONS --------------

- CYP3A Inhibitors and Inducers: Avoid concurrent use of BOSULIF with strong or moderate CYP3A inhibitors and inducers.
- Proton Pump Inhibitors: May decrease bosutinib drug levels. Consider short-acting antacids in place of proton pump inhibitors.

See 17 for PATIENT COUNSELING INFORMATION and FDA-approved patient labeling. Revised: 09/2012

Example 2.10

Read the excerpts of the package insert in Figure 2.27 and fill in the requested information.

1. What is the generic name of the drug?

____

2. For what condition is this drug used?

____

3. What are the most common adverse reactions of this drug?

____

4. What is the recommended dose?

____

5. What should the prescriber do if a person taking Bosulif develops fluid retention?

____

This is what you should have found:

1. bosutinib
2. Treatment of adult clients who have chronic, accelerated, or blast-phase Ph+ chronic myelogenous leukemia
3. Diarrhea, nausea and vomiting, thrombocytopenia, abdominal pain, rash, anemia, pyrexia, and fatigue
4. 500 *mg* once daily by mouth with food
5. Withhold dose, reduce or discontinue Bosulif

Example 2.11

Read the drug information in Figures 2.28 and 2.29 and answer the following questions.

1. What is the generic name of the drug?

____

2. What is the purpose of this drug?

____

3. Who should not use this drug?

____

4. What does this product contain that may cause severe stomach bleeding?

____

5. What should you do if you experience sustained stomach pain after using this drug?

____

Figure 2.28 Information found on Advil packaging.

SOURCE: Courtesy of Pfizer, Inc.

READ AND KEEP CARTON FOR COMPLETE WARNINGS AND INFORMATION

Drug Facts

Active ingredient (in each capsule)	Purpose
Solubilized ibuprofen equal to 200 mg ibuprofen (NSAID)* (present as the free acid and potassium salt)	Pain reliever/ Fever reducer

*nonsteroidal anti-inflammatory drug

Uses
- temporarily relieves minor aches and pains due to:
  - headache
  - toothache
  - backache
  - menstrual cramps
  - the common cold
  - muscular aches
  - minor pain of arthritis
- temporarily reduces fever

Warnings

Allergy alert: Ibuprofen may cause a severe allergic reaction, especially in people allergic to aspirin. Symptoms may include:
- hives
- facial swelling
- asthma (wheezing)
- shock
- skin reddening
- rash
- blisters

If an allergic reaction occurs, stop use and seek medical help right away.

Stomach bleeding warning: This product contains an NSAID, which may cause severe stomach bleeding. The chance is higher if you
- are age 60 or older
- have had stomach ulcers or bleeding problems
- take a blood thinning (anticoagulant) or steroid drug
- take other drugs containing prescription or nonprescription NSAIDs [aspirin, ibuprofen, naproxen, or others]
- have 3 or more alcoholic drinks every day while using this product
- take more or for a longer time than directed

Drug Facts (continued)

Do not use
- if you have ever had an allergic reaction to any other pain reliever/fever reducer
- right before or after heart surgery

Ask a doctor before use if
- stomach bleeding warning applies to you
- you have problems or serious side effects from taking pain relievers or fever reducers
- you have a history of stomach problems, such as heartburn
- you have high blood pressure, heart disease, liver cirrhosis, kidney disease, or asthma
- you are taking a diuretic

Ask a doctor or pharmacist before use if you are
- under a doctor's care for any serious condition
- taking aspirin for heart attack or stroke, because ibuprofen may decrease this benefit of aspirin
- taking any other drug

When using this product
- take with food or milk if stomach upset occurs
- the risk of heart attack or stroke may increase if you use more than directed or for longer than directed

Stop use and ask a doctor if
- you experience any of the following signs of stomach bleeding:
  - feel faint
  - vomit blood
  - have bloody or black stools
  - have stomach pain that does not get better
- pain gets worse or lasts more than 10 days
- fever gets worse or lasts more than 3 days
- redness or swelling is present in the painful area
- any new symptoms appear

If pregnant or breast-feeding, ask a health professional before use. It is especially important not to use ibuprofen during the last 3 months of pregnancy unless definitely directed to do so by a doctor because it may cause problems in the unborn child or complications during delivery.

Drug Facts (continued)

Keep out of reach of children. In case of overdose, get medical help or contact a Poison Control Center right away.

Directions
- **do not take more than directed**
- **the smallest effective dose should be used**
- adults and children 12 years and over: take 1 capsule every 4 to 6 hours while symptoms persist
- if pain or fever does not respond to 1 capsule, 2 capsules may be used
- do not exceed 6 capsules in 24 hours, unless directed by a doctor
- children under 12 years: ask a doctor

Other information
- **each capsule contains:** potassium 20 mg
- read all warnings and directions before use. Keep carton.
- store at 20-25°C (68-77°F)
- avoid excessive heat above 40°C (104°F)

Inactive ingredients FD&C green no. 3, gelatin, light mineral oil, pharmaceutical ink, polyethylene glycol, potassium hydroxide, purified water, sorbitan, sorbitol

Questions or comments? call toll free 1-800-88-ADVIL

Figure 2.29 Advil packaging.

SOURCE: Courtesy of Pfizer, Inc.

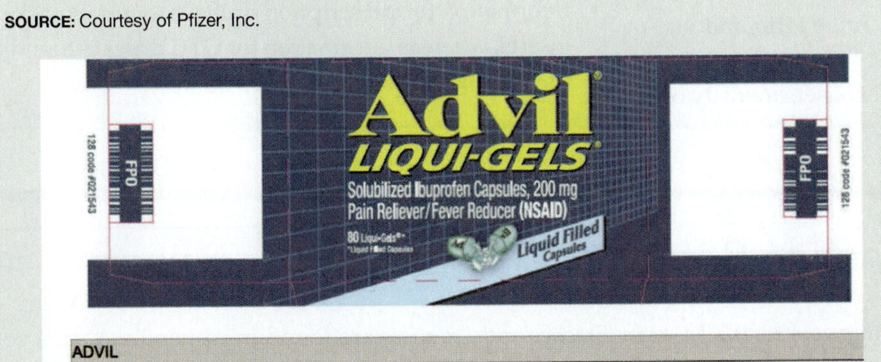

This is what you should have found:

1. ibuprofen
2. Pain reliever/fever reducer
3. People who have ever had an allergic reaction to any other pain reliever/fever reducer or right before or after heart surgery
4. An NSAID
5. Stop taking the drug and consult a doctor

Summary

In this chapter, the medication administration process was discussed, including the people who may administer drugs; the "six rights" and "three checks" of medication administration; and how to interpret prescriptions, medication orders, Medication Administration Records, drug labels, and drug package inserts.

- The six rights of medication administration serve as a guide for *safe* administration of medications to client.
- Failure to achieve any of the six rights constitutes a medication error.
- A person administering medications has a legal and ethical responsibility to report medication errors.
- Medication errors can occur at any point in the medication process.
- More communication between nurses and clients can help prevent medication errors.
- Electronic prescribing of medications can reduce medication errors.
- A drug should be prescribed using its generic name.
- Understanding drug orders requires the interpretation of common abbreviations.
- Never use any abbreviations on The Joint Commission "Official Do Not Use" list.
- Read drug labels carefully; many drugs have look-alike/sound-alike names.
- Carefully read the label to determine dosage strength and check calculations, paying special attention to decimal points.
- Medications must be administered in the form and via the route specified by the prescriber.
- The form of a drug affects its speed of onset, intensity of action, and route of administration.
- The *oral (PO)* route is the one most commonly used.
- *Buccal* and *sublingual* medications must be kept in the mouth until they are completely dissolved.
- *Topical* medications may have local and systemic effects. *Transdermal patches* are applied for their systemic effect.
- *Inhalation* medications may be administered with various devices, such as *nebulizers, dry powder*, and *metered-dose inhalers.*
- *Parenteral* medications are injected into the body. To prevent infection, sterile technique must be used for their administration.
- Before administering any medication, it is essential to identify the client.
- Medications should be documented immediately after, but never before, they are administered.
- No medication should be given without a legal order.
- If persons administering medications have difficulty understanding or interpreting the order, they must clarify the order with the prescriber.
- The medication administration process is rapidly becoming computerized.
- Drug package inserts contain detailed information about the drug indications and usage, dosage and administration, forms and strengths, contraindications, warnings and precautions, adverse reactions, drug interactions, use in special populations, and contact information to report suspected adverse reactions.
- Information for prescription drugs is found in package inserts, whereas information for OTC drugs is found on the packaging itself.

Practice Sets

The answers to *Try These for Practice* and *Exercises* are found in Appendix A. Ask your instructor for the answers to the *Additional Exercises.*

Try These for Practice

Test your comprehension after reading the chapter.

Study the labels in Figures 2.30 to 2.34 and answer the following questions.

1. What is the trade name for alprazolam?

   ____

2. What is the route of administration for clindamycin?

   ____

3. What is the generic name for Crixivan?

   ____

4. How many milligrams of losartan potassium are in one tablet of Hyzaar?

   ____

5. What is the dosage strength for Zemplar injection?

   ____

Figure 2.30 Drug label for Hyzaar.

SOURCE: Reproduced with permission of Merck Sharp & Dohme Corp., a subsidiary of Merck & Co, Inc., Whitehouse Station, New Jersey, USA. All Rights Reserved.

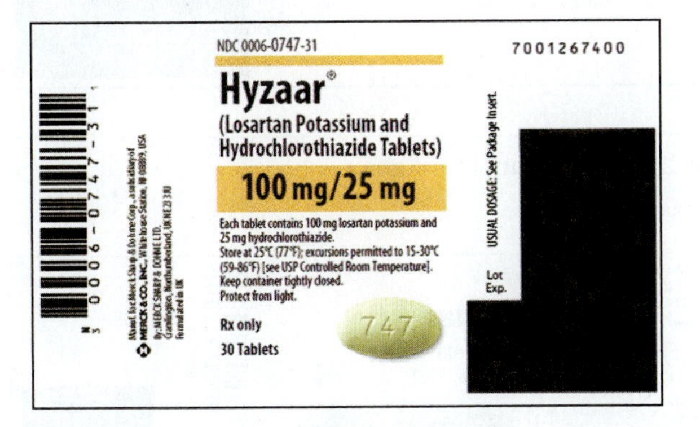

Figure 2.31 Drug label for paricalcitol.

SOURCE: Courtesy of AbbVie

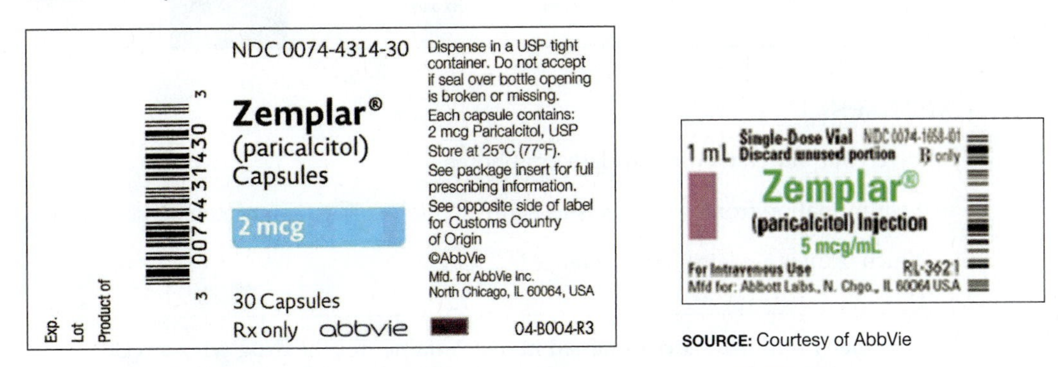

SOURCE: Courtesy of AbbVie

Figure 2.32 Drug label for Cleocin.

SOURCE: Courtesy of Pfizer, Inc.

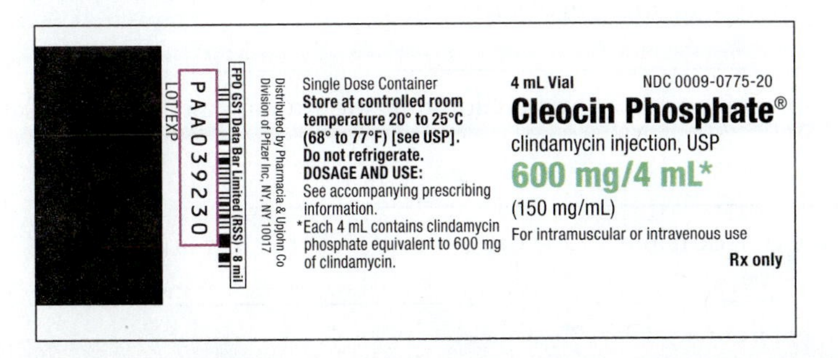

Figure 2.33 Drug label for Crixivan.

SOURCE: Reproduced with permission of Merck Sharp & Dohme Corp., a subsidiary of Merck & Co, Inc., Whitehouse Station, New Jersey, USA. All Rights Reserved.

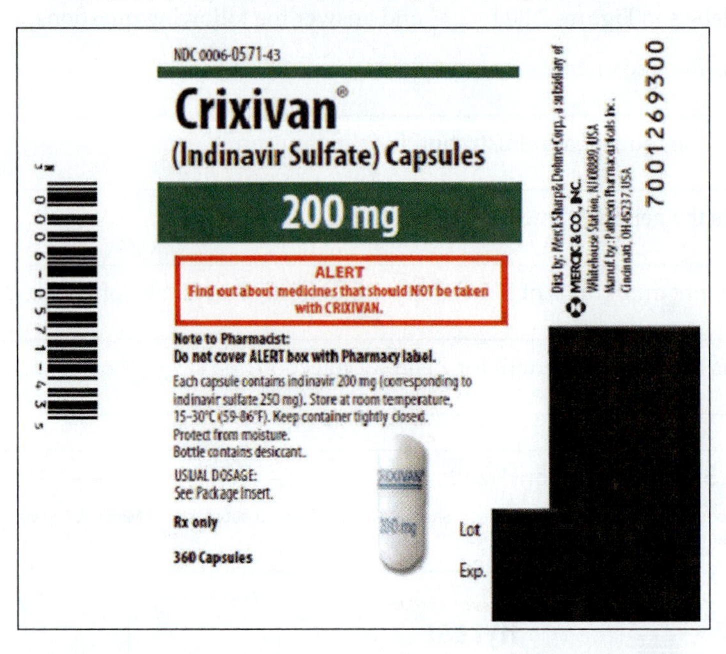

Figure 2.34 Drug label for Xanax.

SOURCE: Courtesy of Pfizer, Inc.

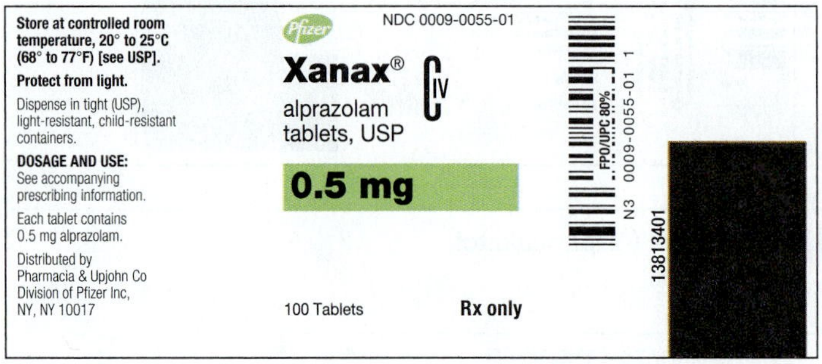

Exercises

Reinforce your understanding in class or at home.

Use the information from drug labels in Figures 2.30 to 2.34 to complete Exercises 1 to 5.

1. Which drug is a controlled substance?

____

2. How many milliliters are contained in the container for the drug whose NDC number is 0009-0775-20?

____

3. What is the dosage strength of Crixivan?

____

4. How many milligrams of hydrochlorothiazide are contained in one tablet of Hyzaar?

____

5. Write the generic name for the drug whose NDC number is 0006-0571-43.

____

6. Study the portions of a MAR in Figures 2.35a, 2.35b, and 2.35c to answer the following questions.

   (a) Which drugs were administered at 10:00 P.M. on 12/10?

   ____

   (b) Using military time, designate the time(s) of day when the client received gabapentin.

   ____

Figure 2.35a Portion of a MAR.

Order Date	Exp Date	Medication Dosage Frequency & Route	Time	12/7	12/8	12/9	12/10	12/11	12/12
12/7	12/13	Neurontin (gabapentin) 100 mg PO t.i.d.	10 AM 2 PM 6 PM	*MC* *MC* *JY*	*MC* *MC* *JY*	*MC* *MC* *JY*	*MC* *MC* *JY*		
12/7	12/16	Vantin (cefpodoxime) 200 mg PO q12h for 10 days	8 AM 8 PM	*SG* *JY*	*SG* *JY*	*SG* *JY*	*SG* *JY*		
12/7	12/13	digoxin 0.125 mg PO daily	10 AM	*MC*	*MC*	*MC*	*MC*		
12/7	12/13	Levemir 7 units subcut at bedtime	10 PM	*JY*	*JY*	*JY*	*JY*		
12/7	12/13	Norvasc (amlodipine) 5 mg PO daily	10 AM	*MC*	*MC*	*MC*	*MC*		

Figure 2.35b Portion of a MAR.

PRN Medication		Medication Dosage Route & Time	Doses Given						
Order Date	Expiration Date		Date	12/10					
12/10	12/13	Tylenol with codeine #3 (300 mg /30 mg) tab 1 PO q4h prn mild-moderate pain	Time	10 PM					
			Init	*JY*					

Figure 2.35c Portion of a MAR.

Initial	Nurse's Signature	Initial	Nurse's Signature
SG	*Sara Gordon RN*		
MC	*Marie Colon RN*		
JY	*Jim Young LPN*		

(c) How many doses of cefpodoxime were administered by nurse Gordon?

____

(d) What is the route of administration for Levemir?

____

(e) Which drugs were administered by nurse Colon on 12/8?

____

7. Study the portion of a physician's order sheet in Figure 2.36 to answer the following questions.

(a) Which drug(s) is/are given four times a day?

____

(b) Which drug(s) is/are given once a day?

____

(c) How many times a day should the client receive Vibramycin?

____

(d) What is the route of administration for Dilaudid?

____

(e) How many times a day can the client receive hydromorphone HCl?

____

Figure 2.36 Portion of a physician's order sheet.

PHYSICIAN'S ORDERS

Order Date	Date Disc	
4/20/2020	4/30/2020	Vibramycin (doxycycline hydrochloride) 100 mg PO q12h
4/20/2020	4/27/2020	digoxin 0.125 mg PO daily
4/20/2020	4/27/2020	Mevacor (lovastatin) 20 mg PO with the evening meal
4/20/2020	4/27/2020	metoclopramide HCl 10 mg PO ac and hs. Give 30 minutes before meals and at bedtime.
4/20/2020	4/23/2020	Dilaudid (hydromorphone hydrochloride) 1 mg IVP (over 2-3 min) q3h prn moderate pain
4/20/2020	4/27/2020	Cozaar (losartan potassium) 25 mg PO daily

8. Use the package insert shown in Figure 2.37 to answer the following questions.

   (a) What is the generic name and form of the drug?

   ____

   (b) For what condition is the intramuscular form of ZyPREXA used?

   ____

Figure 2.37 Excerpt from package insert for ZyPREXA.

HIGHLIGHTS OF PRESCRIBING INFORMATION

These highlights do not include all the information needed to use ZYPREXA safely and effectively. See full prescribing information for ZYPREXA.

ZYPREXA (olanzapine) Tablet for Oral use
ZYPREXA ZYDIS (olanzapine) Tablet, Orally Disintegrating for Oral use
ZYPREXA IntraMuscular (olanzapine) Injection, Powder, For Solution for Intramuscular use

Initial U.S. Approval: 1996

WARNING: INCREASED MORTALITY IN ELDERLY PATIENTS WITH DEMENTIA-RELATED PSYCHOSIS

See full prescribing information for complete boxed warning.

- **Elderly patients with dementia-related psychosis treated with antipsychotic drugs are at an increased risk of death. ZYPREXA is not approved for the treatment of patients with dementia-related psychosis. (5.1, 5.14, 17.2)**
  When using ZYPREXA and fluoxetine in combination, also refer to the Boxed Warning section of the package insert for Symbyax.

--- RECENT MAJOR CHANGES ---

Indications and Usage:

Schizophrenia (1.1)	12/2009
Bipolar I Disorder (Manic or Mixed Episodes) (1.2)	12/2009
Special Considerations in Treating Pediatric Schizophrenia and Bipolar I Disorder (1.3)	12/2009
ZYPREXA IntraMuscular: Agitation Associated with Schizophrenia and Bipolar I Mania (1.4)	12/2009

Dosage and Administration:

Schizophrenia (2.1)	12/2009
Bipolar I Disorder (Manic or Mixed Episodes) (2.2)	12/2009

Warnings and Precautions:

Orthostatic Hypotension (5.8)	05/2010
Leukopenia, Neutropenia, and Agranulocytosis (5.9)	08/2009
Hyperprolactinemia (5.15)	01/2010

--- INDICATIONS AND USAGE ---

ZYPREXA® (olanzapine) is an atypical antipsychotic indicated:

As oral formulation for the:

- Treatment of schizophrenia. (1.1)
  - Adults: Efficacy was established in three clinical trials in patients with schizophrenia: two 6-week trials and one maintenance trial. (14.1)
  - Adolescents (ages 13-17): Efficacy was established in one 6-week trial in patients with schizophrenia (14.1). The increased potential (in adolescents compared with adults) for weight gain and hyperlipidemia may lead clinicians to consider prescribing other drugs first in adolescents. (1.1)
- Acute treatment of manic or mixed episodes associated with bipolar I disorder and maintenance treatment of bipolar I disorder. (1.2)
  - Adults: Efficacy was established in three clinical trials in patients with manic or mixed episodes of bipolar I disorder: two 3- to 4-week trials and one maintenance trial. (14.2)
  - Adolescents (ages 13-17): Efficacy was established in one 3-week trial in patients with manic or mixed episodes associated with bipolar I disorder (14.2). The increased potential (in adolescents compared with adults) for weight gain and hyperlipidemia may lead clinicians to consider prescribing other drugs first in adolescents. (1.2)
- Medication therapy for pediatric patients with schizophrenia or bipolar I disorder should be undertaken only after a thorough diagnostic evaluation and with careful consideration of the potential risks. (1.3)
- Adjunct to valproate or lithium in the treatment of manic or mixed episodes associated with bipolar I disorder. (1.2)
  - Efficacy was established in two 6-week clinical trials in adults (14.2). Maintenance efficacy has not been systematically evaluated.

As ZYPREXA IntraMuscular for the:

- Treatment of acute agitation associated with schizophrenia and bipolar I mania. (1.4)
  - Efficacy was established in three 1-day trials in adults. (14.3)

As ZYPREXA and Fluoxetine in Combination for the:

- Treatment of depressive episodes associated with bipolar I disorder. (1.5)
  - Efficacy was established with Symbyax (olanzapine and fluoxetine in combination) in adults; refer to the product label for Symbyax.
- Treatment of treatment resistant depression (major depressive disorder in patients who do not respond to 2 separate trials of different antidepressants of adequate dose and duration in the current episode). (1.6)
  - Efficacy was established with Symbyax (olanzapine and fluoxetine in combination) in adults; refer to the product label for Symbyax.

--- DOSAGE AND ADMINISTRATION ---

Schizophrenia in adults (2.1)	Oral: Start at 5-10 mg once daily; Target: 10 mg/day within several days
Schizophrenia in adolescents (2.1)	Oral: Start at 2.5-5 mg once daily; Target: 10 mg/day
Bipolar I Disorder (manic or mixed episodes) in adults (2.2)	Oral: Start at 10 or 15 mg once daily
Bipolar I Disorder (manic or mixed episodes) in adolescents (2.2)	Oral: Start at 2.5-5 mg once daily; Target: 10 mg/day
Bipolar I Disorder (manic or mixed episodes) with lithium or valproate in adults (2.2)	Oral: Start at 10 mg once daily
Agitation associated with Schizophrenia and Bipolar I Mania in adults (2.4)	IM: 10 mg (5 mg or 7.5 mg when clinically warranted) Assess for orthostatic hypotension prior to subsequent dosing (max. 3 doses 2-4 hrs apart)
Depressive Episodes associated with Bipolar I Disorder in adults (2.5)	Oral in combination with fluoxetine: Start at 5 mg of oral olanzapine and 20 mg of fluoxetine once daily
Treatment Resistant Depression in adults (2.6)	Oral in combination with fluoxetine: Start at 5 mg of oral olanzapine and 20 mg of fluoxetine once daily

- Lower starting dose recommended in debilitated or pharmacodynamically sensitive patients or patients with predisposition to hypotensive reactions, or with potential for slowed metabolism. (2.1)
- Olanzapine may be given without regard to meals. (2.1)

ZYPREXA and Fluoxetine in Combination:

- Dosage adjustments, if indicated, should be made with the individual components according to efficacy and tolerability. (2.5, 2.6)
- Olanzapine monotherapy is not indicated for the treatment of depressive episodes associated with bipolar I disorder or treatment resistant depression. (2.5, 2.6)
- Safety of co-administration of doses above 18 mg olanzapine with 75 mg fluoxetine has not been evaluated. (2.5, 2.6)

--- DOSAGE FORMS AND STRENGTHS ---

- Tablets (not scored): 2.5, 5, 7.5, 10, 15, 20 mg (3)
- Orally Disintegrating Tablets (not scored): 5, 10, 15, 20 mg (3)
- Intramuscular Injection: 10 mg vial (3)

--- CONTRAINDICATIONS ---

- None with ZYPREXA monotherapy.
- When using ZYPREXA and fluoxetine in combination, also refer to the Contraindications section of the package insert for Symbyax®. (4)
- When using ZYPREXA in combination with lithium or valproate, refer to the Contraindications section of the package inserts for those products. (4)

--- WARNINGS AND PRECAUTIONS ---

- *Elderly Patients with Dementia-Related Psychosis:* Increased risk of death and increased incidence of cerebrovascular adverse events (e.g., stroke, transient ischemic attack). (5.1)
- *Suicide:* The possibility of a suicide attempt is inherent in schizophrenia and in bipolar I disorder, and close supervision of high-risk patients should accompany drug therapy; when using in combination with fluoxetine, also refer to the Boxed Warning and Warnings and Precautions sections of the package insert for Symbyax. (5.2)
- *Neuroleptic Malignant Syndrome:* Manage with immediate discontinuation and close monitoring. (5.3)

Figure 2.37 Excerpt from package insert for ZyPREXA. *(Continued)*

- *Hyperglycemia:* In some cases extreme and associated with ketoacidosis or hyperosmolar coma or death, has been reported in patients taking olanzapine. Patients taking olanzapine should be monitored for symptoms of hyperglycemia and undergo fasting blood glucose testing at the beginning of, and periodically during, treatment. (5.4)
- *Hyperlipidemia:* Undesirable alterations in lipids have been observed. Appropriate clinical monitoring is recommended, including fasting blood lipid testing at the beginning of, and periodically during, treatment. (5.5)
- *Weight Gain:* Potential consequences of weight gain should be considered. Patients should receive regular monitoring of weight. (5.6)
- *Tardive Dyskinesia:* Discontinue if clinically appropriate. (5.7)
- *Orthostatic Hypotension:* Orthostatic hypotension associated with dizziness, tachycardia, bradycardia and, in some patients, syncope, may occur especially during initial dose titration. Use caution in patients with cardiovascular disease, cerebrovascular disease, and those conditions that could affect hemodynamic responses. (5.8)
- *Leukopenia, Neutropenia, and Agranulocytosis:* Has been reported with antipsychotics, including ZYPREXA. Patients with a history of a clinically significant low white blood cell count (WBC) or drug induced leukopenia/neutropenia should have their complete blood count (CBC) monitored frequently during the first few months of therapy and discontinuation of ZYPREXA should be considered at the first sign of a clinically significant decline in WBC in the absence of other causative factors. (5.9)
- *Seizures:* Use cautiously in patients with a history of seizures or with conditions that potentially lower the seizure threshold. (5.11)
- *Potential for Cognitive and Motor Impairment:* Has potential to impair judgment, thinking, and motor skills. Use caution when operating machinery. (5.12)
- *Hyperprolactinemia:* May elevate prolactin levels. (5.15)
- *Use in Combination with Fluoxetine, Lithium or Valproate:* Also refer to the package inserts for Symbyax, lithium, or valproate. (5.16)
- *Laboratory Tests:* Monitor fasting blood glucose and lipid profiles at the beginning of, and periodically during, treatment. (5.17)

------------------------------ ADVERSE REACTIONS ------------------------------

Most common adverse reactions (≥5% and at least twice that for placebo) associated with:

Oral Olanzapine Monotherapy:

- Schizophrenia (Adults) – postural hypotension, constipation, weight gain, dizziness, personality disorder, akathisia (6.1)
- Schizophrenia (Adolescents) – sedation, weight increased, headache, increased appetite, dizziness, abdominal pain, pain in extremity, fatigue, dry mouth (6.1)
- Manic or Mixed Episodes, Bipolar I Disorder (Adults) – asthenia, dry mouth, constipation, increased appetite, somnolence, dizziness, tremor (6.1)
- Manic or Mixed Episodes, Bipolar I Disorder (Adolescents) – sedation, weight increased, increased appetite, headache, fatigue, dizziness, dry mouth, abdominal pain, pain in extremity (6.1)

Combination of ZYPREXA and Lithium or Valproate:

- Manic or Mixed Episodes, Bipolar I Disorder (Adults) – dry mouth, weight gain, increased appetite, dizziness, back pain, constipation, speech disorder, increased salivation, amnesia, paresthesia (6.1)

ZYPREXA and Fluoxetine in Combination: Also refer to the Adverse Reactions section of the package insert for Symbyax. (6)

ZYPREXA IntraMuscular for Injection:

- Agitation with Schizophrenia and Bipolar I Mania (Adults) – somnolence (6.1)

To report SUSPECTED ADVERSE REACTIONS, contact Eli Lilly and Company at 1-800-LillyRx (1-800-545-5979) or FDA at 1-800-FDA-1088 or www.fda.gov/medwatch

------------------------------ DRUG INTERACTIONS ------------------------------

- *Diazepam:* May potentiate orthostatic hypotension. (7.1, 7.2)
- *Alcohol:* May potentiate orthostatic hypotension. (7.1)
- *Carbamazepine:* Increased clearance of olanzapine. (7.1)
- *Fluvoxamine:* May increase olanzapine levels. (7.1)
- *ZYPREXA and Fluoxetine in Combination:* Also refer to the Drug Interactions section of the package insert for Symbyax. (7.1)
- *CNS Acting Drugs:* Caution should be used when taken in combination with other centrally acting drugs and alcohol. (7.2)
- *Antihypertensive Agents:* Enhanced antihypertensive effect. (7.2)
- *Levodopa and Dopamine Agonists:* May antagonize levodopa/dopamine agonists. (7.2)
- *Lorazepam (IM):* Increased somnolence with IM olanzapine. (7.2)
- *Other Concomitant Drug Therapy:* When using olanzapine in combination with lithium or valproate, refer to the Drug Interactions sections of the package insert for those products. (7.2)

----------------------- USE IN SPECIFIC POPULATIONS -----------------------

- *Pregnancy:* ZYPREXA should be used during pregnancy only if the potential benefit justifies the potential risk to the fetus. (8.1)
- *Nursing Mothers:* Breast-feeding is not recommended. (8.3)
- *Pediatric Use:* Safety and effectiveness of ZYPREXA in children <13 years of age have not been established. (8.4)

See 17 for PATIENT COUNSELING INFORMATION and FDA-approved Medication Guide

Revised: 05/2010

(c) What may occur if the drug is taken with diazepam?

____

(d) What is the recommended beginning oral dose for adults with schizophrenia?

____

(e) Should women who are breastfeeding use this drug?

____

9. Fill in the following table with the equivalent times.

Standard Time	Military Time
7:30 A.M.	______
______	1620 *h*
______	0525 *h*
8:10 P.M.	______
______	1259 *h*
12 noon	______
10:30 A.M.	______
______	1741 *h*
7:15 P.M.	______
______	0500 *h*

10. Interpret the following medication orders:
    (a) *aspirin 81 mg PO daily*
    (b) *atorvastatin (Lipitor) 40 mg PO hs*
    (c) *ampicillin 500 mg PO stat, then give 250 mg PO Q.I.D.*
    (d) *gabapentin (Neurontin) four 300-mg cap po q8h*
    (e) *epoetin alfa (Epogen) 40,000 units subcut weekly*
11. Determine the missing component(s) for each of the following medication orders:
    (a) acetaminophen (Tylenol) PO
    (b) sucralfate (Carafate) 1 g
    (c) phenytoin sodium (Dilantin) T.I.D.
    (d) methergine (Ergotrate) 0.2 *mg* q4h for 6 doses
    (e) furosemide (Lasix) 40 *mg* stat
12. (a) A drug is ordered 20 *mg* daily. How many milligrams will you administer?
    (b) A drug is ordered 20 *mg* B.I.D. How many milligrams will you administer?
    (c) A drug is ordered 20 *mg* q12h. How many milligrams will you administer?
    (d) A drug is ordered 20 *mg* daily in two divided doses. How many milligrams will you administer?

Additional Exercises

Now, test yourself!

Use the information from drug labels in Figures 2.38 to 2.42 to complete Exercises 1 to 5.

1. Write the generic name for Singulair.

____

2. Write the trade name for the drug whose NDC number is 0006-0749-54.

____

3. What is the total amount of solution in the bottle of clarithromycin?

____

4. What is the dosage strength of E.E.S. granules?

____

5. What is the dosage strength of the drug whose NDC number is 0074-3956-46?

____

Figure 2.38 Drug label for E.E.S. granules.

SOURCE: Arbor Pharmaceuticals, Inc.

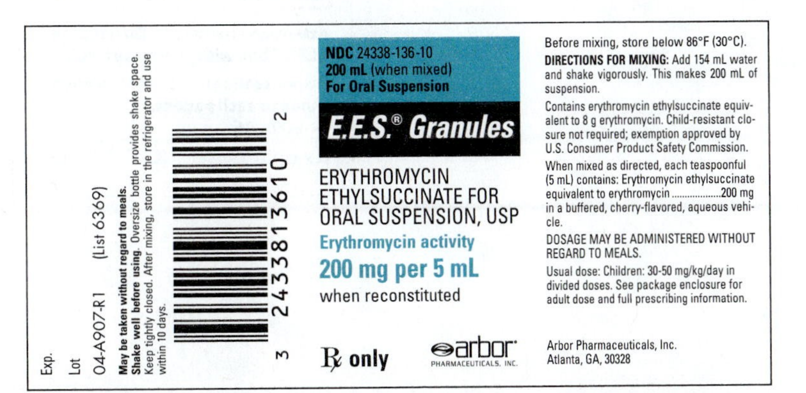

Figure 2.39 Drug label for Zocor.

SOURCE: Reproduced with permission of Merck Sharp & Dohme Corp., a subsidiary of Merck & Co, Inc., Whitehouse Station, New Jersey, USA. All Rights Reserved.

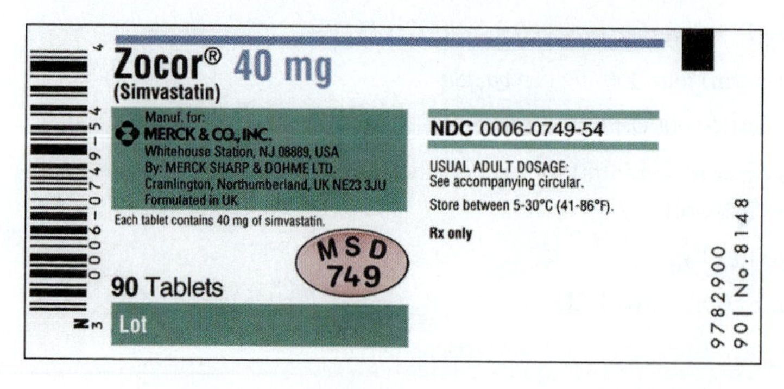

Figure 2.40 Drug label for Singulair.

SOURCE: Reproduced with permission of Merck Sharp & Dohme Corp., a subsidiary of Merck & Co, Inc., Whitehouse Station, New Jersey, USA. All Rights Reserved.

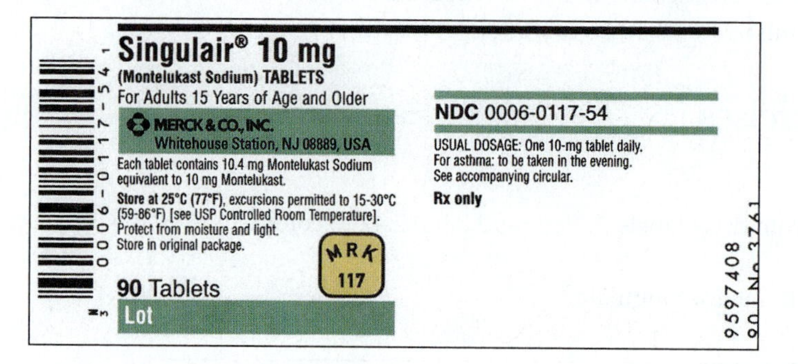

Figure 2.41 Drug label for Biaxin.

SOURCE: Courtesy of AbbVie

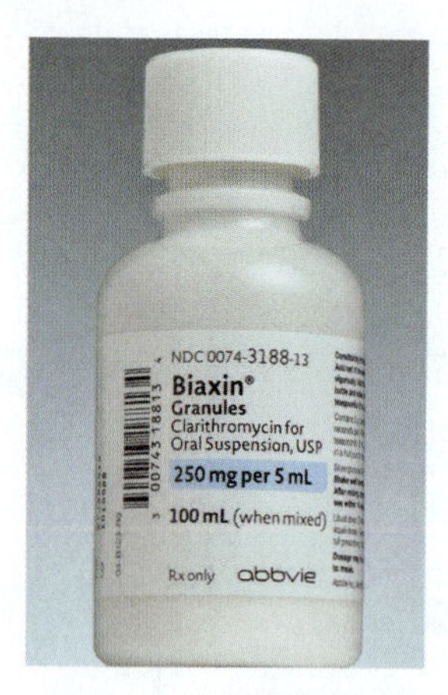

Figure 2.42 Drug label for Kaletra.

SOURCE: Courtesy of AbbVie

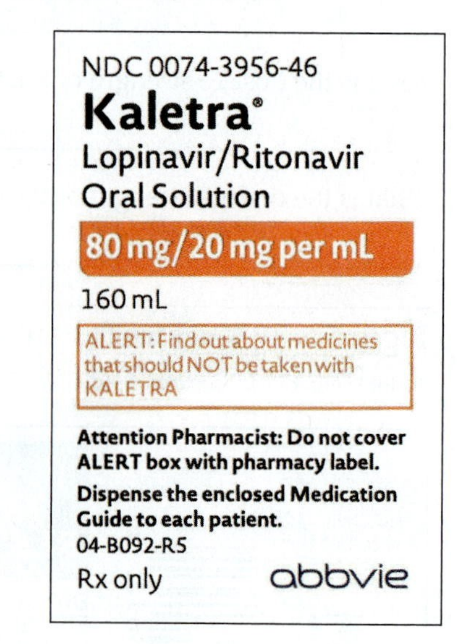

6. Study the MAR in Figures 2.43a and 2.43b and answer the questions.
   (a) Which drugs were administered at 10:00 P.M. on 12/10/2020?

   ____

   (b) Designate the time of the day the client received ibandronate sodium.

   ____

   (c) How many doses of Dilantin were administered to the client by nurse Young?

   ____

   (d) What drugs must be taken before breakfast?

   ____

   (e) What is the last date on which the client will receive Bactrim?

   ____

Figure 2.43a Medication Administration Record for Jane Ambery.

UNIVERSITY HOSPITAL

DAILY MEDICATION ADMINISTRATION RECORD

324689
Jane Ambery
2336 17th Avenue
Brooklyn, NY 10001

12/7/2020
5/01/47
Protestant
HIP

Dr. Mae Ling

PATIENT NAME *Jane Ambery*

ROOM # *112*

ALLERGIC TO (RECORD IN RED): *sulfa, fish*

IF ANOTHER RECORD IS IN USE ☐

DATES GIVEN ↓ MONTH/DAY YEAR: *2020*

RED CHECK INITIAL	ORDER DATE	INITIAL	EXP DATE	MEDICATION, DOSAGE, FREQUENCY AND ROUTE	TIME	12/7	12/8	12/9	12/10	12/11	12/12	12/13
	12/7	MC	12/13	Dilantin (phenytoin) 100 mg	10AM	MC	MC	MC	MC			
				PO t.i.d.	2PM	MC	MC	MC	MC			
					6PM	JY	JY	JY	JY			
	12/7	SG	12/16	Bactrim DS 2tabs PO q12h	8AM	SG	SG	SG	SG			
				for 10 days	8PM	JY	JY	JY	JY			
	12/7	SG	12/13	Bonivar (ibandronate sodium)	6AM	SG	SG	SG	SG			
				2.5 mg PO daily. Take 60 minutes								
				before first food or drink of day								
				(except plain water)								
	12/7	SG	12/13	Humulin N insulin 15 units subcut	7:30AM	SG	SG	SG	SG			
				every morning								
				30 minutes before breakfast								
	12/7	SG	12/13	Humulin R insulin 8 units subcut	7:30AM	SG	SG	SG	SG			
				every morning								
				30 minutes before breakfast								

INT.	NURSES' FULL SIGNATURE AND TITLE	INT.	NURSES' FULL SIGNATURE AND TITLE
SG	Sara Gordon, RN		
MC	Marie Colon, RN		
JY	Jim Young, RN		

Figure 2.43b Medication Administration Record for Jane Ambery.

UNIVERSITY HOSPITAL

DAILY MEDICATION ADMINISTRATION RECORD

324689
Jane Ambery
2336 17th Avenue
Brooklyn, NY

12/7/2020
5/01/47
Protestant
HIP

Dr. Mae Ling, M.D.

PATIENT NAME *Jane Ambery*

ROOM # *112*

ALLERGIC TO (RECORD IN RED): *sulfa, fish*

IF ANOTHER RECORD IS IN USE ☐

DATES GIVEN MONTH/DAY YEAR: *2020*

PRN MEDICATION

ORDER DATE	EXPIRATION DATE/TIME	MEDICATION, DOSAGE, FREQUENCY AND ROUTE		DOSES GIVEN							
12/10	12/17	*Anusol supp 1 PR q4–6h prn*	DATE	12/10							
			TIME	10 PM							
			INIT	JY							
			DATE								
			TIME								
			INIT								

STAT-ONE DOSE-PRE-OPERATIVE MEDICATIONS ◯ Check here if additional sheet in use.

ORDER DATE	MEDICATION–DOSAGE ROUTE	DATE	TIME	INIT	ORDER DATE	MEDICATION–DOSAGE ROUTE	DATE	TIME	INIT

INT.	NURSES' FULL SIGNATURE AND TITLE	INT.	NURSES' FULL SIGNATURE AND TITLE
JY	*Jim Young, RN*		

7. Study the physician's order sheet in Figure 2.44 and then answer the following questions.
   (a) Which drugs are ordered to be given two times a day?

   ____

   (b) How many doses of metoclopramide will the client receive each day?

   ____

Figure 2.44 Physician's order sheet for client Jane Myers.

PHYSICIAN'S ORDERS

ORDER DATE	DATE DISC	
4/20/20	4/30/20	*Omnicef (cefdinir) 300 mg PO q12h for 10 days*
4/20/20	4/27/20	*digoxin 0.125 mg PO daily*
4/20/20	4/27/20	*Glucophage (metformin HCl) 850 mg PO b.i.d. with breakfast and dinner*
4/20/20	4/27/20	*Reglan (metoclopramide) 10 mg PO 30 minutes before meals and at bedtime*
4/20/20	4/23/20	*Duragesic transdermal film ER 25 mg per hour. Remove in 72 hours.*
4/20/20	4/27/20	*Lasix 40 mg PO daily*

PLEASE INDICATE BEEPER # → *222*

Jane Myers
23 College Ave
Salt Lake City
Utah 46022
2/28/52
Episcopal
Aetna
Dr. Juan Rodriguez
#212332
4/20/2020

(c) What is the dose and route of administration of Duragesic?

____

(d) What is the route of administration for metformin?

____

(e) How many doses of cefdinir will the client receive per day?

____

8. Use the package insert shown in Figure 2.45 to answer the following questions.

Figure 2.45 Excerpt from package insert for Savella.

SOURCE: Package Insert for Savella. Copyright © by Forest Laboratories, Inc. Used by permission of Forest Laboratories, Inc.

HIGHLIGHTS OF PRESCRIBING INFORMATION
These highlights do not include all the information needed to use Savella safely and effectively. See full prescribing information for Savella.
Savella® (milnacipran HCl) Tablets
Initial U.S. Approval: 2009

WARNING: SUICIDALITY AND ANTIDEPRESSANT DRUGS
See full prescribing information for complete boxed warning.
- **Increased risk of suicidal ideation, thinking, and behavior in children, adolescents, and young adults taking antidepressants for major depressive disorder (MDD) and other psychiatric disorders. Savella is not approved for use in pediatric patients (5.1)**

------------- RECENT MAJOR CHANGES-------------------
Warnings and Precautions, Serotonin Syndrome or Neuroleptic Malignant Syndrome (NMS)-like Reactions (5.2) 06/2009

-----------------INDICATIONS AND USAGE-----------------
Savella® is a selective serotonin and norepinephrine reuptake inhibitor (SNRI) indicated for the management of fibromyalgia (1)
Savella is not approved for use in pediatric patients (5.1)

-------------DOSAGE AND ADMINISTRATION-------------
- Administer Savella in two divided doses per day (2.1)
- Based on efficacy and tolerability, dosing may be titrated according to the following schedule (2.1):
  Day 1: 12.5 mg once
  Days 2-3: 25 mg/day (12.5 mg twice daily)
  Days 4-7: 50 mg/day (25 mg twice daily)
  After Day 7: 100 mg/day (50 mg twice daily)
- Recommended dose is 100 mg/day (2.1)
- May be increased to 200 mg/day based on individual patient response (2.1)
- Dose should be adjusted in patients with severe renal impairment (2.2)

-----------DOSAGE FORMS AND STRENGTHS-----------
- Tablets: 12.5 mg, 25 mg, 50 mg, 100 mg (3)

-------------------CONTRAINDICATIONS-------------------
- Use of monoamine oxidase inhibitors concomitantly or in close temporal proximity (4.1)
- Use in patients with uncontrolled narrow-angle glaucoma (4.2)

-------------WARNINGS AND PRECAUTIONS-------------
- Suicidality: Monitor for worsening of depressive symptoms and suicide risk (5.1)
- Serotonin Syndrome or Neuroleptic Malignant Syndrome (NMS)-like Reactions: Serotonin syndrome or NMS-like reactions have been reported with SNRIs and SSRIs. Discontinue Savella and initiate supportive treatment (5.2, 7)
- Elevated blood pressure and heart rate: Cases have been reported with Savella. Monitor blood pressure and heart rate prior to initiating treatment with Savella and periodically throughout treatment (5.3, 5.4)
- Seizures: Cases have been reported with Savella therapy. Prescribe Savella with care in patients with a history of seizure disorder (5.5)
- Hepatotoxicity: More patients treated with Savella than with placebo experienced mild elevations of ALT and AST. Rarely, fulminant hepatitis has been reported in patients treated with Savella. Avoid concomitant use of Savella in patients with substantial alcohol use or chronic liver disease (5.6)
- Discontinuation: Withdrawal symptoms have been reported in patients when discontinuing treatment with Savella. A gradual dose reduction is recommended (5.7)
- Abnormal Bleeding: Savella may increase the risk of bleeding events. Caution patients about the risk of bleeding associated with the concomitant use of Savella and NSAIDs, aspirin, or other drugs that affect coagulation (5.9)
- Male patients with a history of obstructive uropathies may experience higher rates of genitourinary adverse events (5.11)

------------------ADVERSE REACTIONS------------------
The most frequently occurring adverse reactions (≥ 5% and greater than placebo) were nausea, headache, constipation, dizziness, insomnia, hot flush, hyperhidrosis, vomiting, palpitations, heart rate increased, dry mouth, and hypertension (6.3)

To report SUSPECTED ADVERSE REACTIONS, contact Forest Pharmaceuticals, Inc., at (800) 678-1605 or FDA at 1-800-FDA-1088 or www.fda.gov/medwatch.

-------------------DRUG INTERACTIONS-------------------
- Savella is unlikely to be involved in clinically significant pharmacokinetic drug interactions (7)
- Pharmacodynamic interactions of Savella with other drugs can occur (7)

-------------USE IN SPECIFIC POPULATIONS-------------
- Pregnancy and nursing mothers: Use only if the potential benefit justifies the potential risk to the fetus or child (8.1, 8.3)
- To enroll in the Savella Pregnancy Registry call 1-877-643-3010 (toll free) or download data forms from the registry website: www.savellapregnancyregistry.com (8.1)

See 17 for PATIENT COUNSELING INFORMATION and Medication Guide.
Revised: May 2010

(a) What is the generic name and form of the drug?

____

(b) What condition is the drug used to treat?

____

(c) What is the initial dose on the first day?

____

(d) Can the drug be used for children?

____

(e) What is the maximum daily dose?

____

9. Fill in the following table with the equivalent times.

Standard time	Military time
9:30 A.M.	______
______	1443 *h*
______	2400 *h*
11:20 P.M.	______
______	0948 *h*
11:40 P.M.	______
______	2042 *h*
2:15 A.M.	______
______	0002 *h*
7:15 A.M.	______

10. Interpret the following medication orders:
    (a) Glucophage (metformin) 500 *mg* PO B.I.D.
    (b) heparin 10,000 *units* subcut q8h
    (c) NITRO-BID 2% (nitroglycerin ointment) one-half inch q6h to chest wall
    (d) Accupril (quinapril hydrochloride) 5 *mg* PO daily
    (e) Tylenol (acetaminophen) 650 *mg* PO q4h prn fever over 101°
11. Determine the missing component(s) for each of the following medication orders:
    (a) Wellbutrin XL® (bupropion hydrochloride) PO
    (b) Glucotrol (glipizide) 1 *tab* before breakfast
    (c) Ambien® (zolpidem tartrate) 10 *mg*
    (d) ibuprofen stat
    (e) Timoptic (timolol maleate) 1 *drop* B.I.D.
12. (a) A drug is ordered 10 *mg* daily. How many milligrams will you administer?
    (b) A drug is ordered 10 *mg* B.I.D. How many milligrams will you administer?
    (c) A drug is ordered 10 *mg* q12h. How many milligrams will you administer?
    (d) A drug is ordered 10 *mg* daily in two divided doses. How many milligrams will you administer?

Chapter 3

Dimensional Analysis and Ratio & Proportion

Learning Outcomes

After completing this chapter, you will be able to

3.1 Solve simple problems by using both Dimensional Analysis and Ratio & Proportion.

3.2 Identify some common units of measurement and their abbreviations.

3.3 Construct unit fractions and ratios from equivalences.

3.4 Convert a quantity expressed with a single unit of measurement to an equivalent quantity with another single unit of measurement.

3.5 Convert a quantity expressed as a rate to another rate.

3.6 Solve complex problems using both Dimensional Analysis and Ratio & Proportion.

This textbook will focus on three different standard mathematical techniques for dosage calculations. In this chapter the *Dimensional Analysis and Ratio & Proportion* methods will be used to perform conversions between units of measurement. In Chapter 6 the third technique, the *Formula* method, will be introduced.

Dimensional Analysis

Introduction to Dimensional Analysis

In courses such as chemistry and physics, students learn to routinely change a quantity in one unit of measurement to an equivalent quantity in a different unit of measurement by cancelling matching units of measurement. The name Dimensional Analysis was chosen because the units of measure (e.g., feet and inches) are called *dimensions*, and these dimensions have to be *analyzed* to see how to do the problems.

The Mathematical Foundation for Dimensional Analysis

Dimensional Analysis relies on two simple mathematical concepts.

Concept 1 **When a nonzero quantity is divided by the same amount, the result is 1.**
For example: $7 \div 7 = 1$

Because you can also write a division problem in fractional form, you get

$$\frac{7}{7} = 1$$

Because $\frac{7}{7}$ is a fraction equal to 1, and the word "unit" means one, the fraction $\frac{7}{7}$ is called a **unit fraction**.

In the preceding unit fraction, you may *cancel* the 7s on the top and bottom. That is, you can divide both numerator and denominator by 7.

$$\frac{\cancel{7}}{\cancel{7}} = \frac{1}{1} = 1$$

Units of measurement are the "labels," such as *inches, feet, minutes,* and *hours,* which are sometimes written after a number. They are also referred to as **dimensions**, or simply **units**. For example, in the quantity *7 days, days* is the unit of measurement.

The equivalent quantities you divide may contain **units of measurement**. For example: 7 days ÷ 7 days = 1

Or in fractional form: $\frac{7\text{ days}}{7\text{ days}} = 1$

In the preceding unit fraction, you may cancel the number 7 and the unit of measurement *days* on the top and bottom and obtain the following:

$$\frac{\cancel{7}\,\cancel{\text{days}}}{\cancel{7}\,\cancel{\text{days}}} = \frac{1}{1} = 1$$

Going one step further, now consider this *equivalence*: **7 days = 1 week.**

Because 7 *days* is the same quantity of time as 1 *week*, when you divide these quantities, you must get 1.

So, both 7 days ÷ 1 week = 1 **and** 1 week ÷ 7 days = 1

Or in unit fractional form: $\frac{7\text{ days}}{1\text{ week}} = 1$ **and** $\frac{1\text{ week}}{7\text{ days}} = 1$

Other unit fractions can be obtained from the equivalences found in Table 3.1.

Table 3.1 Equivalents for Common Units.

12 inches (*in*) = 1 foot (*ft*)
2 pints (*pt*) = 1 quart (*qt*)
16 ounces (*oz*) = 1 pound (*lb*)
60 seconds (*sec*) = 1 minute (*min*)
60 minutes (*min*) = 1 hour (*h* or *hr*)
24 hours (*h* or *hr*) = 1 day
7 days = 1 week (*wk*)
12 months (*mon*) = 1 year (*yr*)

Concept 2 When a quantity is multiplied by 1, the quantity is unchanged.

In the following examples, the quantity 2 *weeks* will be multiplied by the number 1 and also by the unit fractions $\frac{7}{7}$, $\frac{7\text{ days}}{7\text{ days}}$, and $\frac{7\text{ days}}{1\text{ week}}$

2 weeks × 1 = 2 weeks

↓ ↓

$$2\text{ weeks} \times \frac{7}{7} = 2\text{ weeks} \times 1 = 2\text{ weeks}$$

↓ ↓

$$2\text{ weeks} \times \frac{7\text{ days}}{7\text{ days}} = 2\text{ weeks} \times 1 = 2\text{ weeks}$$

↓ ↓

$$2\text{ weeks} \times \frac{7\text{ days}}{1\text{ week}} = 2\text{ weeks} \times 1 = 2\text{ weeks}$$

Consider the previous line again. This time you cancel the *week(s)*!

$$\text{2 weeks} = 2\ \cancel{\text{weeks}} \times \frac{7\ \text{days}}{1\ \cancel{\text{week}}} = (2 \times 7)\ \text{days} = \text{14 days}$$

So, 2 weeks = 14 days.

This shows how to convert a quantity measured in weeks (2 *weeks*) to an equivalent quantity measured in days (14 *days*). With the Dimensional Analysis method, you multiply quantities by unit fractions to convert the units of measure. This procedure demonstrates the basic technique of Dimensional Analysis.

Many of the problems in dosage calculation require changing a quantity with a *single unit of measurement* into an equivalent quantity with a different *single unit of measurement*; for example, changing 2 *weeks* to 14 *days* as was shown above.

Changing a Single Unit of Measurement to Another Single Unit of Measurement

Simple (One-Step) Problems with Single Units of Measurement Using Dimensional Analysis

Suppose you want to express 18 *months* in *years*. That is, you want to convert 18 *months* to an equivalent amount of time in *years*.

This is a **simple** problem. Simple problems have only three elements. The elements in this problem are

The given quantity:	18 months
The quantity you want to find:	? years
An equivalence between them:	1 year = 12 months

To begin the Dimensional Analysis process in a logical way, write the quantity you are given (18 *months*) on the left of an equal sign and the unit you want to change it to (*years*) on the right side, as follows:

$$18\ \text{months} = ?\ \text{years}$$

It may help to write 18 *months* as the fraction $\frac{18\ \text{months}}{1}$

Thus, you now have

$$\frac{18\ \text{months}}{1} = ?\ \text{years}$$

Formulate the Appropriate Unit Fraction To change *months* to *years*, you need an equivalence between *months* and *years*. That equivalence is

$$12\ \text{months} = 1\ \text{year}$$

From this equivalence, you can get two possible unit fractions:

$$\frac{12\ \text{months}}{1\ \text{year}} \quad \text{and} \quad \frac{1\ \text{year}}{12\ \text{months}}$$

But which of these fractions shall you choose? If you multiply $\frac{18\ \text{months}}{1}$ by $\frac{12\ \text{months}}{1\ \text{year}}$, you get

$$\frac{18\ \text{months}}{1} \times \frac{12\ \text{months}}{1\ \text{year}}$$

Notice that both the *months* units are in the numerators of the fractions.

Because no cancellation of the units is possible in this case, do not select this unit fraction.

If, on the other hand, you multiply by $\frac{1 \text{ year}}{12 \text{ months}}$, you get the following:

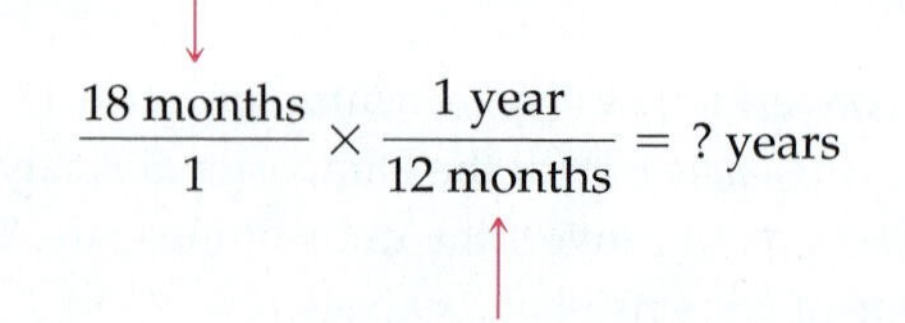

Notice that now *one of the months is in the numerator (top), and the other months is in the denominator (bottom) of a fraction*. Because cancellation of the *months* is now possible, this is the appropriate unit fraction to choose.

Cancel the Units of Measurement $\frac{18 \text{ months}}{1} \times \frac{1 \text{ year}}{12 \text{ months}} = ? \text{ years}$

After you cancel the *months*, notice that *year* (the unit of measurement that you want to find) is the only remaining unit on the left side.

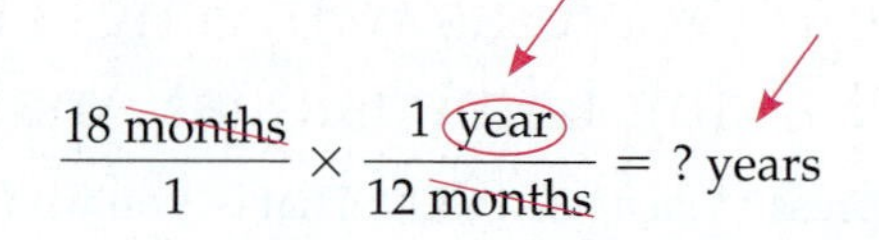

Cancel the Numbers and Finish the Multiplication After you are sure that you have *only the unit of measurement that you want (years) remaining on the left side and that it is on the top of a fraction*, you can complete the cancellation and multiplication of the numbers as follows:

$$\frac{\overset{3}{\cancel{18}} \text{ months}}{1} \times \frac{1 \text{ year}}{\underset{2}{\cancel{12}} \text{ months}} = \frac{3 \text{ years}}{2} \quad \text{or} \quad 1\frac{1}{2} \text{ years}$$

So, 18 *months* is equivalent to $1\frac{1}{2}$ *years*.

Ratio & Proportion

Ratios

A **ratio** compares two quantities. Ratios can be expressed in a variety of ways, including fractional form. For this reason, fractions are sometimes referred to as *ratio*nal numbers.

Suppose a recipe indicates that 1 cup of sugar and 2 cups of flour are needed to make a certain type of cake. The relative amounts of sugar and flour in the cake are crucial to its quality. To compare the amount of sugar to the amount of flour in this recipe, any of the following equivalent *sugar-flour* ratios could be used:

1 cup of sugar *for every* 2 cups of flour
1 cup of sugar *per* 2 cups of flour
1 cup of sugar *to* 2 cups of flour
1 cup to 2 cups
1 to 2
1:2
$\frac{1}{2}$

The order of comparison could be reversed. So, on the other hand, to compare the amount of flour to the amount of sugar in this recipe, the following equivalent *flour-sugar ratios* could be used:

2 cups of flour *for every* 1 cup of sugar
2 cups of flour *per* 1 cup of sugar
2 cups of flour *to* 1 cup of sugar
2 cups to 1 cup
2 to 1
2:1
$\frac{2}{1}$

As you can see, the order of the numbers in the flour-sugar ratio is the reverse of the order in the sugar-flour ratio.

Now, if twice the amount of this cake were needed, the baker would need to double the amount of each of the ingredients in the recipe.

Therefore, instead of

1 cup of sugar and 2 cups of flour,
2 cups of sugar and 4 cups of flour

would be required, and the *sugar-flour ratio* would now be 2 to 4. Although the quantities of sugar and flour have each been increased, the ratio of sugar to flour has not changed; the ratio 1:2 is equivalent to the ratio 2:4. It is easy to see this equivalency when both the ratios are written in fractional form because $\frac{1}{2} = \frac{2}{4}$.

Recall that in Chapter 1 both *building and reducing* fractions were discussed, and $\frac{1}{2}$ could be *"built"* into $\frac{2}{4}$ by multiplying both numerator and denominator by 2, as follows:

$$\frac{1}{2} = \frac{1 \times 2}{2 \times 2} = \frac{2}{4}$$

Similarly, $\frac{2}{4}$ could be *"reduced"* to $\frac{1}{2}$ by dividing both numerator and denominator by 2 as follows:

$$\frac{2}{4} = \frac{2 \div 2}{4 \div 2} = \frac{1}{2}$$

So, $\frac{1}{2}$ and $\frac{2}{4}$ are equivalent ratios.

Now, suppose that three times the amount of the cake were needed. The baker would need to multiply the amount of each ingredient in the recipe by three.

Therefore, instead of using

1 cup of sugar and 2 cups of flour,
3 cups of sugar and 6 cups of flour

would be required.

Continuing this process, a table could be constructed showing the amount of sugar and the corresponding amount of flour needed in order to make various amounts of this cake. See Table 3.2.

Table 3.2 Some Corresponding Amounts of Sugar and Flour for a 1-to-2 Sugar-Flour Ratio.

Cups of Sugar	Cups of Flour
1	2
2	4
3	6
4	8
5	10
6	12

Example 3.1

Suppose a recipe indicates that 1 cup of sugar and 2 cups of flour are needed to make a certain type of cake. If the baker wants to make some of this cake and decides to use 10 cups of flour, how much sugar would be needed?

Cups of Sugar	Cups of Flour
1	2
2	4
3	6
4	8
5 ←	10
6	12

The baker could look at Table 3.2 and see that for 10 cups of flour, 5 cups of sugar are needed.

Another way to solve the problem is to realize that the amount of flour (10 cups) is 5 times the amount of flour (2 cups) in the recipe. Whenever the amount of flour in the recipe is multiplied by 5, the amount of sugar in the recipe must also be multiplied by 5.

So, the terms in the ratio of

1 cup of sugar to 2 cups of flour

are each multiplied by 5 to yield

5 cups of sugar to 10 cups of flour

and 5 cups of sugar would be needed.

Example 3.2

Mary prepares her morning coffee by combining 5 parts black coffee with 2 parts milk.

(a) What is the black coffee-milk ratio expressed in colon [:] form and in fractional form?

(b) Mary wants to make some of her morning coffee and take it along in a thermos bottle. If she used 8 ounces of milk, how much black coffee must be added to the bottle?

(a) The drink has 5 parts black coffee to 2 parts milk. This is a ratio of *5 parts* to *2 parts* or a ratio of *5 to 2*. This ratio can also be written in colon form as *5:2* or in fractional form as $\frac{5}{2}$.

(b) A table could be constructed showing the amount of black coffee and the corresponding amount of milk needed to make various amounts of this drink. See Table 3.3.

Table 3.3 Some Corresponding Amounts of Black Coffee and Milk in a 5-to-2 Ratio.

Ounces of Black Coffee	Ounces of Milk
5	2
10	4
15	6
20	8
25	10
30	12

Mary could look at Table 3.3 and see that for 8 ounces of milk, 20 ounces of black coffee are needed.

Ounces of Black Coffee	Ounces of Milk
5	2
10	4
15	6
20 ←	**8**
25	10
30	12

Rates

Ratios compare quantities with the same units of measurement (for example, ounces with ounces). **Rates** are like ratios except that they compare two quantities with *different units of measurement*.

For example, a car might be traveling on a highway at a constant rate of speed of *50 miles per hour*. This rate has two different units of measurement, *miles* and *hours*. To compare the number of *miles* traveled to the number of *hours* driven, any of the following equivalent *rates of speed* could be used:

50 miles for every 1 hour driven
50 miles per each hour driven
50 miles per hour
50 miles/1 hour
50 miles/hour

Notice that if the car drove twice the number of hours (2 hours), then the car would travel twice the distance (100 miles). However, the rate of speed would be the same.

Now, consider a worker's rate of pay. Suppose the pay rate is $60 for every 2 hours worked. To compare the amount of *dollars* paid to the number of *hours* worked, any of the following equivalent *rates of pay* could be used:

$60 for every 2 hours worked
$60 per 2 hours
$60/2 hours
$30 for every 1 hour worked
$30 per hour
$30/hour

Notice that if a person worked 2 hours for $60, or if the person worked 1 hour for $30, the rate of pay would be equivalent.

Example 3.3

Each can of cola contains 12 ounces.

(a) How many ounces are contained in 6 cans?

(b) How many cans would contain 18 ounces?

(Continued)

(a) A table could be constructed showing the number of 12-ounce cans and the corresponding number of ounces. The last line of the table indicates that 6 cans contain 72 ounces.

Cans of Cola	Ounces of Cola
1	12
2	24
3	36
4	48
5	60
6 →	**72**

Another way to do the problem is to realize that the rate is 12 ounces per 1 can. In this case the number of cans is multiplied by 6, so the number of ounces must also be multiplied by 6.

So, the terms in the rate of

12 ounces per 1 can

are each multiplied by 6 to yield

72 ounces per 6 cans

(b) While 18 ounces is not in the table, 18 oz = 12 oz + 6 oz. If the number of cans in the rate is multiplied by $\frac{1}{2}$, the number of ounces must also be multiplied by $\frac{1}{2}$.

So, the terms in the rate of

12 ounces per 1 can

are each multiplied by $\frac{1}{2}$ to yield

6 *ounces per* $\frac{1}{2}$ *can*

Put these two rates into a table as follows:

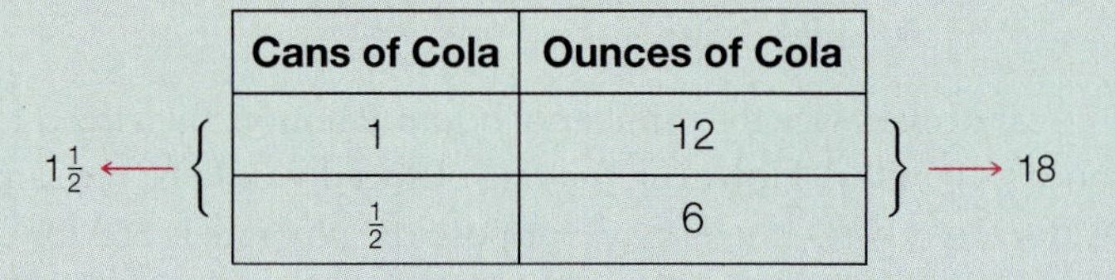

Cans of Cola	Ounces of Cola
1	12
$\frac{1}{2}$	6

$1\frac{1}{2}$ ← { } → 18

By adding the two rows of the preceding table, it can be concluded that 18 ounces of cola are contained in $1\frac{1}{2}$ cans.

Example 3.4

(a) An object is moving at a rate of 72 inches in 2 hours. Express this rate in terms of inches/hour.

(b) An object is moving at a rate of 240 inches per hour. Express this rate in terms of inches/min.

(c) An object is moving at a rate of 2 feet per minute. Express this rate in terms of feet/hour.

You can do this problem in many different ways.

(a) The rate *72 inches in 2 hours*, in fractional form, is $\frac{72\,in}{2\,h}$.

It is already in the form of inches/hour, so merely reduce the fraction as follows:

$$\frac{72\,in}{2\,h} = \frac{72}{2}\frac{in}{h} = 36\,in/h$$

(b) To change *240 inches/hour* to *inches/minute*, substitute 60 minutes for 1 hour as follows:

$$\frac{240\ in}{1\ h} = \frac{240\ in}{60\ min} = \frac{240}{60}\frac{in}{min} = 4\ in/min$$

(c) To change *2 feet/minute* to *feet/hour*, multiply both numerator and denominator by 60 because 60 *min* = 1 *h*.

$$\frac{2\ ft \times 60}{1\ min \times 60} = \frac{120\ ft}{60\ min} = \frac{120\ ft}{1\ h} = 120\ ft/h$$

Proportions

A **proportion** is a statement or equation indicating that two ratios or two rates are equal. For example,

$$\frac{2}{4} = \frac{5}{10} \text{ is a proportion.}$$

True proportions have an interesting property. If the true proportion is written in fractional form, when you cross multiply, the products obtained are equal.

Cross multiply:

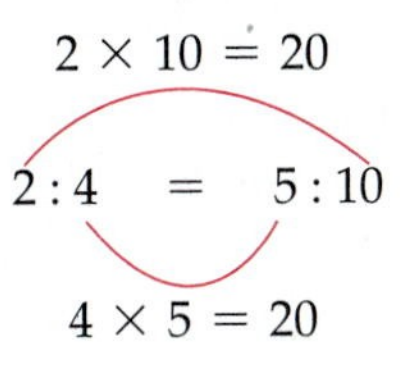

$$(5)(4) = (2)(10)$$

$$20 = 20$$

The products each equal 20.

The proportion $\frac{2}{4} = \frac{5}{10}$ may also be written using the colon form as follows:

$$2:4 = 5:10$$

In this form, the equivalent to cross multiplication is to multiply the means and the extremes (inside numbers and outside numbers) as follows:

$$2 \times 10 = 20$$

$$2:4 \quad = \quad 5:10$$

$$4 \times 5 = 20$$

Again, these products are both equal to 20.

NOTE

This book uses the fractional form of proportions rather than the colon form.

Example 3.5

Verify that $\frac{30}{1,000} = \frac{6}{200}$ is a true proportion.

To verify that this proportion is true, cross multiply. If the products obtained are equal, then the proportion is true.

Cross multiply

$$\frac{30}{1,000} = \frac{6}{200}$$

$$(6)(1000) = (30)(200)$$

$$6,000 = 6,000$$

Because the products are equal, it is a true proportion.

Example 3.6

Is $\frac{30}{120} = \frac{6}{18}$ a true portion?

To determine if this proportion is true, cross multiply. If the products obtained are equal, then the proportion is true.

Cross multiply

$$\frac{30}{120} = \frac{6}{18}$$

$$(6)(120) = (30)(18)$$

$$720 \neq 540$$

Because the products are not equal, $\frac{30}{120} = \frac{6}{18}$ is not a true proportion.

The Mathematics Needed to Solve Proportions

Your first step toward understanding how to solve proportions is a review of a few basic arithmetic and algebraic concepts.

Using Parentheses to Indicate Multiplication

In algebra, letters are used to stand for numbers. The letter x is the symbol most commonly used to represent an unknown number, but the times sign $\times$ is also a symbol for multiplication. To avoid confusion between the two meanings of the same symbol, *the times sign $\times$ is generally avoided* throughout the remainder of the textbook. Instead of using $\times$ to represent multiplication, a pair of parentheses is used.

So, $3 \times 4 = 12$ will often be written as $(3)(4) = 12$.

Multiplying by 1

The rules of algebra are generalizations of the rules of arithmetic. In arithmetic, when 1 is multiplied by 7, the result is 7. When 1 is multiplied by 52, the result is 52. In general, *when 1 is multiplied by any number, the result is that same number*. In algebraic terms, 1 multiplied by x equals x. This can be summarized as:

$$(1)(x) = x$$

Dividing by 1

In arithmetic, when 9 is divided by 1 the result is 9, and when 23 is divided by 1 the result is 23. In general, *when any number is divided by 1 the result is that same number*. In algebraic terms, x divided by 1 equals x. This can be summarized as:

$$\frac{x}{1} = x$$

Shorthand for Multiplication

When a known number is multiplied by an unknown number, 7 times x, for example, this product could be represented as $(7)(x)$. The product of the two numbers (7) and (x) is usually written in the shorthand $7x$. This can be summarized as:

$$(7)(x) = 7x$$

Example 3.7

Simplify the expression: (45)(*x*)

When a known number (45) is multiplied by an unknown number (x), the product may be written in the simplified shorthand form of $45x$.

Commutative Property

In arithmetic, when you multiply numbers, the order of the factors does not matter. You may **commute** the factors (*switch their positions*) without changing the product. For example,

$$3 \times 4 = 12 \quad \text{and} \quad 4 \times 3 = 12,$$

therefore,

$$3 \times 4 = 4 \times 3$$

You may want to use this commutative property when you have to multiply an unknown number by a known number. To multiply an unknown number by 12, you could write $(x)(12)$. But reversing the order of the factors gives $(12)(x)$, and the shorthand for this is $12x$.

Similarly,

$$(x)(37) = (37)(x) = 37x$$

Example 3.8

Simplify the expression: (*x*)(13)

Because the order does not matter when you multiply two numbers, you may write

$$(x)(13) \text{ as } (13)(x)$$

The shorthand for $(13)(x)$ is $13x$.

Cancelling

In arithmetic a fraction can be reduced by cancelling. For example, the fraction $\frac{21}{28}$ could be reduced as follows. Write the numerator and denominator in factored form.

$$\frac{21}{28} = \frac{(7)(3)}{(7)(4)}$$

Now cancel the (7)s.

$$\frac{21}{28} = \frac{(\cancel{7})(3)}{(\cancel{7})(4)} = \frac{3}{4}$$

So, $\frac{21}{28} = \frac{3}{4}$

This cancelling technique will be used in solving simple equations.

Solving Simple Equations

In the process of solving proportions, you will frequently encounter simple equations like:

$$3x = 6$$

This equation states that 3 times a number equals 6. To solve this equation means to find a value of x that will make the equation true. Because 3 times 2 equals 6, the solution is 2.

Not every simple equation can easily be solved mentally. So, the technique for solving such equations is to manipulate them so that x is alone on one side of the equal sign. This can be accomplished by dividing both sides of the equation by the **coefficient of x** (the number multiplying the x).

$$3x = 6$$

coefficient of x

In the term $3x$, the coefficient of x is 3, so you should divide both sides of the equation by 3.

$$\frac{3x}{3} = \frac{6}{3}$$

Now cancel the 3s

$$\frac{\not{3}x}{\not{3}} = \frac{6}{3}$$

This gives

$$x = \frac{6}{3}$$

Simplify $\frac{6}{3}$

$$x = 2$$

Example 3.9

Solve the equation $5x = 35$

To solve this equation means to find the value of x that will make the equation true. The technique is to manipulate the equation so that x is alone on one side of the equation. This can be accomplished by dividing both sides of the equation by the coefficient of x, which is 5 in this case.

$$5x = 35$$

coefficient of x

Divide by 5

$$\frac{5x}{5} = \frac{35}{5}$$

Now cancel

$$\frac{\not{5}x}{\not{5}} = \frac{35}{5}$$

This gives

$$x = 7$$

Solving Proportions

Throughout the textbook you will encounter **proportions** in which one of the four numbers in the proportion is unknown. For example,

$$\frac{2}{?} = \frac{5}{10}$$

In this proportion, the denominator of the first fraction is not known. Unknown numbers are often represented by letters of the alphabet, x in particular. So this equation might also be written as

$$\frac{2}{x} = \frac{5}{10}$$

Finding this unknown number x that makes the proportion true is called "*solving the proportion.*" In general, solving a proportion involves two steps:

1. *Cross multiply* to obtain a simple equation
2. To solve the simple equation, *divide both sides of the equation by the coefficient of x*

Because the proportion is written in fractional form, when you cross multiply, the products obtained are equal.

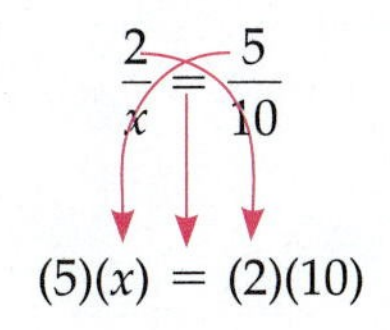

$$(5)(x) = (2)(10)$$

Simplifying, you get the simple equation

$$5x = 20$$

Divide by 5, the coefficient of x

$$\frac{5x}{5} = \frac{20}{5}$$

Cancel

$$\frac{\cancel{5}x}{\cancel{5}} = \frac{20}{5}$$

This gives

$$x = 4$$

So, 4 is the solution of the equation.

You may *check your answer* by substituting 4 for x in the original proportion as follows:

$$\frac{2}{\textcircled{4}} = \frac{5}{10}$$

Now cross multiply

$$\frac{2}{4} = \frac{5}{10}$$

$$(5)(4) = (2)(10)$$

$$20 = 20$$

Because the products are equal, the solution 4 is correct.

NOTE

You should always check your answers to proportion problems by substituting the answer into the proportion, cross multiplying, and seeing if the products are equal.

Example 3.10

Solve the proportion $\frac{5}{12} = \frac{x}{6}$

The first step in solving the proportion is to cross multiply

$$\frac{5}{12} = \frac{x}{6}$$

$$(12)(x) = (5)(6)$$

Simplify

$$12x = 30$$

Divide both sides by 12, the coefficient of x

$$\frac{12x}{12} = \frac{30}{12}$$

Cancel

$$\frac{\cancel{12}x}{\cancel{12}} = \frac{30}{12}$$

This gives

$$x = \frac{30}{12}$$

Simplify

$$x = 2.5$$

Example 3.11

Solve: $\frac{x}{26} = \frac{10.1}{13}$

Cross multiply

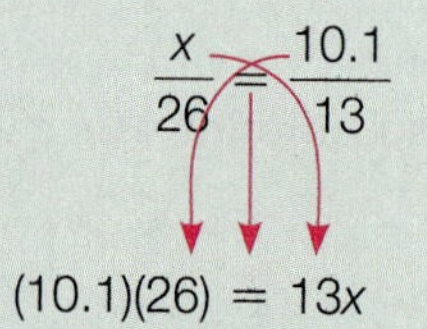

$$(10.1)(26) = 13x$$

At this point, there are two different approaches that may be used to finish the problem.

Method 1: Multiply 10.1 by 26 to obtain 262.6

$$262.6 = 13x$$

Divide both sides by 13, which is the coefficient of x

$$\frac{262.6}{13} = \frac{13x}{13}$$

Cancel

$$\frac{262.6}{13} = \frac{\cancel{13}x}{\cancel{13}}$$

Simplify

$$20.2 = x$$

Method 2: Do not multiply 10.1 by 26 to obtain 262.6, but leave the left side of the equation in factored form as follows:

$$(10.1)(26) = 13x$$

Divide both sides by 13 which is the coefficient of x

$$\frac{(10.1)(26)}{13} = \frac{13x}{13}$$

Cancel

$$\frac{(10.1)(\overset{2}{\cancel{26}})}{\underset{1}{\cancel{13}}} = \frac{\cancel{13}x}{\cancel{13}}$$

$$(10.1)(2) = x$$

Multiply

$$20.2 = x$$

The advantage of *Method 2* in this case is that it avoids the creation of the large number 262.6 and its subsequent division by 13.

Table 3.1 contains equivalents for several common units of measurement, including the equivalence 7 *days* = 1 *week*.

This equivalence can be used to determine the solution to the problem of finding the number of weeks in 21 days. In this problem there are two quantities: *weeks* and *days*. You know that 1 week is equivalent to 7 days, and you need to find the unknown number of weeks that would contain 21 days.

Think of the problem this way:

$$7 \text{ days} = 1 \text{ week}$$

$$21 \text{ days} = ? \text{ weeks}$$

To determine if a proportion exists between *days* and *weeks*, ask yourself the question, "If the number of *weeks* is doubled, is the number of *days* doubled?" If the answer were no, then days and weeks would not be proportional and a proportion would not be used to solve the problem.

But the answer is yes because for a given period of time, whenever the number of weeks is doubled, the number of days would be doubled. So the number of days and the number of weeks are proportional, and a proportion could be used to solve the problem.

The proportion could be set up in either of the following two ways:

$$\frac{weeks}{days} = \frac{weeks'}{days'}$$

or

$$\frac{days}{weeks} = \frac{days'}{weeks'}$$

The same answer will be obtained regardless of which of the two forms is used.

In mathematics the **prime notation** (′) is commonly used to link together two quantities. The primed quantities are linked together, and the unprimed quantities are linked. In this case *days* and *weeks* are associated together, whereas *days′* (read, *days prime*) is associated with *weeks′*.

Because you know that 1 week equals 7 days, you can substitute those numbers, *1* and *7*, for *weeks* and *days*, respectively. Because you need to find the number of weeks (x) containing 21 days, you can substitute those quantities, x and *21*, for *weeks′* and *days′*, respectively.

Substituting into the second form $\frac{days}{weeks} = \frac{days'}{weeks'}$

you obtain

$$\frac{7\ days}{1\ week} = \frac{21\ days}{x\ weeks}$$

Eliminate the units of measurement

$$\frac{7}{1} = \frac{21}{x}$$

Cross multiply

$$\frac{7}{1} = \frac{21}{x}$$

$$(21)(1) = (7)(x)$$

Simplify

$$21 = 7x$$

Divide both sides by 7, the coefficient of x

$$\frac{21}{7} = \frac{7x}{7}$$

Cancel

$$\frac{21}{7} = \frac{\cancel{7}x}{\cancel{7}}$$

Simplify

$$3 = x$$

You have just used the ratio and proportion method to convert a given amount of time measured in one unit of measurement (21 days) to an equivalent amount of time measured in another unit of measurement (3 weeks).

Simple (One-Step) Problems with Single Units of Measurement Using Ratio & Proportion

Suppose that you want to express 30 months as an equivalent amount of time measured in years. That is,

30 months = ? years

Both 30 *months* and ? *years* are quantities that have single units of measurement. This problem can be solved by using a proportion. The steps to follow in solving a proportion problem are:

1. *Identify the two units of measurement in the problem.*
   In this problem there are two quantities: *months* and *years*.
2. *Write a known equivalence between the units of measurement.*
   You need to know that 12 months is equivalent to 1 year.
3. *Let x stand for the amount you are trying to find and write an equivalence involving x.*
   You have to find the unknown number of years (x) that would contain 30 months.
   So, think of the problem this way:

12 months = 1 year

30 months = x years

4. *Write a proportion using the two units of measurement.*
Because the number of months and the number of years are proportional, a proportion could be used to solve the problem. The proportion could be set up in either of the following two ways:

$$\frac{yr}{mon} = \frac{yr'}{mon'}$$

or

$$\frac{mon}{yr} = \frac{mon'}{yr'}$$

You will get the same answer regardless of which of the two forms you use.

5. *Substitute into the proportion.*
Because you know that 1 year equals 12 months, you can substitute those numbers, 1 and 12, for *years* and *months*, respectively. And because you need to find the number of years (x) containing 30 months, you can substitute those quantities (x and 30) for *years'* and *months'*, respectively.

Substituting into the second form $\frac{mon}{yr} = \frac{mon'}{yr'}$

you obtain

$$\frac{12\ mon}{1\ yr} = \frac{30\ mon}{x\ yr}$$

6. *Eliminate the units of measurement*

$$\frac{12}{1} = \frac{30}{x}$$

7. *Cross multiply*

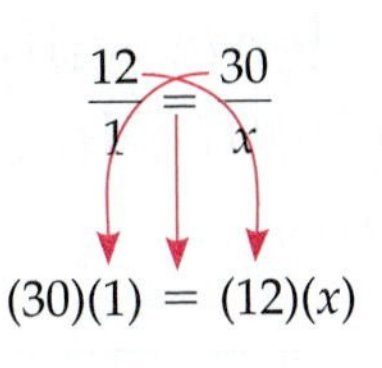

$$(30)(1) = (12)(x)$$

Simplify

$$30 = 12x$$

8. *Divide both sides of the equation by 12, the coefficient of x.*

$$\frac{30}{12} = \frac{12x}{12}$$

9. *Cancel*

$$\frac{30}{12} = \frac{\cancel{12}\,x}{\cancel{12}}$$

Simplify

$$2\tfrac{1}{2} = x$$

So, 30 months is equivalent to $2\frac{1}{2}$ years.

10. *Check your answer.*
In the proportion, replace x by $2\frac{1}{2}$, cross multiply, and see if the cross products are equal.

$$\frac{12}{1} = \frac{30}{2\frac{1}{2}}$$

Cross multiply

$$\frac{12}{1} = \frac{30}{2\frac{1}{2}}$$

$$(30)(1) = (12)(2\tfrac{1}{2})$$

Simplify

$$30 = 30$$

Because the products are equal, the answer is verified. In summary, the steps in solving a proportion are:

1. Identify the two units of measurement in the problem.
2. Write a known equivalence between the units of measure.
3. Let x stand for the amount you are trying to find and write an equivalence involving x.
4. Write a proportion using the two units of measurement.
5. Substitute into the proportion.
6. Eliminate the units.
7. Cross multiply.
8. Divide both sides of the equation by the coefficient of x (unless it is 1).
9. Cancel and simplify.
10. Check your answer by substituting and cross multiplying.

For each of the following examples, both Dimensional Analysis and Ratio & Proportion methods are shown side by side for comparison purposes.

Simple (One-Step) Problems with Single Units of Measurement using both Dimensional Analysis and Ratio & Proportion

NOTE

When a unit of measure follows a numeric fraction, write the unit of measure in the numerator (top) of the fraction. For example, write $\frac{1}{2}$ *hour* as $\frac{1\ hour}{2}$.

Example 3.12

Change $2\frac{1}{4}$ *hours* to an equivalent amount of time in *minutes*.

DIMENSIONAL ANALYSIS

Elements in this problem are

Given quantity: $2\frac{1}{4}$ *hours*

Quantity you want to find: ? *minutes*

Equivalence between them: 1 *hour* = 60 *minutes*

$$2\frac{1}{4}\,hours = ?\ minutes$$

RATIO & PROPORTION

In this problem there are two quantities: *minutes* and *hours*. You need to know that 60 minutes is equivalent to 1 hour, and you have to find the unknown number of minutes that would contain $2\frac{1}{4}$ *hours*.

So, think of the problem this way:

60 *minutes* = 1 *hour*

? *minutes* = $2\frac{1}{4}$ *hours*

Avoid doing multiplication with mixed numbers; change them to improper fractions or decimal numbers. In this case, you can write $2\frac{1}{4}$ *hours* as the improper fraction $\frac{9}{4}$ *hours*. It is better to write the quantity $\frac{9}{4}$ *hours* as $\frac{9 \text{ hours}}{4}$ to make it clear that the unit of measurement (*hours*) is in the numerator of the fraction, not in the denominator.

So, the problem becomes $\frac{9 \text{ hours}}{4} = ? \text{ minutes}$.

Formulate the Appropriate Unit Fraction. You want to change *hours* to *minutes*, so you need an equivalence between *hours* and *minutes*. That equivalence is

$$1 \text{ hour} = 60 \text{ minutes}$$

Because you want to eliminate (cancel) the *hours*, and because *hours* are on the top, as follows:

$$\frac{9 \text{ hours}}{4} = ? \text{ minutes}$$

you need to multiply by the unit fraction with *hour* on the bottom, as follows:

$$\frac{9 \text{ hours}}{4} \times \frac{60 \text{ minutes}}{1 \text{ hour}} = ? \text{ minutes}$$

Cancel the Units

$$\frac{9 \cancel{\text{hours}}}{4} \times \frac{60 \text{ minutes}}{1 \cancel{\text{hour}}} = ? \text{ minutes}$$

NOTE

To eliminate a particular unit of measurement in the numerator, use a unit fraction with that same unit of measurement in the denominator.

After you cancel the *hour(s)*, make sure that *minutes* (the unit you want) is the only remaining unit of measurement and that it is in a numerator (top) of a fraction.

$$\frac{9 \cancel{\text{hours}}}{4} \times \frac{60 \text{ minutes}}{1 \cancel{\text{hour}}} = ? \text{ minutes}$$

Cancel the Numbers and Finish the Multiplication

$$\frac{9 \cancel{\text{hours}}}{\cancelto{1}{4}} \times \frac{\cancelto{15}{60} \text{ minutes}}{1 \cancel{\text{hour}}} = 135 \text{ minutes}$$

Because the number of minutes and the number of hours are proportional, a proportion could be used to solve the problem. The proportion could be set up as

$$\frac{min}{hr} = \frac{min'}{hr'}$$

Because 60 minutes equals 1 hour, you can substitute the numbers *60* and *1* for *minutes* and *hours*, respectively. And because you need to find the number of minutes (x) equal to $2\frac{1}{4}$ hours, you can substitute those quantities
(x and $2\frac{1}{4}$) for *minutes'* and *hours'*, respectively.

Substituting, you get

$$\frac{60 \text{ min}}{1 \text{ hr}} = \frac{x \text{ min}}{2\frac{1}{4} \text{ hr}}$$

Eliminate the units of measurement

$$\frac{60}{1} = \frac{x}{2\frac{1}{4}}$$

Cross multiply

$$(x)(1) = (60)(2\tfrac{1}{4})$$

Simplify

$$x = 135$$

So, $2\frac{1}{4}$ hours is equivalent to 135 minutes.

Example 3.13

Change 4.5 *feet* to an equivalent length measured in *inches*.

DIMENSIONAL ANALYSIS

Given quantity:	4.5 *feet*
Quantity you want to find:	? *inches*
Equivalence between the two quantities:	1 *foot* = 12 *inches*

$$4.5 \textit{ feet} = ? \textit{ inches}$$

You want to cancel the *feet* and get the answer in *inches*, so choose a fraction with *feet* (or *foot*) on the bottom and *inches* on the top. You need a fraction in the form of $\frac{? \textit{ inches}}{? \textit{ feet}}$.

Because 1 *foot* = 12 *inches*, the fraction you need is $\frac{12 \textit{ inches}}{1 \textit{ foot}}$

$$\frac{4.5 \cancel{\textit{feet}}}{1} \times \frac{12 \textit{ inches}}{1 \cancel{\textit{foot}}} = 54 \textit{ inches}$$

RATIO & PROPORTION

In this problem there are two quantities: *inches* and *feet*. You need to know that 12 inches is equivalent to 1 foot, and you have to find the unknown number of inches that would be equivalent to 4.5 feet.

So, think of the problem this way:

$$12 \textit{ inches} = 1 \textit{ feet}$$
$$x \textit{ inches} = 4.5 \textit{ feet}$$

Because the number of inches and the number of feet are proportional, a proportion could be used to solve the problem. The proportion could be set up as

$$\frac{in}{ft} = \frac{in'}{ft'}$$

Because 12 inches equals 1 foot, you can substitute those numbers, *12* and *1*, for *feet* and *inches*, respectively. And because you need to find the number of inches (x) containing 4.5 feet, you can substitute those quantities, x and 4.5, for *inches′* and *feet′*, respectively.

Substituting you get

$$\frac{12 \textit{ in}}{1 \textit{ ft}} = \frac{x \textit{ in}}{4.5 \textit{ ft}}$$

Eliminate the units of measurement

$$\frac{12}{1} = \frac{x}{4.5}$$

Cross multiply

$$\frac{12}{1} = \frac{x}{4.5}$$

$$(x)(1) = (12)(4.5)$$

Simplify

$$x = 54$$

So, 4.5 feet is equivalent to 54 inches.

Example 3.14

An infant weighs 6 pounds. What is the weight of the infant in ounces?

DIMENSIONAL ANALYSIS

Given quantity:	6 *pounds*
Quantity you want to find:	? *ounces*
Equivalence between them:	1 *pound* = 16 *ounces*

$$6 \textit{ pounds} = ? \textit{ ounces}$$

$$\frac{6 \textit{ pounds}}{1} = ? \textit{ ounces}$$

RATIO & PROPORTION

You have to find the number of ounces that would be equivalent to 6 pounds.

So, think of the problem this way:

$$16 \textit{ ounces} = 1 \textit{ pound}$$

$$x \textit{ ounces} = 6 \textit{ pounds}$$

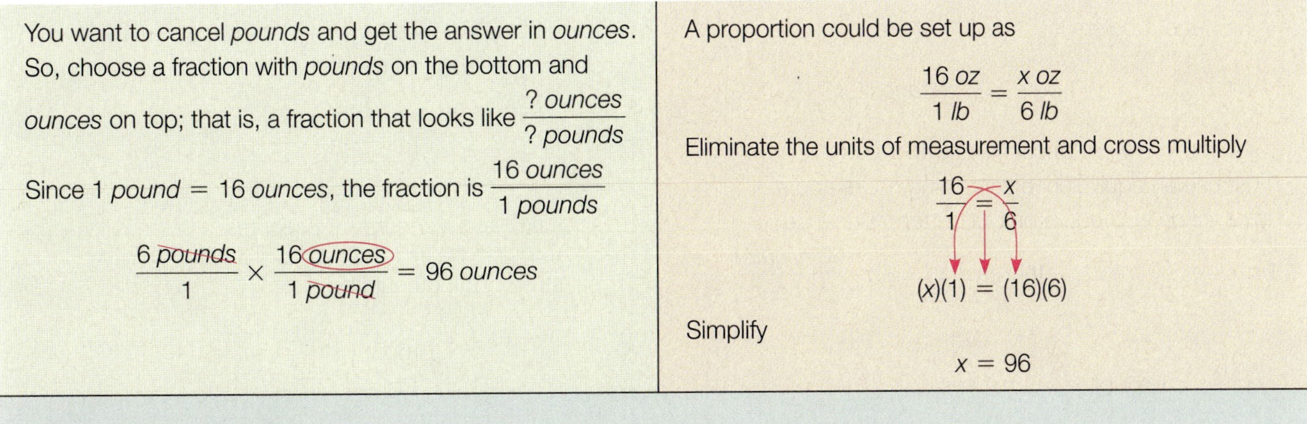

So, the infant weighs 96 ounces.

In Example 3.14, the number of ounces that is equivalent to 6 pounds was found. The proportion used was in the form:

(1) $$\frac{oz}{lb} = \frac{oz'}{lb'}$$

Other proportions that students may choose to use to solve the problem are:

(2) $$\frac{lb}{oz} = \frac{lb'}{oz'}$$

(3) $$\frac{oz}{oz'} = \frac{lb}{lb'}$$

(4) $$\frac{lb}{lb'} = \frac{oz}{oz'}$$

Any of these forms will give the correct answer. However, for consistency this textbook uses only types 1 and 2.

Complex (Multi-Step) Problems with Single Units of Measurement

Sometimes you will encounter problems that will require the procedures used previously to be repeated one or more times. We call such problems **complex**. In a complex problem, multiplication by more than one unit fraction is required. The method is very similar to that used with simple problems.

Example 3.15

Convert 4 *hours* to an equivalent time in *seconds*.

DIMENSIONAL ANALYSIS

Given quantity:	4 *hours*
Quantity you want to find:	? *seconds*
Equivalence between hours and seconds:	?

Most people do not know the direct equivalence between hours and seconds. But you do know the following two equivalences: 1 *hour* = 60 *minutes* and 1 *minute* = 60 *seconds*.

RATIO & PROPORTION

In this problem there are two quantities: *seconds* and *hours*. Most people have not memorized the direct equivalence between seconds and hours. But they do know equivalences between *hours* and *minutes* and between *minutes* and *seconds*, namely,

1 *hour* = 60 *minutes*

and

1 *minute* = 60 *seconds*

(Continued)

So the problem is

$$4 \textit{ hours} = ? \textit{ seconds}$$

First, you want to cancel *hours*. To do this, you must use an equivalence containing *hours* and a unit fraction with *hours* on the bottom. Because 1 *hour* = 60 *minutes*, this fraction will be $\frac{60 \textit{ minutes}}{1 \textit{ hour}}$

$$\frac{4 \textit{ hours}}{1} \times \frac{60 \textit{ minutes}}{1 \textit{ hour}} = ? \textit{ seconds}$$

After the *hours* are cancelled, as shown previously, only *minutes* remain on the left side. So, what you have done at this point is changed 4 *hours* to (4 × 60 = 240) *minutes*, but you want to obtain the answer in *seconds*.

Therefore, the *minutes* must now be cancelled. Because *minutes* is in the numerator, a fraction with *minutes* in the denominator is required.

Because 1 *minute* = 60 *seconds*, the fraction is $\frac{60 \textit{ seconds}}{1 \textit{ minute}}$

Now multiplying by this unit fraction, you get

$$\frac{4 \textit{ hours}}{1} \times \frac{60 \textit{ minutes}}{1 \textit{ hour}} \times \frac{60 \textit{ seconds}}{1 \textit{ minute}} = ? \textit{ seconds}$$

Cancel the *minutes* and notice that the only unit of measurement remaining on the left side is *seconds*, the unit that you want to find!

$$\frac{4 \textit{ hours}}{1} \times \frac{60 \textit{ minutes}}{1 \textit{ hour}} \times \frac{60 \textit{ seconds}}{1 \textit{ minute}} = ? \textit{ seconds}$$

Now that you have the unit of measurement that you want (seconds) on the left side, cancel the numbers (not possible in this example) and finish the multiplication:

$$\frac{4 \textit{ hours}}{1} \times \frac{60 \textit{ minutes}}{1 \textit{ hour}} \times \frac{60 \textit{ seconds}}{1 \textit{ minute}} = 14{,}400 \textit{ seconds}$$

This problem is done in two steps; first change the 4 *hours* to *minutes*, and then change the resulting *minutes* to *seconds*.

Think of *Step 1* this way:

$$1 \textit{ hour} = 60 \textit{ minutes}$$
$$4 \textit{ hours} = x \textit{ minutes}$$

The first proportion could be

$$\frac{60 \textit{ min}}{1 \textit{ h}} = \frac{x \textit{ min}}{4 \textit{ h}}$$

Eliminate the units of measurement and cross multiply

$$\frac{60}{1} = \frac{x}{4}$$

$$(x)(1) = (60)(4)$$

$$x = 240$$

So, 4 hours is equivalent to 240 minutes.

In *Step 2*, change *240 minutes to seconds*.

Think of *Step 2* this way:

$$1 \textit{ minute} = 60 \textit{ seconds}$$

$$240 \textit{ minutes} = x \textit{ seconds}$$

The second proportion could be

$$\frac{1 \textit{ min}}{60 \textit{ sec}} = \frac{240 \textit{ min}}{x \textit{ sec}}$$

Eliminate the units of measurement and cross multiply

$$\frac{1}{60} = \frac{240}{x}$$

$$(240)(60) = (1)(x)$$

$$14{,}400 = x$$

So, 4 hours is equivalent to 14,400 *seconds*.

Example 3.16

Convert 50,400 *minutes* to an equivalent time in *days*.

DIMENSIONAL ANALYSIS

Given quantity: 50,400 *minutes*

Quantity you want to find: ? *days*

Equivalence between minutes and days: ?

You might not know the direct equivalence between minutes and days. But you do know the following two equivalences: 60 *minutes* = 1 *hour* and 24 *hours* = 1 *day*.

$$50{,}400 \textit{ minutes} = ? \textit{ days}$$

You want to cancel *minutes*. To do this, you must use an equivalence containing *minutes* and make a unit fraction with *minutes* on the bottom. Because 60 *minutes* = 1 *hour*, this fraction will be $\frac{1 \textit{ hour}}{60 \textit{ minutes}}$.

$$50{,}400 \cancel{\textit{minutes}} \times \frac{1 \textit{ hour}}{60 \cancel{\textit{minutes}}} = ? \textit{ days}$$

After the *minutes* are cancelled as shown, only *hour* remains on the left side, but you want to obtain the answer in *days*. Therefore, the *hour* must now be cancelled. This will require a unit fraction with *hours* in the denominator. Because 1 *day* = 24 *hours*, this fraction is $\frac{1 \textit{ day}}{24 \textit{ hours}}$.

After cancelling the *hours*, you now have

$$50{,}400 \cancel{\textit{minutes}} \times \frac{1 \cancel{\textit{hour}}}{60 \cancel{\textit{minutes}}} \times \frac{1 \textit{ day}}{24 \cancel{\textit{hours}}} = ? \textit{ days}$$

Because only *day* (in the numerator) is on the left side, the numbers can be cancelled.

$$\overset{840}{\cancel{50{,}400}} \cancel{\textit{minutes}} \times \frac{1 \cancel{\textit{hour}}}{\underset{1}{\cancel{60}} \cancel{\textit{minutes}}} \times \frac{1 \textit{ day}}{24 \cancel{\textit{hours}}}$$

$$= \frac{840}{24} \textit{ days} = 35 \textit{ days}$$

RATIO & PROPORTION

In this problem, there are two quantities: *minutes* and *days*. Most people have not memorized the direct equivalence between minutes and days. But they do know that

60 *minutes* is equivalent to 1 *hour*

and

24 *hours* is equivalent to 1 *day*

This problem is done in two steps; first change the *50,400 minutes to hours*, and then change the resulting *hours to days*.

Think of *Step 1* this way:

$$60 \textit{ minutes} = 1 \textit{ hour}$$
$$50{,}400 \textit{ minutes} = x \textit{ hours}$$

The first proportion could be

$$\frac{60 \textit{ min}}{1 \textit{ h}} = \frac{50{,}400 \textit{ min}}{x \textit{ h}}$$

Eliminate the units of measurement and cross multiply

$$\frac{60}{1} = \frac{50{,}400}{x}$$

$$(50{,}400)(1) = (60)(x)$$
$$50{,}400 = 60x$$

Divide by 60 and cancel

$$\frac{50{,}400}{60} = \frac{\cancel{60} x}{\cancel{60}}$$
$$840 = x$$

So 50,400 minutes is equivalent to 840 hours.

In *Step 2* you change the *840 hours* to *days*

Think of *Step 2* this way:

$$24 \textit{ hours} = 1 \textit{ day}$$
$$840 \textit{ hours} = x \textit{ days}$$

The second proportion could be

$$\frac{1 \textit{ day}}{24 \textit{ h}} = \frac{x \textit{ day}}{840 \textit{ h}}$$

Eliminate the units of measurement and cross multiply

$$\frac{1}{24} = \frac{x}{840}$$

$$(x)(24) = (1)(840)$$
$$24x = 840$$

Divide by 24 and cancel.

$$\frac{\cancel{24} x}{\cancel{24}} = \frac{840}{24}$$
$$x = 35$$

So, 50,400 minutes is equivalent to 35 days.

Changing One Rate to Another Rate

A *rate* is a fraction with different units of measurement on top and bottom. For example, 50 *miles* per *hour* written as 50 miles/hour and 3 *pounds* per *week* written as 3 pounds/week are rates. In dosage calculation, the bottom unit of measurement is frequently time (e.g., *hours* or *minutes*). We sometimes want to change one rate into another rate. These problems are done in a manner similar to the method that was used to do the single-unit-to-single-unit problems.

Rate conversion is not needed in this textbook until flow rates are encountered beginning in Chapter 10. Therefore, some students may prefer to study the rest of this chapter at that time.

Simple (One-Step) Problems with Rates

In dealing with rate conversions, students generally find it easier to use Dimensional Analysis or other techniques rather than Ratio & Proportion. However, in the following examples both methods are shown along with some of the other techniques.

Example 3.17

Convert 5 *feet per hour* to an equivalent rate of speed in *inches per hour*.

DIMENSIONAL ANALYSIS

Given rate: 5 *feet* per *hour*

Rate you want to find: ? *inches* per *hour*

Because you are looking for a rate, you start with the *given* rate:

$$5 \textit{ feet} \text{ per hour} = ? \textit{ inches} \text{ per } \textit{hour}$$

Write these rates as fractions:

$$\frac{5 \textit{ feet}}{\textit{hour}} = \frac{? \textit{ inches}}{\textit{hour}}$$

Notice that you are given a rate with *hour* in the denominator, and the rate you are looking for also has *hour* in the denominator. Therefore, *the denominator does not have to be changed!*

But the given rate has *feet* in the numerator, and the rate you want has a different unit, *inches*, in the numerator. Therefore, *feet* must be changed.

To cancel *feet*, you must use an equivalence containing *feet*, namely, 12 *inches* = 1 *foot*. Because *feet* is in the numerator, you need a unit fraction with *feet* in the denominator. This unit fraction is $\frac{12 \textit{ inches}}{1 \textit{ foot}}$.

After the *feet* are cancelled, *inches* remain on top and *hour* remains on the bottom, and those are the units you want. Finally, do the multiplication of the numbers.

$$\frac{5 \cancel{\textit{feet}}}{\textit{hour}} \times \frac{12 \textit{ inches}}{1 \cancel{\textit{foot}}} = \frac{60 \textit{ inches}}{\textit{hour}}$$

RATIO & PROPORTION

In this problem, there are two rates.

Think of the problem this way:

$$\frac{5 \textit{ feet}}{\textit{hour}} = \frac{? \textit{ inches}}{\textit{hour}}$$

Notice that the given rate and the rate you are looking for both have the same denominator, *hour*. Therefore, the denominator does not have to be changed. But the given rate has *feet* in the numerator, and the rate you want has a different unit, *inches*, in the numerator. Therefore, the problem becomes

$$5 \textit{ feet} = x \textit{ inches}$$

and you know that

$$1 \textit{ foot} = 12 \textit{ inches}$$

So, the proportion can be written as

$$\frac{1 \textit{ ft}}{12 \textit{ in}} = \frac{5 \textit{ ft}}{x \textit{ in}}$$

Eliminate the units of measurement and cross multiply

$$\frac{1}{12} = \frac{5}{x}$$

$$(5)(12) = (1)(x)$$

Simplify

$$60 = x$$

Therefore, 5 *feet per hour* equals *60 inches per hour*.

Example 3.18

Convert 90 *feet per hour* to an equivalent rate in *feet per minute*.

DIMENSIONAL ANALYSIS

Given rate: 90 *ft/h*

Rate you want to find: ? *ft/min*

Because you are looking for a rate, you start with the given rate,

$$90 \text{ ft per h} = ? \text{ ft/min}$$

$$\frac{90 \text{ ft}}{\text{h}} = \frac{? \text{ ft}}{\text{min}}$$

Notice that you are given a rate with *ft* in the numerator, and the answer you are looking for also has *ft* in the numerator. Therefore, the numerator does not have to be changed!

But the given rate has *h* in the denominator, and the rate you want has a different unit, *min*, in the denominator. Therefore, *h* must be eliminated. Since *h* is in the denominator, you need a fraction with *h* in the numerator.

Use the equivalence 1 h = 60 min. This unit fraction is $\frac{1 \text{ h}}{60 \text{ min}}$.

$$\frac{90 \text{ ft}}{\cancel{\text{h}}} \times \frac{1 \cancel{\text{h}}}{60 \text{ min}} = \frac{? \text{ ft}}{\text{min}}$$

After the *h* is cancelled, *ft* remains on top and *min* is on the bottom, and those are the units you want. Cancel the numbers and finish the multiplication.

$$\frac{\overset{3}{\cancel{90}} \text{ ft}}{\cancel{\text{h}}} \times \frac{1 \cancel{\text{h}}}{\underset{2}{\cancel{60}} \text{ min}} = \frac{3 \text{ ft}}{2 \text{ min}} = \frac{1.5 \text{ ft}}{\text{min}}$$

SUBSTITUTION

In this problem, there are two rates. Think of the problem this way:

$$\frac{90 \text{ feet}}{1 \text{ hour}} = ? \frac{\text{ft}}{\text{min}}$$

Notice that the given rate and the rate you are looking for both have the same numerator, *feet*. Therefore, the numerator does not have to be changed. But the given rate has *hour* in the denominator, and the rate you want has a different unit, *minute*, in the denominator.

This change can be accomplished by substituting 60 minutes for 1 hour in the rate $\frac{90 \text{ ft}}{1 \text{ h}}$ as follows:

$$\frac{90 \text{ ft}}{1 \text{ h}} = \frac{90 \text{ ft}}{60 \text{ min}} = \frac{90}{60} \frac{\text{ft}}{\text{min}}$$

Because $\frac{90}{60} = 1.5$

$$\frac{90}{60} \frac{\text{ft}}{\text{min}} = 1.5 \frac{\text{ft}}{\text{min}}$$

So, *90 feet/hour* is equivalent to *1.5 feet per minute*.

Example 3.19

Convert 3 *ounces per day* to an equivalent rate measured in *ounces per week*.

DIMENSIONAL ANALYSIS

Given rate: 3 *oz/day*

Rate you want to find: ? *oz/wk*

You want to change one rate to another rate.

$$\frac{3 \text{ oz}}{\text{day}} = ? \frac{\text{oz}}{\text{wk}}$$

MULTIPLYING NUMERATOR AND DENOMINATOR OF A RATE BY THE SAME NUMBER

You want to change one rate to another rate.

$$\frac{3 \text{ oz}}{\text{day}} = ? \frac{\text{oz}}{\text{wk}}$$

(Continued)

The numerators are both in *ounces*. The denominators do not match, therefore the *day must be changed to wk*. Because *day* is in the denominator, you must use an equivalent unit fraction with *day* in the numerator. This fraction will be $\frac{7\ days}{1\ wk}$

$$\frac{3\ oz}{\cancel{day}} \times \frac{7\ \cancel{day}}{1\ wk} = \frac{21\ oz}{wk}$$

The numerators are both in *ounces*. The denominators do not match, therefore the *day must be changed to wk*. Because 7 days = 1 week, an easy way to do this example is to multiply the given rate by $\frac{7}{7}$.

$$\frac{3\ oz}{day} \times \frac{7}{7} = \frac{21\ oz}{7\ days} \text{ or } \frac{21\ oz}{wk}$$

So, *3 ounces per day* is equivalent to *21 ounces per week*.

Example 3.20

Convert *4 pints per day* to an equivalent rate measured in *quarts per day*.

DIMENSIONAL ANALYSIS

You want to change one rate to another rate.

$$\frac{4\ pt}{day} = ?\ \frac{qt}{day}$$

The denominators are both in *days*. The numerators do not match, therefore the *pt must be changed to qt*. Because *pt* is in the numerator, you must use an equivalent unit fraction with *pt* in the denominator. This fraction will be $\frac{1\ qt}{2\ pt}$

$$\frac{4\ \cancel{pt}}{day} \times \frac{1\ qt}{2\ \cancel{pt}} = \frac{2\ qt}{day}$$

RATIO & PROPORTION

You want to change one rate to another rate.

$$\frac{4\ pt}{day} = ?\ \frac{qt}{day}$$

Because the denominators are the same, you need only change 4 *pints* to *quarts*.

Think of the problem as

$$4\ pt = x\ qt$$
$$2\ pt = 1\ qt$$

Use the proportion,

$$\frac{x\ qt}{4\ pt} = \frac{1\ qt}{2\ pt}$$

Eliminate the units of measurement and cross multiply

$$\frac{x}{4} = \frac{1}{2}$$

$$(1)(4) = (x)(2)$$
$$4 = 2x$$
$$2 = x$$

So, *4 pints per day* is equivalent to *2 quarts per day*.

Complex (Multi-Step) Problems with Rates

When using Dimensional Analysis these examples involve more than one unit fraction, and when using Ratio & Proportion they require more than one proportion or other technique.

Example 3.21

Convert $10\frac{1}{2}$ *feet/hour* to an equivalent rate in *inches/minute*.

DIMENSIONAL ANALYSIS

Given rate: $10\frac{1}{2}$ *feet/hour*

Rate you want to find: ? *inches/minute*

Since you are looking for a rate, you should start with a rate.

$$10\tfrac{1}{2} \textit{ feet/hour} = ? \textit{ inches/minute}$$

Write $10\frac{1}{2}$ as the improper fraction $\frac{21}{2}$

$$\frac{21 \textit{ ft}}{2 \textit{ h}} = \frac{? \textit{ in}}{\textit{min}}$$

You want to cancel *ft*. To do this, you must use an equivalence containing *ft* on the bottom. Because you want to convert to *inches*, use the equivalence 12 *inches* = 1 *foot*, and the unit fraction will be $\frac{12 \textit{ in}}{1 \textit{ ft}}$.

$$\frac{21 \textit{ ft}}{2 \textit{ h}} \times \frac{12 \textit{ in}}{1 \textit{ ft}} = \frac{? \textit{ in}}{\textit{min}}$$

After the *ft* are cancelled, *in* is on top, which is what you want. But *h* is on the bottom and it must be cancelled. This will require a fraction with *h* in the numerator. From the equivalence 1 *hour* = 60 *minutes*, the unit fraction is $\frac{1 \textit{ h}}{60 \textit{ min}}$.

After cancelling the hours, you now have

$$\frac{21 \textit{ ft}}{2 \textit{ h}} \times \frac{12 \textit{ in}}{1 \textit{ ft}} \times \frac{1 \textit{ h}}{60 \textit{ min}} = \frac{? \textit{ in}}{\textit{min}}$$

You now have *in* on top and *min* on the bottom, so do the cancelling and multiplications of the numbers.

$$\frac{21 \textit{ ft}}{2 \textit{ h}} \times \frac{\overset{1}{\cancel{12}} \textit{ in}}{1 \textit{ ft}} \times \frac{1 \textit{ h}}{\underset{5}{\cancel{60}} \textit{ min}} = \frac{21 \textit{ in}}{10 \textit{ min}} \quad \textit{or} \quad \frac{2.1 \textit{ in}}{\textit{min}}$$

RATIO & PROPORTION

In this problem there are two rates.

$$\frac{10\frac{1}{2} \textit{ feet}}{1 \textit{ hour}} = ?\frac{\textit{inches}}{\textit{minute}}$$

Notice that the given rate and the rate you are looking for both have different numerators and different denominators. Therefore, both must be changed: $10\frac{1}{2}$ *feet* must be changed to inches, and 1 hour must be changed to minutes.

First change $10\frac{1}{2}$ *feet* to *inches*

Think of the problem as

$$10\tfrac{1}{2} \textit{ feet} = x \textit{ inches}$$
$$1 \textit{ foot} = 12 \textit{ inches}$$

Substituting into a proportion you get

$$\frac{1 \textit{ foot}}{12 \textit{ inches}} = \frac{10\frac{1}{2} \textit{ feet}}{x \textit{ inches}}$$

Eliminate the units of measurement and cross multiply

$$\frac{1}{12} = \frac{10\frac{1}{2}}{x}$$

$$(10\tfrac{1}{2})(12) = (1)(x)$$

$$126 = x$$

So, $10\frac{1}{2}$ feet equals 126 inches, and the problem becomes

$$\frac{126 \textit{ inches}}{1 \textit{ hour}} = ?\frac{\textit{inches}}{\textit{minute}}$$

Now you need to change 1 hour to minutes. You replace 1 hour by 60 minutes

$$\frac{126 \textit{ inches}}{1 \textit{ hour}} = \frac{126 \textit{ inches}}{60 \textit{ minutes}} = \frac{126}{60} \frac{\textit{inches}}{\textit{minute}}$$

but $\frac{126}{60} = 2.1$

So, $10\frac{1}{2}$ *feet/hour* is equivalent to 2.1 *inches/minute*.

Example 3.22

Write 3.2 *inches/second* in *feet/minute*.

DIMENSIONAL ANALYSIS

Given rate: 3.2 *in/sec*

Rate you want to find: ? *ft/min*

RATIO & PROPORTION

In this problem there are two rates. Think of the problem this way:

$$\frac{3.2 \textit{ in}}{1 \textit{ sec}} = ?\frac{\textit{ft}}{\textit{min}}$$

(Continued)

Since you are looking for a **rate**, you should start with a **rate**.

$$\frac{3.2\ in}{sec} = \frac{?\ ft}{min}$$

You want to cancel *in*. To do this, you must use an equivalence containing *in* on the bottom.

This fraction will be $\frac{1\ ft}{12\ in}$

$$\frac{3.2\ in}{sec} \times \frac{1\ ft}{12\ in} = \frac{?\ ft}{min}$$

Now, *ft* is on top, which is what you want. But *sec* is on the bottom and it must be cancelled. This will require a fraction with *sec* in the numerator: $\frac{60\ sec}{1\ min}$.

Now cancel and multiply the numbers.

$$\frac{3.2\ \cancel{in}}{\cancel{sec}} \times \frac{1\ ft}{\cancel{12}_{1}\ \cancel{in}} \times \frac{\cancel{60}^{5}\ \cancel{sec}}{1\ min} = \frac{16\ ft}{min}$$

Notice that the given rate and the rate you want have different numerators and different denominators. Therefore, both must be changed. The inches must be changed to feet, and the seconds must be changed to minutes.

You can change the denominator (1 *sec*) to minutes by multiplying both numerator and denominator by 60 as follows:

$$\frac{3.2\ in}{1\ sec} \times \frac{60}{60} = \frac{192\ in}{60\ sec}$$

Replace 60 seconds with 1 minute

$$\frac{192\ in}{60\ sec} = \frac{192\ in}{1\ min}$$

Now the problem becomes

$$\frac{192\ in}{1\ min} = \frac{?\ feet}{min}$$

Now, only the numerator must be changed. Change 192 inches to feet.

Think of the problem as

$$x\ feet = 192\ inches$$

$$1\ foot = 12\ inches$$

Substituting into a proportion you get

$$\frac{1\ foot}{12\ inches} = \frac{x\ feet}{192\ inches}$$

Eliminate the units of measurement and cross multiply

$$\frac{1}{12} = \frac{x}{192}$$

$$(x)(12) = (1)(192)$$

$$12x = 192$$

Divide by 12 and cancel

$$\frac{\cancel{12}\,x}{\cancel{12}} = \frac{192}{12}$$

$$x = 16$$

Therefore, *3.2 inches/second* equals *16 feet/minute*.

Example 3.23

A person drinks water at *2 qt per day*. Convert this to an equivalent rate measured in *pints per week*.

DIMENSIONAL ANALYSIS

Given rate: *2 qt/day*

Rate you want to find: *? pt/wk*

You want to change one rate to another rate.

$$\frac{2\ qt}{day} = ?\frac{pt}{wk}$$

RATIO & PROPORTION

We need to change one rate to another.

$$\frac{2\ qt}{day} = ?\frac{pt}{wk}$$

Notice that the given rate and the rate you are looking for both have the different numerators

Neither the units on the tops (*qt* and *pt*), nor those on the bottoms (*day* and *wk*) match, therefore both the *pt* and the *sec* must be changed (cancelled). Suppose you start with *qt*. Because *qt* is on the top, you must use an equivalent unit fraction with *qt* on the bottom.

This fraction will be $\frac{2\ pt}{1\ qt}$

$$\frac{2\ qt}{day} \times \frac{2\ pt}{1\ qt} = ?\frac{pt}{wk}$$

Now, *pt* is on the top, which is what you want. But *day* is on the bottom and it must be cancelled. This will require a unit fraction with *day* in the numerator. This fraction will be $\frac{7\ days}{1\ wk}$

After you cancel all the units, multiply the numbers

$$\frac{2\ qt}{day} \times \frac{2\ pt}{1\ qt} \times \frac{7\ days}{wk} = 28\ \frac{pt}{wk}$$

and different denominators. Therefore, both must be changed; 2 *quarts* must be changed to *pints*, and 1 *day* must be changed to *weeks*.

We know the equivalence: 7 *days* = 1 *week*

If you multiply the given rate by the fraction $\frac{7}{7}$, you get

$$\frac{2\ qt}{day} \times \frac{7}{7} = \frac{14\ qt}{7\ days} \quad or \quad \frac{14\ qt}{wk}$$

So the problem becomes

$$\frac{14\ qt}{wk} = ?\frac{pt}{wk}$$

Now change *14 quarts* to *pints*.

Think of the problem as

$$14\ quarts = x\ pints$$
$$1\ quarts = 2\ pints$$

Use the proportion

$$\frac{14\ qt}{x\ pt} = \frac{1\ qt}{2\ pt}$$

Eliminate the units of measurement and cross multiply

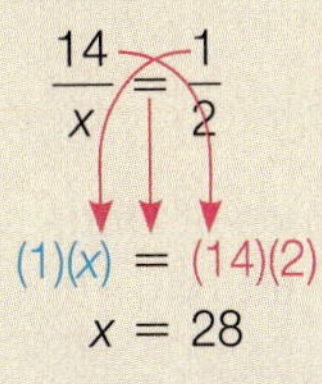

$$x = 28$$

So, *2 quarts per day* is equivalent to *28 pints per week*.

Example 3.24

A person gains *96 ounces per year*. Convert this rate to *pounds per month*.

DIMENSIONAL ANALYSIS

Given rate: 96 *oz/yr*

Rate you want to find: ? *lb/mon*

You want to change one rate to another rate.

$$\frac{96\ oz}{yr} = ?\frac{lb}{mon}$$

Neither the units on the tops (*lb* and *oz*) nor those on the bottoms (*mon* and *yr*) match, therefore both the *oz* and the *yr* must be changed (cancelled). Suppose you start with *oz*. Because *oz* is on the top, you must use an equivalent unit fraction with *oz* on the bottom. This fraction will be $\frac{16\ oz}{1\ lb}$

$$\frac{96\ oz}{yr} \times \frac{1\ lb}{16\ oz} = ?\frac{lb}{mon}$$

RATIO & PROPORTION

We need to change one rate to another:

$$\frac{96\ oz}{1\ yr} = ?\frac{lb}{mon}$$

Notice that the given rate and the rate you are looking for both have the different numerators and different denominators. Therefore, both must be changed; 96 *ounces* must be changed to *pounds*, and 1 *year* must be changed to *months*.

We know the equivalence: 12 *months* = 1 *year*

If you replace 1 year by 12 months in the given rate, the problem becomes

$$\frac{96\ oz}{12\ mon} = ?\frac{lb}{mon}$$

(Continued)

Now, *lb* is on the top, which is what you want. But *yr* is on the bottom and it must be cancelled. This will require a unit fraction with *yr* in the numerator. This fraction will be $\frac{1\ yr}{12\ mon}$

After you cancel all the units, then cancel and multiply the numbers.

$$\frac{96\ \cancel{oz}}{\cancel{yr}} \times \frac{1\ lb}{16\ \cancel{oz}} \times \frac{1\ \cancel{yr}}{12\ mon} = 0.5\frac{lb}{mon}$$

or reducing you get

$$\frac{8\ oz}{1\ mon} = ?\ \frac{lb}{mon}$$

The denominators now match, so now change *8 ounces* to *pounds*.

Think of the problem as

$$8\text{ oz} = x\ lb$$
$$16\text{ oz} = 1\ lb$$

Substituting into a proportion you get

$$\frac{8\ oz}{x\ lb} = \frac{16\ oz}{1\ lb}$$

Eliminate the units of measurement and cross multiply

$$\frac{8}{x} = \frac{16}{1}$$

$$(16)(x) = (8)(1)$$
$$x = 0.5$$

So, *96 ounces per year* is equivalent to 0.5 *pounds per month*.

Summary

In this chapter the methods of Dimensional Analysis and Ratio & Proportion were introduced.

For Dimensional Analysis:

Mathematical concepts were reinforced:

- A nonzero number divided by itself equals 1.
- A fraction equal to 1 is called a unit fraction.
- When a quantity is multiplied (or divided) by 1, the quantity is unchanged.
- Cancellation always involves a quantity in a numerator and another quantity in a denominator.

Simple (one-step) single-unit-to-single-unit problems:

- Start with the **given** single unit of measure on the left side of the = sign.
- Write the single unit of measure you want to **find** on the right side of the = sign.
- Identify an **equivalence** containing the units of measure in the problem.
- Use the equivalence to make a unit fraction with the **given** unit of measure in the **denominator.**
- Multiply by the unit fraction.
- Cancel the units of measure. The only unit of measurement remaining on the left side (in a numerator) will match the unit of measure on the right side.
- Cancel the numbers and finish the multiplication.

Simple (one-step) rate-to-rate problems:

- Start with the given rate on the left side of the equal sign.
- Write the rate you want to **find** on the right side of the equal sign.
- Identify a unit of measure that must be cancelled.
- Find an **equivalence** containing the unwanted unit of measure you want to cancel.
- Choose a unit fraction that leads to cancellation of the unwanted unit of measurement.
- Cancel the units of measurement. The only units of measurement remaining on the left side (in a numerator) will match the units of measure on the right side.
- Cancel the numbers and finish the multiplication.
- In medical dosage calculations involving rates of flow, time (in minutes or hours) will always be in the denominator.

Complex (multi-step) problems:

- Repeat the preceding steps until the only unit of measurement(s) remaining on the left side is the same as the unit of measurement(s) on the right side.

For Ratio & Proportion:

- A ratio is a comparison of two numbers.
- A ratio can be written as a fraction.
- Ratios are equal if their fractional forms are equivalent fractions.
- Order matters: a ratio of *2 to 3* is not the same as a ratio of *3 to 2*.
- A rate compares two quantities that have different units of measurement.

- Rates often have a unit of time in the denominator.
- A proportion can be written as an equation with a ratio on each side of the equal sign.
- A proportion is true if the products of cross multiplication are equal.
- Two quantities are proportional if, whenever you double one of the quantities, you double the other.
- The steps in solving a proportion are:

  1. Identify the two units of measurement in the problem.
  2. Write a known equivalence between the units of measure.
  3. Let x stand for the unit you are trying to find and write an equivalence involving x.
  4. Write a proportion using the two units of measurement.
  5. Substitute into the proportion.
  6. Eliminate the units.
  7. Cross multiply.
  8. Divide both sides of the equation by the coefficient of x (unless the coefficient is 1).
  9. Cancel and simplify if possible.
  10. Check the answer by substituting and cross multiplying.

Practice Sets

The answers to *Try These for Practice* and *Exercises* are found in Appendix A. Ask your instructor for the answers to the *Additional Exercises*.

Try These for Practice

Test your comprehension after reading the chapter.

1. How many seconds are in 6.5 *minutes*? ________
2. What is the weight in ounces of an infant who weighs 10 *pounds* 10 *ounces*?

   ____
3. How many hours are equivalent to 5,400 *seconds*?
4. Water is dripping at the rate of 12 *drops every* 15 *seconds*. Find this drip rate measured in *drops per minute*.
5. A man is losing 8 *ounces per day*. Express this rate of weight loss in *pounds per week*.

Exercises

Reinforce your understanding in class or at home.

1. $0.2\ h =$ ________ *min*
2. $1\frac{1}{2}\ yr =$ ________ *mon*
3. $2\frac{3}{4}\ days =$ ________ *h*
4. $5.25\ lb =$ ________ *oz*
5. $\frac{1}{4}\ h =$ ________ *sec*
6. $\dfrac{1\ ft}{min} = \_\_\_\_\_\_\_\_ \dfrac{in}{min}$
7. $\dfrac{1\ ft}{min} = \_\_\_\_\_\_\_\_ \dfrac{ft}{h}$
8. How many *hours* are equivalent to 720 *minutes*?
9. A faucet is running water at the rate of one-half *pint every minute*. What is this flow rate expressed in *pints per hour*?
10. A neonate weighs 4 *pounds* and 6 *ounces*. Express the weight of this baby in *ounces*.
11. What fraction of an *hour* is 900 *seconds*?
12. If 1 *quart* equals 2 *pints* and 1 *pint* equals 2 *cups*, then how many *cups* are in one and a half *quarts*?
13. How many *seconds* are in 1 *week*?

14. A child is 3 *feet* 6 *inches* tall. What is the child's height in *inches*?
15. Water leaks out of a hose at the rate of 2 *qt/min*. Find this rate of flow measured in *pt/min*.
16. Water leaks out of a hose at the rate of 2 *qt/min*. Find this rate of flow measured in *qt/h*.
17. Water leaks out of a hose at the rate of 2 *qt/min*. Find this rate of flow in *pt/h*.
18. 15 ft/h = ? in/min
19. 12 oz/day = ? lb/wk
20. If 2 *t* of a drug are administered *q4h*, how many *tablespoons* are administered *per day*?

Additional Exercises

Now, test yourself!

1. 0.25 *hours* = __________ *minutes*
2. $5\frac{1}{4}$ *years* = __________ *months*
3. $2\frac{1}{3}$ *days* = __________ *hours*
4. 2.5 *lb* = __________ *oz*
5. $\frac{3}{4}h$ = __________ *min*
6. 18 *mon* = __________ *yr*
7. 36 *in* = __________ *ft*
8. 40 *oz* = __________ *lb*
9. An infant weighs 6 *pounds* 5 *ounces* at birth. What is the weight in *ounces*? __________.
10. The diameter of a human hair is 0.075 *millimeter*. If 1 *millimeter* equals 1,000 *micrometers* (also called microns), and 1 *micron* equals 1,000 *nanometers*, then how many *nanometers* equal the diameter of a human hair? __________
11. What fraction of an *hour* is 1,350 *seconds*? __________
12. What is the height in *inches* of a person who is 6 *feet* 2 *inches* tall? __________
13. Write 604,800 *seconds* as an equivalent amount of time in *weeks*. __________
14. If a person is 70 *inches* tall, express this *height* in *feet* and *inches*.
15. 4 pt/min = ? qt/min
16. 2 pt/min = ? pt/h
17. 0.2 pt/min = ? qt/h
18. 2 in/min = ? ft/h
19. 2 oz/day = ? lb/wk
20. 0.02 *inches per second* is equivalent to how many *feet per hour*?

Unit 2

Systems of Measurement

Chapter 4
The Household and Metric Systems

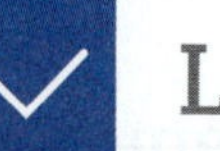

Learning Outcomes

After completing this chapter, you will be able to

4.1 Identify the units of measurement in the household and metric systems.

4.2 Recognize the abbreviations for the units of measurement in the two systems.

4.3 State the equivalents for the units of volume.

4.4 State the equivalents for the units of weight.

4.5 State the equivalents for the units of length.

4.6 Convert from one unit to another within each of the two systems.

Historically, the United States has used three different systems to measure drugs: the apothecary, household, and metric systems.

The **apothecary** system is the oldest of the three systems, and it is difficult to use. Because its use led to many medication errors, The Joint Commission, FDA, and ISMP have suggested that it be discontinued. Package inserts and other drug references no longer use the apothecary system for recommended medication dosages. Therefore, the apothecary system is not included in this chapter.

The **household** system was originally designed so that medication dosages could be measured at home using ordinary kitchen utensils. However, because the capacity of kitchen teaspoons and tablespoons is not standardized, using them may result in dosing errors. In 2014 the National Council for Prescription Drug Programs (NCPDP) recommended that dosages prescribed in teaspoons and tablespoons "may encourage the use of non-calibrated household spoons for dosing medications" and that "milliliters should be the standard unit of measure used on prescription container labels for oral medications."* So, while the household system is still in use, like the apothecary system, it may also be on the way out!

Only devices calibrated in household units (e.g., droppers and medication cups) should be used to administer medications prescribed in household units of measurement.

The **metric** system is the most logically organized and easiest to use of all the systems of measurement. It was first adopted by France a few years after the French revolution of 1789. It is also referred to as the *International System of Units*. It can be abbreviated as SI, which are the first two initials of its French name, *Système International d'Unités*. The metric system will eventually replace all other systems of measurement used in health care.

In this chapter you are introduced to the household and metric systems.

*National Council for Prescription Drug Programs (NCPDP).

The Household System

Liquid Volume in the Household System

Occasionally, household measurements are used when prescribing liquid medication. Table 4.1 lists equivalent values, with their abbreviations, for units of liquid measurement in the household system.

Table 4.1 Household Equivalents of Liquid Volume.

1 quart (*qt*) = 2 pints (*pt*)
1 pint (*pt*) = 2 measuring cups
1 measuring cup = 8 ounces (*oz*)
1 ounce (*oz*) = 2 tablespoons (T)
1 tablespoon (T) = 3 teaspoons (t)

ALERT

Using ordinary tableware to measure medications may constitute a safety risk because ordinary tableware does not come in standard sizes. Therefore, clients and their families should be advised to use the measuring device provided with the medication rather than the kitchen tablespoon, for example.

NOTE

The unit *ounce*, which is used to measure liquid volumes, is sometimes referred to as *fluid ounce* (*fl oz*).

You can use dimensional analysis or ratio & proportion to convert from one unit of measurement to an equivalent unit of measurement within the household system the same way you converted units of measurement in Chapter 3. The following examples show both methods of converting units of measurement within the household system.

Example 4.1

In preparation for a colonoscopy the prescriber writes the following order: *polyethylene glycol (MiraLAX) 17g PO daily for 3 days*. The label states "Stir and dissolve one 17*g* packet in 4 ounces of any beverage and drink." How many cups of the polyethylene glycol solution will the client drink over the 3 days?

The daily dose (17 *g*) is contained in approximately 4 ounces of solution. So, each day the client must drink 4 ounces for a total of 12 ounces over the 3 days. You need to change the 12 ounces to cups.

DIMENSIONAL ANALYSIS

$$12\ oz = ?\ cups$$

You want to cancel the *ounces* and get the answer in *cups*. You need a unit fraction in the form of $\frac{?\ cups}{?\ oz}$

Because 1 *cup* = 8 *ounces*, the unit fraction is $\frac{1\ cup}{8\ oz}$

$$\frac{12\ \cancel{oz}}{1} \times \frac{1\ cup}{8\ \cancel{oz}} = 1\frac{1}{2}\ cups$$

RATIO & PROPORTION

Think of the problem this way:

8 *ounces* = 1 *cup* [known equivalent]
12 *ounces* = *x cups* [what we are looking for]

One way to set up the proportion is

$$\frac{8\ oz}{1\ cup} = \frac{12\ oz}{x\ cup}$$

Eliminate the units of measurement

$$\frac{8}{1} = \frac{12}{x}$$

Cross multiply

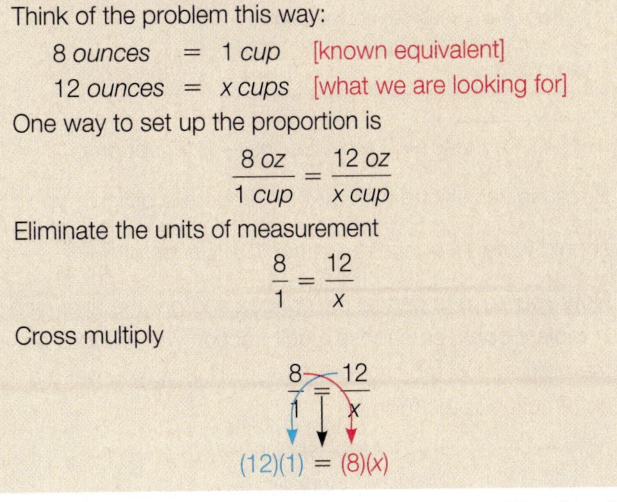

$$(12)(1) = (8)(x)$$

(Continued)

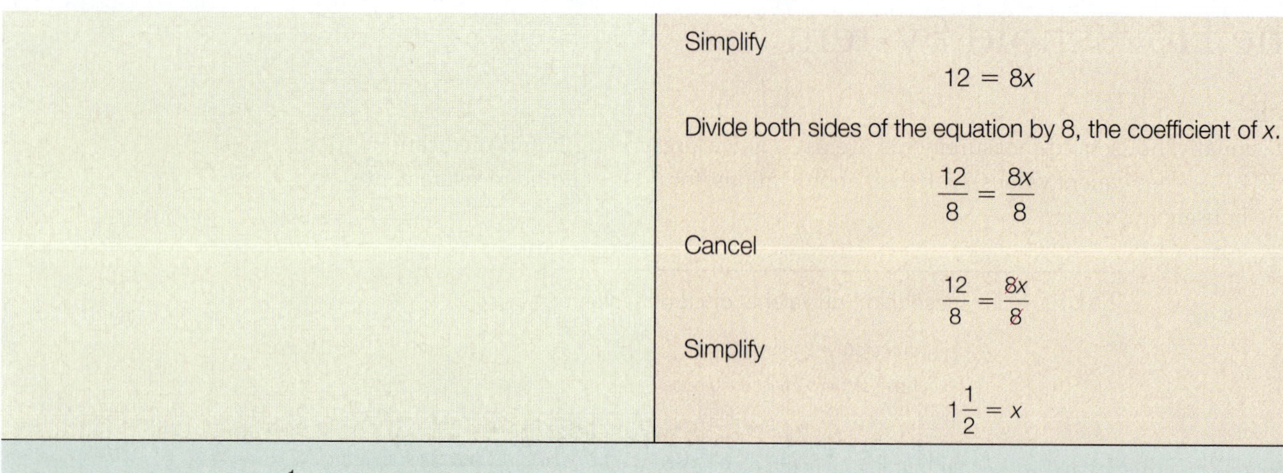

Simplify

$$12 = 8x$$

Divide both sides of the equation by 8, the coefficient of x.

$$\frac{12}{8} = \frac{8x}{8}$$

Cancel

$$\frac{12}{8} = \frac{\cancel{8}x}{\cancel{8}}$$

Simplify

$$1\frac{1}{2} = x$$

So, the client will drink $1\frac{1}{2}$ cups of the solution.

NOTE

In the household system for quantities less than 1, either decimal numbers or fractions may be used. However, fractions are preferred. For example, $\frac{1}{2}$ *qt* is preferred over 0.5 *qt*.

Example 4.2

A client needs to drink $1\frac{1}{2}$ *ounces* of an elixir per day. How many teaspoons would be equivalent to this dosage?

DIMENSIONAL ANALYSIS

$$1\tfrac{1}{2}\ ounces = ?\ teaspoons$$

If you do not know a direct equivalence between *ounces* and *teaspoons*, then this will be a complex (multistep) problem, which requires first changing *ounces* to *tablespoons* and then changing *tablespoons* to *teaspoons*.

NOTE

Teaspoon is sometimes abbreviated as *tsp*, and tablespoon is sometimes abbreviated as *tbs*.

$$1\tfrac{1}{2}\ ounces \rightarrow ?\ tablespoons \rightarrow ?\ teaspoons$$

Because calculating with mixed numbers is difficult, you should write $1\frac{1}{2}$ *ounces* as either 1.5 *ounces* or $\frac{3\ ounces}{2}$

Now you want to cancel the *ounces* and get the answer in *tablespoons*, so choose a unit fraction with *ounces* on the bottom and *tablespoons* on top. That is, you need a unit fraction in the form of

$$\frac{?\ tablespoons}{?\ ounces}$$

RATIO & PROPORTION

In this problem, there are two quantities: *ounces* and *teaspoons*.

Because you may not know the direct equivalence between ounces and teaspoons, you will first change $1\frac{1}{2}$ ounces to an equivalent number of tablespoons, and then change the resulting tablespoons to teaspoons. This problem, then, requires two steps.

Step 1 *Change $1\frac{1}{2}$ ounces to tablespoons*

1 ounce = 2 tablespoons [known equivalence]

$1\frac{1}{2}$ ounces = x tablespoons

One way to set up the proportion is

$$\frac{1\ oz}{2\ T} = \frac{1\frac{1}{2}\ oz}{x\ T}$$

Eliminate the units of measurement

$$\frac{1}{2} = \frac{1\frac{1}{2}}{x}$$

Because 1 *ounce* = 2 *tablespoons*, the fraction you need is $\frac{2\ tablespoons}{1\ ounce}$

Cancel the *ounces*

$$\frac{3\ \cancel{ounces}}{2} \times \frac{2\ tablespoons}{1\ \cancel{ounce}} = ?\ teaspoons$$

After cancelling the *ounces* as shown, only *tablespoons* remain in the numerator on the left side. But you want the answer to be in *teaspoons*, so you must cancel the *tablespoons*. This requires a second unit fraction with *tablespoons* in the denominator. The fraction is $\frac{3\ teaspoons}{1\ tablespoon}$

$$\frac{3\ \cancel{oz}}{2} \times \frac{2\ \cancel{T}}{1\ \cancel{oz}} \times \frac{3\ t}{1\ \cancel{T}} = ?\ t$$

After cancelling the *tablespoons* as shown below, only *teaspoons* remain in the numerator on the left side. *Teaspoons* is the unit you want on the left side, so now focus on the numbers. Cancel the twos and multiply as shown below:

$$\frac{3\ \cancel{oz}}{\cancel{2}} \times \frac{\cancel{2}\ \cancel{T}}{1\ \cancel{oz}} \times \frac{3\ t}{1\ \cancel{T}} = 9\ t$$

Cross multiply

$$\frac{1}{2} = \frac{1\frac{1}{2}}{x}$$

$$(1\tfrac{1}{2})(2) = (1)(x)$$

$$3 = x$$

So, $1\frac{1}{2}$ oz is equivalent to 3 tablespoons.

Step 2 *Change 3 tablespoons to teaspoons*

1 tablespoon = 3 teaspoons [known equivalence]

3 tablespoons = *x* teaspoons

One way to set up the proportion is

$$\frac{3\ t}{1\ T} = \frac{x\ t}{3\ T}$$

Eliminate the units of measurement

$$\frac{3}{1} = \frac{x}{3}$$

Cross multiply

$$\frac{3}{1} = \frac{x}{3}$$

$$x = 9$$

So, $1\frac{1}{2}$ oz is equivalent to 9 teaspoons.

Weight in the Household System

The only units of weight used in the household system of medication administration are ounces (*oz*) and pounds (*lb*), as shown in Table 4.2.

Table 4.2 Household Equivalents of Weight.

1 pound (*lb*) = 16 *ounces* (*oz*)

NOTE

Ounces used for weight should not be confused with ounces used for volume. However, one fluid ounce of water weighs one ounce.

Recall that the above equivalence was stated in Chapter 3.

Example 4.3

An infant weighs 5 *lb* 8 *oz*. What is the weight of the infant in ounces?

Remember that 5 *lb* 8 *oz* means 5 *lb* + 8 *oz*.

DIMENSIONAL ANALYSIS

First change the 5 *lb* to ounces

$$5\ lb = ?\ oz$$

Cancel the pounds and obtain the equivalent amount in ounces

$$5\ lb \times \frac{?\ oz}{?\ lb} = ?\ oz$$

RATIO & PROPORTION

First change the 5 *lb* to ounces. Think:

16 *ounces* = 1 pound [known equivalence]

x ounces = 5 pounds

One way to set up the proportion is

$$\frac{16\ oz}{1\ lb} = \frac{x\ oz}{5\ lb}$$

(Continued)

Because 16 *oz* = 1 *lb*, the unit fraction is $\frac{16\ oz}{1\ lb}$

$$5\ lb \times \frac{16\ oz}{1\ lb} = 80\ oz$$

Eliminate the units of measurement and cross multiply

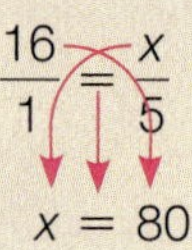

$x = 80$

Now add the extra 8 ounces 80 *oz* + 8 *oz* = 88 *oz*
So, the 5 *lb* 8 *oz* infant weighs 88 *oz*.

Length in the Household System

The only units of length used in the household system for medication administration are feet (*ft*) and inches (*in*), as shown in Table 4.3.

Table 4.3 Household Equivalents for Length.

1 *foot (ft)* = 12 *inches (in)*

Recall that the above equivalence was stated in Chapter 3.

Example 4.4

A child is 3 *ft* 2 in tall. Find the child's height in inches.

Remember that 3 *ft* 2 *in* means 3 *ft* + 2 *in*.

DIMENSIONAL ANALYSIS

First, change the 3 feet to inches.

3 *feet* = ? *inches*

You want to cancel the *feet* and get the answer in *inches*, so choose a fraction with *feet* on the bottom and *inches* on top. You need a unit fraction in the form of $\frac{?\ inches}{?\ feet}$

Because 1 *foot* = 12 *inches*, the fraction you need is $\frac{12\ inches}{1\ foot}$

$$\frac{3\ feet}{1} \times \frac{12\ inches}{1\ foot} = 36\ inches$$

RATIO & PROPORTION

First, change the 3 feet to inches.
Think of the problem this way:

1 *ft* = 12 *in* [known equivalent]
3 *ft* = *x in*

One way to set up the proportion is

$$\frac{1\ ft}{12\ in} = \frac{3\ ft}{x\ in}$$

Eliminate the units of measurement

$$\frac{1}{12} = \frac{3}{x}$$

Cross multiply

$$\frac{1}{12} = \frac{3}{x}$$

$$(12)(3) = (1)(x)$$

Simplify

$$36 = x$$

So, 3 *feet* is equivalent to 36 *inches*. Now add the extra 2 *inches* 36 *in* + 2 *in* = 38 *inches*
So, the 3 *feet* 2 *inches* child is 38 *inches* tall.

Decimal-Based Systems

As seen in Chapter 1, our *place-value number system* is a *decimal* system, that is, it is based on the number 10. The *U.S. monetary system* and the *metric system* are also decimal systems.

The *U.S. monetary system* uses the dollar as its fundamental unit. All other denominations are decimal multiples or fractions of the dollar.

hundred-dollar bill	ten-dollar bill	dollar bill	dime	penny

An amount of money measured in one denomination can be easily converted to another denomination by merely moving the decimal point the appropriate number of places.

For example, to convert *60 dimes* to *pennies*, see in the chart that *dime* to *penny* is one jump to the *right*.

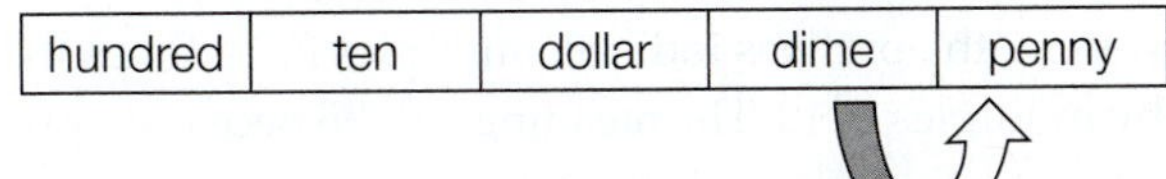

So, move the decimal point in 60 dimes one place to the *right* as follows:

60 dimes = 60.0 dimes = 6 0 0 . pennies, or 600 pennies

To convert *80 dollars* to *ten dollar bills*, see in the chart that *dollar* to *ten* is one jump to the *left*.

hundred	ten	dollar	dime	penny

So, move the decimal point in 80 dollars one place to the *left*, as follows:

80 dollars = 80. dollars = 8 . 0 tens = 8 tens

To convert 4 *hundred-dollar bills* to *dimes*, see in the chart that *hundred* to *dime* is a jump of 3 *places to the right*.

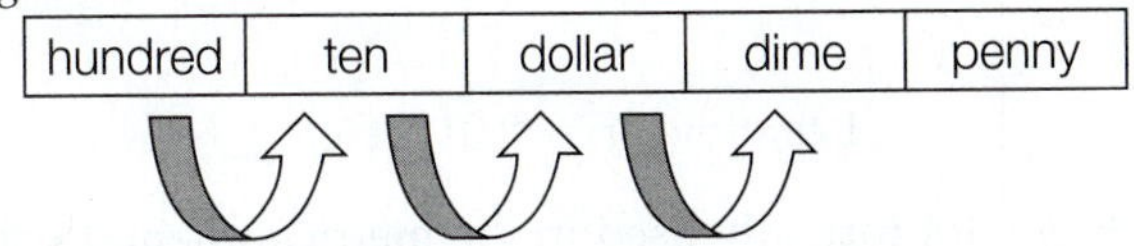

So, move the decimal point in 4 hundreds 3 *places to the right*.

4 hundreds = 4.000 hundreds = 4 0 0 0 . dimes or 4,000 dimes.

The Metric System

The metric system is the most widely used general system of measurement in the world today, with the United States being the only exception among developed countries. However, in all countries, the metric system is the preferred system for prescribing medications.

Because the *metric system* is based on 10, converting quantities in this system can also be accomplished by merely shifting the decimal point. The simplicity of its decimal basis has encouraged the proliferation of the metric system.

At the heart of the *metric* system are the *fundamental* or *base units*. The **base units** needed for medical dosages are *gram (g)*, *liter (L)*, and *meter (m)*; these base units are used to measure weight, liquid volume, and length, respectively.

Decimal multiples of any of the base units are obtained by appending standard *metric prefixes* to the base unit. Table 4.4 shows both the base units and their **metric prefixes** with their abbreviations. Note that only the prefixes in blue are used in dosage calculation.

Table 4.4 Format of the Metric System.

Name	kilo	hecto	deka	BASE UNIT	deci	centi	milli	*	*	micro
Abbreviation	k	h	da	g, L, m	d	c	m	*	*	mc
Multiple of the Base	1,000	100	10	1	0.1	0.01	0.001	*	*	0.000001

NOTE

To help remember the important metric prefixes, various mnemonics may be employed. Two are: King Henry Doesn't Usually Drink Cold Malted Milk, or Kids Hate Drudgery Until Dawn Calculating Many Metrics (kilo, hecto, deka, unit, deci, centi, milli, micro).

In the metric system, the prefixes indicate multiples of 10 times the base unit, or the base unit divided by multiples of 10. The meanings of the necessary prefixes are found in Table 4.5.

NOTE

Depending on the country, spellings may be *meter/metre, liter/litre, or deca/deka*.

Table 4.5 Metric Prefixes Used in Health Care.

Metric Prefixes			
kilo	means	one thousand	(1,000 times the base)
deci	means	one tenth	(0.1 times the base)
centi	means	one hundredth	(0.01 times the base)
milli	means	one thousandth	(0.001 times the base)
micro	means	one millionth	(0.000001 times the base)

The metric prefixes are appended to the base units. For example,

1 kilogram = 1,000 grams

and

1 centimeter = 0.01 meter.

Fractions, such as $\frac{1}{2}$, are not formally used in the metric system. Decimal numbers are preferred, for example, $3\frac{1}{2}$ grams is written as 3.5 grams.

Liquid Volume in the Metric System

Drugs in liquid form are measured by volume. The volume of a liquid is the amount of space it occupies. In dosage calculations for liquid volumes only, *liters* and *milliliters* are used (see Table 4.6).

Table 4.6 Metric Equivalents of Liquid Volume.

1 cubic centimeter (*cc* or cm^3) = 1 milliliter (*mL*)
1,000 milliliters (*mL*) = 1 liter (*L*)

Milliliters are used for smaller amounts of fluids. The prefix *milli-* means $\frac{1}{1,000}$, so

$$1 \text{ liter } (L) = 1{,}000 \text{ milliliters } (mL)$$

Milliliters are equivalent to *cubic centimeters* (cm^3 or *cc*), so

$$1\ mL = 1\ cm^3 = 1 \text{ cc}$$

ALERT

The abbreviation *mL* should be used instead of the abbreviation *cc* because "c" may be confused with "u" (units) or "cc" with "00" (double zero).

You must be able to convert from one unit of measurement to another within the metric system. With liquids in the metric system you need to make conversions only between *liters* and *milliliters*. Of course, you could make such conversions by using *dimensional analysis* or *ratio and proportion*. However, conversions involving metric-system units can be done by merely *moving the decimal point*. The metric system for liquid volume has the following format, but only the units in blue are used to calculate liquid volumes. *Liters (L)* and *milliliters (mL)* are the only metric units for liquid volume used in this textbook. An IV bag may contain *1 liter* of a saline solution, and a syringe may contain *5.3 mL* of a drug.

NOTE

Deciliters (*dL*) may be encountered in lab reports. However, deciliters are not used in calculating medical dosages.

kilo	hecto	deka	Base Unit	deci	centi	milli
kL	*hL*	*daL*	*L*	*dL*	*cL*	*mL*

3 jumps

Because *liters* and *milliliters* are 3 places apart, conversions between them will require a movement of three decimal places. In Example 4.5, two of the three methods are compared.

In the remaining examples of this chapter, the methods of solution shown alternate between *Dimensional Analysis* and *Ratio & Proportion*. The method of *Moving the Decimal Point* is also shown for each example.

NOTE

In Example 4.5 when converting 0.5 *L* to 500 *mL*, the unit of measurement got smaller, whereas the number got larger.

Example 4.5

If the prescriber ordered *0.5 L of 5% dextrose in water*, how many milliliters were ordered?

RATIO & PROPORTION

In this problem there are two quantities: *liters* and *milliliters*. Think of the problem like this:

$$1\ L = 1{,}000\ mL \text{ [known equivalence]}$$
$$0.5\ L = x\ mL$$

One way to set up the proportion is

$$\frac{1\ L}{1{,}000\ mL} = \frac{0.5\ L}{x\ mL}$$

Eliminate the units of measurement and cross multiply

$$\frac{1}{1{,}000} = \frac{0.5}{x}$$

$$500 = x$$

MOVING THE DECIMAL POINT

Base Unit	deci	centi	milli
L	*dL*	*cL*	*mL*

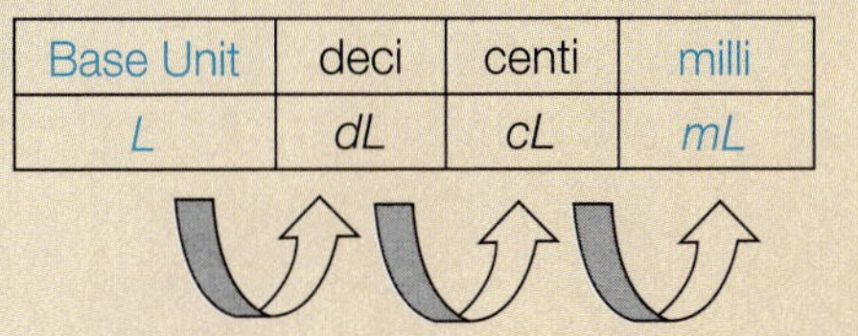

For this example, to convert *liters* to *milliliters* is a jump of *3 places to the right*, so, in the quantity 0.5 L, move the decimal point *3 places to the right*, as follows:

$$0.5\ L = 0.500\ L = 0\,5\,0\,0.\ mL = 500.\ mL = 500\ mL.$$

ALERT

Write 0.5 *L* instead of $\frac{5}{10}L$ or $\frac{1}{2}L$ because in the metric system, quantities are written as decimal numbers instead of fractions.

So, the prescriber ordered 500 milliliters of 5% dextrose in water.

Example 4.6

The client is to receive *1,750 milliliters of 0.9% NaCl IV q12h.* What is this volume in liters?

DIMENSIONAL ANALYSIS

$$1{,}750\ mL = ?\ L$$

Cancel the milliliters and obtain the equivalent amount in liters.

$$\frac{1{,}750\ mL}{1} \times \frac{?\ L}{?\ mL} = ?\ L$$

Because 1,000 *mL* = 1 *L*, the unit fraction you want is $\frac{1\ L}{1{,}000\ mL}$

$$\frac{1{,}750\ \cancel{mL}}{1} \times \frac{1\ L}{1{,}000\ \cancel{mL}} = \frac{1{,}750\ L}{1{,}000} = 1.75\ L$$

MOVING THE DECIMAL POINT

For this example, to convert *milliliters* to *liters* is a jump of *3 places to the left*.

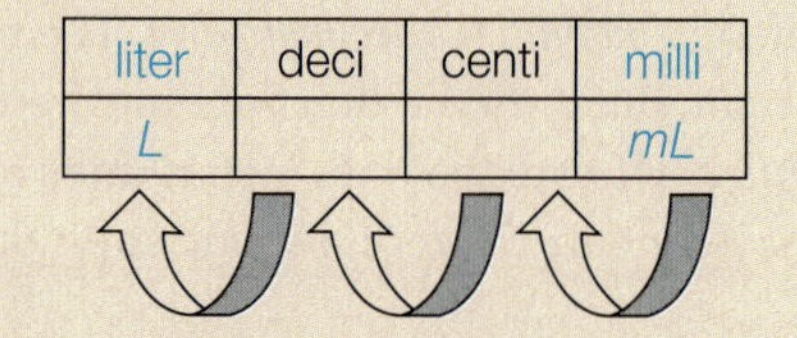

So, in 1,750 mL move the decimal point *3 places to the left* as follows:

1,750 *mL* = 1,750. *mL* = 1 . 7 5 0 *L* = 1.750 *L* = 1.75 *L*

So, 1,750 *mL* of 0.9% NaCl is the same amount as 1.75 *L* of 0.9% NaCl.

NOTE

When converting 1,750 *mL* to 1.75 *L*, notice that the units of measurement get larger (*mL* to *L*) while the numbers get smaller (1,750 to 1.75).

Weight in the Metric System

Drugs in dry form are generally measured by weight. In dosage calculations, *kilograms, grams, milligrams*, and *micrograms* (written in order of size) are used to measure weight. *Kilograms* are the largest of these units of measurement, and *micrograms* are the smallest (see Table 4.7).

Table 4.7 Metric Equivalents of Weight.

1 kilogram (*kg*) = 1,000 grams (*g*)
1 gram (*g*) = 1,000 milligrams (*mg*)
1 milligram (*mg*) = 1,000 micrograms (*mcg*)

Kilograms are used for the weight of clients. The prefix *kilo-* means 1,000, so

1 kilogram (*kg*) = 1,000 *grams* (*g*)

Milligrams are used for measuring the weight of drugs, and *micrograms* are used for very small weights of drugs.

The prefix *milli-* means $\frac{1}{1{,}000}$, and *micro-* means $\frac{1}{1{,}000{,}000}$, so

1 gram (*g*) = 1,000 milligrams (*mg*)

1 milligram (*mg*) = 1,000 micrograms (*mcg*)

ALERT

The abbreviation for microgram, *mcg*, is preferred instead of the formerly used abbreviation µ*g* because µ*g* may be mistaken for the abbreviation for milligram, *mg*. This error would result in a dose that would be 1,000 times greater than the prescribed dose.

The metric system for weight (grams) features the following format. Only the units in blue are needed for dosage calculations involving weight:

kilo	hecto	deka	Base Unit	deci	centi	milli	*	*	micro
kg	*hg*	*dag*	*gram (g)*	*dg*	*cg*	*mg*			*mcg*

For weight, the only units needed for medical dosage calculations are *kilogram (kg), gram (g), milligram (mg),* and *microgram (mcg).* Because these units are all 3 places apart, the jumps between them will always be 3 jumps. The following shortened version of the metric weight chart will be useful in the next few examples:

kilogram	gram	milligram	micro-gram
kg	*g*	*mg*	*mcg*

3 jumps   3 jumps   3 jumps

Example 4.7

The order reads *125 mcg of Lanoxin (digoxin) PO daily.* How many milligrams of this cardiac medication would you administer to the client?

RATIO & PROPORTION

Think of the problem like this:

1,000 *mcg* = 1 *mg* [known equivalence]
125 *mcg* = *x mg*

One way to set up the proportion is

$$\frac{1{,}000\ mcg}{1\ mg} = \frac{125\ mcg}{x\ mg}$$

Eliminate the units of measurement and cross multiply

$$\frac{1{,}000}{1} = \frac{125}{x}$$

$$125 = 1{,}000\,x$$

Divide both sides by 1,000

$$\frac{125}{1{,}000} = \frac{1{,}000\,x}{1{,}000}$$

$$0.125 = x$$

MOVING THE DECIMAL POINT

In this problem, you convert from *mcg* to *mg*. The movement from *mcg* to *mg* in the following chart is a movement of one column to the left.

Therefore, the conversion is accomplished by moving the decimal point 3 places to the left.

Kilo-	Fundamental Unit	Milli-	Micro-
kilogram (*kg*)	**gram** (*g*)	**milli**gram (*mg*)	**micro**gram (*mcg*)

125 *mcg* = 125. *mcg* = .1 2 5 *mg*

= .125 *mg* = 0.125 *mg*

So, 125 *mcg* is the same amount as 0.125 *mg*, and you would administer 0.125 *mg* of digoxin.

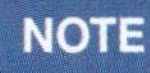

NOTE

A dose is always expressed in the form of a number and a unit of measure. Both are important. For example:
150 *mcg*, 2.5 *mg*, 3 tablets, 1.5 *mL*, 0.5 *L*.
When you write your answer, be sure to include the appropriate unit of measurement.

Example 4.8

The order reads *Glucotrol (glipizide) 15 mg PO daily ac breakfast.* How many grams of this hypoglycemic agent would you administer?

DIMENSIONAL ANALYSIS

$$15\ mg = ?\ g$$

Cancel the milligrams and obtain the equivalent amount in grams.

$$15\ mg \times \frac{?\ g}{?\ mg} = ?\ g$$

$$15\ \cancel{mg} \times \frac{1\ g}{1{,}000\ \cancel{mg}} = \frac{15}{1{,}000}g$$

$$\frac{15}{1{,}000}g = 0.015\ g$$

MOVING THE DECIMAL POINT

In this problem, you convert from *mg* to *g*. The movement from *mg* to *g* in the following chart is a movement of one column to the left. Therefore, the conversion is accomplished by moving the decimal point 3 places to the left.

Kilo-	Fundamental Unit	Milli-	Micro-
kilogram (*kg*)	**gram** (*g*)	**milli**gram (*mg*)	**micro**gram (*mcg*)

$$15\ mg = 15.\ mg = .0\,1\,5\ g$$

$$= .015\ g = 0.015\ g$$

So, 15 *mg* is the same amount as 0.015 *g*, and you would administer 0.015 *g* of Glucotrol.

Example 4.9

An infant weighs 4.5 kilograms. Convert this weight to grams.

RATIO & PROPORTION

Think of the problem like this:

$1\ kg = 1{,}000\ g$ [known equivalence]

$4.5\ kg = x\ g$

One way to set up the proportion is

$$\frac{1\ kg}{1{,}000\ g} = \frac{4.5\ kg}{x\ g}$$

Eliminate the units of measurement and cross multiply

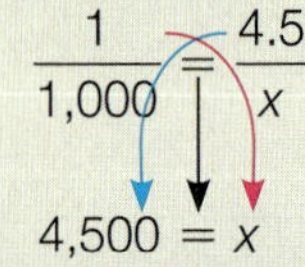

$$\frac{1}{1{,}000} = \frac{4.5}{x}$$

$$4{,}500 = x$$

MOVING THE DECIMAL POINT

To convert *kg* to *g*, jump *3 places to the right*.

kilogram	gram	milligram	microgram
kg	*g*	*mg*	*mcg*

Move the decimal point *3 places to the right*.

$$4.5\ kg = 4.500\ kg = 4\,5\,0\,0.\ g = 4{,}500\ g$$

So, 4.5 kilograms is equivalent to 4,500 grams.

Length in the Metric System

The metric system for meters has the following format, but only the units in blue are used in measuring lengths.

Centimeters (cm) and *millimeters (mm)* are the only metric units of length used in this textbook. A client's height might be measured in *centimeters*, and the diameter of a tumor might be measured in *centimeters* or *millimeters*.

kilo	hecto	deka	Base Unit	deci	centi	milli
km	*hm*	dam	meter(*m*)	*dm*	*cm*	*mm*

1 jump

Because *centimeters* and *millimeters* are adjacent units, conversion between them will require a movement of one decimal place. See Table 4.8.

Table 4.8 Metric Equivalents of Length.

1 centimeter (*cm*) = 10 millimeters (mm)

NOTE

In metric conversions of liquid volumes and weights, the decimal point is always moved 3 places. However, in metric conversions of length (*cm* and *mm*), the decimal point is moved only one place.

Example 4.10

A wound has a length of 0.7 centimeters. What is the length of this wound in millimeters?

DIMENSIONAL ANALYSIS

0.7 *centimeters* = ? *millimeters*

You want to cancel the *centimeters* and get the answer in *millimeters*, so choose a unit fraction with *centimeters* on the bottom and *millimeters* on top. You need a fraction in the form of $\frac{?\ mm}{?\ cm}$

Because 1 *centimeter* = 10 *millimeters*, the fraction you need is $\frac{10\ mm}{1\ cm}$

$$\frac{0.7\ \cancel{cm}}{1} \times \frac{10\ mm}{1\ \cancel{cm}} = 7\ mm$$

MOVING THE DECIMAL POINT

To convert *centimeters* to *millimeters*, jump *1 place to the right*.

meter	decimeter	centimeter	millimeter
m	dm	cm	mm

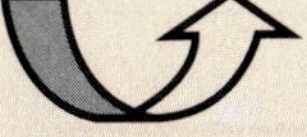

So, in *0.7 cm* move the decimal point *1 place to the right*.

0.7 *cm* = 0 7 . *mm* = 7. *mm* = 7 *mm*

So, the wound has a length of 7 millimeters.

Example 4.11

A baby's wet diaper weighs 41 grams. Estimate the volume of urine in the wet diaper if a dry diaper weighs 30 grams.

To find the weight of urine in the diaper, subtract the weight of the dry diaper from the weight of the wet diaper as follows: $41\ g - 30\ g = 11\ g$

Because 1 gram of urine has a volume of 1 milliliter, 11 grams of urine has a volume of 11 milliliters.

So, the volume of urine in the diaper is 11 *mL*.

NOTE

The basic metric units of meter, liter, and gram have the following relationship: 1 cubic centimeter of water has a volume of 1 milliliter and weighs 1 gram.

Summary

In this chapter, the household and metric systems of measurement were introduced.

- The metric system is the dominant system used in health care.
- The apothecary system is being phased out.
- It is important to memorize the equivalences between the various units of measurement of the household and metric systems.
- It is important to memorize the abbreviations for the various units of measurement.
- To convert units of measure in the household system, use dimensional analysis or ratio & proportion.
- To convert units of measure in the metric system, use dimensional analysis, ratio & proportion, or the shortcut method of moving the decimal point. Always jump 3 places except for *cm-mm* conversions, which use a one-place jump.
- Remember, each jump is 3 places in this chart:

kilogram	gram	milligram	microgram
kg	*g, L*	*mg, mL*	*mcg*

- Abbreviations for units of measurement are not followed by periods.
  Example: *40 mg* and *5 t* (not 40 *mg*. and 5 t.).
- Abbreviations for units of measurement are not made plural by adding the letter *s*.
  Example: *70 mcg* and *3 oz* (not 70 *mcg*s and 3 *ozs*).
- Insert a leading zero for decimal numbers less than 1.
  Example: *0.05 g* and *0.34 mL* (not .05 *g* and .34 *mL*).
- Omit trailing zeros for decimal numbers.
  Example: *7.3 mL* and *0.07 g* (not 7.30 *mL* and 0.070 *g*).
- Numbers greater than 999 need commas.
  Example: *2,500 mL* and *20,000 mcg* (not 2500 *mL* and 20000 *mcg*).
- Leave space between the number and the unit of measurement.
  Example: *60 mL* and *100 g* (not 60*mL* and 100*g*).
- Avoid the use of fractions with metric units of measurement.
  Example: *0.5 mL* and *1.5 g* (not $\frac{1}{2}$ *mL* and $1\frac{1}{2}$ *g*).

Practice Sets

The answers to *Try These for Practice*, *Exercises*, and *Cumulative Review Exercises* are found in Appendix A. Ask your instructor for the answers to the *Additional Exercises*.

Try These for Practice

Test your comprehension after reading the chapter.

1. You need to memorize all the metric and household equivalents. To test yourself, fill in the missing numbers in the following chart.

Metric System

(a) 1 *L* = ________ *mL*

(b) 1 *mL* = ________ *cc*

(c) 1 *L* = ________ cm^3

(d) 1 *kg* = ________ *g*

(e) 1 *g* = ________ *mg*

(f) 1 *mg* = ________ *mcg*

(g) 1 *cm* = ________ *mm*

Household System

(h) 1 *qt* = ________ *pt*

(i) 1 *pt* = ________ *cups*

(j) 1 *measuring cup* = ________ *oz*

(k) 1 *oz* = ________ *T*

(l) 1 *T* = ________ *t*

(m) 1 *ft* = ________ *in*

(n) 1 *lb* = ________ *oz*

2. How many *micrograms* of a drug are contained in one 15-*milligram* tablet of the drug?
3. Avonex (interferon beta-1a) is a drug used to treat multiple sclerosis (MS). A client is to receive a 30 *mcg* injection of this drug once a week. How many *milligrams* of Avonex will the client receive in one week?
4. A client with HIV is to receive *nelfinavir mesylate* (Viracept) *750 mg PO t.i.d.* How many grams of this protease inhibitor will the client receive in 4 days?
5. A man drinks *one cup* of water q6h. At this rate how many ounces of water will he drink in 3 days?

Exercises

Reinforce your understanding in class or at home.

1. 56 *mg* = ________ *mcg*
2. 600 *mg* = ________ *g*
3. 16 *cups* = ________ *qt*
4. 5.6 *cm* = ________ *mm*
5. 4.5 *lb* = ________ *oz*
6. Use the label on the bottle in Figure 4.1 to determine the number of *micrograms* in one tablet of the drug.

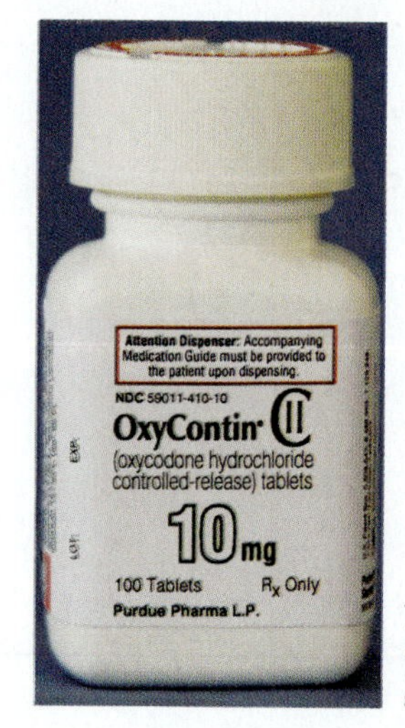

Figure 4.1 Bottle of OxyContin.

SOURCE: © Purdue, used with permission.

7. The prescriber ordered *ProBanthine (propantheline bromide) 30 mg PO ac and hs*. How many *grams* of ProBanthine will the client receive in one week?
8. Order: *Benlysta (belimumab) 650 mg IV q 4 wk*. How many *grams* will the client receive?
9. The urinary output of a client with an indwelling Foley catheter is 1,400 *milliliters*. How many *liters* of urine are in the bag?
10. 42,000 $mcg = ?\ mg$
11. 2,650 $g = ?\ kg$
12. $4\frac{1}{2} qt = ?\ pt$
13. Read the label in Figure 4.2 to determine the number of micrograms of methylprednisolone acetate that is contained in 1 milliliter of Depo-Medrol.

Figure 4.2 Drug label for Depo-Medrol.

SOURCE: Courtesy of Pfizer, Inc.

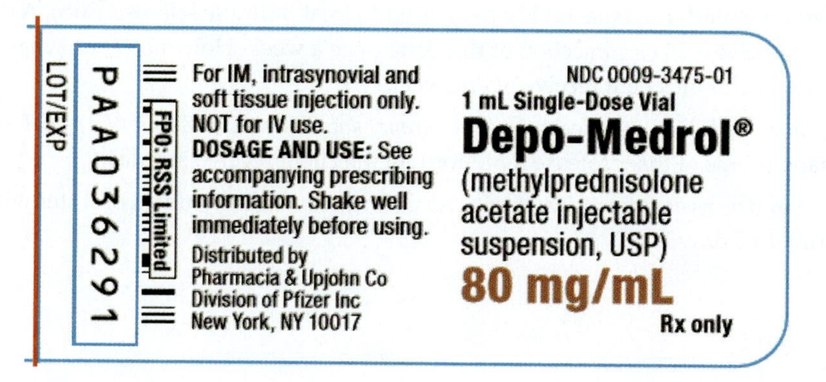

14. A client with a bacterial infection must receive ***ciprofloxacin HCl*** *(Cipro) 750 mg PO q12h*. How many grams of Cipro will the client receive in one day?
15. According to the portion of the physician's order sheet shown in Figure 4.3, how many *mcg* of Halcion will the client receive per day?

Figure 4.3 Portion of a physician's order sheet.

Date	Time	Order
7/7/2020	0800h	***triazolam*** *(Halcion) 0.125 mg PO hs*

16. Order: ***oxacillin sodium*** *0.25 g po q8h*. How many *mg* will the client receive?
17. Read the label in Figure 4.4 and determine the number of grams of **trimethoprim** that are contained in one tablet.

Figure 4.4 Drug label for **sulfamethoxazole and trimethoprim.**

SOURCE: Copyright TEVA, Used with permission

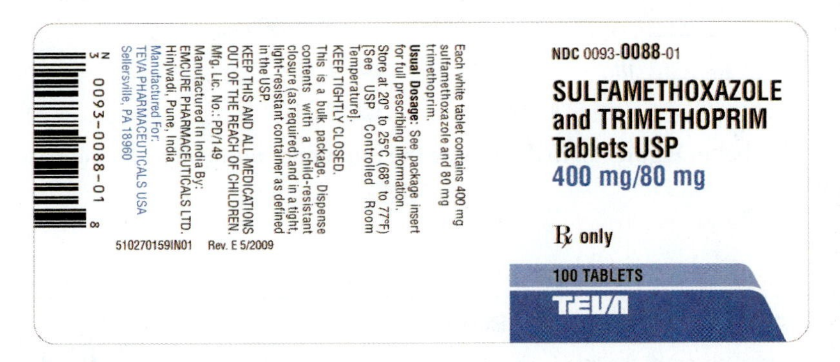

18. Read the label in Figure 4.5 and determine how many grams of **anidulafungin** are contained in the vial.

Figure 4.5 Drug label for **anidulafungin.**

SOURCE: Courtesy of Pfizer, Inc.

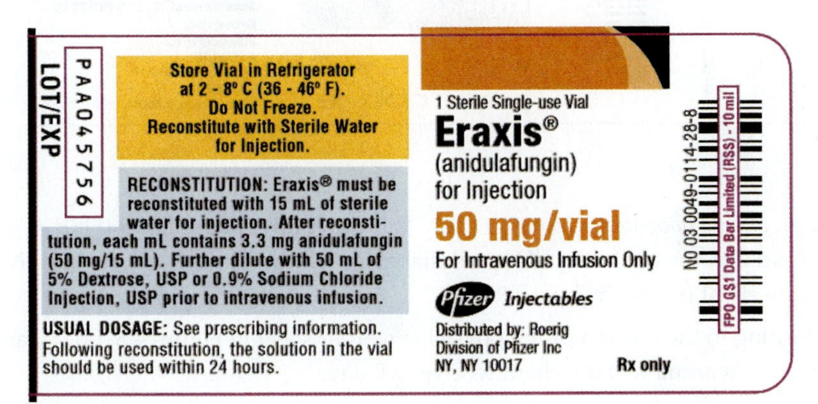

19. How many kilograms does an infant weigh if the infant weighs 3,200 *g*?
20. Order: ***captopril*** *450 mg PO daily in three divided doses*. Read the excerpt from the *Nurse's Drug Guide* in Figure 4.6 and determine whether or not the following order is safe for an adult client with heart failure.

ROUTE & DOSAGE

Hypertension

Adult/Adolescent: **PO** 12.5–25 mg b.i.d. or t.i.d., may increase to 50 mg t.i.d. (max: 450 mg/day)

Heart Failure

Adult: **PO** 25 mg b.i.d.; may increase to 50 mg t.i.d. if needed (max: 450 mg/day)

Proteinuria with Diabetic Nephropathy

Adult: **PO** 25 mg t.i.d.

Left Ventricular Function Post MI

Adult: **PO** 6.25–12.5 mg t.i.d.

Renal Insufficiency Dosage Adjustment

CrCl 10–50 mL/min: 75% of dose; *less than 10 mL/min:* 50% of dose

Figure 4.6 Excerpt for **captopril** from the *Nurse's Drug Guide.*

SOURCE: From Pearson Nurses's Drug Guide. Published by Pearson Education.

Additional Exercises

Now, test yourself!

1. 9.6 *mg* = ________ *mcg*
2. 0.06 *g* = ________ *mg*
3. 40 *mg* = ________ *g*
4. 6.25 *L* = ________ *mL*
5. 21 *mm* = ________ *cm*
6. $2\frac{1}{2}$ *pt* = ________ *cups*
7. 24 *mL* = ________ *cc*
8. 250,000 *mcg* = ________ *mg*
9. 3.5 *qt* = ________ *pt*
10. 4 *T* = ________ *t*
11. 2 *cups* = ________ *oz*
12. 0.35 *kg* = ________ *g*
13. Use the label in Figure 4.7 to determine the number of *micrograms* in one Biaxin tablet.

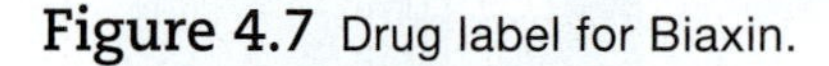

Figure 4.7 Drug label for Biaxin.

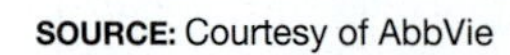

SOURCE: Courtesy of AbbVie

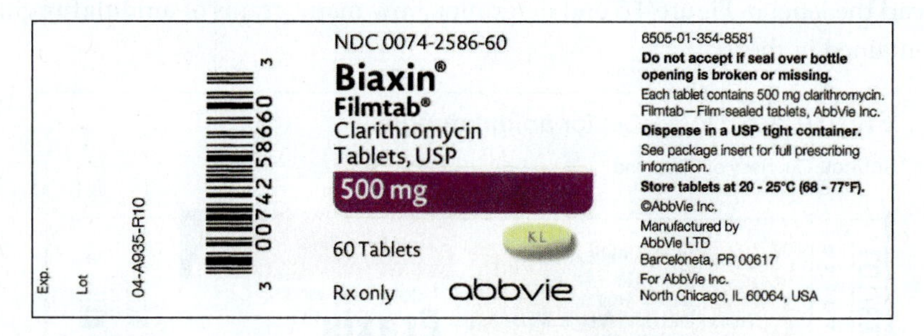

14. Order: *Nesina (alogliptin) 25 mg po daily*. This dipeptidyl peptidase-4 (DPP-4) inhibitor is used in the treatment of type II diabetes mellitus. How many *grams* of Nesina will the client receive in 1 week?
15. According to the portion of the physician's order sheet in Figure 4.8, how many grams of Avandia will the client receive in 7 days?

Figure 4.8 Portion of a physician's order sheet.

Date	Time	Order
8/9/2016	1430 *h*	Avandia (rosiglitazone maleate) 2 *mg po b.i.d.*

16. Order: *Amoxil (amoxicillin) oral susp 1 tsp po q8h*. How many *tablespoons* of Amoxil will the client receive in 3 full days?
17. Read the label in Figure 4.9 to determine the number of *grams* of Norvir contained in 1 *mL* of the Norvir solution.

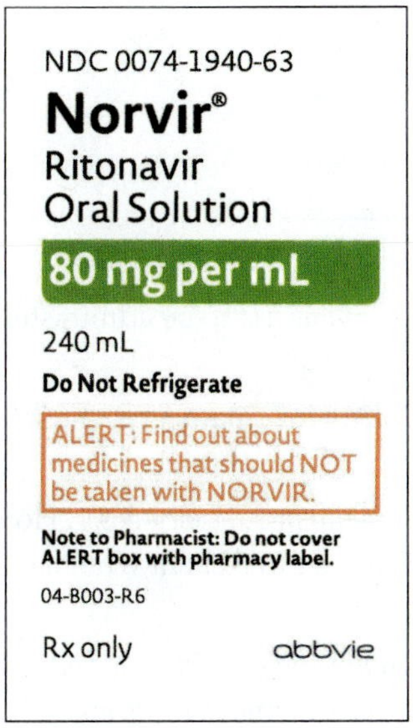

NDC 0074-1940-63
Norvir®
Ritonavir
Oral Solution
80 mg per mL
240 mL
Do Not Refrigerate
ALERT: Find out about medicines that should NOT be taken with NORVIR.
Note to Pharmacist: Do not cover ALERT box with pharmacy label.
04-B003-R6
Rx only
abbvie

Figure 4.9 Drug label for Norvir.

18. Read the label in Figure 4.10 and determine how many *grams* of Isentress are contained in one tablet.

Figure 4.10 Drug label for Isentress.

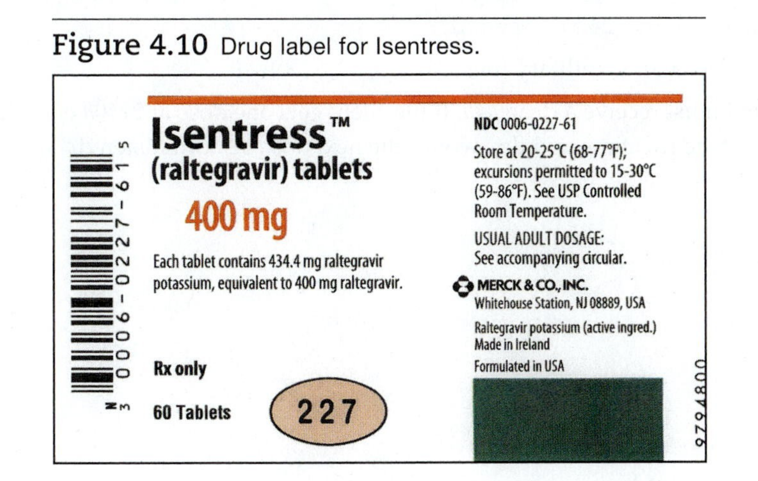

19. An infant weighs 3.1 *kg*. How much does the infant weigh in *grams*?
20. Read the portion of the package insert in Figure 4.11 and determine whether or not this order is a safe starting dose: *Dilaudid (hydromorphone HCl) 1.7 mg IM q6h prn for pain.*

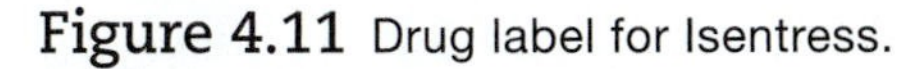
Figure 4.11 Drug label for Isentress.

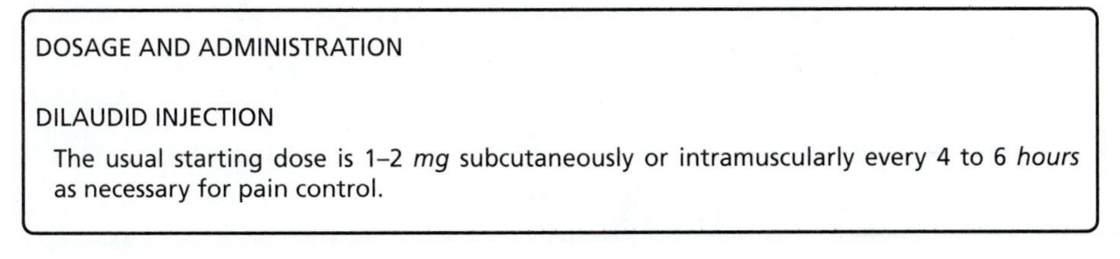
DOSAGE AND ADMINISTRATION

DILAUDID INJECTION

The usual starting dose is 1–2 *mg* subcutaneously or intramuscularly every 4 to 6 *hours* as necessary for pain control.

Cumulative Review Exercises

Reinforce your mastery of previous chapters.

1. 88 *mm* = ________ *cm*
2. 40 oz = ________ *lb*
3. 3.7 *L* = ________ *mL*
4. 5 *T* = ________ *t*
5. 5 *ft* = ________ *in*
6. $2\frac{1}{2}$ *cups per day* = ? *ounces per week*
7. Order: *Dilantin (phenytoin) 300 mg po t.i.d.* How many *grams* are to be administered to the client in the course of one day?
8. A client must drink 16 *ounces* of the laxative GoLYTELY. How many *cups* must the client drink?
9. Order: *Ritalin (methylphenidate hydrochloride) 20 mg po daily in 2 divided doses.* How many *mg* of this psychostimulant drug will you administer to a client who has attention-deficit hyperactivity disorder (ADHD)?
10. What is missing from this order? *Sitavig (acyclovir) 50 mg apply within one hour after the onset of symptoms and before the appearance of any signs of herpes labialis lesions.*
11. If a client receives a drug *25 mg po b.i.d.*, how many *mg* are administered in a 24-hour period?
12. If a client receives a drug *25 mg po q12h*, how many *mg* are administered in a 24-hour period?
13. If a client receives a drug *25 mg po daily in two divided doses*, how many *mg* are administered in a 24-hour period?
14. Write 10:44 A.M. in military time.
15. A client must receive a drug *q4h*. If the client gets one dose at 2140*h* on Monday, at what (standard) time and day would the next dose be administered?

Pearson Nursing Student Resources Find additional review materials at: **nursing.pearsonhighered.com**

Chapter 5

Converting from One System of Measurement to Another

Learning Outcomes

After completing this chapter, you will be able to

5.1 State the equivalent units of weight between the metric and household systems.

5.2 State the equivalent units of volume between the metric and household systems.

5.3 State the equivalent units of length between the metric and household systems.

5.4 Convert a quantity measured in metric units to its equivalent measured in household units.

5.5 Convert a quantity measured in household units to its equivalent measured in metric units.

When calculating drug dosages, you will sometimes need to convert a quantity expressed in one system of measurement to an equivalent quantity expressed in a different system of measurement. For example, you might need to convert a quantity measured in ounces (household system) to the same quantity measured in milliliters (metric system). This chapter shows you how to accomplish such conversions.

Equivalents of Common Units of Measurement

You will need to learn the basic equivalents between the units of measurement in the household and metric systems. The units of measurement in the two systems do not match up nicely with each other. For example, 1 quart (rounded off to the nearest hundred thousandth of a milliliter) is equal to 946.35295 milliliters. It would be impractical to use such an equivalence. So to make computations easier, 1 quart is approximated by 1,000 milliliters. All of the equivalents in the tables below are approximations. Table 5.1 lists some common equivalent values for weight, volume, and length in the two systems of measurement. An expanded summary of the relationships that you should know among all the equivalents of liquid volume is provided in Table 5.2.

NOTE

Some books use these alternative approximations:

250 *mL* ≈ 1 *cup*

480 *mL* ≈ 1 *pt*

Table 5.1 Approximate Equivalents (Metric to Household) for Volume, Weight, and Length.

	Metric		Household
Volume	5 milliliters (*mL*)	≈	1 teaspoon (*t*)
	15 milliliters (*mL*)	≈	1 tablespoon (*T*)
	30 milliliters (*mL*)	≈	1 ounce (*oz*)
	240 milliliters (*mL*)	≈	1 cup
	500 milliliters (*mL*)	≈	1 pint (*pt*)
	1,000 milliliters (*mL*)	≈	1 quart (*qt*)
Weight	1 kilogram (*kg*)	≈	2.2 pounds (*lb*)
Length	2.5 centimeters (*cm*)	≈	1 inch (*in*)

NOTE

In dosage calculations 2.5 centimeters is an adequate approximation for 1 inch. However, the exact relationship is 2.54 *cm* = 1 *in*.

Table 5.2 Approximate Equivalents (Household to Metric) for Volume.

1 teaspoon	≈	5 *mL*
1 tablespoon = 3 teaspoons	≈	15 *mL*
1 ounce = 2 tablespoons = 6 teaspoons	≈	30 *mL*
1 cup = 8 ounces = 16 tablespoons	≈	240 *mL*
1 pint = 2 cups = 16 ounces	≈	500 *mL*
1 quart = 2 pints = 4 cups = 32 ounces	≈	1,000 *mL* = 1*L*

You can convert quantities from one system to another in exactly the same way you converted from one unit to another within the same system.

Figure 5.1 depicts medication cups with units of measurement from household and metric systems.

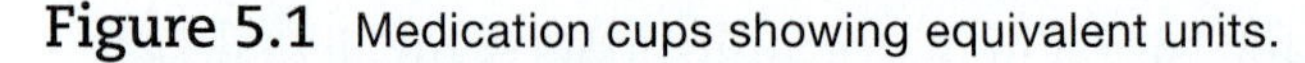

Figure 5.1 Medication cups showing equivalent units.

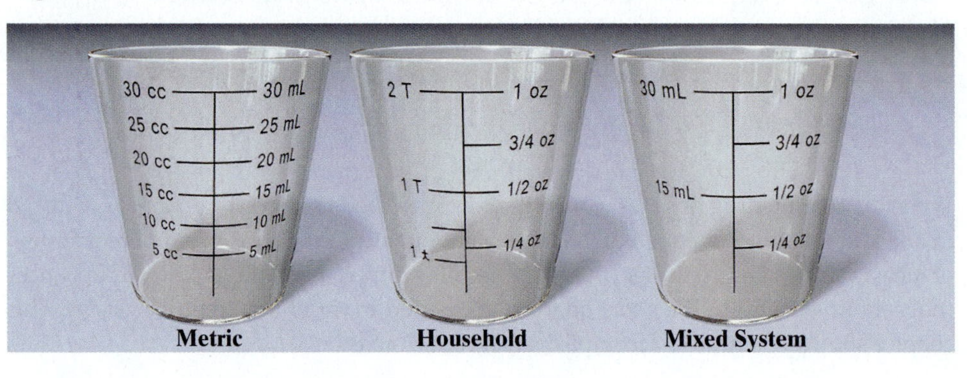

The surface, called the *meniscus*, of a liquid in a medication cup is not flat (Figure 5.2). It is curved. Place the medication cup on a flat surface and move your eye to the level of the meniscus to read the amount of liquid at the level of the bottom of the meniscus.

Figure 5.2 Medication cup filled to 10 mL.

SOURCE: Pearson Education, Inc.

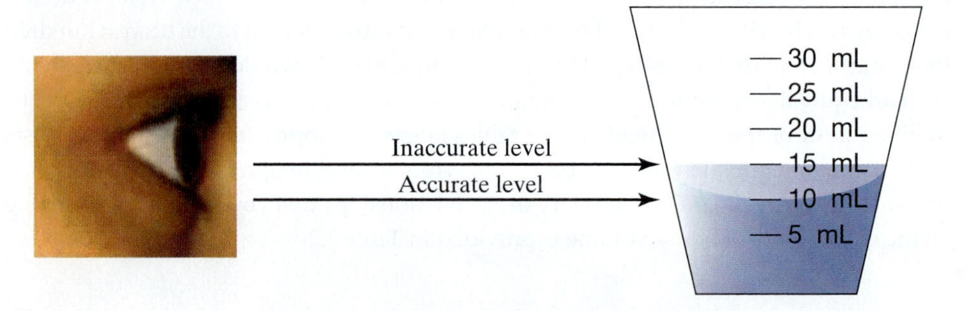

Metric-Household Conversions

Volume Conversions

Example 5.1

Convert 8 teaspoons to an equivalent volume measured in milliliters.

DIMENSIONAL ANALYSIS

$$8\ t = ?\ mL$$

You want to cancel the teaspoons and obtain the equivalent in milliliters.

$$8\ t \times \frac{?\ mL}{?\ t} = ?\ mL$$

You use the equivalence $5\ mL = 1\ t$.

So, the unit fraction is $\frac{5\ mL}{1\ t}$

$$8\ \cancel{t} \times \frac{5\ mL}{1\ \cancel{t}} = 40\ mL$$

NOTE

Although 1 *t* is approximately equal to 5 *mL*, in Example 5.1, for simplicity, the equal sign is used. This practice will be followed throughout the textbook.

RATIO & PROPORTION

$$8\ t = ?\ mL$$

In this problem, there are two quantities: *teaspoons* and *milliliters*.

Think of the problem this way:

$8\ t = x\ mL$

$1\ t = 5\ mL$ [known equivalent]

One way to set up the proportion is

$$\frac{8t}{x\ mL} = \frac{1t}{5\ mL}$$

Eliminate the units of measurement

$$\frac{8}{x} = \frac{1}{5}$$

Cross multiply and simplify

$$\frac{8}{x} = \frac{1}{5}$$

$$(x)(1) = (8)(5)$$

$$x = 40$$

So, 8 teaspoons is equivalent to 40 milliliters.

Example 5.2

Change $1\frac{1}{2}$ pints to milliliters.

DIMENSIONAL ANALYSIS

$$1\tfrac{1}{2}\ pt = ?\ mL$$

You want to cancel the pints and obtain the equivalent amount in milliliters.

$$\frac{3\ pt}{2} \times \frac{?\ mL}{?\ pt} = ?\ mL$$

Because $500\ mL = 1\ pt$, the unit fraction is $\frac{500\ mL}{1\ pt}$

$$\frac{3\ \cancel{pt}}{\underset{1}{\cancel{2}}} \times \frac{\overset{250}{\cancel{500}}\ mL}{1\ \cancel{pt}} = 750\ mL$$

RATIO & PROPORTION

$$1\frac{1}{2} pt = ?\ mL$$

Think of the problem this way:

$1\frac{1}{2} pt = x\ mL$

$1\ pt = 500\ mL$ [known equivalent]

One way to set up the proportion is

$$\frac{1\frac{1}{2}\ pt}{x\ mL} = \frac{1\ pt}{500\ mL}$$

Eliminate the units of measurement

$$\frac{1\frac{1}{2}}{x} = \frac{1}{500}$$

(Continued)

Cross multiply and simplify

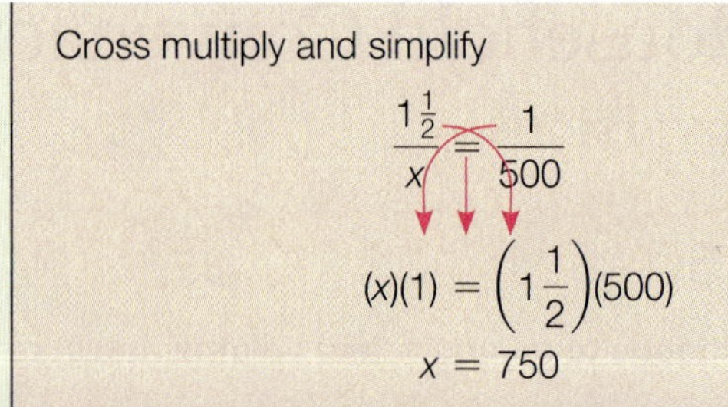

$$(x)(1) = \left(1\frac{1}{2}\right)(500)$$

$$x = 750$$

So, $1\frac{1}{2}$ pints is equivalent to 750 milliliters.

Example 5.3

A client is to receive 60 *milliliters* of a medication. How many ounces will the client receive?

DIMENSIONAL ANALYSIS

60 *milliliters* = ? *ounces*

You want to cancel the *milliliters* and get the answer in *ounces*, so choose a fraction with *milliliters* on the bottom and *ounces* on top.

You need a fraction in the form of $\frac{?\,oz}{?\,mL}$

Because 1 *oz* = 30 *mL*, the unit fraction you need is $\frac{1\,oz}{30\,mL}$

$$\frac{\overset{2}{\cancel{60}}\,\cancel{mL}}{1} \times \frac{1\,oz}{\underset{1}{\cancel{30}}\,\cancel{mL}} = 2\,oz$$

RATIO & PROPORTION

Think of the problem this way:

60 *mL* = *x oz*

30 *mL* = 1 *oz* [known equivalent]

One way to set up the proportion is

$$\frac{60\,mL}{x\,oz} = \frac{30\,mL}{1\,oz}$$

Eliminate the units of measurement

$$\frac{60}{x} = \frac{30}{1}$$

Cross multiply and simplify

$$\frac{60}{x} = \frac{30}{1}$$

$$(x)(30) = (1)(60)$$

$$30x = 60$$

Divide by 30 and cancel

$$\frac{\cancel{30}x}{\cancel{30}} = \frac{60}{30}$$

$$x = 2$$

So, the client will receive 2 *ounces* of the medication.

NOTE

Example 5.3 could be done mentally by understanding that, because 1 ounce = 30 milliliters, then twice as many ounces (2 oz) will equal twice as many milliliters (60 mL). That is, 2 *oz* = 60 *mL*.

Example 5.4

A medication cup contains 22.5 milliliters of a solution. How many tablespoons are in the medication cup?

DIMENSIONAL ANALYSIS

$$22.5 \textit{ milliliters} = ? \textit{ tablespoons}$$

You want to cancel the *milliliters* and get the answer in *tablespoons*, so choose a fraction with *milliliters* on the bottom and *tablespoons* on top. You need a fraction in the form of $\frac{?\,T}{?\,mL}$

Because 15 *milliliters* = 1 *tablespoon*, the unit fraction you need is $\frac{1\,T}{15\,mL}$

$$\frac{22.5\,\cancel{mL}}{1} \times \frac{1\text{ T}}{15\,\cancel{mL}} = 1.5\,T$$

RATIO & PROPORTION

Think of the problem this way:

$$22.5\,mL = x\,T$$
$$15\,mL = 1\,T \quad \text{[known equivalent]}$$

One way to set up the proportion is

$$\frac{22.5\,mL}{x\,T} = \frac{15\,mL}{1\,T}$$

Eliminate the units of measurement, cross multiply, and simplify

$$\frac{22.5}{x} = \frac{15}{1}$$

$$(x)(15) = (1)(22.5)$$
$$15x = 22.5$$

Divide by 15 and cancel

$$\frac{\cancel{15}x}{\cancel{15}} = \frac{22.5}{15}$$
$$x = 1.5$$

So, the medication cup contains $1\frac{1}{2}$ *tablespoons*.

Weight Conversions

Example 5.5

A client weighs 150 *pounds*. What is the client's weight measured in kilograms?

DIMENSIONAL ANALYSIS

$$150 \textit{ pounds} = ? \textit{ kilograms}$$

You want to cancel the *pounds* and get the answer in *kilograms*, so choose a fraction with *pounds* on the bottom and *kilograms* on top.

You need a fraction in the form of $\frac{?\,kg}{?\,lb}$

Because 2.2 *pounds* = 1 *kilogram*, the unit fraction you need is $\frac{1\,kg}{2.2\,lb}$

$$\frac{150\,\cancel{lb}}{1} \times \frac{1\text{ kg}}{2.2\,\cancel{lb}} = 68.18\,kg$$

RATIO & PROPORTION

Think of the problem this way:

$$150\,lb = x\,kg$$
$$2.2\,lb = 1\,kg \quad \text{[known equivalent]}$$

One way to set up the proportion is

$$\frac{150\,lb}{x\,kg} = \frac{2.2\,lb}{1\,kg}$$

Eliminate the units of measurement, cross multiply, and simplify

$$\frac{150}{x} = \frac{2.2}{1}$$

$$(x)(2.2) = (1)(150)$$
$$2.2x = 150$$

Divide by 2.2 and cancel

$$\frac{\cancel{2.2}x}{\cancel{2.2}} = \frac{150}{2.2}$$
$$x = 68.18$$

So, the client weighs 68 *kilograms*.

Example 5.6

Jennifer weighs 115 *pounds* 8 *ounces*. What is her weight in kilograms?

DIMENSIONAL ANALYSIS

$$115\ lb\ 8\ oz \quad \text{means} \quad 115\ lb + 8\ oz$$

First determine Jennifer's weight in pounds. To do this, convert 8 ounces to pounds.

$$8\ oz = ?\ lb$$

You want to cancel ounces and obtain the equivalent amount in pounds.

$$8\ oz \times \frac{?\ lb}{?\ oz} = ?\ lb$$

Because $1\ lb = 16\ oz$, the unit fraction is $\frac{1\ lb}{16\ oz}$

$$\overset{1}{\cancel{8}}\ \cancel{oz} \times \frac{1\ lb}{\underset{2}{\cancel{16}}\ \cancel{oz}} = \frac{1}{2}\ lb$$

So, Jennifer weighs $115\ lb + \frac{1}{2}\ lb$ or 115.5 pounds. Now, convert 115.5 pounds to kilograms

$$115.5\ lb = ?\ kg$$

You want to cancel pounds and obtain the equivalent amount in kilograms

$$115.5\ lb \times \frac{?\ kg}{?\ lb} = ?\ kg$$

Because $1\ kg = 2.2\ lb$, the unit fraction is $\frac{1\ kg}{2.2\ lb}$

$$115.5\ \cancel{lb} \times \frac{1\ kg}{2.2\ \cancel{lb}} = 52.5\ kg$$

RATIO & PROPORTION

$$115\ lb\ 8\ oz \quad \text{means} \quad 115\ lb + 8\ oz$$

First, determine Jennifer's weight in pounds. To do this, convert 8 ounces to pounds.
Think of the problem this way:

$$8\ oz = x\ lb$$
$$16\ oz = 1\ lb \quad \text{[known equivalent]}$$

One way to set up the proportion is

$$\frac{8\ oz}{x\ lb} = \frac{16\ oz}{1\ lb}$$

Eliminate the units of measurement, cross multiply, and simplify

$$\frac{8\ oz}{x\ lb} = \frac{16\ oz}{1\ lb}$$
$$(16)(x) = (8)(1)$$
$$16x = 8$$

Divide by the coefficient of x, cancel, and simplify

$$\frac{\cancel{16}x}{\cancel{16}} = \frac{8}{16}$$
$$x = \frac{1}{2}$$

Jennifer weighs $115\frac{1}{2}$ pounds.
Now, to change 115.5 pounds to kilograms, think of the problem as

$$115.5\ lb = x\ kg$$
$$2.2\ lb = 1\ kg \quad \text{[known equivalent]}$$

One way to set up the proportion is

$$\frac{115.5\ lb}{x\ kg} = \frac{2.2\ lb}{1\ kg}$$

Eliminate the units of measurement, cross multiply, and simplify

$$\frac{115.5}{x} = \frac{2.2}{1}$$
$$(2.2)(x) = (115.5)(1)$$
$$2.2x = 115.5$$

Divide by the coefficient of x, cancel, and simplify

$$\frac{\cancel{2.2}x}{\cancel{2.2}} = \frac{115.5}{2.2}$$
$$x = 52.5$$

So, Jennifer weighs 52.5 *kilograms*.

NOTE

In Example 5.6, the 8 ounces could have been changed to $\frac{1}{2}$ pound mentally by understanding that because 16 ounces = 1 pound, then one-half as many ounces (8 oz) will equal one-half as many pounds ($\frac{1}{2}$ *lb*). That is, 8 oz = $\frac{1}{2}$ *lb*.

Example 5.7

An infant weighs 4 *kilograms*. What is the infant's weight measured in pounds and ounces?

DIMENSIONAL ANALYSIS

4 *kilograms* = ? *pounds*

You want to cancel the *kilograms* and get the answer in *pounds*, so choose a fraction with *kilograms* on the bottom and *pounds* on top.

You need a fraction in the form of $\frac{?\ lb}{?\ kg}$

Because 1 *kilogram* = 2.2 *pounds*, the unit fraction you need is $\frac{2.2\ lb}{1\ kg}$

$$\frac{4\ \cancel{kg}}{1} \times \frac{2.2\ lb}{1\ \cancel{kg}} = 8.8\ lb$$

So, the infant weighs 8 *lb* + 0.8 *lb*

Next, change the 0.8 lb to ounces.

0.8 *lb* = ? *ounces*

You want to cancel the *pounds* and get the answer in *ounces*, so choose a fraction with *pounds* on the bottom and *ounces* on top.

Because 1 *pound* = 16 *ounces*, the unit fraction you need is $\frac{16\ oz}{1\ lb}$

$$\frac{0.8\ \cancel{lb}}{1} \times \frac{16\ oz}{1\ \cancel{lb}} = 12.8\ oz \approx 13\ oz$$

RATIO & PROPORTION

First change the weight to pounds.

Think of the problem this way:

4 *kg* = *x lb*

1 *kg* = 2.2 *lb* [known equivalent]

One way to set up the proportion is

$$\frac{x\ lb}{4\ kg} = \frac{2.2\ lb}{1\ kg}$$

Eliminate the units of measurement, cross multiply, and simplify

$$\frac{x}{4} = \frac{2.2}{1}$$

$$(4)(2.2) = (1)(x)$$

$$8.8 = x$$

The infant weighs 8.8 pounds (8 *pounds* + 0.8 *pounds*). To change the 0.8 pound to ounces, think of the problem as

0.8 *lb* = *x oz*

1 *lb* = 16 *oz* [known equivalent]

One way to set up the proportion is

$$\frac{0.8\ lb}{x\ oz} = \frac{1\ lb}{16\ oz}$$

Eliminate the units of measurement, cross multiply, and simplify

$$\frac{0.8}{x} = \frac{1}{16}$$

$$(1)(x) = (0.8)(16)$$

$$x = 12.8 \approx 13$$

So, the infant weighs 8 pounds 13 ounces.

Length Conversions

EXAMPLE 5.8

Adam is 6 *feet* 3 *inches* tall. What is his height in centimeters?

(Continued)

DIMENSIONAL ANALYSIS

$$6\ ft\ 3\ in \quad \text{means} \quad 6\ ft + 3\ in$$

First determine Adam's height in inches. To do this, convert 6 feet to inches

$$6\ ft = ?\ in$$

You want to cancel feet and obtain the equivalent height in inches

$$6\ ft \times \frac{?\ in}{?\ ft} = ?\ in$$

Because 1 ft = 12 in, the unit fraction is $\frac{12\ in}{1\ ft}$

$$6\ \cancel{ft} \times \frac{12\ in}{1\ \cancel{ft}} = 72\ in$$

Next, add the extra 3 inches

$$72\ in + 3\ in = 75\ in$$

Now convert 75 inches to centimeters

$$75\ in = ?\ cm$$

You want to cancel inches and obtain the equivalent length in centimeters

$$75\ in \times \frac{?\ cm}{?\ in} = ?\ cm$$

Because 1 in = 2.5 cm, the unit fraction is $\frac{2.5\ cm}{1\ in}$

$$75\ \cancel{in} \times \frac{2.5\ cm}{1\ \cancel{in}} = 187.5\ cm$$

RATIO & PROPORTION

$$6\ ft\ 3\ in \quad \text{means} \quad 6\ ft + 3\ in$$

First, determine Adam's height in inches. To do this, convert 6 feet to inches.

Think of the problem this way:

$$6\ ft = x\ in$$
$$1\ ft = 12\ in \quad \text{[known equivalent]}$$

One way to set up the proportion is

$$\frac{6\ ft}{x\ in} = \frac{1\ ft}{12\ in}$$

Eliminate the units of measurement, cross multiply, and simplify

$$\frac{6\ ft}{x\ in} = \frac{1\ ft}{12\ in}$$
$$(1)(x) = (6)(12)$$
$$x = 72$$

Now, add the extra 3 inches

$$72\ in + 3\ in = 75\ in$$

Adam is 75 inches tall.

To change 75 inches to centimeters, think of the problem as

$$75\ in = x\ cm$$
$$1\ in = 2.5\ cm \quad \text{[known equivalent]}$$

One way to set up the proportion is

$$\frac{75\ in}{x\ cm} = \frac{1\ in}{2.5\ cm}$$

Eliminate the units of measurement, cross multiply, and simplify

$$\frac{75\ in}{x\ cm} = \frac{1\ in}{2.5\ cm}$$
$$(1)(x) = (75)(2.5)$$
$$x = 187.5 \approx 188$$

So, Adam is 188 centimeters tall.

NOTE

In Example 5.8, the 6 feet could have been changed to 72 inches by understanding that because 1 foot = 12 inches, then 6 times as many feet (6 ft) will equal six times as many inches (72 in). That is, 6 ft = 72 in.

Example 5.9

A tumor has a diameter of 2 inches. What is the diameter of the tumor measured in millimeters?

DIMENSIONAL ANALYSIS

First change from *inches* to *centimeters*, and then from *centimeters* to *millimeters*.

2 inches → ? *centimeters* → ? *millimeters*

You want to cancel the *inches* and get the answer in *centimeters*, so choose a fraction with *inches* on the bottom and *centimeters* on top.

Because 1 *inch* = 2.5 *centimeters*, the unit fraction you need is $\frac{2.5\ cm}{1\ in}$

$$\frac{2\ in}{1} \times \frac{2.5\ cm}{1\ in} = ?\ mm$$

Next, you want to cancel the *cm* and get the answer in *mm*, so choose a unit fraction with *cm* on the bottom and *mm* on top.

Because 1 *centimeter* = 10 millimeters, the unit fraction you need is $\frac{10\ mm}{1\ cm}$

$$\frac{2\ in}{1} \times \frac{2.5\ cm}{1\ in} \times \frac{10\ mm}{1\ cm} = 50\ mm$$

RATIO & PROPORTION

First use the equivalence 2.5 centimeters= 1 inch.

Think of the problem this way:

$2\ in = x\ cm$

$1\ in = 2.5\ cm$ [known equivalent]

One way to set up the proportion is

$$\frac{2\ in}{x\ cm} = \frac{1\ in}{2.5\ cm}$$

Eliminate the units of measurement, cross multiply, and simplify

$$\frac{2}{x} = \frac{1}{2.5}$$

$$(x)(1) = (2)(2.5)$$

$$x = 5$$

So, the diameter of the tumor is 5 centimeters.

Now change to millimeters

5 cm = ? mm

To convert *centimeters* to *millimeters* is a jump of 1 *place to the right*.

meter	decimeter	centimeter	millimeter
m	*dm*	*cm*	*mm*

So, in 5 cm, move the decimal point *1 place to the right*.

5 *cm* = 5.0 *cm* = 5 0 . *mm* = 50. *mm* = 50 *mm*

So, the tumor has a diameter of 50 *millimeters*.

Summary

In this chapter, quantities measured in one system of measurement were converted to equivalent quantities measured in a different system of measurement.

- It is important to memorize all the equivalences for volume, weight, and length between the metric and household systems of measurement.
- Both Dimensional Analysis and Ratio & Proportion can be used to perform conversions between the metric and household systems.
- The equivalences between systems are not exact; they are approximate.
- When performing conversions between two systems, your answers are not exact; they are approximate.
- When performing conversions between two systems, answers may differ somewhat, depending on which approximate equivalences are used.

Practice Sets

The answers to *Try These for Practice, Exercises,* and *Cumulative Review Exercises* are found in Appendix A. Ask your instructor for the answers to the *Additional Exercises.*

Try These for Practice

Test your comprehension after reading the chapter.

1. To do the exercises at the end of this chapter, you need to memorize all the equivalents presented so far. To test yourself, fill in the missing numbers in the following chart.

Metric System

(a) 1 *L* = ____________ *mL*

(b) 1 *kg* = ____________ *g*

(c) 1 *g* = ____________ *mg*

(d) 1 *mg* = ____________ *mcg*

(e) 1 *cm* = ____________ *mm*

Household System

(f) 1 *qt* = ____________ *pt*

(g) 1 *pt* = ____________ *cups*

(h) 1 *cup* = ____________ *oz*

(i) 1 *oz* = ____________ *T*

(j) 1 *T* = ____________ *t*

(k) 1 *lb* = ____________ *oz*

(l) 1 *ft* = ____________ *in*

Mixed Systems

(m) 1 *in* ≈ ____________ *cm*

(n) 1 *kg* ≈ ____________ *lb*

(o) 1 *t* ≈ ____________ *mL*

(p) 1 *T* ≈ ____________ *mL*

(q) 1 *oz* ≈ ____________ *mL*

(r) 1 *cup* ≈ ____________ *mL*

(s) 1 *pt* ≈ ____________ *mL*

(t) 1 *qt* ≈ ____________ *mL*

(u) 1 *oz* = ____________ *T* = ____________ *t* ≈ ____________ *mL*

(v) 1 *qt* = ______ *pt* = ______ *cups* = ______ *oz* ≈ ______ *mL*

2. Harold is 5 *feet* 3 *inches* tall. What is his height rounded off to the nearest whole *centimeter*?

3. Order: *Ravicti (glycerol phenylbutyrate) 15 mL po in three equally divided dosages, each rounded up to the nearest 0.5 mL.* How many *teaspoons* will you administer?
4. How many milliliters are in an 8-ounce cup of coffee?
5. A client is told to drink *2,500* milliliters of fluid. How many quarts of fluid should the client drink?

Exercises

Reinforce your understanding in class or at home.

1. 4 *t* ≈ ____________ *mL*
2. 8 *oz* ≈ ____________ *mL*
3. 45 *mL* ≈ ____________ *T*
4. 120 *mL* ≈ ____________ *cup*
5. 150 *lb* ≈ ____________ *kg* (round off to tenth of a *kg*)
6. Order: *albuterol sulfate 2 mg po t.i.d.* Read the label in Figure 5.3 and determine the number of teaspoons of syrup that are contained in one dose.

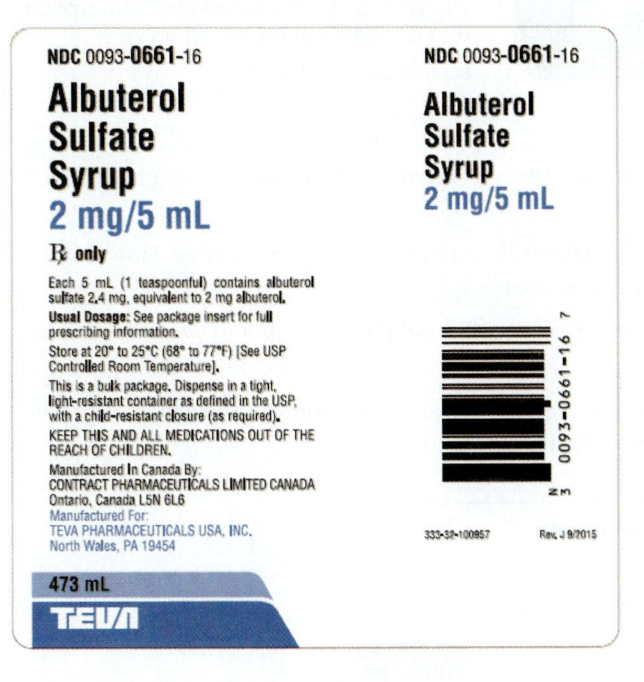

Figure 5.3 Drug label for Albuterol Sulfate Syrup.

SOURCE: Copyright TEVA, Used with permission

7. The diameter of a wound is 50 *mm*. What is the diameter of the wound measured in *inches*?
8. 24 *t* = ? *T*
9. 120 *mL* ≈ ? *oz*
10. Read the label in Figure 5.4 and determine how many *teaspoons* of dextromethorphan are in the container.

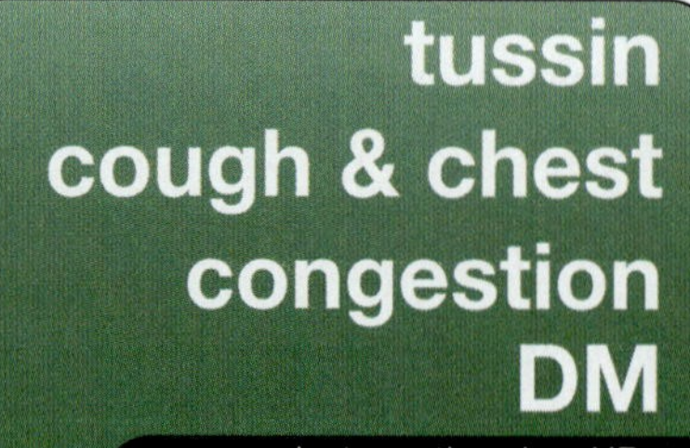

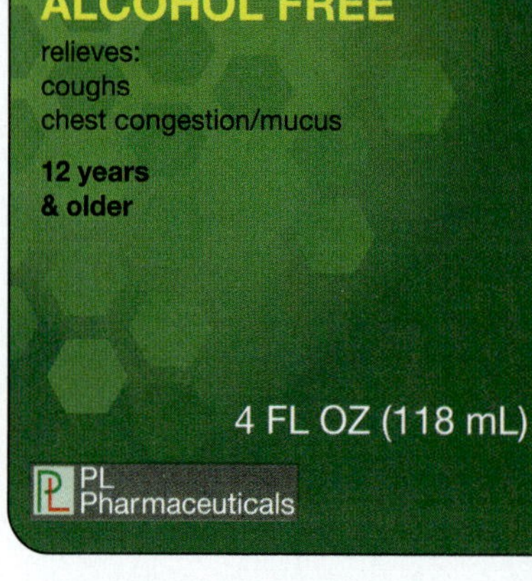

Figure 5.4 Box for dextromethorphan. (For educational purposes only)

SOURCE: Courtesy of Pfizer, Inc.

11. General George Washington was 185 *centimeters* tall. What was his height in *feet* and *inches*?
12. Order: *Kynamro (mipomersen sodium) 200 milligrams subcut once weekly*. How many *grams* will the client receive each week?
13. A neonate weighs 3,100 *grams*. Convert this weight to *pounds* and *ounces* (rounded off to the nearest *ounce*).
14. How many teaspoons of the antiepileptic oral suspension whose label is shown in Figure 5.5 contain 600 *mg* of felbamate?

Figure 5.5 Drug label for **felbamate**.

SOURCE: Meda Pharmaceuticals Inc.

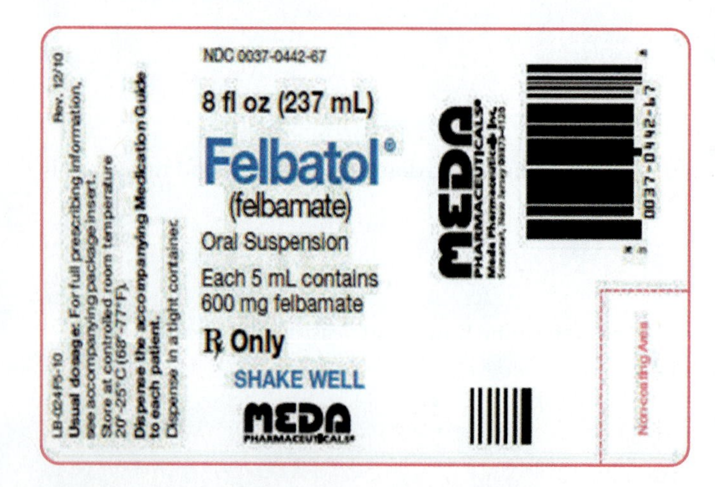

15. Order: *Nuplazid (**pimavanserin**) 34 mg PO daily*. The strength of the drug is *17 mg per tablet*. How many tablets of this selective serotonin inverse antagonist should be given to the client?
16. An indwelling urinary catheter drains into a collection bag that contains *1,200 mL* of urine. How many ounces of urine are in the collection bag?
17. *Percocet (oxycodone/acetaminophen)* is a combination drug with strength of *2.5 mg/325 mg per tablet*. How many grams of acetaminophen are contained in one tablet?
18. Harold is producing urine at the rate of *40 milliliter/hour*, and Thomas is producing urine at *1.5 quart/day*. Which person is producing urine at the faster rate?
19. A bottle of *acetaminophen and codeine phosphate* has a volume of *473 mL*. The adult dose of this drug is *1 tablespoon*. How many full adult doses are contained in the bottle?
20. A morbidly obese client weighs *420 pounds*. What is the client's weight in kilograms?

Additional Exercises

Now, test yourself!

1. 4.7 *mg* = ____________ *mcg*
2. 400 *mL* = ____________ *L*
3. 60 *mL* ≈ ____________ *t*
4. 4 *T* ≈ ____________ *mL*
5. 50 *lb* ≈ ____________ *kg* (round off to the nearest tenth)
6. 50 *kg* ≈ ____________ *lb*
7. 3.5 *pt* ≈ ____________ *oz*
8. 4 *T* = ____________ *oz*
9. 7.5 *cm* ≈ ____________ *in*
10. How many *tablespoons* are contained in the Lexapro container whose label is shown in Figure 5.6?

Figure 5.6 Drug label for Lexapro.

SOURCE: Forest Pharmaceuticals

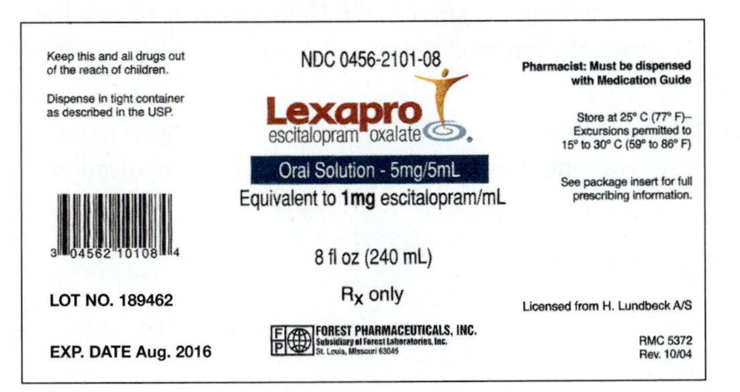

11. A client is 5 *feet* 9 *inches* tall. Find the height of the client in *centimeters*.
12. Find the weight in *grams* of a 7-*pound* infant (round off to the nearest *gram*).
13. Harold weighs 250 *pounds* now. If Harold goes on a diet and loses 30 *pounds*, then how many *kilograms* will he weigh?
14. Use Figure 5.7 to determine the total number of *grams* of pseudoephedrine that are in the entire container.

Figure 5.7 Drug box for Alavert.

SOURCE: Courtesy of Pfizer, Inc.

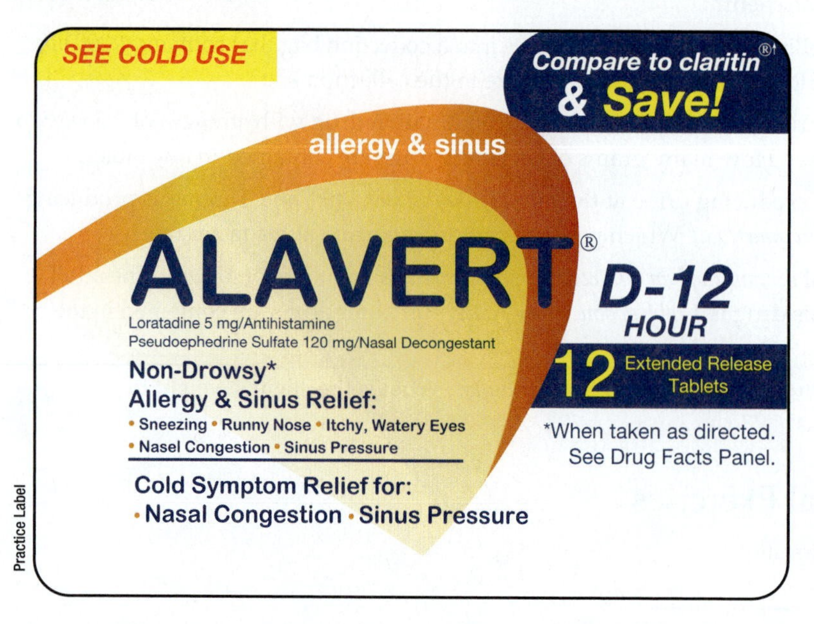

15. A nurse administers 30 *mL* of a drug by mouth t.i.d. to a client. This client is to be discharged and must continue to take the medication at home. How many *tablespoons* should the client be advised to take daily?
16. The client is required to take *Allegra (fexofenadine) 60 mg po b.i.d.* How many *grams* of this drug will the client take in 3 days?
17. What is the client's total fluid intake in *milliliters* for the day if he had the following fluid intake:

    Breakfast: 8 *oz* milk, 8 *oz* water
    Lunch: 6 *oz* juice, 3 *T* medication
    Dinner: 6 *oz* soup, 12 *oz* soda, 4 *oz* jello

18. The order for a client is *Robitussin syrup (guaifenesin) 10 mL po q4h*. How many *ounces* of Robitussin would the client have received by 10 P.M. if the first dose was administered at noon?
19. The client must receive *Cipro (ciprofloxacin hydrochloride)* 500 *mg b.i.d.* × 10 *days* for acute sinusitis. How many *grams* of Cipro will the client have received in total at the end of the 10 days?
20. A school nurse administers 2 *teaspoons* of Children's Tylenol to a child who has a fever. How many such doses are contained in an 8-*ounce* bottle of this medication?

Cumulative Review Exercises

Reinforce your mastery of previous chapters.

1. 176 *lb* ≈ ____________ *kg*
2. 80 *mg* = ____________ *g*
3. 2 *qt* ≈ ____________ *mL*
4. 120 *mL* = ____________ *L*
5. 5 *lb* ≈ ____________ *g* (round off to the nearest whole gram)
6. 24 *oz/day* = ? *pt/day*
7. 3 *t/day* ≈ ? *mL/wk*

8. Order: *Osphena (ospemifene) 60 mg po with food daily.* How many *grams* of this estrogen agonist/antagonist will the client receive in total in 2 weeks?
9. A client enters the ICU at 5:30 A.M. and leaves 8 hours later. At what time did the client leave the ICU (in military time)?
10. The maximum dose of VariZIG (varicella zoster immune globulin [human]) is 625 *International Units* for all clients greater than 40 *kilograms* in weight. Harold weighs 70 *lb*. May Harold receive 625 *International Units* of this drug?
11. Write *8:35 P.M.* in military time.
12. Convert the rate of *2 cups/day* to an equivalent rate measured in *mL/h*.
13. Order: *chlorpheniramine maleate 24 mg po in three divided doses per day.* How many milligrams do you give the client?
14. Order: *levocetirizine 15 mg po b.i.d.* The safe dose range for this client with chronic urticaria is *10–20 mg/day*. Is the ordered dose safe?
15. Convert a length of *30 millimeters* to centimeters.

Unit 3

Oral and Parenteral Medications

Chapter 6

Oral Medications

Learning Outcomes

After completing this chapter, you will be able to

6.1 Use the Formula method to calculate dosages.

6.2 Calculate Simple (one-step) problems for oral medications in solid and liquid form.

6.3 Calculate Complex (multi-step) problems for oral medications in solid and liquid form.

6.4 Calculate doses for medications measured in milliequivalents.

6.5 Interpret drug labels in order to calculate doses for oral medication.

6.6 Calculate doses based on body weight.

6.7 Calculate body surface area.

6.8 Calculate doses based on body surface area.

In this chapter you learn how to calculate doses of oral medications both in solid and liquid form. You are introduced to *client-specific* dosages that use the *size of the client* (body weight or body surface area [BSA]) to determine the appropriate dose. In the previous chapters you have used the **Dimensional Analysis** and **Ratio & Proportion** methods. In this chapter you learn another method for calculating dosages, the **Formula** method.

Simple (One-Step) Problems

In the calculations you have done in previous chapters, all the equivalents have come from standard tables, for example, $1t = 5\ mL$. In this chapter, the equivalent used will depend on the *strength of the drug* that is available; for example, $1\ tab = 15\ mg$. In the following examples, the equivalent is found on the label of the drug container.

Medication in Solid Form

Oral medications are the most common type of prescription. As discussed in Chapter 2, oral medications come in many forms (tablets, capsules, caplets, and liquid), and drug manufacturers prepare oral medications in commonly prescribed dosages. Oral medications are often supplied in a variety of strengths.

Whenever possible, it is preferable to obtain the medication in the same strength as the dose ordered, or if that is not available, choose a strength that equals a multiple of the prescribed dose. For example, if the order requires 100 *mg* to be administered, tablets with a strength of 100 *mg*/tab would make dosage computation unnecessary, and 1 tablet would be administered. However, tablets with a strength of 50 *mg*/tab would make dosage computation necessary, and 2 tablets would be administered.

It is best to *administer the fewest number of tablets or capsules possible*. For example, if a prescriber orders *ampicillin 750 mg po q12h* and you have both the 250-*mg* and 500-*mg* capsules available, then you would administer one 500-*mg* capsule and one 250-*mg* capsule rather than three 250-*mg* capsules.

In clinical settings, unit-dose medications are usually supplied by the pharmacist.

NOTE

If your calculations indicate a large number of tablets (or capsules) per dose, you should verify your calculations with another health professional. Also check the usual dosage of the medication with a pharmacist and/or a drug reference.

Formula Method

In Chapters 3, 4, and 5 three different methods for converting one unit of measurement to another were illustrated: *dimensional analysis, ratio & proportion*, and *moving the decimal point*. Now these three methods are used to calculate dosages along with the *formula* method. The formula method is used only for *dosage calculation*; it is not used for *unit conversion*, which was the focus of the last three chapters.

$$\frac{D}{H} \times Q = X$$

The formula is commonly used to calculate dosages. To use this formula, you must be able to identify what the four symbols represent.

D stands for the DESIRED dose that the prescriber ordered.

H stands for the amount of the drug on HAND, the strength available in *mg*, *mL*, etc.

Q stands for the QUANTITY containing the amount of the drug on hand, the number of tablets, capsules, *milliliters*, etc.

X stands for the UNKNOWN amount to be administered.

For example, if 50 *mg* of drug is to be administered to a client and the strength of the drug is 25 *mg* per tablet, then the client would receive 2 tablets. The formula method uses a shorthand for the elements of this illustration: the desired dose is 50 *mg* (*D*); the strength of the drug is 25 *mg*/tablet (H/Q) so the amount on hand is 25 *mg* (*H*) and the quantity containing the 25 *mg* is 1 tablet (*Q*); and finally the amount to be administered is 2 tablets (*X*).

Read the following chart and identify D, H, Q, and X for the formula method.

A. warfarin sodium (Coumadin) 5 *mg* PO daily. How many tablets will you give? The label states 2.5 *mg/tab*.	D = H = Q = X =
B. nifedipine (Procardia) 20 *mg* PO T.I.D. How many capsules will you give? The label states 10 *mg/cap*.	D = H = Q = X =
C. amoxicillin 75 *mg* PO Q.I.D. How many *milliliters* will you give? The label states 125 *mg*/5 *mL*.	D = H = Q = X =

D. digoxin (Lanoxin) 5 *mg* PO daily. How many tablets will you give? The label states 250 *mcg/tab*.	D = H = Q = X =
E. potassium chloride 15 *mEq* PO daily. How many milliequivalents will you give? The label states 20 *mEq*/15 *mL*.	D = H = Q = X =

Here are the answers:

A. warfarin sodium (Coumadin) 5 *mg* PO daily. How many tablets will you give? The label states 2.5 *mg*/*tab*.	D = 5 *mg* H = 2.5 *mg* Q = 1 *tab* X = ? *tab*
B. nifedipine (Procardia) 20 *mg* PO T.I.D. How many capsules will you give? The label states 10 *mg*/*cap*.	D = 20 *mg* H = 10 *mg* Q = 1 *cap* X = ? *cap*
C. amoxicillin 75 *mg* PO Q.I.D. How many *milliliters* will you give? The label states 125 *mg*/5 *mL*.	D = 75 *mg* H = 125 *mg* Q = 5 *mL* X = ? *mL*
D. digoxin (Lanoxin) 5 *mg* PO daily. How many tablets will you give? The label states 250 *mcg*/*tab*.	D = 5 *mg* H = 250 *mcg* Q = 1 *tab* X = ? *tab*
E. potassium chloride 15 *mEq* PO daily. How many milliequivalents will you give? The label states 20 *mEq*/15 *mL*.	D = 15 *mEq* H = 20 *mEq* Q = 15 *mL* X = ? *mL*

For comparison purposes, here is a typical oral medication problem that is done by using the **formula, ratio & porportion,** and **dimensional analysis methods**. Suppose the order is *Tegretol 400 mg po b.i.d.* The Tegretol on hand is in the form of 200-*mg* tablets. How many tablets will you administer?

Using the Formula Method

D: The desired dose is **400** ***mg***.

H & Q: To find *H* and *Q*, the strength of the drug $\frac{200\ mg}{1\ tablet}$ is thought of as $\frac{H}{Q}$. The amount of the drug on hand (H) is **200** ***mg***, and the quantity (Q) containing 200 *mg* of drug is **1 tablet**.

X: The unknown amount to be administered is**? tablets**.

Fill in the formula $\frac{D}{H} \times Q = X$

$$\frac{400\ mg}{200\ mg} \times 1\ tab = ?\ tab$$

Cancel $$\frac{\overset{2}{\cancel{400}}\ \cancel{mg}}{\underset{1}{\cancel{200}}\ \cancel{mg}} \times 1\ tab = ?\ tab$$

Multiply $2 \times 1\ tab = 2\ tab$

Using Ratio & Proportion

You want to convert the prescribed dose of 400 *mg* to the number of tablets to be administered.

Think of the problem this way:

$$400\ mg = x\ tab \quad \text{(dose)}$$
$$200\ mg = 1\ tab \quad \text{(strength)}$$

Substitute into the proportion

$$\frac{400\ mg}{x\ tab} = \frac{200\ mg}{1\ tab}$$

Eliminate the units of measurement, cross multiply, and simplify

$$\frac{400}{x} = \frac{200}{1}$$
$$(200)(x) = (400)(1)$$
$$200x = 400$$

Divide both sides of the equation by 200, the coefficient of x

$$\frac{200x}{200} = \frac{400}{200}$$

Simplify

$$\frac{\cancel{200}x}{\cancel{200}} = \frac{400}{200}$$
$$x = 2$$

Using Dimensional Analysis

You must convert the dose of 400 *mg* to tablets.

$$400\ mg = ?\ tab$$

Cancel the *milligrams* and obtain the equivalent amount in tablets

$$400\ mg \times \frac{?\ tab}{?\ mg} = \textbf{? tab}$$

Use the strength to obtain the unit fraction. Because 1 *tab* = 200 *mg*, the fraction is $\frac{1\ tab}{200\ mg}$

$$\frac{400\ \cancel{mg}}{1} \times \frac{1\ tab}{200\ \cancel{mg}} = \textbf{2 tab}$$

Each of the above three methods gives the same answer of 2 tablets. In this chapter all of the examples can be solved by any one of these methods. The formula method, along with one of the other methods, are illustrated in most of the remaining examples in this chapter.

Example 6.1

The order reads *butabarbital sodium (Butisol Sodium) 60 mg PO 60 min before surgery*. Read the drug label shown in Figure 6.1. How many tablets of this preoperative sedative will you administer to the client?

(Continued)

Figure 6.1 Drug label for butabarbital sodium (Butisol Sodium).

SOURCE: Meda Pharmaceuticals Inc.

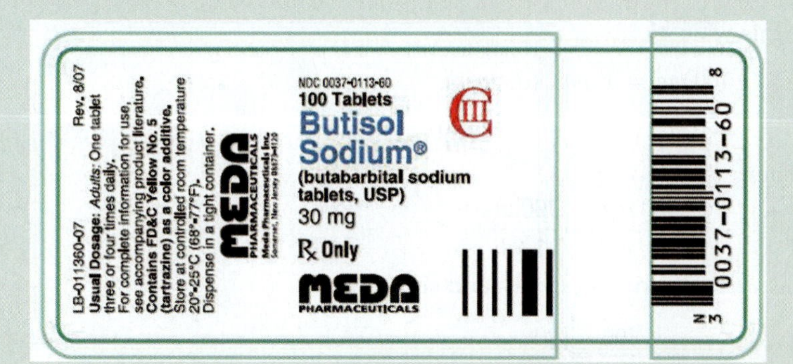

FORMULA METHOD

D (desired dose) = 60 *mg*

H (dose on hand) = 30 *mg*

Q (dosage unit) = 1 *tab*

X (unknown) = ? *tab*

Fill in the formula $\frac{D}{H} \times Q = X$

$$\frac{60\ mg}{30\ mg} \times 1\ tab = ?\ tab$$

Cancel

$$\frac{\overset{2}{\cancel{60}}\ \cancel{mg}}{\underset{1}{\cancel{30}}\ \cancel{mg}} \times 1\ tab = ?\ tab$$

Multiply $2 \times 1\ tab = 2\ tab$

DIMENSIONAL ANALYSIS

Convert 60 *mg* to tablets

$$60\ mg = ?\ tab$$

Cancel the *milligrams* and calculate the equivalent amount in capsules

$$60\ mg \times \frac{?\ tab}{?\ mg} = ?\ tab$$

Because the label indicates that each tablet contains 30 *mg*, use the unit fraction $\frac{1\ tab}{30\ mg}$

$$\overset{2}{\cancel{60}}\ \cancel{mg} \times \frac{1\ tab}{\underset{1}{\cancel{30}}\ \cancel{mg}} = 2\ tab$$

So, you would give 2 tablets by mouth 60 *minutes* before surgery.

NOTE

D and *H* must always be the same unit of measurement, and *Q* and *X* must always be the same unit of measurement before you can use the formula method.

NOTE

Throughout this textbook, when calculating dosages to be administered to the client, do your calculations for *one dose* of medication, unless otherwise directed.

Example 6.2

Each day a client receives 40 *mg* of duloxetine (Cymbalta). Read the drug label shown in Figure 6.2 and determine how many capsules of this drug for the treatment of a major depressive disorder are given to the client each day.

Figure 6.2 Drug label for duloxetine (Cymbalta).

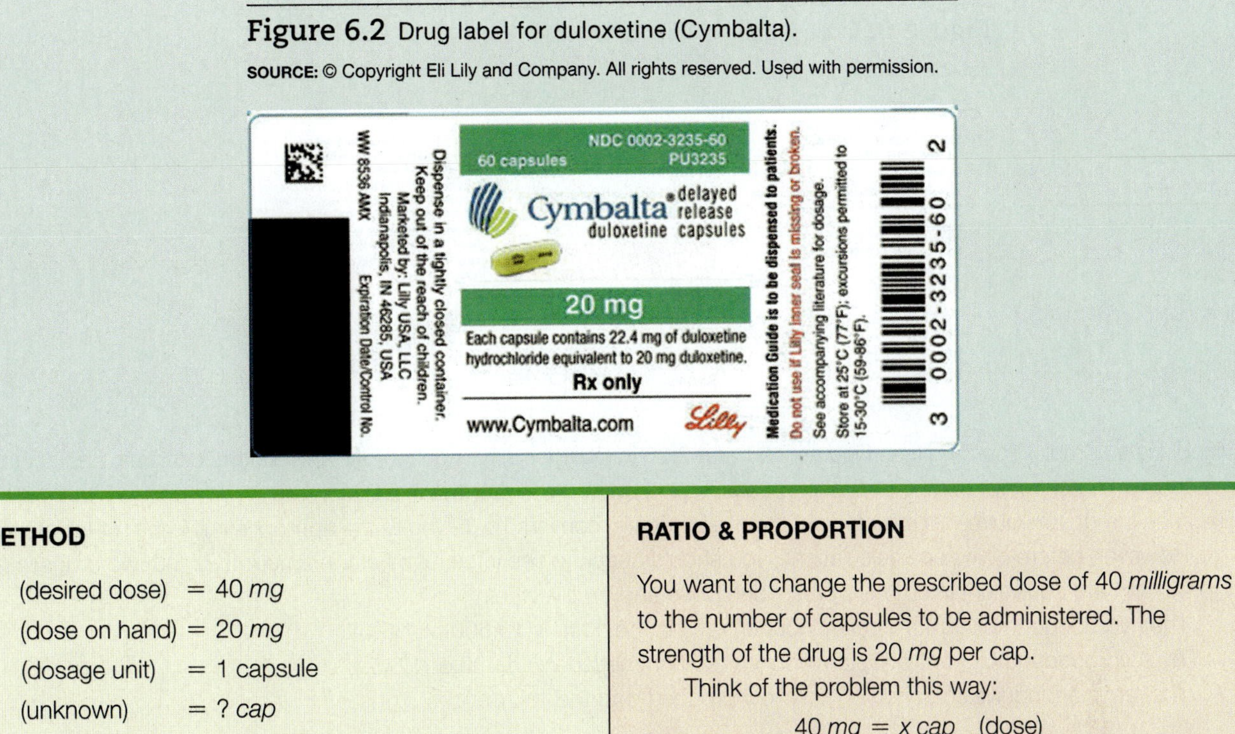

METHOD

D (desired dose) = 40 *mg*

H (dose on hand) = 20 *mg*

Q (dosage unit) = 1 capsule

X (unknown) = ? *cap*

Fill in the formula $\frac{D}{H} \times Q = X$

$$\frac{40\ mg}{20\ mg} \times 1\ cap = ?\ cap$$

Cancel $\frac{\overset{2}{\cancel{40}}\ \cancel{mg}}{\underset{1}{\cancel{20}}\ \cancel{mg}} \times 1\ cap = ?\ cap$

Multiply $2 \times 1\ cap = 2\ cap$

RATIO & PROPORTION

You want to change the prescribed dose of 40 *milligrams* to the number of capsules to be administered. The strength of the drug is 20 *mg* per cap.

Think of the problem this way:

$40\ mg = x\ cap$ (dose)

$20\ mg = 1\ cap$ (strength)

One way to set up the proportion is

$$\frac{40\ mg}{x\ cap} = \frac{20\ mg}{1\ cap}$$

Eliminate the units of measurement, cross multiply, and simplify

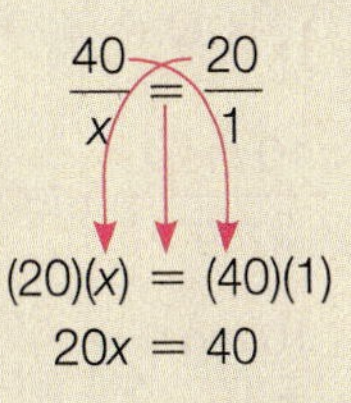

$$\frac{40}{x} = \frac{20}{1}$$

$$(20)(x) = (40)(1)$$

$$20x = 40$$

Divide both sides of the equation by 20, the coefficient of x

$$\frac{20x}{20} = \frac{40}{20}$$

Simplify

$$\frac{\cancel{20}x}{\cancel{20}} = \frac{40}{20}$$

$$x = 2$$

So, 2 capsules are given to the client each day.

Example 6.3

Read the label in Figure 6.3. How many tablets of this narcotic analgesic will be needed for a dose containing 10 *mg* of hydrocodone bitartrate and 600 *mg* of acetaminophen?

(Continued)

Figure 6.3 Drug label for Vicodin.

SOURCE: Courtesy of AbbVie

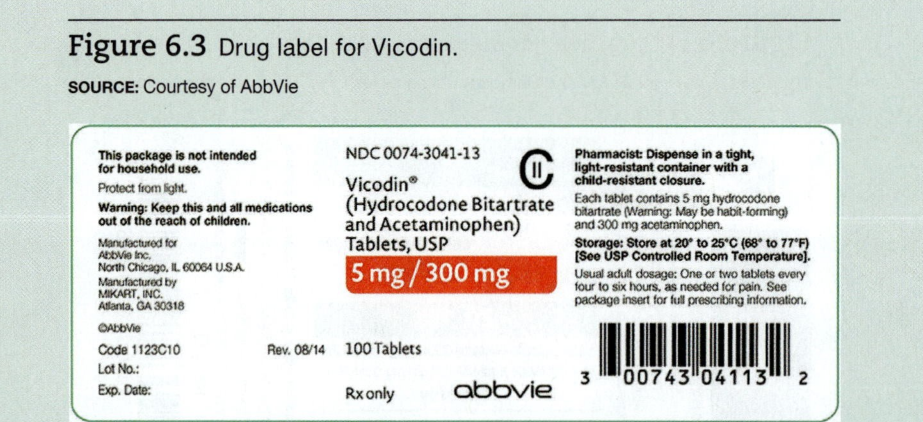

Vicodin is a combination drug (see Figures 2.24 and 2.25 in Chapter 2) composed of hydrocodone bitartrate and acetaminophen. Therefore, for computational purposes, you need address only the first listed drug (hydrocodone bitartrate). Because the dose requires 10 *mg* of hydrocodone bitartrate, convert the 10 *mg* to the appropriate number of tablets.

However, before doing any calculations, you should check to see if the ratios of the amounts of the two drugs in Vicodin are equivalent in *both* the prescribed *dose* and on the *label*.

The hydrocodone bitartrate–acetaminophen ratio in the *dose* is 10:600 or 1:60.

The hydrocodone bitartrate–acetaminophen ratio on the *label* is 5:300 or 1:60.

The ratios are equivalent, and you can now proceed with the calculations.

FORMULA METHOD

D (desired dose) = 10 *mg*

H (dose on hand) = 5 *mg*

Q (dosage unit) = 1 tablet

X (unknown) = ? tab

Fill in the formula $\frac{D}{H} \times Q = X$

$$\frac{10\ mg}{5\ mg} \times 1\ tab = ?\ tab$$

Cancel $$\frac{\overset{2}{\cancel{10}}\ \cancel{mg}}{\underset{1}{\cancel{5}}\ \cancel{mg}} \times 1\ tab = ?\ tab$$

Multiply $2 \times 1\ tab = 2\ tab$

DIMENSIONAL ANALYSIS

$$10\ mg = ?\ tab$$

Cancel the *milligrams* and obtain the equivalent amount in tablets

$$10\ \cancel{mg} \times \frac{?\ tab}{?\ \cancel{mg}} = ?\ tab$$

The label indicates that one tablet contains 5 *mg* of hydrocordone bitartrate.

Because 1 tab = 5 *mg*, the unit fraction is $\frac{1\ tab}{5\ mg}$

$$\overset{2}{\cancel{10}}\ \cancel{mg} \times \frac{1\ tab}{\underset{1}{\cancel{5}}\ \cancel{mg}} = 2\ tab$$

Because 2 tablets contain 10 *mg* of hydrocordone bitartrate and 600 *mg* of acetaminophen, 2 tablets would be needed for this dose.

NOTE

The chance of medication error increases as the number of tablets to be administered increases. Also, you need to consider the comfort of the client who is required to swallow a large number of tablets. Many individuals do not like to take medication, and they may be reluctant to swallow large quantities of tablets.

Example 6.4

The order is for *valsartan (Diovan) 160 mg PO daily*. The medication is available in three different strengths, see Figure 6.4. Determine how you would administer this dose using the fewest number of the available tablets.

Figure 6.4 valsartan (Diovan) drug labels of three different strengths.

SOURCE: Courtesy of Novartis Pharma AG

NDC 0078-0423-15	NDC 0078-0358-34	NDC 0078-0359-34
Diovan® 40 mg	Diovan® 80 mg	Diovan® 160 mg
valsartan	valsartan	valsartan
30 Scored Tablets	90 Tablets	90 Tablets
Rx only	Rx only	Rx only
NOVARTIS	NOVARTIS	NOVARTIS

The 160 *mg* dose could be administered in any of the following ways:

- One 160 *mg* tablet
- Two 80 *mg* tablets
- One 80 *mg* tablet and two 40 *mg* tablets
- Four 40 *mg* tablets

Because you want to administer the fewest number of tablets, you would choose to administer one 160 *mg* tablet.

Medication in Liquid Form

Because pediatric and geriatric clients, as well as clients with neurological conditions, may be unable to swallow medication in tablet form, sometimes oral medications are ordered in liquid form. The label states how much drug is contained in a given amount of liquid.

For medications supplied in liquid form, you must calculate the volume of the liquid that contains the prescribed drug dosage. Medication cups, oral syringes, or calibrated droppers are used to measure the dose. See Figure 6.5.

Figure 6.5 Measuring drugs in liquid form (calibrated droppers, oral syringe, and measuring cups).

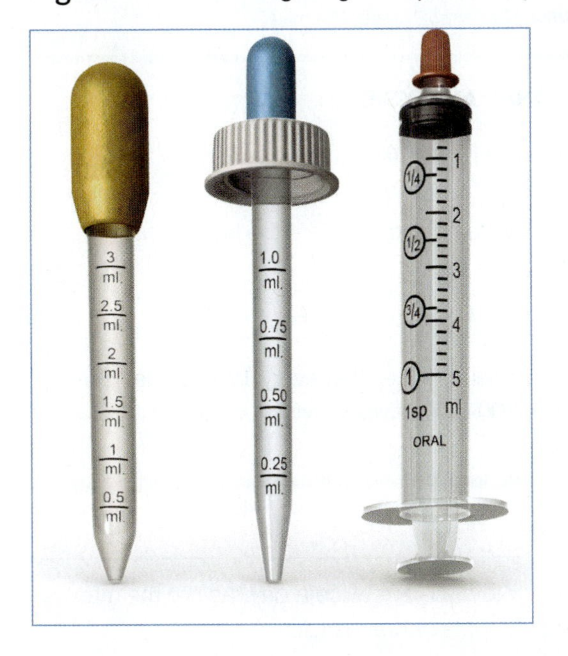

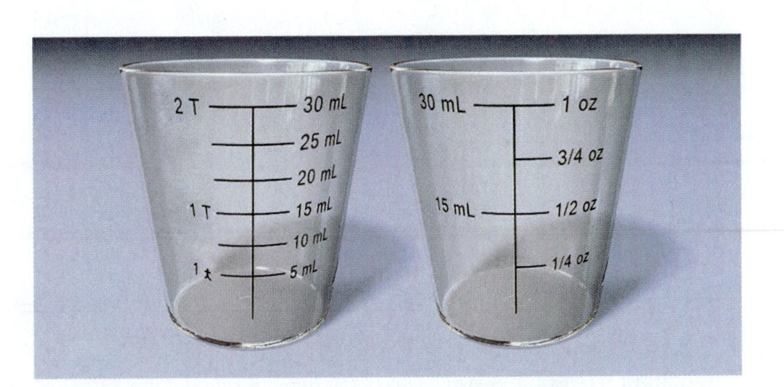

NOTE

Some liquid oral medications are supplied with special calibrated droppers or oral syringes that are used *only* for these medications (e.g., digoxin and Lasix). Some medication cups do not accurately measure amounts less than 5 *mL*.

Example 6.5

The prescriber orders *cyclosporine oral solution (Neoral Oral Solution) 140 mg PO b.i.d.* Read the label in Figure 6.6 and determine how many *milliliters* you will prepare.

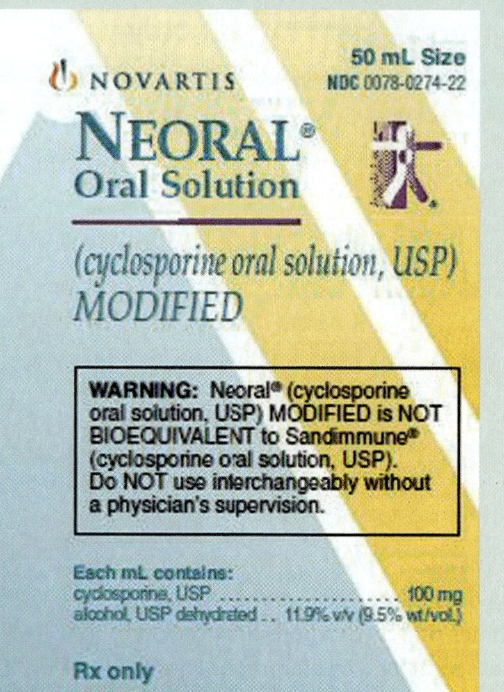

Figure 6.6 Drug label for cyclosporine.

SOURCE: Courtesy of Novartis Pharma AG

FORMULA METHOD

D (desired dose) = 140 *mg*

H (dose on hand) = 100 *mg*

Q (dosage unit) = 1 *mL*

X (unknown) = ? *mL*

Fill in the formula $\frac{D}{H} \times Q = X$

$$\frac{140\ mg}{100\ mg} \times 1\ mL = ?$$

Cancel $\frac{140\ \cancel{mg}}{100\ \cancel{mg}} \times 1\ mL = ?\ mL$

Multiply $1.4 \times 1\ mL = 1.4\ mL$

DIMENSIONAL ANALYSIS

Convert 140 *mg* to *milliliters*

$$140\ mg = ?\ mL$$

Cancel the *milligrams* and calculate the equivalent amount in *mL*

$$140\ mg \times \frac{?\ mL}{?\ mg} = ?\ mL$$

Because the label indicates that every 1 *mL* of the solution contains 100 *mg* of cyclosporine, use the unit fraction $\frac{1\ mL}{100\ mg}$.

$$140\ \cancel{mg} \times \frac{1\ mL}{100\ \cancel{mg}} = 1.4\ mL$$

So, you would administer 1.4 *mL* of this immunosuppressive drug by mouth to the client twice a day. As per the manufacturer's directions you would add the 1.4 *mL* of cyclosporine to 30 *mL* of apple or orange juice.

Example 6.6

The prescriber orders *azithromycin oral suspension 500 mg PO stat, then 250 mg for four days*. Read the label in Figure 6.7 and determine the number of *milliliters* you will administer to the client for the stat dose.

Figure 6.7 Drug label for azithromycin.

SOURCE: Copyright TEVA, Used with permission

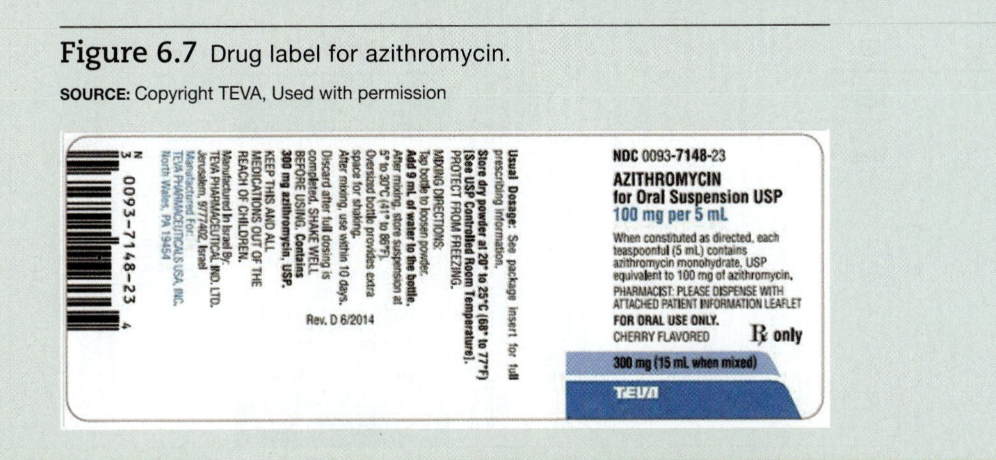

FORMULA METHOD

D (desired dose) = 500 *mg*
H (dose on hand) = 100 *mg*
Q (dosage unit) = 5 *mL*
X (unknown) = ? *mL*

Fill in the formula $\frac{D}{H} \times Q = X$

$$\frac{500\ mg}{100\ mg} \times 5\ mL = ?\ mL$$

Cancel $\frac{500\ \cancel{mg}}{100\ \cancel{mg}} \times 5\ mL = ?\ mL$

Multiply $5 \times 5\ mL = 25\ mL$

DIMENSIONAL ANALYSIS

Convert 500 *milligrams* to *milliliters*

$$500\ mg = ?\ mL$$

Cancel the *milligrams* and calculate the equivalent amount in *mL*

$$500\ \text{mg} \times \frac{?\ mL}{?\ mg} = ?\ mL$$

Because the label indicates that every 5 *mL* of the solution contains 100 *mg* of azithromycin, use the unit fraction $\frac{5\ mL}{100\ mg}$.

$$500\ \cancel{mg} \times \frac{5\ ml}{100\ \cancel{mg}} = 25\ mL$$

So, you would give 25 *mL* of this antibiotic by mouth to the client immediately. See Figure 6.8.

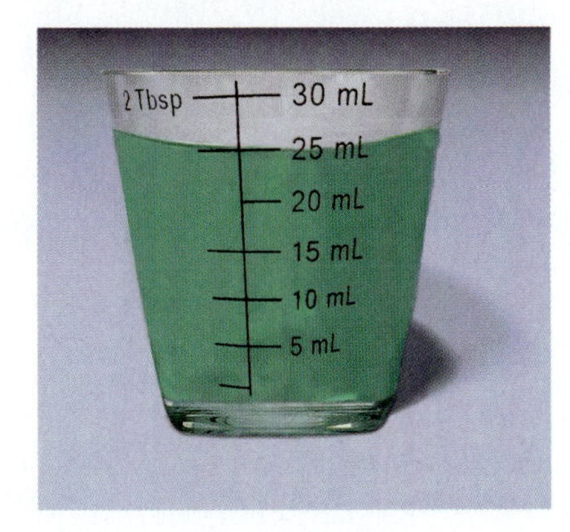

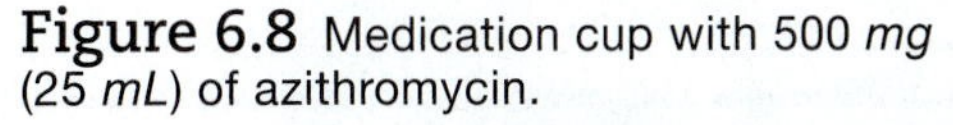
Figure 6.8 Medication cup with 500 *mg* (25 *mL*) of azithromycin.

Example 6.7

The physician orders *Omnicef (cefdinir) 500 mg PO q12h*. Read the label in Figure 6.9. Determine the number of *mL* you would administer to the client.

(Continued)

Figure 6.9 Drug label for Omnicef.

SOURCE: Courtesy of AbbVie

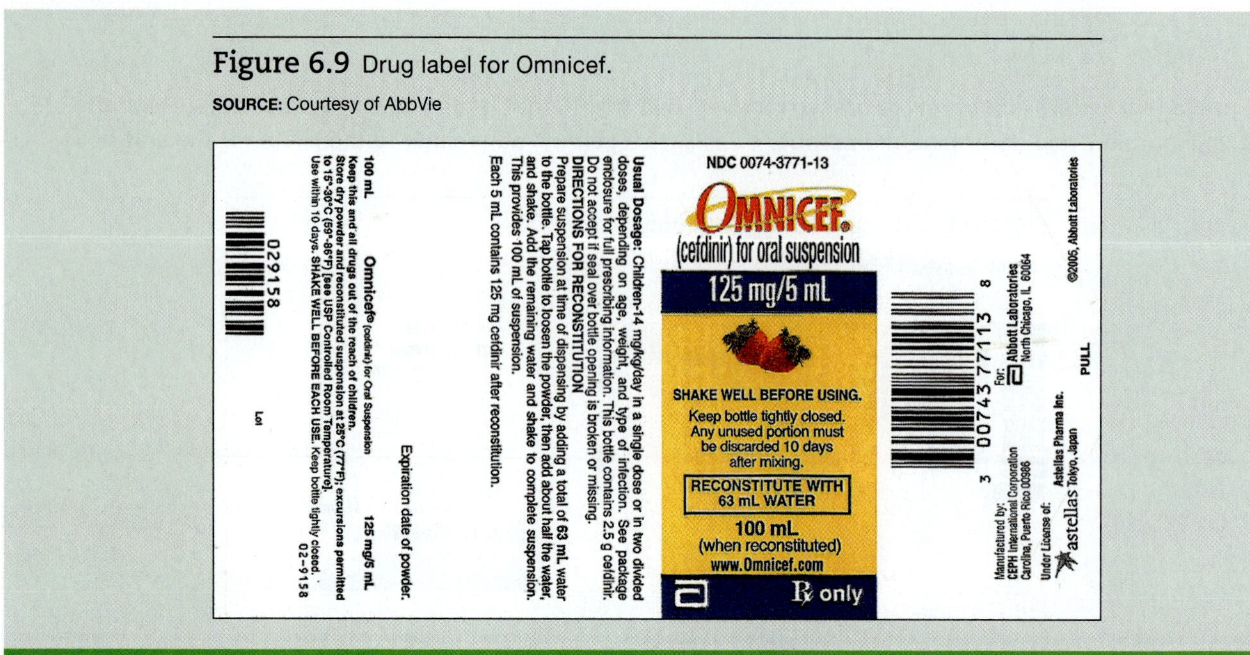

FORMULA METHOD

D (desired dose) = 500 *mg*

H (dose on hand) = 125 *mg*

Q (dosage unit) = 5 *mL*

X (unknown) = ? *mL*

Fill in the formula $\frac{D}{H} \times Q = X$

$$\frac{500\ mg}{125\ mg} \times 5\ mL = ?\ mL$$

Cancel $$\frac{\overset{4}{\cancel{500\ mg}}}{\underset{1}{\cancel{125\ mg}}} \times 5\ ml = ?\ mL$$

Multiply $4 \times 5\ mL = 20\ mL$

RATIO & PROPORTION

You want to change the 500 *mg* dose prescribed to *milliliters*. The strength of the drug is 12.5 *mg* per 5 *mL*.

Think of the problem this way:

$$500\ mg = x\ mL \quad \text{(dose)}$$
$$125\ mg = 5\ mL \quad \text{(strength)}$$

One way to set up the proportion is

$$\frac{500\ mg}{x\ mL} = \frac{125\ mg}{5\ mL}$$

Eliminate the units of measurement, cross multiply, and simplify

$$\frac{500}{x} = \frac{125}{5}$$

$$(125)(x) = (500)(5)$$
$$125x = 2{,}500$$
$$x = \frac{2{,}500}{125}$$
$$x = 20$$

So, you would give 20 *mL* of this antibiotic by mouth every 12 *hours* to the client. See Figure 6.10.

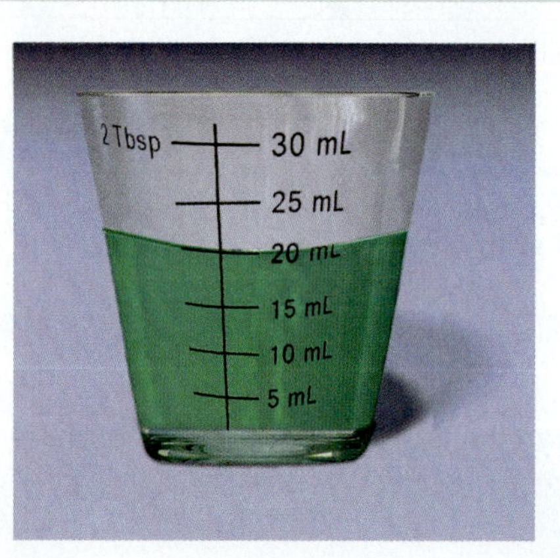

Figure 6.10 Medication cup with 500 *mg* (20 *mL*) of Omnicef.

Medications Measured in Milliequivalents

Some drugs are measured in **milliequivalents**, which are abbreviated as *mEq*. A milliequivalent is an expression of the number of *grams* of a drug contained in one milliliter of solution. Pharmaceutical companies label electrolytes (sodium chloride, potassium chloride, and calcium chloride, for example) in *milligrams* as well as in milliequivalents.

NOTE

In Example 6.8, the order states "in three divided doses." This instructs the practitioner to separate the total daily dose into 3 equal parts over a 24-hour period. To ensure even distribution of the medication, the frequency of the doses should also be regular and consistent, so the drug is administered every 8 *hours*.

Example 6.8

Order: *potassium chloride 30 mEq PO daily in three divided doses.* Read the label in Figure 6.11 and determine how many tablets of this electrolyte supplement you should administer.

Figure 6.11 Drug label for K-Tab.

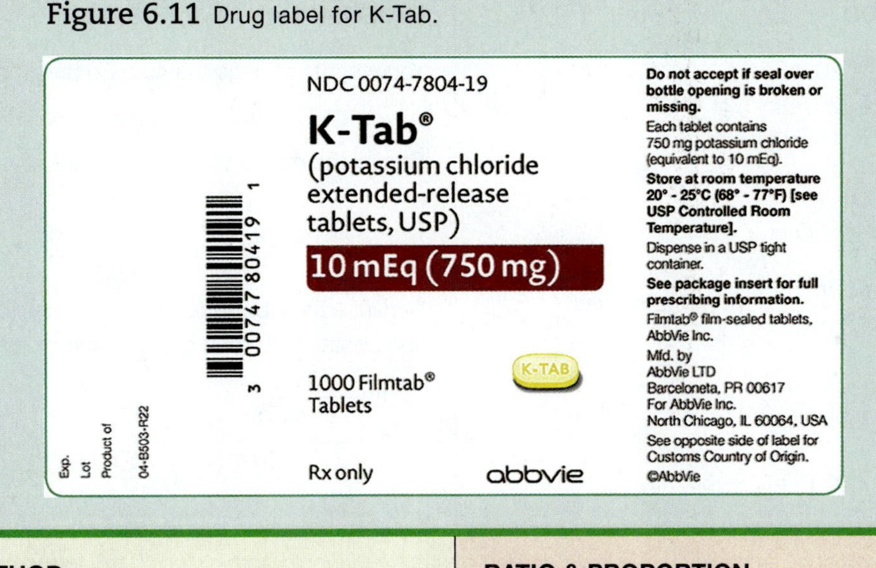

FORMULA METHOD

D (desired dose) = 30 *mEq*
H (dose on hand) = 10 *mEq*
Q (dosage unit) = 1 tab
X (unknown) = ? tab

Fill in the formula $\frac{D}{H} \times Q = X$

$$\frac{30\ mEq}{10\ mEq} \times 1\ tab = ?\ tab$$

Cancel $$\frac{\overset{3}{\cancel{30}}\ \cancel{mEq}}{\underset{1}{\cancel{10}}\ \cancel{mEq}} \times 1\ tab = ?\ tab$$

Multiply $$3 \times 1\ tab = 3\ tab$$

RATIO & PROPORTION

Think of the problem this way:

30 *mEq* = *x* tab (dose)
10 *mEq* = 1 tab (strength)

One way to set up the proportion is

$$\frac{30\ mEq}{x\ tab} = \frac{10\ mEq}{1\ tab}$$

Eliminate the units of measurement, cross multiply, and simplify

$$\frac{30}{x} = \frac{10}{1}$$

$$10x = 30$$

$$x = 3$$

Because the order indicates "three divided doses," you would administer 1 tablet of K-Tab every 8 *hours*.

Example 6.9

The prescriber ordered *potassium chloride 40 mEq po daily in two divided doses.* Read the label in Figure 6.12 and determine the number of *milliliters* of this electrolyte supplement that you would administer.

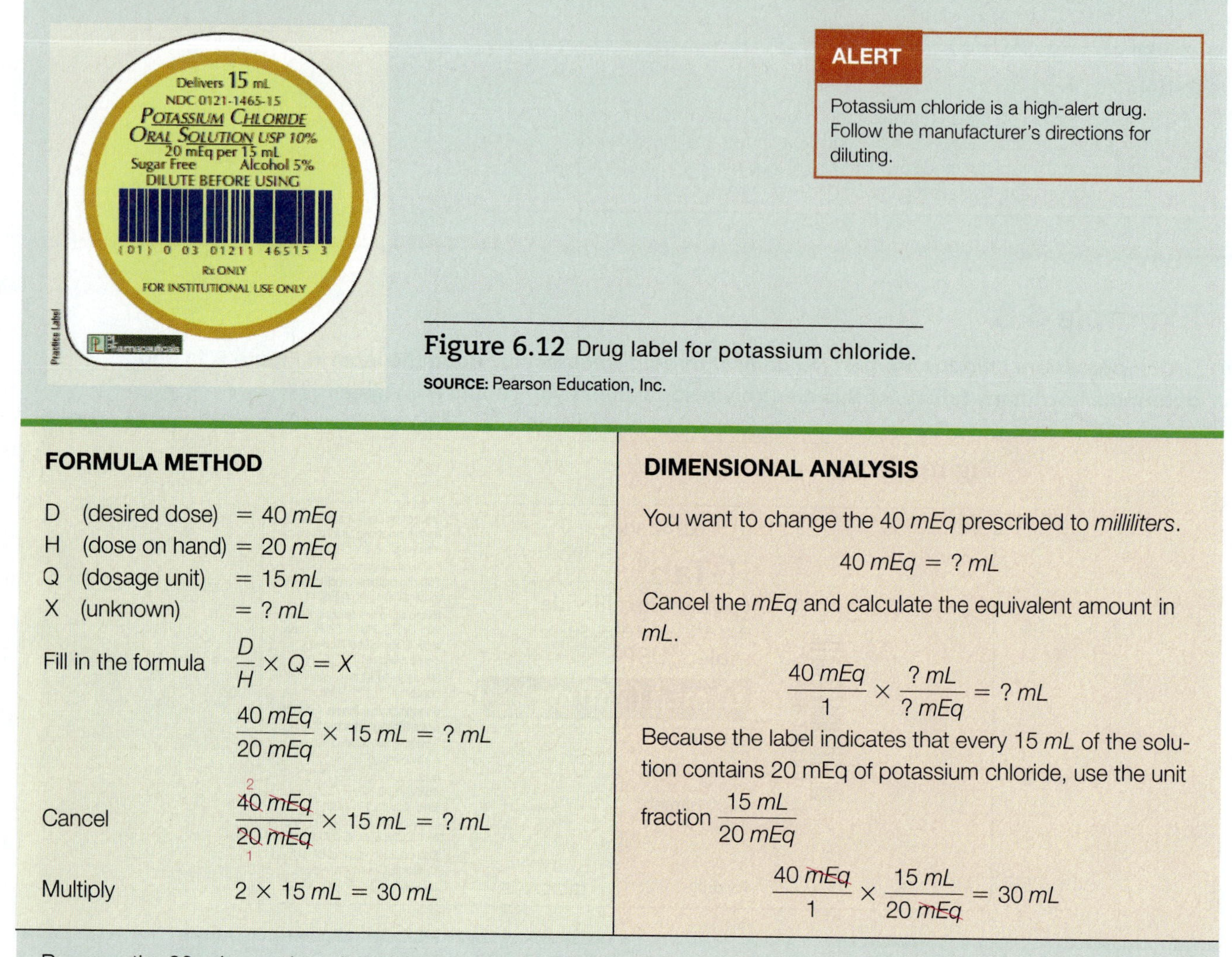

Figure 6.12 Drug label for potassium chloride.

SOURCE: Pearson Education, Inc.

ALERT

Potassium chloride is a high-alert drug. Follow the manufacturer's directions for diluting.

FORMULA METHOD

D (desired dose) = 40 *mEq*
H (dose on hand) = 20 *mEq*
Q (dosage unit) = 15 *mL*
X (unknown) = ? *mL*

Fill in the formula $\frac{D}{H} \times Q = X$

$$\frac{40\ mEq}{20\ mEq} \times 15\ mL = ?\ mL$$

Cancel $\frac{\overset{2}{\cancel{40}}\ \cancel{mEq}}{\underset{1}{\cancel{20}}\ \cancel{mEq}} \times 15\ mL = ?\ mL$

Multiply $2 \times 15\ mL = 30\ mL$

DIMENSIONAL ANALYSIS

You want to change the 40 *mEq* prescribed to *milliliters.*

$$40\ mEq = ?\ mL$$

Cancel the *mEq* and calculate the equivalent amount in *mL*.

$$\frac{40\ mEq}{1} \times \frac{?\ mL}{?\ mEq} = ?\ mL$$

Because the label indicates that every 15 *mL* of the solution contains 20 mEq of potassium chloride, use the unit fraction $\frac{15\ mL}{20\ mEq}$

$$\frac{40\ \cancel{mEq}}{1} \times \frac{15\ mL}{20\ \cancel{mEq}} = 30\ mL$$

Because the 30 *mL* must be administered in "two divided doses," you would administer 15 *mL* to the client.

Complex (Multistep) Problems

Sometimes dosage calculations will require that multiplication by unit fractions be repeated one or more times. Recall that we examined complex problems in Chapter 3.

For example, if each tablet of a drug contains 1.25 *mg*, how many tablets would contain 0.0025 gram? This problem is done below using three different approaches.

Using Dimensional Analysis

For complex problems, it helps to organize the information you will need for the computation as follows:

Given quantity	0.0025 *g* [*single unit of measurement*]
Strength	1 *tab* = 1.25 *mg* [*equivalence*]
Quantity you want to find	? *tab* [*single unit of measurement*]

Because you want to find a *single unit of measurement* (? tablets), you must start with a *single unit of measurement* (0.0025 *g*). The *equivalence* (1 *tab* = 1.25 *mg*) will be used to form a unit fraction. So, the problem is

$$0.0025\ g = ?\ tab$$

You do not know the direct equivalence between *grams* and tablets. This is a **complex** problem because you need to first convert 0.0025 *grams* to *milligrams*, and then convert the *milligrams* to tablets.

$$0.0025\ g \longrightarrow ?\ mg \longrightarrow ?\ tab$$

First, you want to cancel *grams (g)*. To do this you must use an equivalence containing *grams* to make a unit fraction with *grams* in the denominator. Because the equivalence is 1 *g* = 1,000 *mg*, the unit fraction is $\frac{1{,}000\ mg}{1\ g}$

$$0.0025\ \cancel{g} \times \frac{1{,}000\ mg}{1\ \cancel{g}} = ?\ tab$$

After the *grams* are cancelled, only *milligrams* remain on the left side. Now you need to change the *milligrams* to *tablets*. Because the strength is 1.25 *mg* = 1 *tab*, the unit fraction is $\frac{1\ tab}{1.25\ mg}$

$$0.0025\ \cancel{g} \times \frac{1{,}000\ \cancel{mg}}{1\ \cancel{g}} \times \frac{1\ tab}{1.25\ \cancel{mg}} = ?\ tab$$

After cancelling the *milligrams*, only tablets remain on the left side. Now complete your calculation by multiplying the numbers.

$$0.0025\ \cancel{g} \times \frac{1{,}000\ \cancel{mg}}{1\ \cancel{g}} \times \frac{1\ tab}{1.25\ \cancel{mg}} = \frac{2.5\ tab}{1.25} = 2\ tab$$

Using Ratio & Proportion and Moving the Decimal Point

You want to change 0.0025 *g* to tablets. The strength of the tablets is 1.25 *mg* per tab.

Think of the problem this way:

0.0025	*g*	= *x tab*	(dose)
1.25	*mg*	= 1 *tab*	(strength)

Notice that the *g* and *mg* do not match. Therefore, a conversion must be done before you can set up a proportion. In this case, change 0.0025 *g* to an equivalent amount of *milligrams*.

kilogram	gram	milligram	microgram
kg	g	mg	mcg

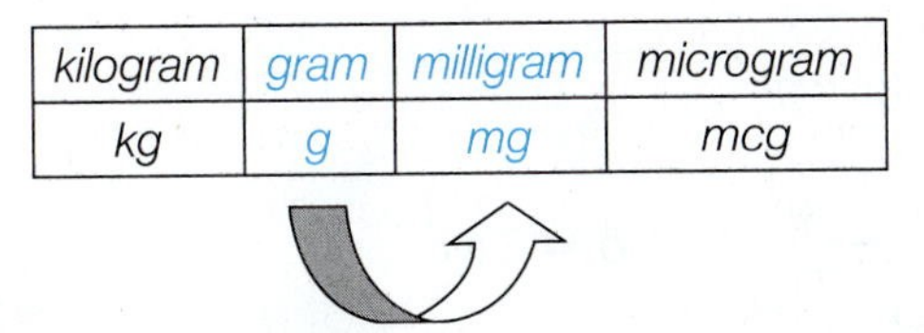

Move the decimal point *3 places to the right*

$$0.0025\ g = 0.0025\ g = 0002.5\ mg = 2.5\ mg$$

Now, think of the problem this way:

$$2.5\ mg = x\ tab \quad \text{(dose)}$$

$$1.25\ mg = 1\ tab \quad \text{(strength)}$$

One way to set up the proportion is

$$\frac{2.5\ mg}{x\ tab} = \frac{1.25\ mg}{1\ tab}$$

Eliminate the units of measurement, cross multiply, and simplify

$$\frac{2.5}{x} = \frac{1.25}{1}$$

$$1.25x = 2.5$$

$$x = 2$$

Using Moving the Decimal Point and the Formula Method

D (desired dose) = 0.0025 *g*

H (dose on hand) = 1.25 *mg*

Q (dosage unit) = 1 *tab*

X (unknown) = ? *tab*

D and H are not in the same units of measurement. To use the formula method, the units of measurement of D and H must match. Also, the units of measurement of Q and X must match.

This is a complex problem because first you need to convert 0.0025 *grams* to an equivalent amount of *milligrams* before you can apply the formula. You can do this by moving the decimal point *3 places to the right*.

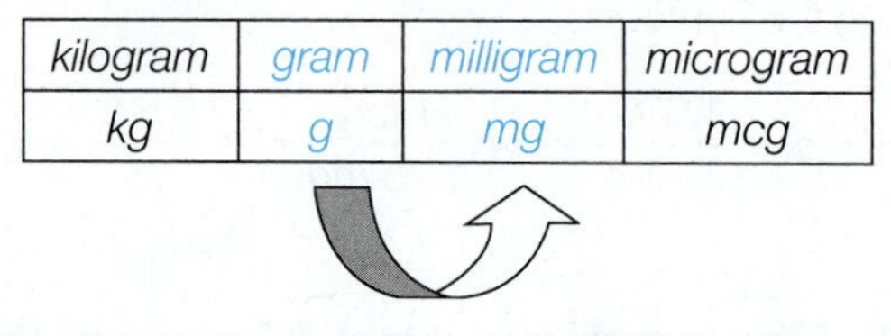

kilogram	gram	milligram	microgram
kg	g	mg	mcg

$$0.0025\ g = 0.002.5\ g = 000.25\ mg = 2.5\ mg$$

Now, both D and H match; they are in *milligrams*, and you have:

D (desired dose) = 2.5 *mg*

H (dose on hand) = 1.25 *mg*

Q (dosage unit) = 1 *tab*

X (unknown) = ? *tab*

Fill in the formula $\frac{D}{H} \times Q = X$

$$\frac{2.5\ mg}{1.25\ mg} \times 1\ tab = ?\ tab$$

Cancel $\frac{\overset{2}{\cancel{2.5\ mg}}}{\underset{1}{\cancel{1.25\ mg}}} \times 1\ tab = ?\ tab$

Multiply $2 \times 1\ tab = 2\ tab$

So, two 1.25 *mg* tablets contains 0.0025 *grams*.

Example 6.10

How many 300-*mg* Ziagen (abacavir sulfate) tablets contain 0.9 *g* of Ziagen?

FORMULA METHOD

D (desired dose) = 0.9 *g*
H (dose on hand) = 300 *mg*
Q (dosage unit) = 1 *tab*
X (unknown) = ? *tab*

D and H do not match. This is a complex problem because you first need to convert 0.9 *g* to an equivalent amount of *milligrams*.

kilogram	gram	milligram	microgram
kg	g	mg	mcg

Move the decimal point *3 places to the right*

0.9 *g* = 0.900 *g* = **0. 9 0 0 *g*** = 0900. *mg* = 900 *mg*

D (desired dose) = 900 *mg*
H (dose on hand) = 300 *mg*
Q (dosage unit) = 1 *tab*
X (unknown) = ? *tab*

Now, D and H match.

Fill in the formula $\frac{D}{H} \times Q = X$

$$\frac{900\ mg}{300\ mg} \times 1\ tab = ?\ tab$$

Cancel $\frac{\overset{3}{\cancel{900}}\ \cancel{mg}}{\underset{1}{\cancel{300}}\ \cancel{mg}} \times 1\ tab = ?\ tab$

Multiply $3 \times 1\ tab = 3\ tab$

RATIO & PROPORTION

You want to change 0.9 *g* to tablets. The strength of the tablets is 300 *mg* per tab.

Think of the problem this way:

0.9 *g* = *x tab* (dose)
300 *mg* = 1 *tab* (strength)

Notice that the *g* and *mg* do not match. Therefore, a conversion must be done before you can set up a proportion. In this case, change 0.09 *g* to an equivalent amount of *milligrams*.

kilogram	gram	milligram	microgram
kg	g	mg	mcg

Move the decimal point *3 places to the right*

0.9 *g* = 0.900 *g* = **0. 9 0 0 *g*** = 0900. *mg* = 900 *mg*

Now, think of the problem this way:

900 *mg* = *x tab* (dose)
300 *mg* = 1 *tab* (strength)

One way to set up the proportion is

$$\frac{900\ mg}{x\ tab} = \frac{300\ mg}{1\ tab}$$

Eliminate the units of measurement, cross multiply, and simplify

$$\frac{900}{x} = \frac{300}{1}$$

$$300x = 900$$

$$x = 3$$

So, three 300-*mg* tablets contain 0.9 *g* of Ziagen.

Example 6.11

Read the label in Figure 6.13 to determine the number of carbamazepine (Tegretol) tablets that would contain a dose of 0.4 *g*.

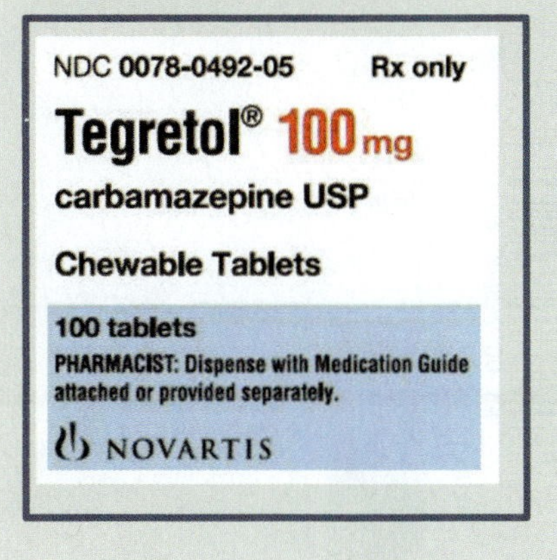

Figure 6.13 Drug label for carbamazepine (Tegretol).

SOURCE: Courtesy of Novartis Pharma AG

(Continued)

FORMULA METHOD

D (desired dose) = 0.4 *g*
H (dose on hand) = 100 *mg*
Q (dosage unit) = 1 *tab*
X (unknown) = ? *tab*

You need to first convert 0.4 *g* to an equivalent amount of *milligrams*.

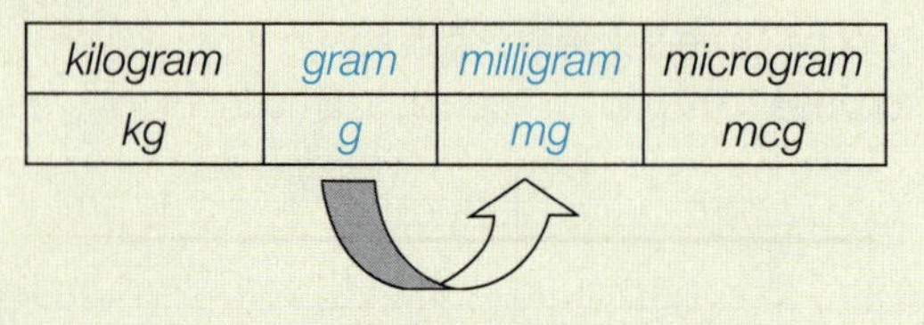

kilogram	*gram*	*milligram*	*microgram*
kg	*g*	*mg*	*mcg*

Move the decimal point *3 places to the right*

0.4 *g* = 0.400 *g* = **0. 4 0 0 *g*** = 0400. *mg* = 400 *mg*

Fill in the formula 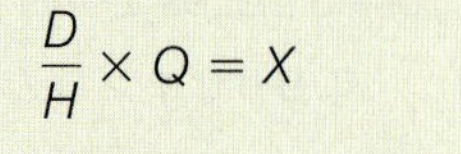 $\frac{D}{H} \times Q = X$

$$\frac{400\ mg}{100\ mg} \times 1\ tab = ?\ tab$$

Cancel $\frac{\cancel{400\ mg}}{\cancel{100\ mg}} \times 1\ tab = ?\ tab$

Multiply $4 \times 1\ tab = 4\ tab$

DIMENSIONAL ANALYSIS

Given quantity: 0.4 *g*
Strength: 1 *tab* = 100 *mg*
Quantity you want to find: ? *tab*

In this problem you want to convert 0.4 gram to *milligrams* and then convert *milligrams* to tablets.

$$0.4\ g \longrightarrow ?\ mg \longrightarrow ?\ tab$$

You can do this on one line as follows

$$0.4\ g \times \frac{?\ mg}{?\ g} \times \frac{?\ tab}{?\ mg} = ?\ tab$$

Because 1,000 *mg* = 1 *g*, the first unit fraction is $\frac{1{,}000\ mg}{1\ g}$

Because 100 *mg* = 1 *tab*, the second unit fraction is $\frac{1\ tab}{100\ mg}$

$$0.4\ \cancel{g} \times \frac{\overset{10}{\cancel{1{,}000\ mg}}}{1\ \cancel{g}} \times \frac{1\ tab}{\underset{1}{\cancel{100\ mg}}} = 4\ tab$$

So, 4 tablets will contain 0.4 *g* of the drug.

NOTE

Although Example 6.12 would be simpler using *milligrams*, we do the calculation using *micrograms* to practice complex problems. For safety purposes, drug manufacturers often place both microgram and *milligram* concentrations on drug labels.

Example 6.12

The order is *Tikosyn (dofetilide) 0.5 mg PO b.i.d*. Read the label shown in Figure 6.14. Calculate how many capsules of this antiarrythmic drug should be given to the client. Although there are two strengths on the label (*mcg* and *mg*), calculate the problem using microgram strength.

Figure 6.14 Drug label for Tikosyn.

(Reg. trademark of Pfizer Inc. Reproduced with permission.)

Store at controlled room temperature, 15° to 30°C (59° to 86°F).
PROTECT FROM MOISTURE AND HUMIDITY.
Dispense in tight containers (USP).
DOSAGE AND USE
See accompanying prescribing information.
Each capsule contains 125 mcg (0.125 mg) dofetilide.
NDC 0069-5800-60
60 Capsules Rx only
Tikosyn®
(dofetilide)
125
125 mcg (0.125 mg)
Pfizer Pfizer Labs
Division of Pfizer Inc, NY, NY 10017
N3 0069-5800-60 3
7400
MADE IN USA
05-5549-32-2

FORMULA METHOD

D (desired dose) = *0.5 mg*
H (dose on hand) = *125 mcg*
Q (dosage unit) = 1 *cap*
X (unknown) = ? *cap*

You need to first convert 0.5 *milligrams* to an equivalent amount of *micrograms*.

kilogram	*gram*	*milligram*	*microgram*
kg	*g*	*mg*	*mcg*

Move the decimal point *3 places to the right*

0.5 *g* = 0.500 *g* = **0.5 0 0 *g*** = 0500. *mcg* = 500 *mcg*

Fill in the formula $\frac{D}{H} \times Q = X$

$$\frac{500\ mcg}{125\ mcg} \times 1\ cap = ?\ cap$$

Cancel $$\frac{\overset{4}{\cancel{500\ mcg}}}{\underset{1}{\cancel{125\ mcg}}} \times 1\ cap = ?\ cap$$

Multiply $4 \times 1\ cap = 4\ cap$

RATIO & PROPORTION

Think of the problem this way:

0.5 *mg* = *x cap* (dose)
125 *mcg* = 1 *cap* (strength)

Notice that the *mg* and *mcg* do not match. Therefore, a conversion must be done before you can set up a proportion. In this case, change 0.5 *mg* to an equivalent amount of *micrograms*.

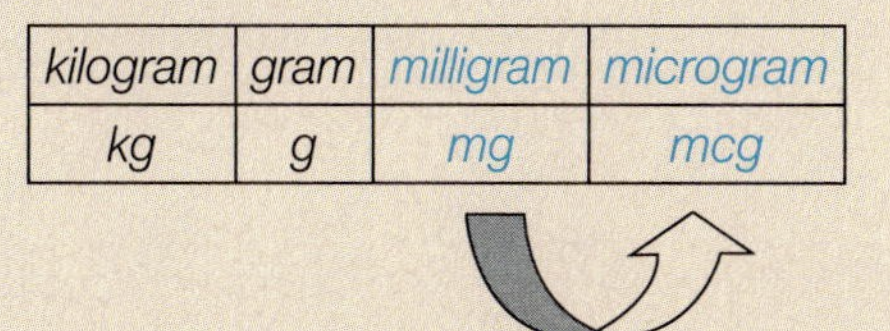

kilogram	*gram*	*milligram*	*microgram*
kg	*g*	*mg*	*mcg*

Move the decimal point *3 places to the right*

0.5 *mg* = 0.500 *mg* = **0.5 0 0 *mg*** = **0500. *mcg*** = 500 *mcg*

Now, think of the problem this way:

500 *mcg* = *x cap* (dose)
125 *mcg* = 1 *cap* (strength)

One way to set up the proportion is

$$\frac{500\ mcg}{x\ cap} = \frac{125\ mcg}{1\ cap}$$

Eliminate the units of measurement, cross multiply, and simplify

$$\frac{500}{x} = \frac{125}{1}$$

$$125x = 500$$
$$x = 4$$

So, you should give 4 capsules by mouth twice a day to the client.

Example 6.13

The order is *Daypro (oxaprozin) 1.8 g PO once daily each morning*. The drug is supplied as 600 *mg* per caplet. How many caplets of this anti-inflammatory drug should be given to the client?

FORMULA METHOD

D (desired dose) = *1.8 g*
H (dose on hand) = *600 mg*
Q (dosage unit) = 1 cap
X (unknown) = cap

You need to first convert 1.8 *g* to an equivalent amount of *milligrams*.

DIMENSIONAL ANALYSIS

Given quantity: 1.8 *g*
Strength: 1 cap = 600 *mg*
Quantity you want to find: ? cap

In this problem you want to convert 1.8 *grams* to *milligrams* and then convert *milligrams* to caplets.

1.8 *g* ⟶ ? *mg* ⟶ ? cap

(Continued)

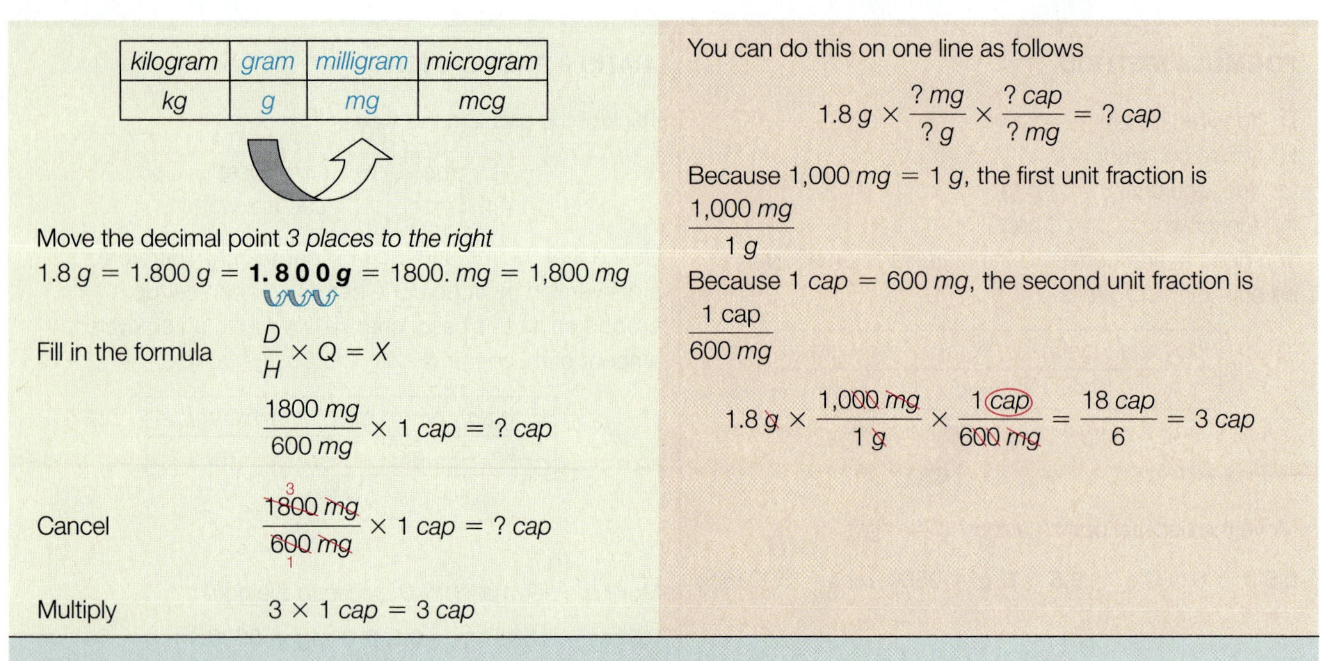

kilogram	*gram*	*milligram*	*microgram*
kg	*g*	*mg*	*mcg*

Move the decimal point *3 places to the right*

$1.8\ g = 1.800\ g = \mathbf{1.800\ g} = 1800.\ mg = 1{,}800\ mg$

Fill in the formula $\frac{D}{H} \times Q = X$

$$\frac{1800\ mg}{600\ mg} \times 1\ cap = ?\ cap$$

Cancel $$\frac{\overset{3}{\cancel{1800}}\ \cancel{mg}}{\underset{1}{\cancel{600}}\ \cancel{mg}} \times 1\ cap = ?\ cap$$

Multiply $3 \times 1\ cap = 3\ cap$

You can do this on one line as follows

$$1.8\ g \times \frac{?\ mg}{?\ g} \times \frac{?\ cap}{?\ mg} = ?\ cap$$

Because $1{,}000\ mg = 1\ g$, the first unit fraction is $\frac{1{,}000\ mg}{1\ g}$

Because $1\ cap = 600\ mg$, the second unit fraction is $\frac{1\ cap}{600\ mg}$

$$1.8\ \cancel{g} \times \frac{1{,}00\cancel{0}\ \cancel{mg}}{1\ \cancel{g}} \times \frac{1\ cap}{60\cancel{0}\ \cancel{mg}} = \frac{18\ cap}{6} = 3\ cap$$

So, you should give 3 caplets by mouth to the client once a day in the morning.

Example 6.14

The physician orders *Norvir (ritonavir) 0.6 g PO b.i.d.* Read the label in Figure 6.15 and determine the number of *mL* of this protease inhibitor your client would receive.

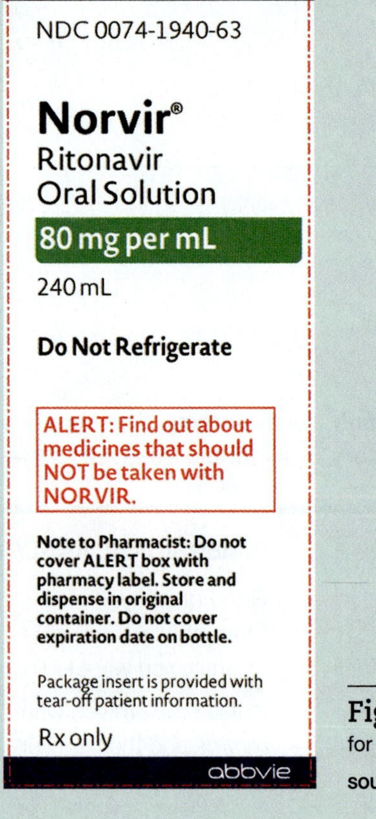

Figure 6.15 Drug label for Norvir.

SOURCE: Courtesy of AbbVie

FORMULA METHOD

D (desired dose) = 0.6 *g*
H (dose on hand) = 80 *mg*
Q (dosage unit) = 1 *mL*
X (unknown) = ? *mL*

You need to first convert 0.6 *g* to an equivalent amount of *milligrams*.

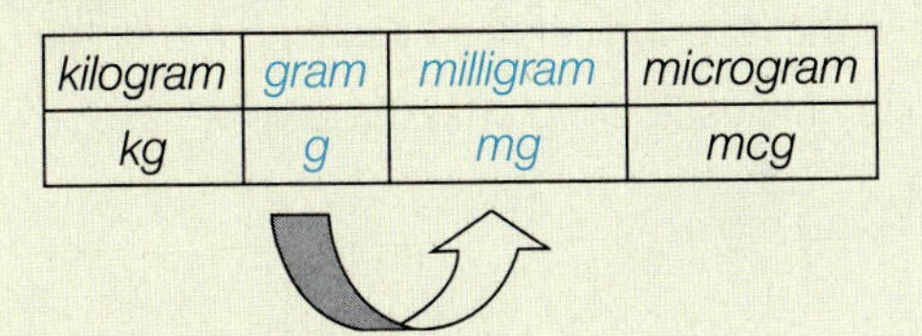

kilogram	gram	milligram	microgram
kg	g	mg	mcg

Move the decimal point *3 places to the right*

$0.6\ g = 0.600\ g = \mathbf{0.6\,0\,0\ g} = \mathbf{600.}\ mg = 600\ mg$

Fill in the formula $\frac{D}{H} \times Q = X$

$$\frac{600\ mg}{80\ mg} \times 1\ mL = ?\ mL$$

Cancel $\frac{\overset{15}{\cancel{600}}\ \cancel{mg}}{\underset{2}{\cancel{80}}\ \cancel{mg}} \times 1\ mL = ?\ mL$

Multiply $\frac{15}{2} \times 1\ mL = 7.5\ mL$

RATIO & PROPORTION

Think of the problem this way:

0.6 | g | = *x mL* (dose)
80 | mg | = 1 *mL* (strength)

Notice that the *g* and *mg* do not match. Therefore, a conversion must be done before you can set up a proportion. In this case, change 0.6 *g* to an equivalent amount of *milligrams*.

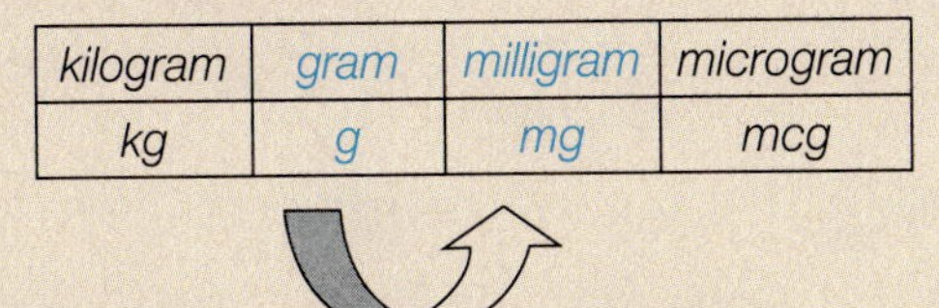

kilogram	gram	milligram	microgram
kg	g	mg	mcg

Move the decimal point *3 places to the right*

$0.6\ g = 0.600\ g = \mathbf{0.6\,0\,0\ g} = \mathbf{600.\ mg} = 600\ mg$

Now, think of the problem this way:

600 *mg* = *x mL* (dose)
80 *mg* = 1 *mL* (strength)

One way to set up the proportion is

$$\frac{600\ mg}{x\ mL} = \frac{80\ mg}{1\ mL}$$

Eliminate the units of measurement, cross multiply, and simplify

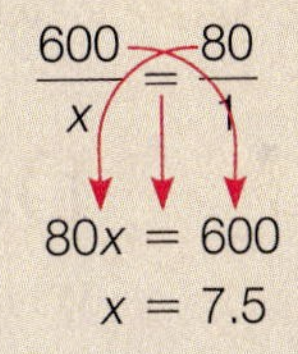

$$\frac{600}{x} = \frac{80}{1}$$

$$80x = 600$$

$$x = 7.5$$

So, you would give 7.5 *mL* by mouth to the client.

Example 6.15

For a client with bronchitis the prescriber orders *clarithromycin oral suspension (Biaxin) 500 mg PO q12h for 14 days*. Read the label in Figure 6.16 and determine the number of *milliliters* you will administer to the client.

Figure 6.16 Drug label for clarithromycin oral suspension (Biaxin).

SOURCE: Courtesy of AbbVie

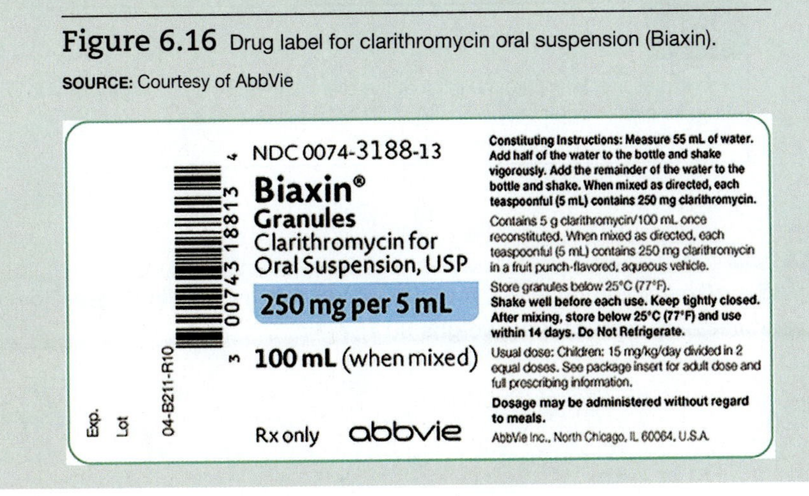

(Continued)

FORMULA METHOD

D (desired dose) = 500 *mg*
H (dose on hand) = 250 *mg*
Q (dosage unit) = 5 *mL*
X (unknown) = ? *mL*

Fill in the formula $\frac{D}{H} \times Q = X$

$$\frac{500\ mg}{250\ mg} \times 5\ mL = ?\ mL$$

Cancel $\frac{500\ \cancel{mg}}{250\ \cancel{mg}} \times 5\ mL = ?\ mL$

Multiply $2 \times 5\ mL = 10\ mL$

DIMENSIONAL ANALYSIS

Convert 500 *milligrams* to *milliliters*

$$500\ mg = ?\ mL$$

Cancel the *milligrams* and calculate the equivalent amount in *mL*

$$500\ mg \times \frac{?\ mL}{?\ mg} = ?\ mL$$

Because the label indicates that every 5 *mL* of the solution contains 250 *mg* of azithromycin, use the unit fraction $\frac{5\ mL}{250\ mg}$.

$$500\ \cancel{mg} \times \frac{5\ ml}{250\ \cancel{mg}} = 10\ mL$$

So, you would give 10 *mL* by mouth to the client every 12 *hours*.

Dosages Based on the Size of the Client

Sometimes the amount of medication prescribed is based on the client's size. A client who is larger will receive a larger dose of the drug, and a client who is smaller will receive a smaller dose of the drug. The size of a client is measured by either *body weight* or *body surface area* (*BSA*). In general, when the order is based on the size of the client, if you multiply the *size of the client* by the *order*, you will obtain the *dose*. This can be expressed by the shortcut formula:

Size of client × *Order* = *Dose*

Dosages Based on Body Weight

When an order is based on the body weight of the client, the client's weight is expressed in *kilograms*. For example, an order might indicate that the client should receive "*5 g/kg*," which is read "*5 grams per kilogram*," and it means that the client should receive *5 grams* of the drug for each *kilogram* of the client's body weight. Based on such an order, a neonate weighing *1 kg* should receive *5 g* of the drug, another weighing *2 kg* should receive *10 g* of the drug, a baby weighing *3 kg* should receive *15 g* of the drug, and so on.

Whether you use *dimensional analysis*, *ratio & proportion*, or *formula* methods to do the following problems, it is best to start out with **Size of the client × Order** to obtain the Dose.

NOTE

The expression 15 *mg/kg* means that the client is to receive 15 *milligrams* of the drug for each *kilogram* of body weight. Therefore, you will use the equivalent 15 *mg* (of drug) = 1 *kg* (of body weight).

Example 6.16

Order: *Dilantin (phenytoin) 15 mg/kg loading dose PO, then 300 mg/d*. For the loading dose, how many *mg* of this anticonvulsant would you administer to a client who weighs 80 *kg*?

Body weight: 80 *kg*
Order: 15 *mg/kg*
Dose: ? *mg*

FORMULA METHOD

You want to "change" the body weight of the client (80 *kg*) to *milligrams* of drug. The order is 15 *mg/kg*, so use the formula

Size of client × *Order* = *Dose*

$$80\ \cancel{kg} \times \frac{15\ mg}{1\ \cancel{kg}} = 1{,}200\ mg$$

RATIO & PROPORTION

Think of the problem this way:

80 *kg* (body weight) = *x mg* (drug) (dose)
1 *kg* (body weight) = 15 *mg* (drug) (order)

One way to set up the proportion is

$$\frac{80\ kg}{x\ mg} = \frac{1\ kg}{15\ mg}$$

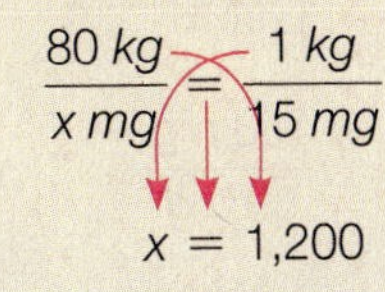

$$x = 1{,}200$$

Therefore, the client should receive 1,200 *mg* of Dilantin for the loading dose.

Example 6.17

Order: *Vibramycin (doxycycline calcium) 2 mg/lb daily PO for 10 days.* Read the label in Figure 6.17 and determine how many *milliliters* of this antibiotic you would administer to a client who weighs 90 *lb*.

Figure 6.17 Drug label for Vibramycin.

SOURCE: Courtesy of Pfizer, Inc.

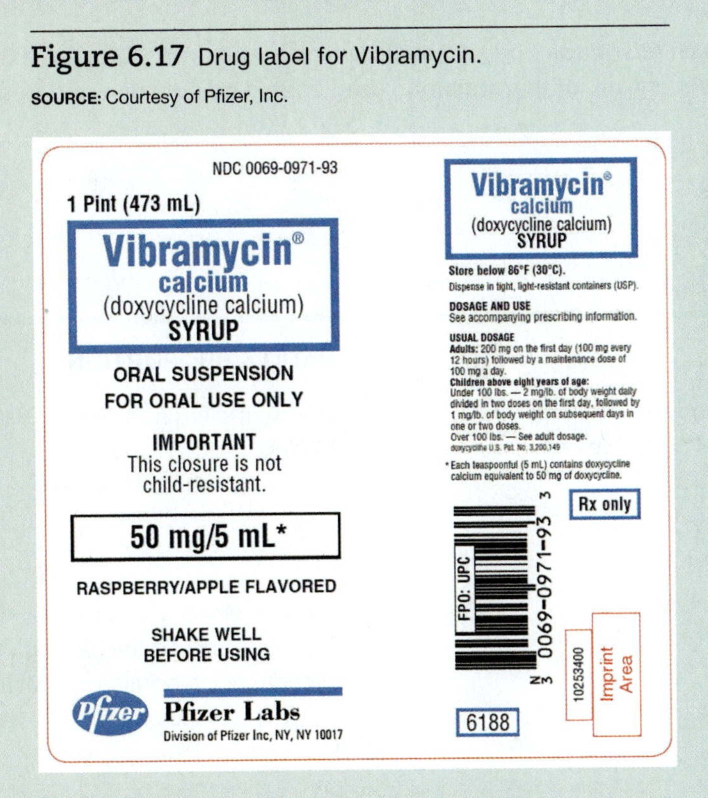

Client weight: 90 *lb*

Order: 2 *mg/lb*

Strength: 50 *mg*/5 *mL*

Administer: ? *mL*

When an order is based on the size of the client, you can use this formula:

Size of the client × Order = Dose

$$\frac{90\ \cancel{lb}}{1} \times \frac{2\ mg}{\cancel{lb}} = 180\ mg$$

(Continued)

FORMULA METHOD

D (desired dose) = 180 *mg*
H (dose on hand) = 50 *mg*
Q (dosage unit) = 5 *mL*
X (unknown) = ? *mL*

Fill in the formula $\frac{D}{H} \times Q = X$

$$\frac{180\ mg}{50\ mg} \times 5\ mL = ?\ mL$$

Cancel and multiply $\frac{180\ \cancel{mg}}{50\ \cancel{mg}} \times 5\ mL = 18\ mL$

DIMENSIONAL ANALYSIS

Now convert the dose of 180 *mg* to *mL*.

$$180\ mg = ?\ mL$$

Because each 5 *mL* of the solution contains 50 *mg* of the drug, the unit fraction is $\frac{5\ mL}{50\ mg}$

$$\frac{180\ \cancel{mg}}{1} \times \frac{5\ mL}{50\ \cancel{mg}} = 18\ mL$$

So, the client should receive 18 *mL* of Vibramycin daily for 10 days.

Example 6.18

The physician orders *Biaxin (clarithromycin) 7.5 milligrams per kilogram PO q12h*. If the drug strength is 250 *milligrams* per 5 *mL*, how many *mL* of this antibiotic drug should be administered to a client who weighs 70 *kilograms*?

Body weight 70 *kg*
Order 7.5 *mg/kg*
Strength 250 *mg*/5 *mL*
Find ? *ml*

FORMULA METHOD

You want to "change" the body weight of the client (70 *kg*) to *milligrams* of drug. The order is 7.5 *mg/kg*, so use the formula

Size of client × Order = Dose

$$70\ \cancel{kg} \times \frac{7.5\ mg}{1\ \cancel{kg}} = 525\ mg$$

Therefore, the client should receive 525 *mg*

D (desired dose) = 525 *mg*
H (dose on hand) = 250 *mg*
Q (dosage unit) = 5 *mL*
X (unknown) = ? *mL*

Fill in the formula $\frac{D}{H} \times Q = X$

$$\frac{525\ mg}{250\ mg} \times 5\ mL = ?\ mL$$

Cancel $\frac{\overset{21}{\cancel{525}}\ \cancel{mg}}{\underset{10}{\cancel{250}}\ \cancel{mg}} \times 5\ mL = ?\ mL$

Multiply $2.1 \times 5\ mL = 10.5\ mL$

RATIO & PROPORTION

The client's weight is 70 *kg* and the order is for 7.5 *mg/kg*. Multiply the *size of the client* by the *order* to determine how many *milligrams* of Biaxin to give the client.

$$70\ \cancel{kg} \times \frac{7.5\ mg}{\cancel{kg}} = 525\ mg$$

So, the client must receive 525 *mg* of Biaxin.

Now, convert the 525 *mg* of Biaxin to *milliliters*. The strength of the solution is 250 *mg*/5 *mL*.

Think of the problem this way:

525 *mg* = *x mL* (dose)
250 *mg* = 5 *mL* (strength)

One way to set up the proportion is

$$\frac{525\ mg}{x\ mL} = \frac{250\ mg}{5\ mL}$$

$$250x = 2{,}626$$
$$x = 10.5$$

The client should receive 10.5 *mL* of Biaxin by mouth every 12 *hours*.

Dosages Based on Body Surface Area

In some cases, **body surface area (BSA)** may be used rather than **weight** in determining appropriate drug dosages. This is particularly true when calculating dosages for children, those receiving cancer therapy, burn clients, and clients requiring critical care. A client's BSA can be estimated by using formulas.

NOTE

Use a search engine, such as Google, to search the Web for "Body Surface Area Calculators" to obtain links to online BSA calculators.

BSA Formulas

Body surface area can be approximated by formula using either a handheld calculator or an online website. BSA, which is measured in square meters (m^2), can be determined by using either of the following two mathematical formulas:

Formula for metric units:

$$BSA = \sqrt{\frac{\text{weight in kilograms} \times \text{height in centimeters}}{3{,}600}}$$

Formula for household units:

$$BSA = \sqrt{\frac{\text{weight in pounds} \times \text{height in inches}}{3{,}131}}$$

Example 6.19

Find the BSA of an adult who is 183 *cm* tall and weighs 92 *kg*.

Because this example has metric units (*kilograms* and *centimeters*), we use the following formula:

$$BSA = \sqrt{\frac{\text{weight in kilograms} \times \text{height in centimeters}}{3{,}600}}$$

$$= \sqrt{\frac{92 \times 183}{3{,}600}}$$

At this point we need a calculator with a square-root key.

$$= \sqrt{4.6767}$$

$$= 2.16256$$

Therefore, the BSA of this adult is 2.16 m^2.

NOTE

In Example 6.19, the metric formula for BSA is used, and in Example 6.20, the household formula for BSA is used. However, each formula provided the BSA measured in square meters (m^2). In this book, we round off BSA to two decimal places.

Example 6.20

What is the BSA of a man who is 5 *feet* 5 *inches* tall and weighs 150 *pounds*?

First you convert 5 *feet* 5 *inches* to 65 *inches*.

(Continued)

Because the example has household units (pounds and inches), we use the following formula:

$$BSA = \sqrt{\frac{\text{weight in pounds} \times \text{height in inches}}{3{,}131}}$$

$$= \sqrt{\frac{150 \times 65}{3{,}131}}$$

$$= \sqrt{3.11402}$$

$$= 1.7646$$

Therefore, the BSA of this adult is 1.76 m^2.

Example 6.21

The physician orders 40 *mg/m*² of a drug PO once daily. How many *milligrams* of the drug would you administer to an adult client weighing 88 *kg* with a height of 150 *cm*?

The first step is to determine the BSA of the client.

Using the formula, you get

$$BSA = \sqrt{\frac{88 \times 150}{3{,}600}}$$

$$= \sqrt{3.6667}$$

$$= 1.91\ m^2$$

BSA: 1.91 m^2
Order: 40 mg/m^2
Find: ? *mg*

The client's BSA is 1.91 m^2, and the order is for 40 mg/m^2. Multiply the *size of the client* by the *order* to determine how many *milligrams* of the drug to give the client.

$$1.91\ \cancel{m^2} \times \frac{40\ mg}{\cancel{m^2}} = 76.4\ mg$$

You would administer 76.4 *mg* of the drug to the client.

ALERT

Before a medication is administered, it is the responsibility of the health care practitioner administering the medication to check the *safe dosage and administration range* for the drug in the *Physicians' Desk Reference* (PDR), in a designated drug book, on the manufacturer's website, or with the pharmacist.

Example 6.22

The prescriber ordered 30 *mg/m*² of a drug PO stat for a client who has a BSA of 1.65 *m*². The "safe dose range" for this drug is 20 to 40 *mg* per day. Calculate the prescribed dose in *milligrams* and determine if it is within the safe range.

BSA: $1.65\ m^2$
Order: $30\ mg/m^2$
Find: $?\ mg$

The client's BSA is $1.65\ m^2$, and the order is for $30\ mg/m^2$. Multiply the *size of the client* by the *order* to determine how many *milligrams* of the drug to give the client.

$$1.65\ m^2 \times \frac{30\ mg}{m^2} = 49.5\ mg$$

The safe dose range is 20–40 *mg* per day.

So, the dose prescribed, 49.5 *mg*, is higher than the upper limit (40 *mg*) of the daily "safe dose range." It is an overdose. Therefore, the prescribed dose is not safe, and you may not administer this drug. You must consult with the prescriber.

Example 6.23

Order: *leucovorin calcium* 10 *mg/m*^{2} *PO q6h until serum methotrexate level is less than* 10^{-8} *M.* Read the label in Figure 6.18 and calculate how many *tablets* you will administer to a client who has a BSA of 1.49 *m*^{2}. The package information states that these are scored *tablets*.

Figure 6.18 Drug label for leucovorin calcium.

SOURCE: Pearson Education, Inc.

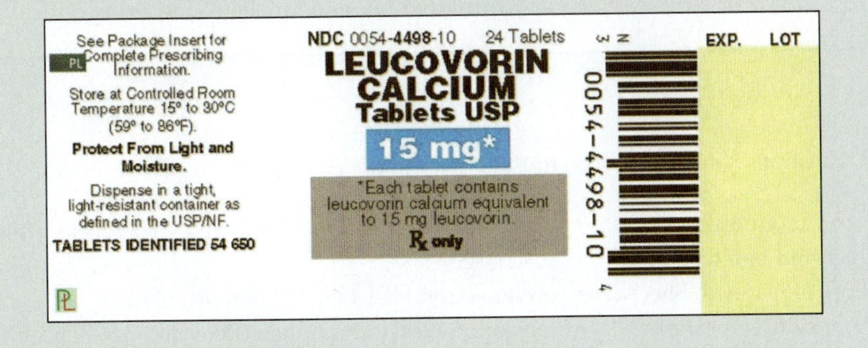

BSA: $1.49\ m^2$ [single unit of measurement]
Order: $10\ mg/m^2$ [equivalence]
Strength: $1\ tab = 15\ mg$ [equivalence]
Administer: $?\ tab$ [single unit of measurement]

The client's BSA is $1.49\ m^2$, and the order is $10\ mg/m^2$. First, multiply the *size of the client* by the *order* to determine how many *milligrams* of the drug to give the client, and then use the strength to change the resulting *milligrams* to tablets. This can be done in one line as follows:

$$1.49\ m^2 \times \frac{10\ mg}{m^2} \times \frac{1\ tab}{15\ mg} = 0.993\ tab$$

So, you will administer 1 *tablet* to the client by mouth every 6 *hours*.

Summary

In this chapter, you learned the computations necessary to calculate dosages of oral medications in liquid and solid form. You also learned about the equipment used to accurately measure liquid medication.

- It is crucial to ensure that every medication administered is within the recommended safe dosage range.

Calculating doses for oral medications in solid and liquid form

- The label states the strength of the drug (e.g., 10 *mg*/tab, 15 *mg*/*mL*).
- Sometimes oral medications are ordered in liquid form for special populations such as pediatrics, geriatrics, and clients with neurological conditions.
- Some medication cups cannot accurately measure volumes less than 5 *mL*.
- Special calibrated droppers or oral syringes that are supplied with some liquid oral medications may be used to administer *only those medications*.
- Some drugs, such as electrolytes, are measured in milliequivalents (mEq).

Calculating dosages using the formula method

- The formula $\frac{D}{H} \times Q = X$ can be used to calculate dosages.
- Always include the units of measurement when setting up the formula.
- *D and H* must always have the same units of measurement, and *Q and X* must have the same units of measurement.
- If the desired dose ordered is in a different unit of measurement than the dose on hand, convert them to the same unit of measurement before using the formula.

Calculating doses based on body weight

- Dosages based on body weight are generally measured in *milligrams* per *kilogram* (*mg*/*kg*).
- Start calculations with the weight of the client.
- Multiply the size of the client (kg) by the order to obtain the dose.
- Size of the Client × Order = Dose
- Medications may be prescribed by body weight in special populations such as pediatrics and geriatrics.

Calculating doses based on body surface area

- Body surface area (BSA) is measured in square meters (m^2).
- Start calculations with the BSA of the client.
- Multiply the size of the client (m^2) by the order to obtain the dose.
- Size of the Client × Order = Dose
- BSA is estimated by using a formula.
- BSA may be utilized to determine dosages for special client populations such as those receiving cancer therapy, burn therapy, and for clients requiring critical care.

Case Study 6.1

Read the case study and answer the questions. Answers can be found in Appendix A.

A 67-year-old female is admitted to the ambulatory surgery center for a repair of her fractured patella. An ORIF (open reduction external fixation) is planned. She has a history of heart failure, hypertension, hyperlipidemia, osteoarthritis, and Parkinson's dementia. She has a past surgical history of four caesarean sections and a cholecystectomy. She is 5 feet 7 inches tall and weighs 150 pounds. She denies any allergies to food or drugs, does not smoke, and drinks wine socially. Her vital signs on admission were: T 98.8° F; B/P 148/94; P 104 R 22. She received a regional block anesthesia, progressed well in the recovery room, and is preparing for discharge home.

Discharge orders

- Knee immobilizer, elevate leg, move toes as much as possible
- Ice to knee 20 *minutes* every hour
- Crutches, non-weight-bearing
- Observe for increased swelling or sudden severe pain
- Make appointment for follow-up care 2 weeks after discharge
- ondansetron HCl 4 *mg* PO q6h prn nausea
- oxycodone/acetaminophen (Percocet) 2.5/325 *mg* PO one or two tab q6h for pain. Take Percocet before becoming too uncomfortable.
- Resume pre-admission medications
  - diltiazem HCl (Cardizem LA) extended-release 180 *mg* PO daily
  - rivastigmine tartrate (Exelon) 3 *mg* PO B.I.D. with meals
  - valsartan (Diovan) 80 *mg* PO daily
  - atorvastatin (Lipitor) 20 *mg* PO daily
  - docusate sodium (Colace) 100 *mg* PO T.I.D.

1. Select the appropriate label and calculate how many tablets of diltiazem HCl the client will take each day.
2. Select the appropriate rivastigmine tartrate label and calculate how many capsules the client will take in 24 *hours*.

3. Select the appropriate valsartan label and calculate the number of tablets the client will take each day.
4. How many tablets of atorvastatin will the client take?
5. The strength on the Colace is 50 *mg* per capsule. How many capsules will the client take each day?
6. Select the appropriate pain medication label and calculate the maximum amount of acetaminophen the client may take in a 24 *h* period.
7. Select the appropriate ondansetron HCl label and determine how many tablets the client would take.

Case Study 6.1 Drug labels.

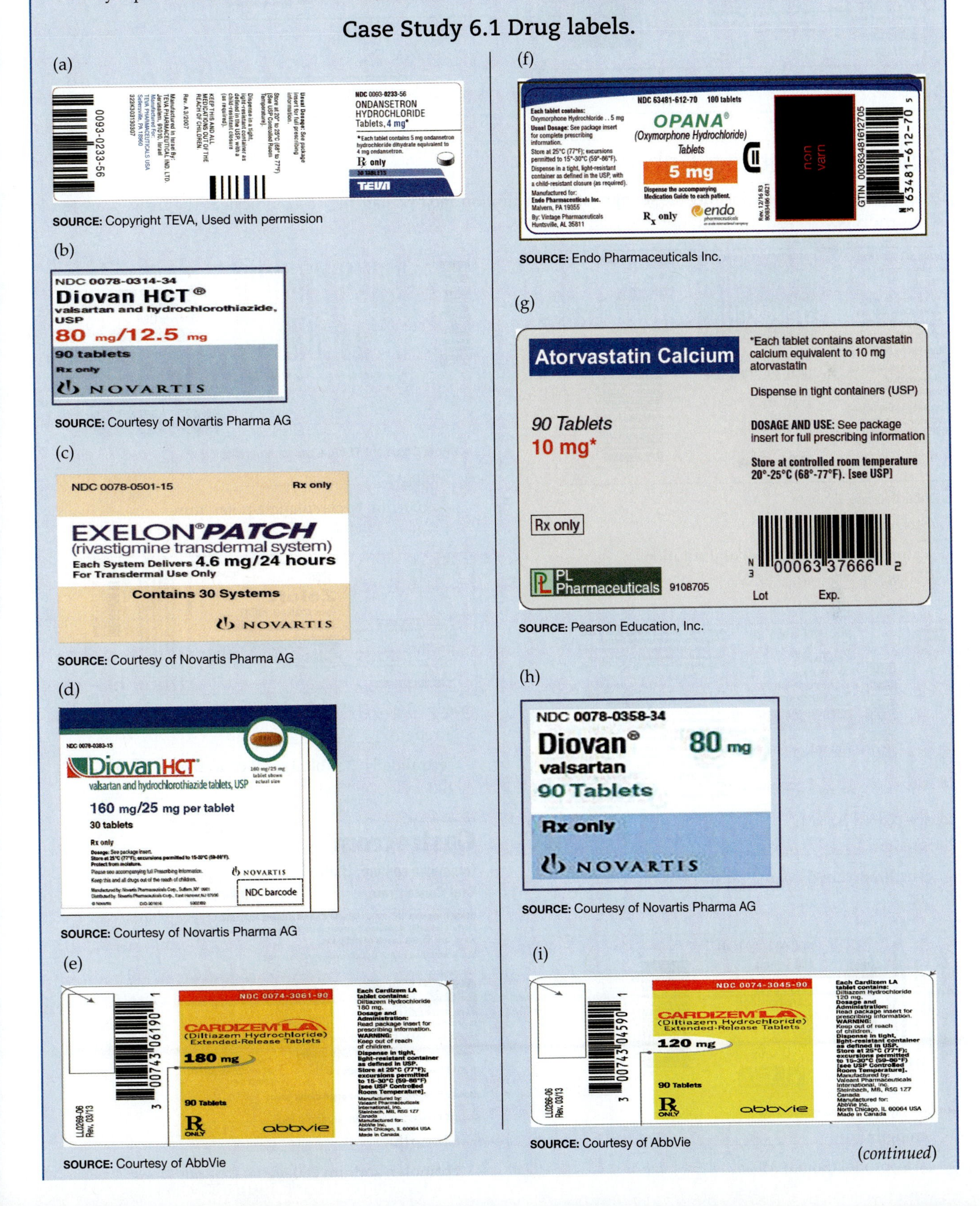

SOURCE: Copyright TEVA, Used with permission

SOURCE: Courtesy of Novartis Pharma AG

SOURCE: Courtesy of Novartis Pharma AG

SOURCE: Courtesy of Novartis Pharma AG

SOURCE: Courtesy of AbbVie

SOURCE: Endo Pharmaceuticals Inc.

SOURCE: Pearson Education, Inc.

SOURCE: Courtesy of Novartis Pharma AG

SOURCE: Courtesy of AbbVie

(continued)

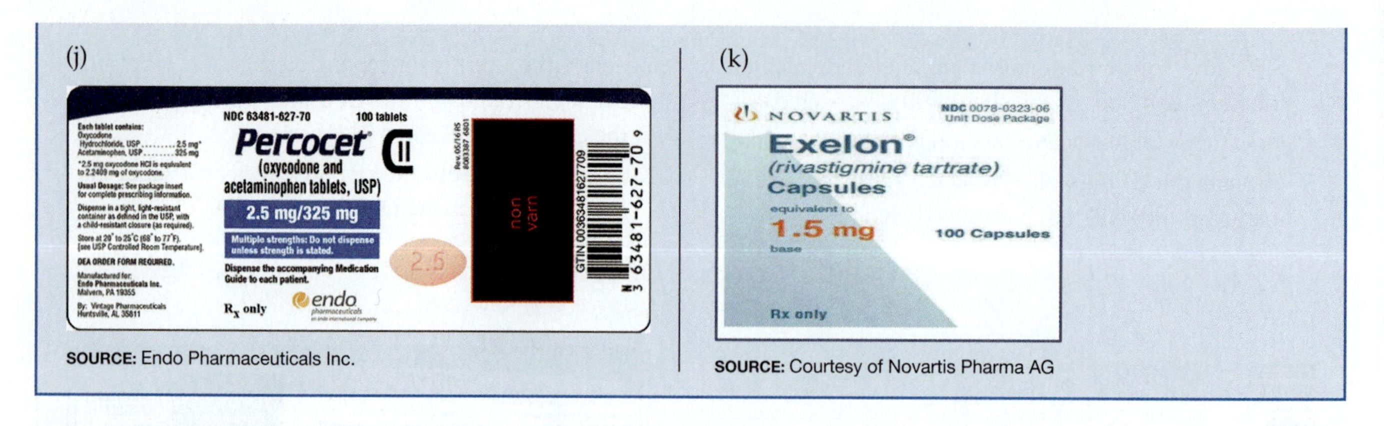

SOURCE: Endo Pharmaceuticals Inc.

SOURCE: Courtesy of Novartis Pharma AG

Practice Reading Labels

Using the following labels, identify the strength of the medication and calculate the doses indicated. The answers are found in Appendix A.

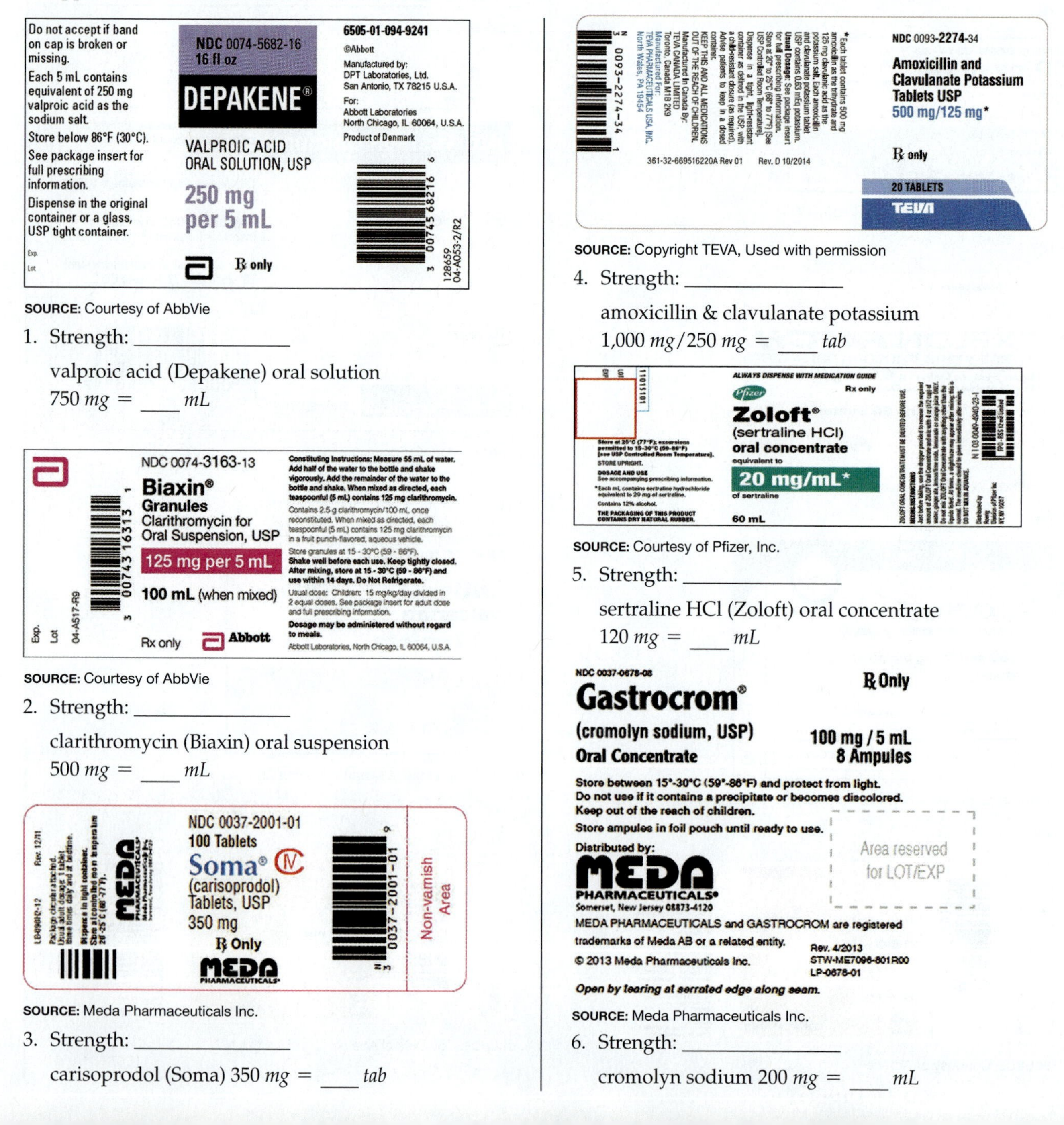

SOURCE: Courtesy of AbbVie

1. Strength: ______________

   valproic acid (Depakene) oral solution

   750 *mg* = ____ *mL*

SOURCE: Courtesy of AbbVie

2. Strength: ______________

   clarithromycin (Biaxin) oral suspension

   500 *mg* = ____ *mL*

SOURCE: Meda Pharmaceuticals Inc.

3. Strength: ______________

   carisoprodol (Soma) 350 *mg* = ____ *tab*

SOURCE: Copyright TEVA, Used with permission

4. Strength: ______________

   amoxicillin & clavulanate potassium

   1,000 *mg*/250 *mg* = ____ *tab*

SOURCE: Courtesy of Pfizer, Inc.

5. Strength: ______________

   sertraline HCl (Zoloft) oral concentrate

   120 *mg* = ____ *mL*

SOURCE: Meda Pharmaceuticals Inc.

6. Strength: ______________

   cromolyn sodium 200 *mg* = ____ *mL*

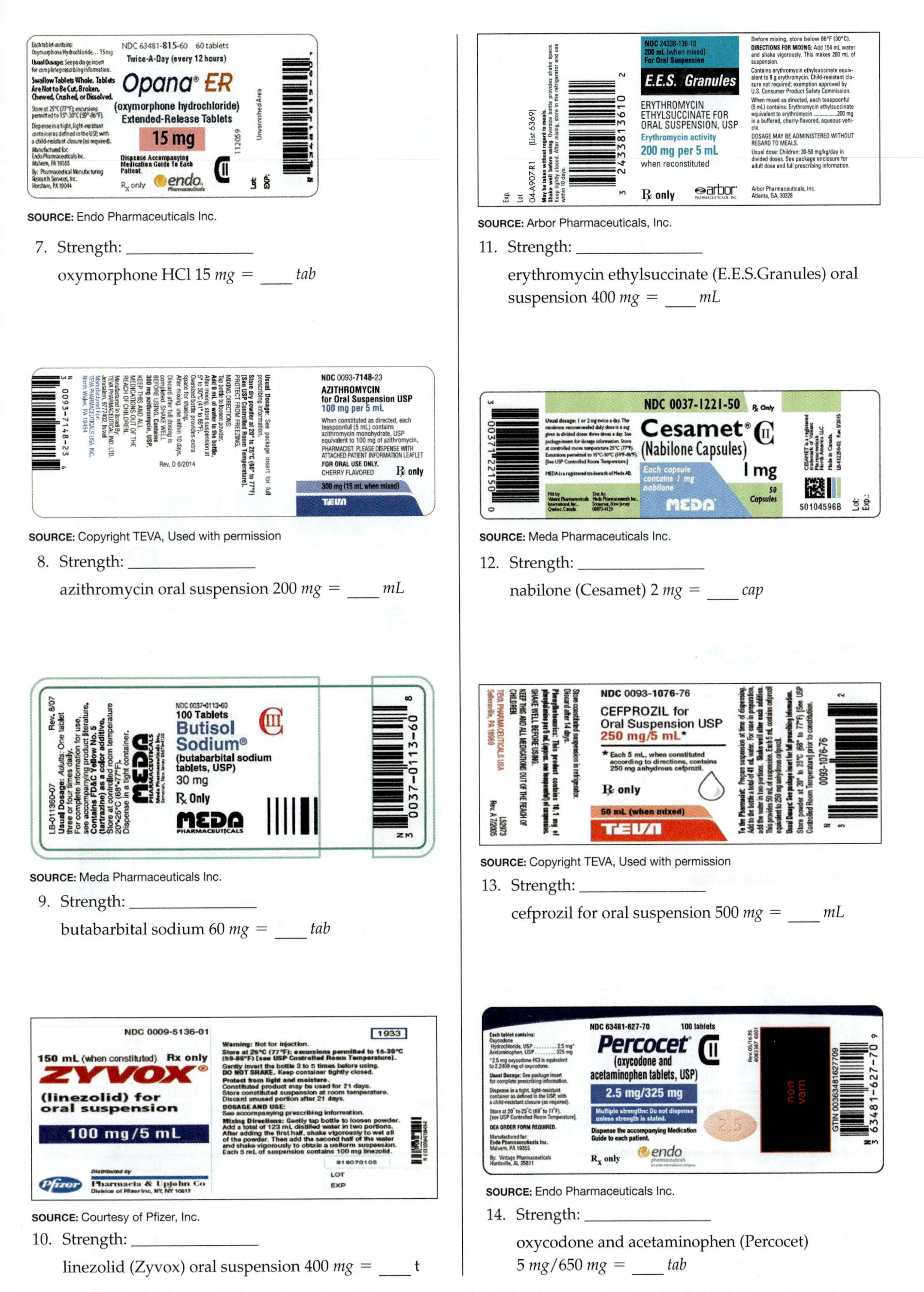

SOURCE: Endo Pharmaceuticals Inc.

7. Strength: ______________

oxymorphone HCl 15 *mg* = ___ *tab*

SOURCE: Copyright TEVA, Used with permission

8. Strength: ______________

azithromycin oral suspension 200 *mg* = ___ *mL*

SOURCE: Meda Pharmaceuticals Inc.

9. Strength: ______________

butabarbital sodium 60 *mg* = ___ *tab*

SOURCE: Courtesy of Pfizer, Inc.

10. Strength: ______________

linezolid (Zyvox) oral suspension 400 *mg* = ___ t

SOURCE: Arbor Pharmaceuticals, Inc.

11. Strength: ______________

erythromycin ethylsuccinate (E.E.S.Granules) oral suspension 400 *mg* = ___ *mL*

SOURCE: Meda Pharmaceuticals Inc.

12. Strength: ______________

nabilone (Cesamet) 2 *mg* = ___ *cap*

SOURCE: Copyright TEVA, Used with permission

13. Strength: ______________

cefprozil for oral suspension 500 *mg* = ___ *mL*

SOURCE: Endo Pharmaceuticals Inc.

14. Strength: ______________

oxycodone and acetaminophen (Percocet) 5 *mg*/650 *mg* = ___ *tab*

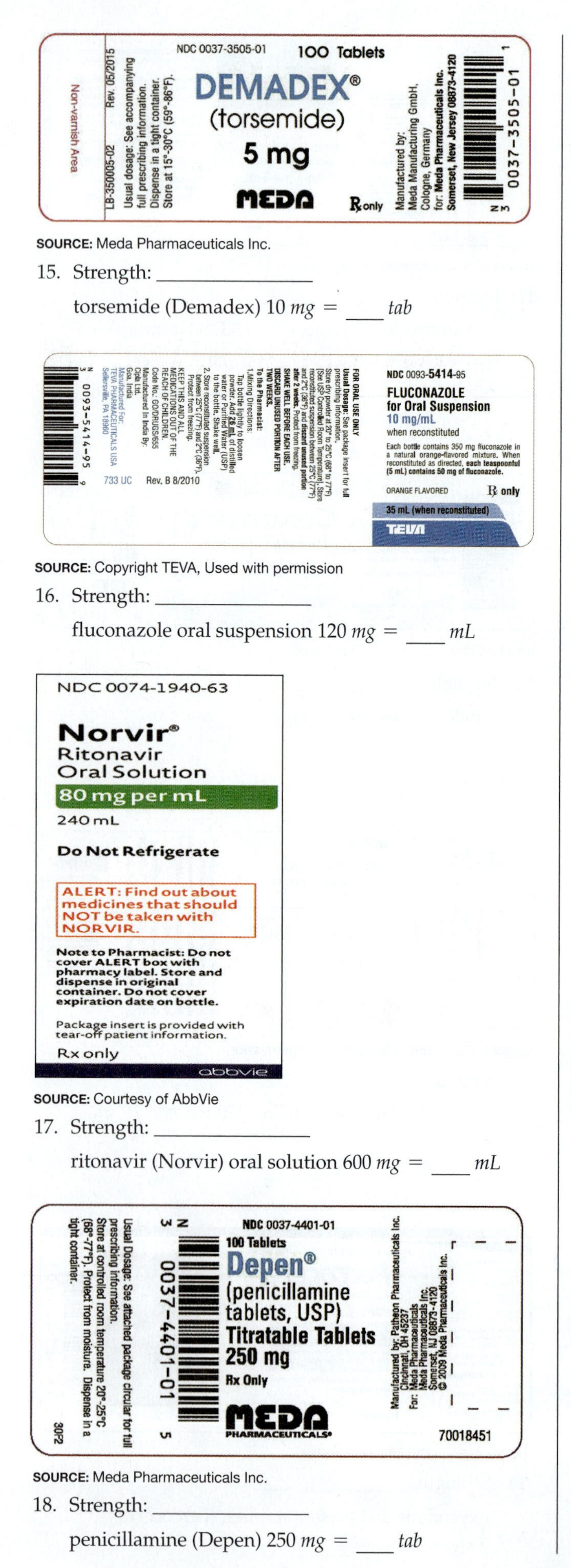

SOURCE: Meda Pharmaceuticals Inc.

15. Strength: ______________

torsemide (Demadex) 10 *mg* = ____ *tab*

SOURCE: Copyright TEVA, Used with permission

16. Strength: ______________

fluconazole oral suspension 120 *mg* = ____ *mL*

SOURCE: Courtesy of AbbVie

17. Strength: ______________

ritonavir (Norvir) oral solution 600 *mg* = ____ *mL*

SOURCE: Meda Pharmaceuticals Inc.

18. Strength: ______________

penicillamine (Depen) 250 *mg* = ____ *tab*

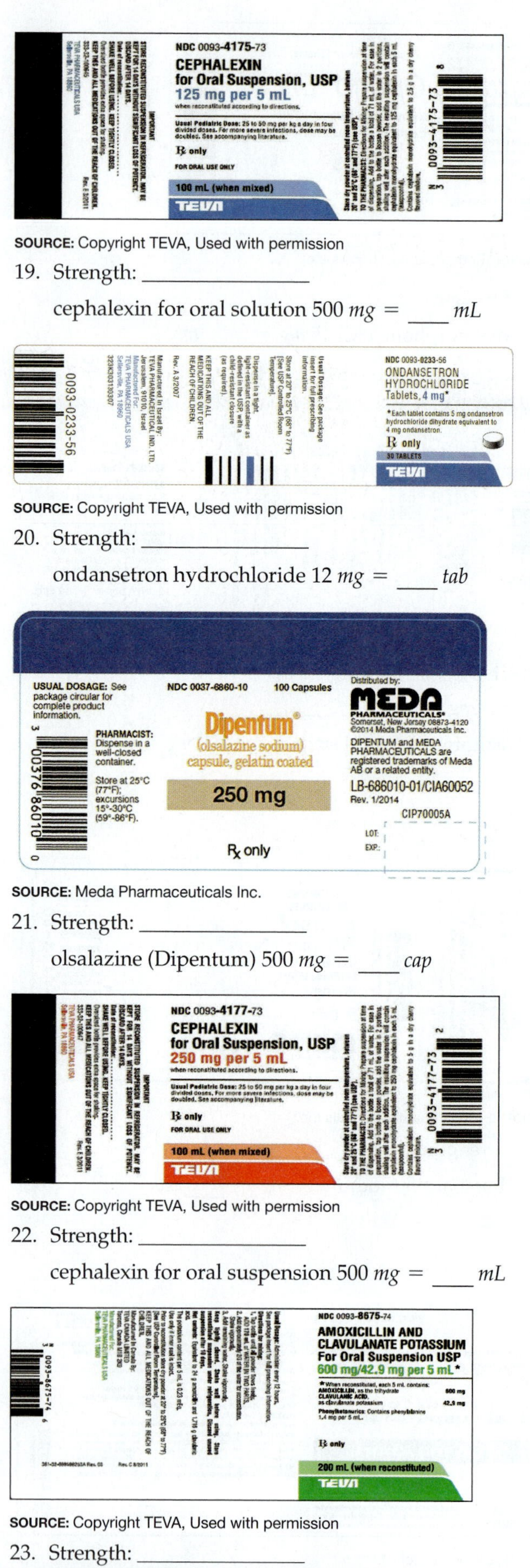

SOURCE: Copyright TEVA, Used with permission

19. Strength: ______________

cephalexin for oral solution 500 *mg* = ____ *mL*

SOURCE: Copyright TEVA, Used with permission

20. Strength: ______________

ondansetron hydrochloride 12 *mg* = ____ *tab*

SOURCE: Meda Pharmaceuticals Inc.

21. Strength: ______________

olsalazine (Dipentum) 500 *mg* = ____ *cap*

SOURCE: Copyright TEVA, Used with permission

22. Strength: ______________

cephalexin for oral suspension 500 *mg* = ____ *mL*

SOURCE: Copyright TEVA, Used with permission

23. Strength: ______________

amoxicillin and clavulanate potassium 1,200 *mg*/85.8 *mg* = ____ *mL*

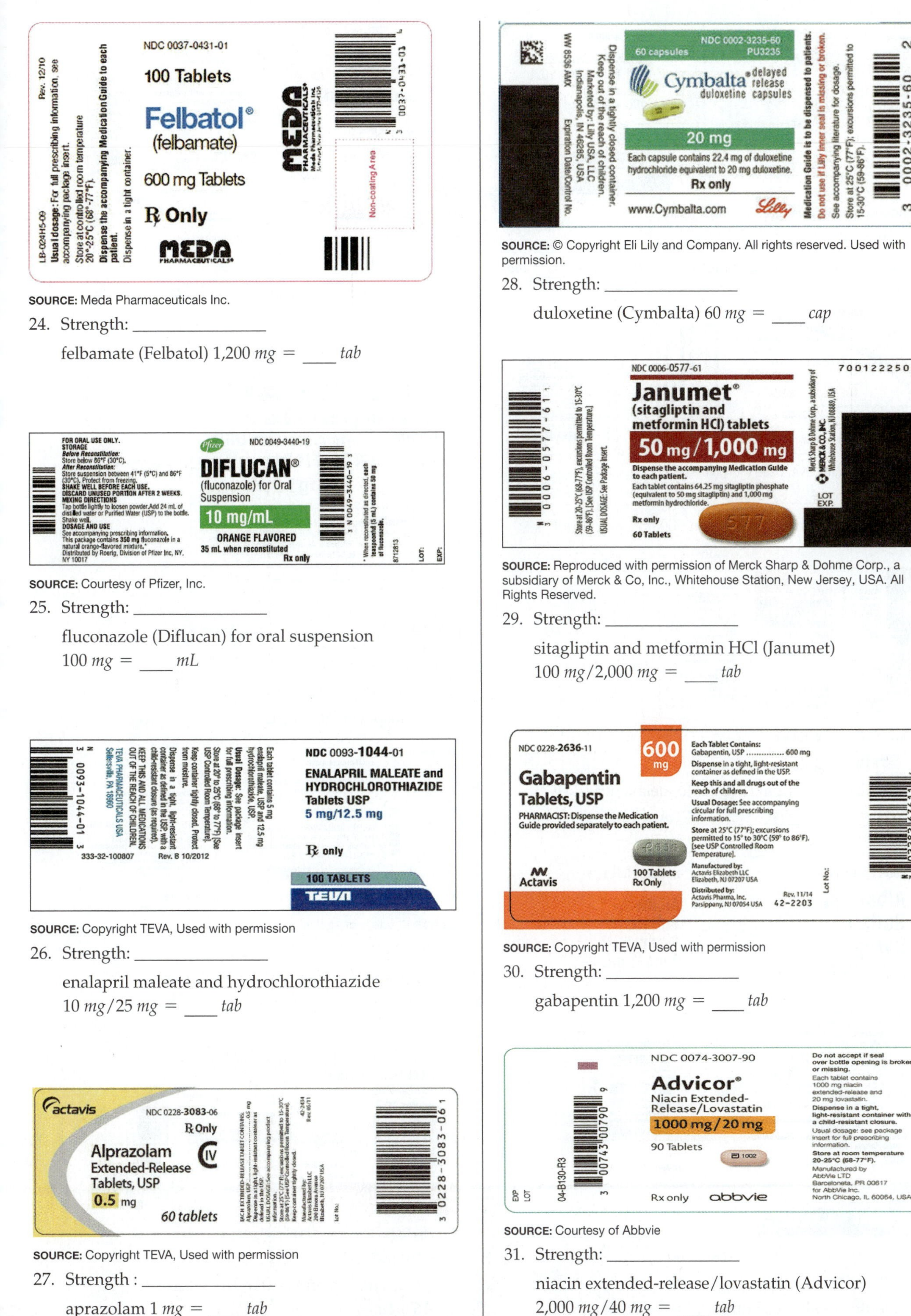

SOURCE: Meda Pharmaceuticals Inc.

24. Strength: _______________

    felbamate (Felbatol) 1,200 *mg* = ____ *tab*

SOURCE: Courtesy of Pfizer, Inc.

25. Strength: _______________

    fluconazole (Diflucan) for oral suspension 100 *mg* = ____ *mL*

SOURCE: Copyright TEVA, Used with permission

26. Strength: _______________

    enalapril maleate and hydrochlorothiazide 10 *mg*/25 *mg* = ____ *tab*

SOURCE: Copyright TEVA, Used with permission

27. Strength : _______________

    aprazolam 1 *mg* = ____ *tab*

SOURCE: © Copyright Eli Lily and Company. All rights reserved. Used with permission.

28. Strength: _______________

    duloxetine (Cymbalta) 60 *mg* = ____ *cap*

SOURCE: Reproduced with permission of Merck Sharp & Dohme Corp., a subsidiary of Merck & Co, Inc., Whitehouse Station, New Jersey, USA. All Rights Reserved.

29. Strength: _______________

    sitagliptin and metformin HCl (Janumet) 100 *mg*/2,000 *mg* = ____ *tab*

SOURCE: Copyright TEVA, Used with permission

30. Strength: _______________

    gabapentin 1,200 *mg* = ____ *tab*

SOURCE: Courtesy of Abbvie

31. Strength: _______________

    niacin extended-release/lovastatin (Advicor) 2,000 *mg*/40 *mg* = ____ *tab*

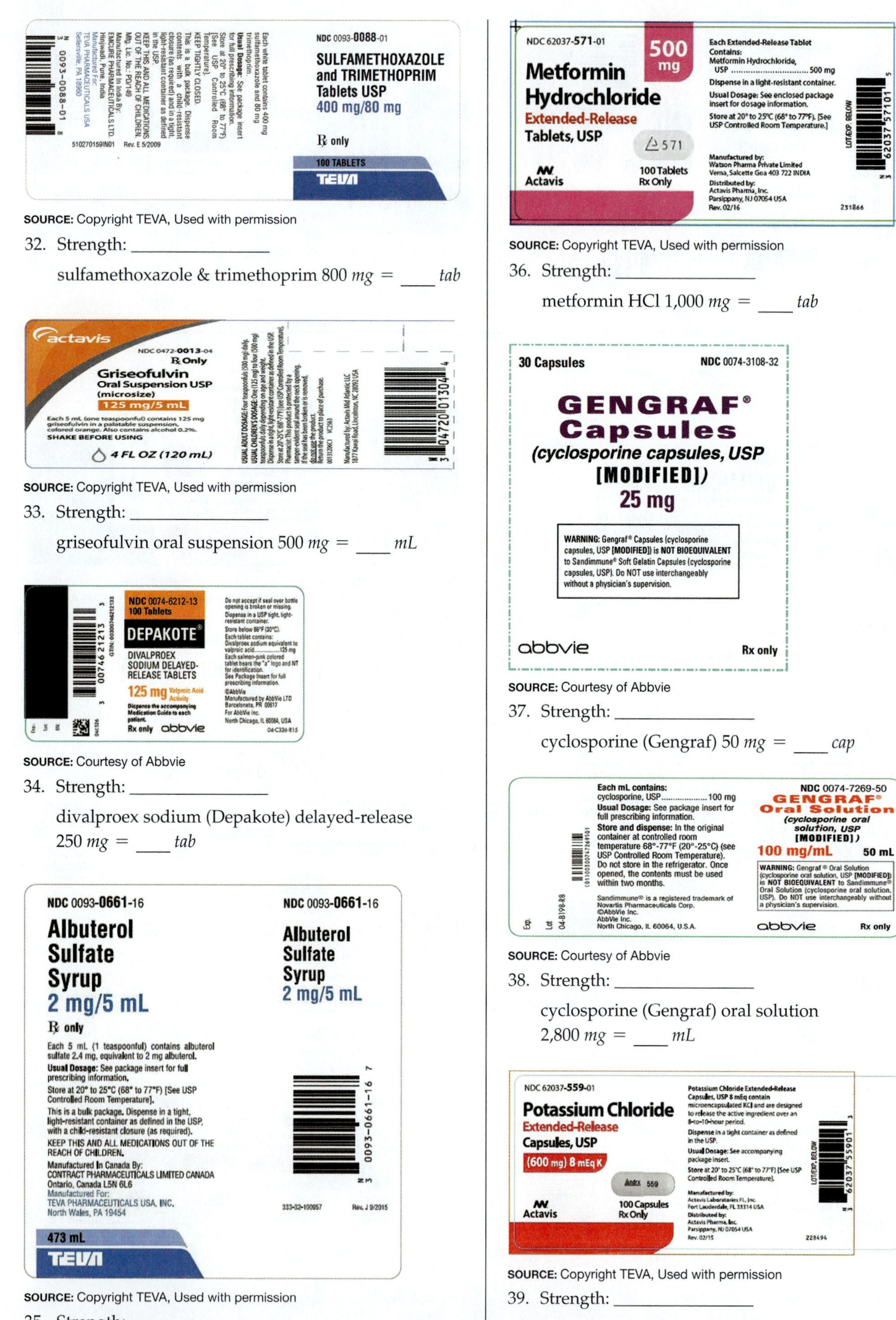

SOURCE: Copyright TEVA, Used with permission

32. Strength: ______________

sulfamethoxazole & trimethoprim 800 *mg* = ___ *tab*

SOURCE: Copyright TEVA, Used with permission

33. Strength: ______________

griseofulvin oral suspension 500 *mg* = ___ *mL*

SOURCE: Courtesy of Abbvie

34. Strength: ______________

divalproex sodium (Depakote) delayed-release 250 *mg* = ___ *tab*

SOURCE: Copyright TEVA, Used with permission

35. Strength: ______________

albuterol sulfate syrup 6 *mg* = ___ *mL*

SOURCE: Copyright TEVA, Used with permission

36. Strength: ______________

metformin HCl 1,000 *mg* = ___ *tab*

SOURCE: Courtesy of Abbvie

37. Strength: ______________

cyclosporine (Gengraf) 50 *mg* = ___ *cap*

SOURCE: Courtesy of Abbvie

38. Strength: ______________

cyclosporine (Gengraf) oral solution 2,800 *mg* = ___ *mL*

SOURCE: Copyright TEVA, Used with permission

39. Strength: ______________

potassium chloride extended-release 16 *mEq* = ___ *cap*

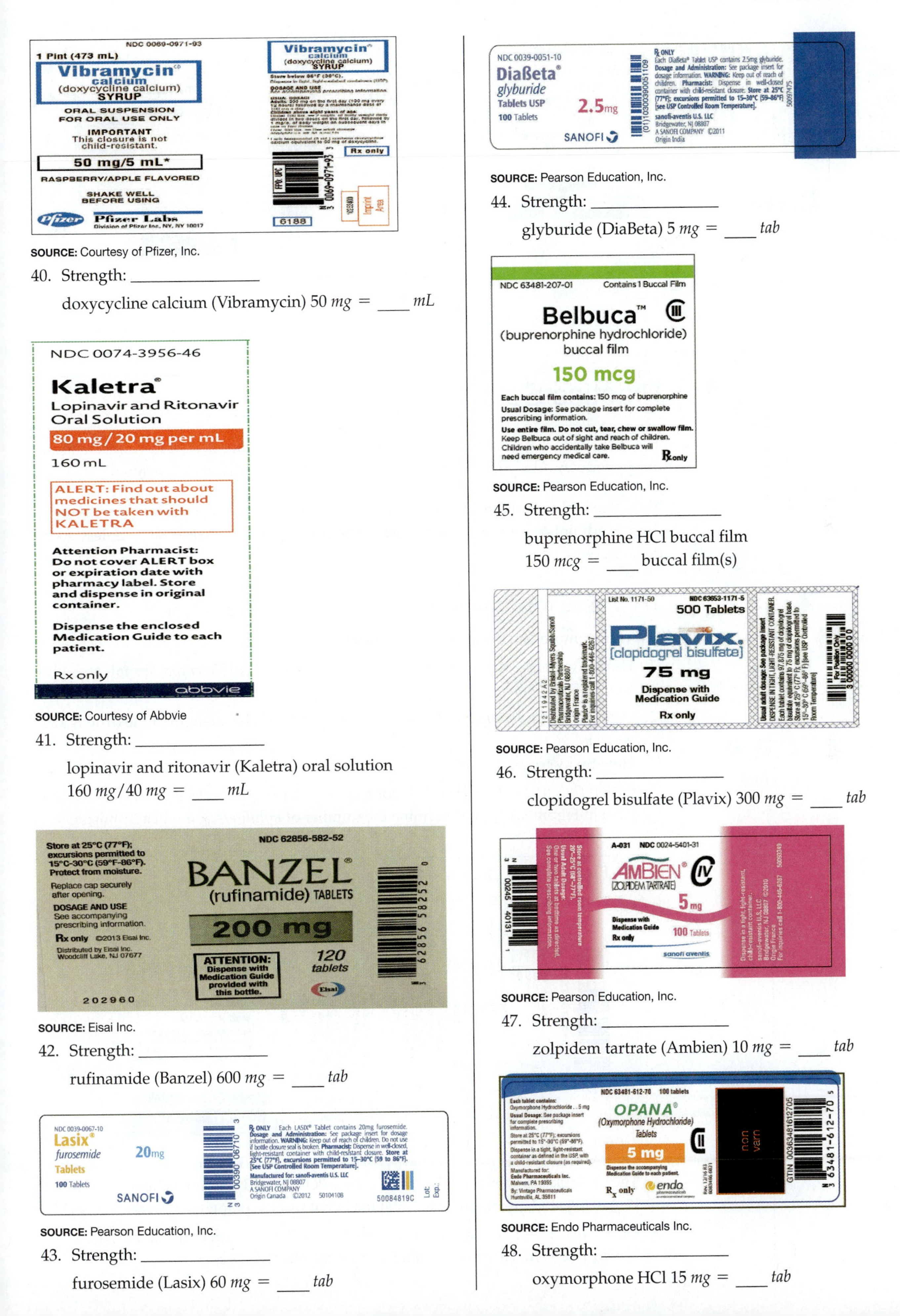

SOURCE: Courtesy of Pfizer, Inc.

40. Strength: ____________

doxycycline calcium (Vibramycin) 50 *mg* = ____ *mL*

SOURCE: Courtesy of Abbvie

41. Strength: ____________

lopinavir and ritonavir (Kaletra) oral solution 160 *mg*/40 *mg* = ____ *mL*

SOURCE: Eisai Inc.

42. Strength: ____________

rufinamide (Banzel) 600 *mg* = ____ *tab*

SOURCE: Pearson Education, Inc.

43. Strength: ____________

furosemide (Lasix) 60 *mg* = ____ *tab*

SOURCE: Pearson Education, Inc.

44. Strength: ____________

glyburide (DiaBeta) 5 *mg* = ____ *tab*

SOURCE: Pearson Education, Inc.

45. Strength: ____________

buprenorphine HCl buccal film 150 *mcg* = ____ buccal film(s)

SOURCE: Pearson Education, Inc.

46. Strength: ____________

clopidogrel bisulfate (Plavix) 300 *mg* = ____ *tab*

SOURCE: Pearson Education, Inc.

47. Strength: ____________

zolpidem tartrate (Ambien) 10 *mg* = ____ *tab*

SOURCE: Endo Pharmaceuticals Inc.

48. Strength: ____________

oxymorphone HCl 15 *mg* = ____ *tab*

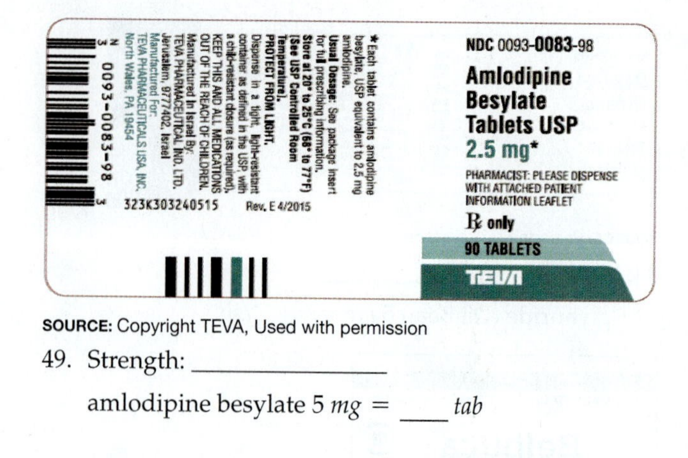

SOURCE: Copyright TEVA, Used with permission

49. Strength: ______________

    amlodipine besylate 5 *mg* = ____ *tab*

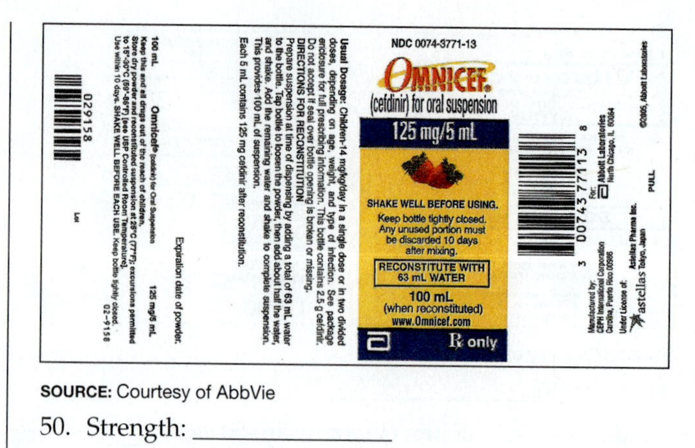

SOURCE: Courtesy of AbbVie

50. Strength: ______________

    cefdinir (Omnicef) oral suspension 500 *mg* = ____ *mL*

Practice Sets

The answers to *Try These for Practice*, *Exercises*, and *Cumulative Review Exercises* are found in Appendix A. Ask your instructor for the answers to the *Additional Exercises*.

Note: Remember that throughout this text when you are asked to calculate the amount of drug to administer, it is assumed to be the amount "per administration"—unless specified otherwise.

Try These for Practice

Test your comprehension after reading the chapter.

1. Use the formula to estimate the BSA of a person who is 153 *centimeters* tall and who weighs 72 *kilograms*.
2. Order: *Dilantin (phenytoin suspension) 250 mg po t.i.d*. The strength of the drug is 125 *mg*/5 *mL*.

   How many *teaspoons* will you administer?
3. Order: *fluconazole 200 mg po daily* for a client with esophageal candidiasis. Read the label in Figure 6.19 and determine the number of *milliliters* you will administer.

Figure 6.19 Drug label for fluconazole.

SOURCE: Copyright TEVA, Used with permission

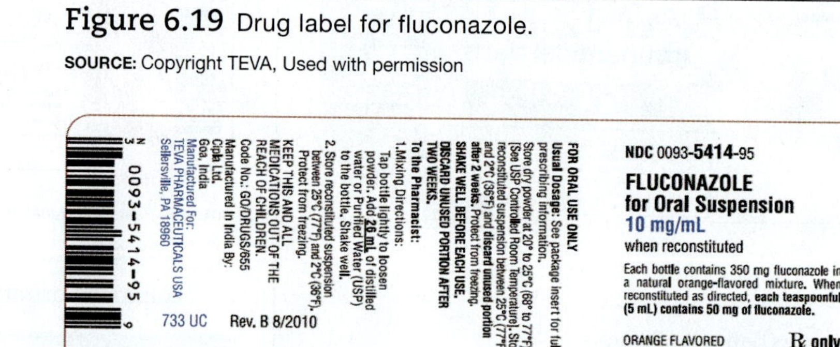

4. The prescriber ordered 125 *mg*/*m*^{2} *of a drug PO q6h for 3 days* for a client who has a BSA of 1.4 *m*^{2}. How many *grams* will the client receive in total for the three days?
5. Order: *amoxicillin 375 mg oral suspension po q8h*. The strength of this antibiotic is 125 *mg* per 5 *mL*. How many *milliliters* will the client receive?

Exercises

Reinforce your understanding in class or at home.

1. Order: *Coumadin (warfarin sodium) 7.5 mg po daily*. The strength of the scored *tablets* is 2.5 *mg/tablet*. How many *tablets* of this vitamin K antagonist would be given to the client who has venous thrombosis?
2. Order: *Dynapen (dicloxacillin sodium) 250 mg po q6h for 7 days*. The strength of the oral suspension is 62.5 *mg/5 mL*. How many *teaspoons* will you administer to the client who has an upper respiratory tract infection?
3. The dosage range for the antineoplastic agent Mithracin (plicamycin) is 25–30 *mcg/kg* daily. What is the safe dosage range in *mg* per day for a client who weighs 190 *pounds* and has a malignant tumor?
4. The daily safe dose range for a certain drug is 1–5 mg/m^2. A 6-foot-tall client who weighs 200 *pounds* is scheduled to receive 40 *mg* of the drug each day. Is the scheduled dose safe for this client?
5. Order: *Tegretol (carbamazepine) 200 mg po b.i.d.* The strength of the oral suspension is 100 *mg/5 mL*. How many *teaspoons* will you give the client who has bipolar disorder?
6. Use the formula to estimate the BSA of a person who is 160 *cm* tall and weighs 83 *kg*.
7. Order: *Anadrol-50 (oxymetholone) 200 mg po daily*. The recommended dose for this anabolic steroid is 1–5 *mg/kg/d*. Is the prescribed order in the recommended range for a client who has aplastic anemia and weighs 75 *kg*?
8. The prescribed order is 120 $mg/m^2/d \times 14$ *days PO*. How many *grams* will the client who has a BSA of 1.4 m^2 receive in total after this two-week regimen?
9. See Figure 6.20 to determine the number of capsules of Cymbalta (duloxetine hydrochloride) that you would administer each day after the first week to a client who has fibromyalgia.

ROUTE & DOSAGE

Depression
Adult: PO 40–60 mg/d in one or two divided doses

Generalized Anxiety/Diabetic Neuropathy
Adult: PO 60 mg once daily

Fibromyalagia
Adult: PO 30 mg/d in × 1 wk then 60 mg/d

Figure 6.20 Excerpt from a drug guide and the drug label for Cymbalta.

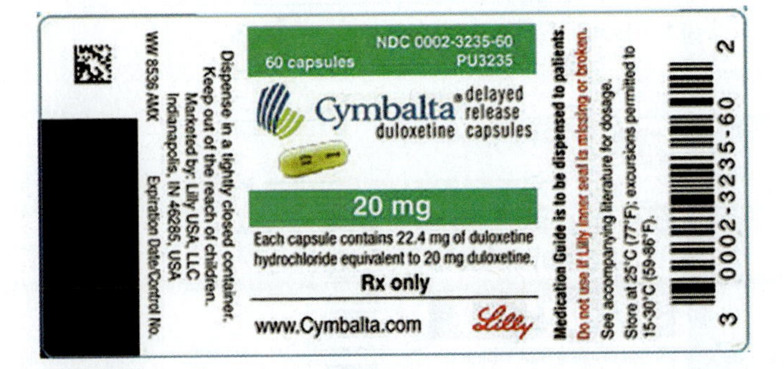

10. A drug is ordered 100 mg/m^2 PO B.I.D. How many *milliliters* will a client receive if her BSA is 1.80 m^2 and the concentration of the solution is 100 *mg/5 mL*?

11. Order: *Aldactazide (spironolactone and hydrochlorothiazide) 100 mg/100 mg PO B.I.D.* Read the label in Figure 6.21 and determine how many *tablets* of this diuretic you will administer.

____

Figure 6.21 Drug label for Aldactazide.

SOURCE: Courtesy of Pfizer, Inc.

Store below 25°C (77°F).
Protect from light.
Dispense in a tight, light-resistant, child-resistant container.
DOSAGE AND USE
See accompanying prescribing information.
Each tablet contains
50 mg spironolactone and
50 mg hydrochlorothiazide.
Distributed by
G.D. Searle
Division of Pfizer Inc
NY, NY 10017
MADE IN USA
(includes foreign content)

Pfizer NDC 0025-1021-31
Aldactazide®
spironolactone and hydrochlorothiazide tablets
50 mg / 50 mg
100 Tablets **Rx only**

FPO: UPC NDC (80%)
N 3 0025-1021-31 2
13702600

12. Order: *alprazolam 0.25 mg PO T.I.D.* Read the label in Figure 6.22 and determine how many *milliliters* of this antianxiety drug you will administer.

____

Figure 6.22 Drug label for alprazolam. (For educational purposes only)

SOURCE: Pearson Education, Inc.

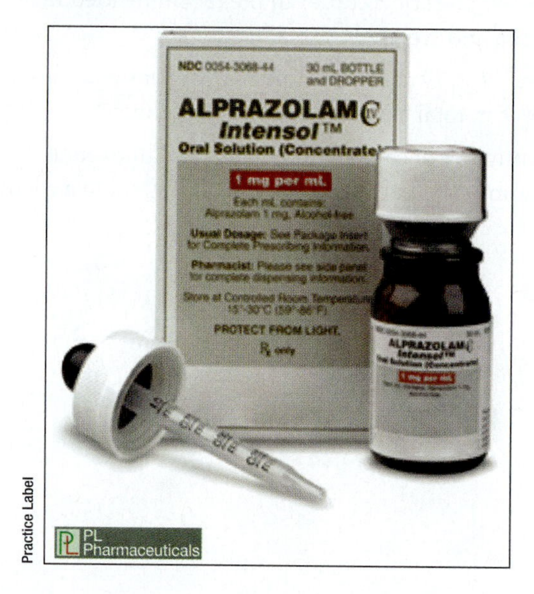

13. The prescriber ordered *Bosulif (bosutinib) 500 mg PO daily to be given with food for a client who has chronic myelogenous leukemia (CML).* Read the label in Figure 6.23 and determine how many *tablets* to administer.

____

Figure 6.23 Drug label for Bosulif.

SOURCE: Courtesy of Pfizer, Inc.

Store at 20°C to 25°C (68°F to 77°F); excursions permitted to 15°C to 30°C (59°F to 86°F) [see USP Controlled Room Temperature].
Dispense in tight (USP), child-resistant containers.
DOSAGE AND USE
See accompanying prescribing information.
*Each tablet contains 516.98 mg of bosutinib monohydrate equivalent to 500 mg of bosutinib.
Distributed by Pfizer Labs
Division of Pfizer Inc
NY, NY 10017
MADE IN SPAIN

Pfizer NDC 0069-0136-01
Bosulif®
(bosutinib) tablets
500 mg*
Do not crush or cut tablet
For Oncology Use Only
30 Tablets **Rx only**

N3 0069-0136-01 1
413278
Exp.
Lot

14. For a client with diarrhea the recommended dosage of neomycin sulfate is *50 mg/kg po in 4 divided doses for 2-3 days*. If an order for an 80 *kg* client with diarrhea is *neomycin sulfate 1g po q.i.d. for 3 days*, is the order safe?
15. Read the label in Figure 6.24 and determine the number of *grams* of valsartan (Diovan) that are contained in the entire bottle.

Figure 6.24 Drug label for Diovan.

SOURCE: Courtesy of Novartis Pharma AG

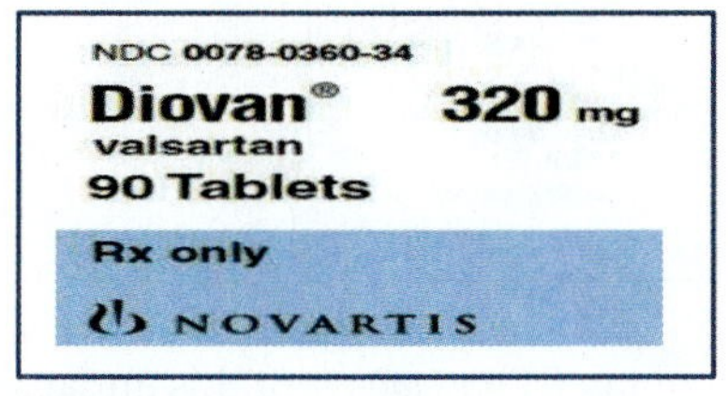

16. Estimate the body surface area of a client who is 6 *feet* tall and weighs 210 *pounds.*
17. A drug is ordered 40 mg/m^2 *po b.i.d.* How many *milliliters* will a client receive if her BSA is 1.33 m^2 and the strength of the drug is 2 *mg/mL*?
18. Order: *pancrelipase (Creon) 1,000 lipase units/kg per meal*. Read the label in Figure 6.25 and determine the number of capsules a client who weighs 50 *kg* will receive.

Figure 6.25 Drug label for pancrelipase (Creon).

SOURCE: Courtesy of Abbvie

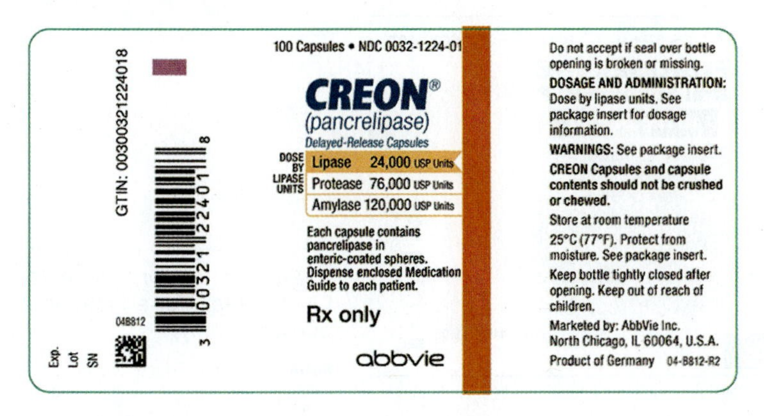

19. Order: *fluoxetine hydrochloride (Prozac) 40 mg PO in two divided doses*. The strength of the drug is 20 *mg* per cap. How many capsules of this antidepressant will you administer to the client?
20. Order: *oxycodone and acetaminophen 10 mg/650 mg PO q4h prn severe pain.* How many 5 *mg*/325 *mg* tablets of this opioid analgesic will you administer to the client.

Additional Exercises

Now, test yourself!

1. Order: *Depakene (valproic acid) 750 mg/day po in three divided doses.* Read the label in Figure 6.26. How many *capsules* of this anticonvulsant will you administer to the client who has mania?

Figure 6.26 Drug label for Depakene.

SOURCE: Courtesy of AbbVie

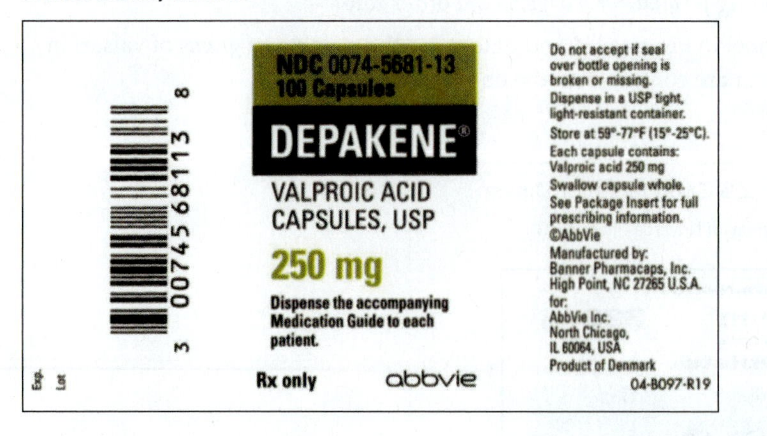

2. Order: *Xanax (alprazolam) 1.5 mg po t.i.d.* How many 0.5 *mg tablets* of this antianxiety drug will you administer to the client who suffers from panic attacks?
3. Order: *amoxicillin oral suspension 500 mg po q8h*. The concentration of the amoxicillin solution is 125 *mg*/5 *mL*. How many *milliliters* of this antibiotic will you administer to the client who has a mild infection?
4. Order: *potassium chloride 80 mEq po in two divided doses daily*. The concentration of the potassium chloride is *40 mEq/15 mL*. How many *milliliters* of this electrolytic replacement solution will you administer to the client who has hypokalemia?
5. Order: *furosemide 50 mg po b.i.d.* Read the label in Figure 6.27. How many teaspoons of this diuretic will you administer to the client who has high blood pressure?

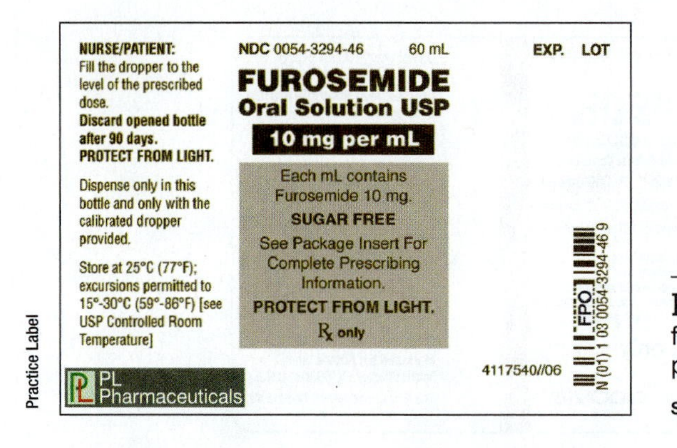

Figure 6.27 Drug label for furosemide. (For educational purposes only)

SOURCE: Pearson Education, Inc.

6. Order: *Xyrem (sodium oxybate) 2.25 g po given at bedtime while in bed and repeat 4 hours later*. How many *milliliters* of this central nervous system depressant will you administer to the client who has cataplexy if the strength of the Xyrem solution is 500 *mg/mL*?
7. Basketball player Shaquille O'Neal stands 7 *feet* 1 *inch* in height and weighs 325 *pounds*. Estimate his BSA.
8. Entertainer Madonna weighs 52 *kg* and is 160 *cm* in height. Estimate her BSA.
9. A drug is ordered *6 mg/kg po b.i.d.* How many *tablets* will a client receive if he weighs 148 *pounds* and the strength of the *tablet* is 200 *mg/tab*?
10. A drug is ordered 200 mg/m^2 *po b.i.d.* How many *mL* will a client receive if her BSA is 1.34 m^2 and the concentration of the solution is 5 *mg/mL*?
11. Order: *ERY-TAB (erythromycin) 333 mg po q8h*. Read the label in Figure 6.28. How many *tablets* of this macrolide antibiotic will you administer to the client who has a severe infection?

Figure 6.28 Drug label for ERY-TAB.

SOURCE: Arbor Pharmaceuticals, Inc.

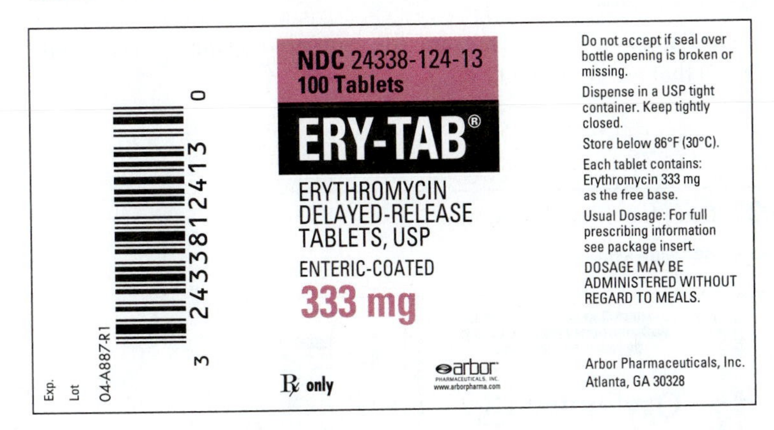

12. Order: *Kaletra (lopinavir/ritonavir) 800/200 mg po daily*. Read the label in Figure 6.29. How many *mL* of this antiretroviral agent will you administer to the client who has HIV?

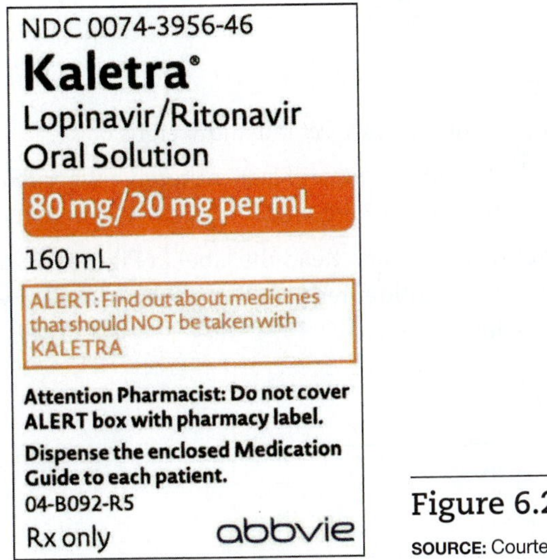

Figure 6.29 Drug label for Kaletra.

SOURCE: Courtesy of AbbVie

13. Order: *metformin hydrochloride 750 mg po b.i.d. with meals*. Read the label in Figure 6.30. How many *tablets* of this antidiabetic drug will you administer to the client?

Figure 6.30 Drug label for metformin HCl.

SOURCE: Copyright TEVA, Used with permission

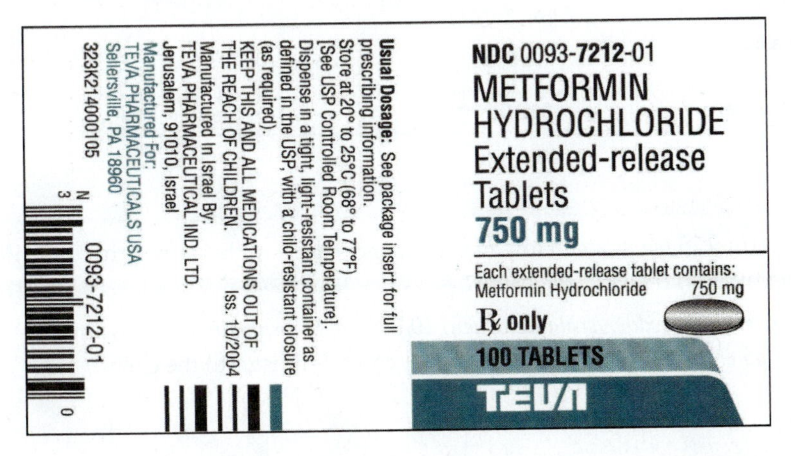

14. Order: *phenobarbitol sodium 400 mg po in two divided doses daily*. The recommended dosage of this anticonvulsant is 1–3 *mg/kg/d*. Is the prescribed dose safe for the client who weighs 203 *pounds*?

15. Read the label in Figure 6.31 and determine the number of *grams* of OxyContin (oxycodone HCl) that are contained in the entire bottle.

Figure 6.31 Drug label for OxyContin.

SOURCE: © Purdue, used with permission.

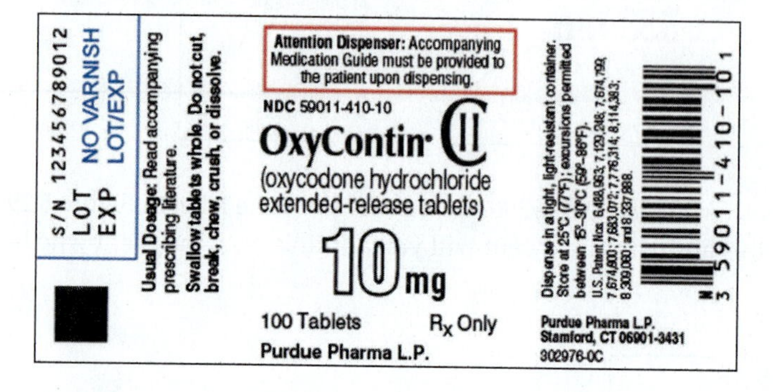

16. Estimate the body surface area of a client who is 5 *feet* tall and weighs 60 *kg*.

17. A drug is ordered $50\ mg/m^2$ *po b.i.d.* How many *mL* will a client receive if her BSA is $1.44\ m^2$ and the concentration of the solution is 2 *mg/mL*?

18. Order: *Lexapro (escitalopram oxalate) 10 mg po daily*. Read the label in Figure 6.32 and determine the number of *milliliters* of this antidepres-sant that a geriatric client who has generalized anxiety will receive in a week.

Figure 6.32 Drug label for Lexapro.

SOURCE: Forest Pharmaceuticals

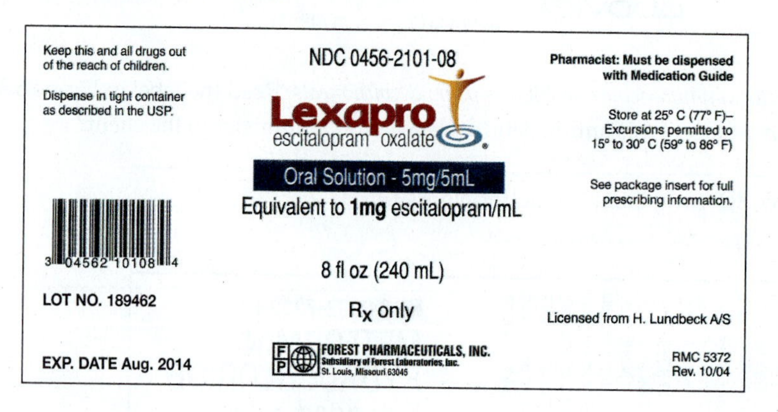

19. Order: *digoxin 0.75 mg po stat*. How many 0.25 *mg tablets* of this antiar-rhythmic drug will you administer to the client?

20. Order: *Percocet (oxycodone/acetaminophen) 10/650 mg po prn pain q6h*. How many 5/325 *mg tablets* of this opioid analgesic will you administer to the client?

Cumulative Review Exercises

Review your mastery of previous chapters.

1. 4 *T* = ? *mL*
2. 44 *lb* = ? *kg*
3. 480 *oz* = ? *pt*
4. 47 *mm* = ? *cm*
5. Order: *Ceclor (cefaclor) 100 mg po q.i.d.* The label states 125 *mg* per 5 *mL*. How many *milliliters* of this antibiotic will you administer?
6. Order: *sulfamethoxazole and trimethoprim 800 mg/160 mg PO q12h x 14 days.* See the label in Figure 6.33. How many tablets of this synthetic antibacterial combination product will you administer to a client with a urinary tract infection?

Figure 6.33 Drug label for sulfamethoxazole and trimethoprim.

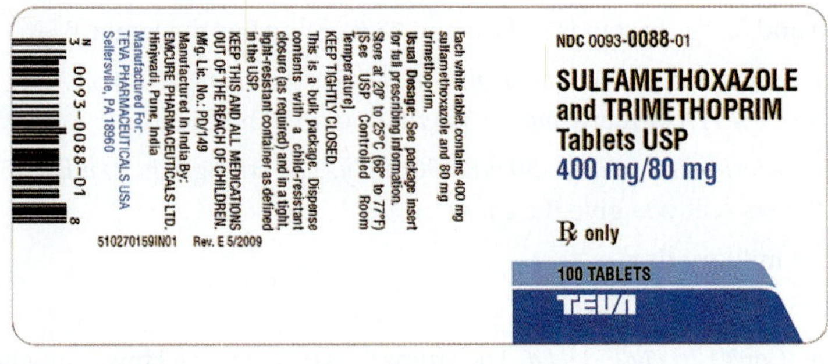

SOURCE: Copyright TEVA, Used with permission

7. Order: *Augmentin* (amoxicillin and clavulanate potassium) *500 mg PO q12h.* The strength on the label is 125 *mg* per 5 *mL*. How many *milliliters* of this antibiotic will you administer? Draw a line at the correct measurement on the medication cup in Figure 6.34.

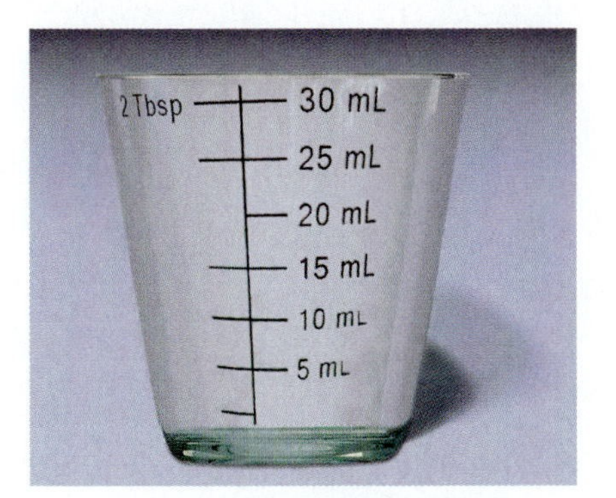

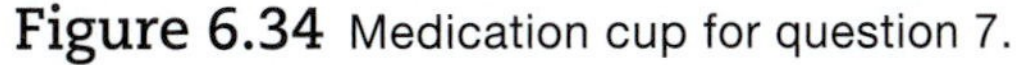

Figure 6.34 Medication cup for question 7.

8. Order: *felbamate (Felbatol) 1200 mg po daily in three divided doses.* See the label in Figure 6.35. How many *milliliters* of this antiepileptic drug will you administer to a client whose epilepsy is so severe that there is a substantial risk of aplastic anemia and/or liver failure?

Figure 6.35 Drug label for felbamate (Felbatol).

SOURCE: Meda Pharmaceuticals Inc.

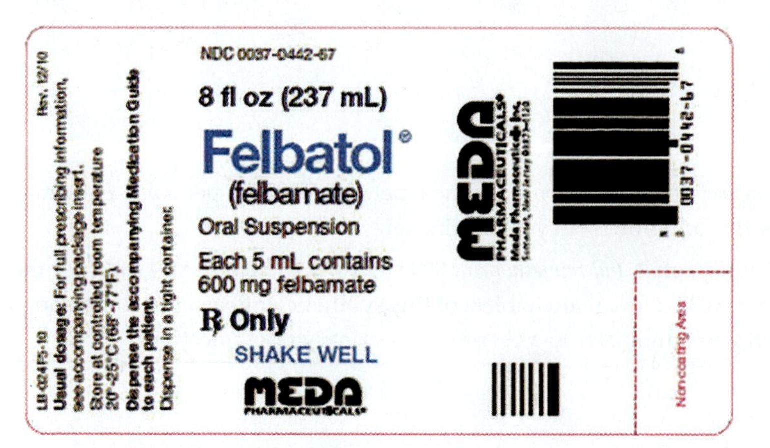

9. Estimate the BSA for a person who is 6 *ft* 3 *in* tall and weighs 200 *lb*.
10. James is 150 *cm* and 85 *kg*; Tristan is 165 *cm* and 93 *kg*. Who has the larger BSA?
11. Order: *doxycycline monohydrate (Vibramycin) oral suspension 100 mg PO q12h*. The strength is 25 *mg*/5*mL*. How many *milliliters* will you give the client?
12. Order: *potassium chloride oral solution 30 mEq PO daily*. The strength is 20 *mEq*/15 *ml*. How many *milliliters* will you give the client?
13. Write 2:07 AM in military time.
14. Convert 6,000 *g* to *kg*.
15. Order: *carvedilol (Coreg) 25 mg PO b.i.d.* The strength is 6.25 *mg/tab*. How many tablets of this antihypertensive drug will you give the client?

Chapter 7

Syringes

Learning Outcomes

After completing this chapter, you will be able to

7.1 Identify the parts of a syringe and needle.

7.2 Identify various types of syringes.

7.3 Interpret the calibrations on syringes of various sizes.

7.4 Select the most appropriate syringe to administer a prescribed dose.

7.5 Measure single insulin dosages.

7.6 Combine two different types of insulin in one syringe.

7.7 Interpret insulin labels.

In this chapter you learn how to use various types of syringes to measure medication dosages. You also discuss the difference between the types of insulin and how to measure single insulin dosages and combined insulin dosages.

A **syringe** is a device used to draw in or eject either air or liquid. When fitted with a needle, it is called a hypodermic syringe and may be used to inject medication into the body. Oral syringes (without the needles) are used to administer medication orally. Syringes are made of plastic or glass, designed for one-time use, and packaged either separately or together with needles of appropriate sizes. After use, syringes must be discarded in special puncture-resistant containers. See Figure 7.1.

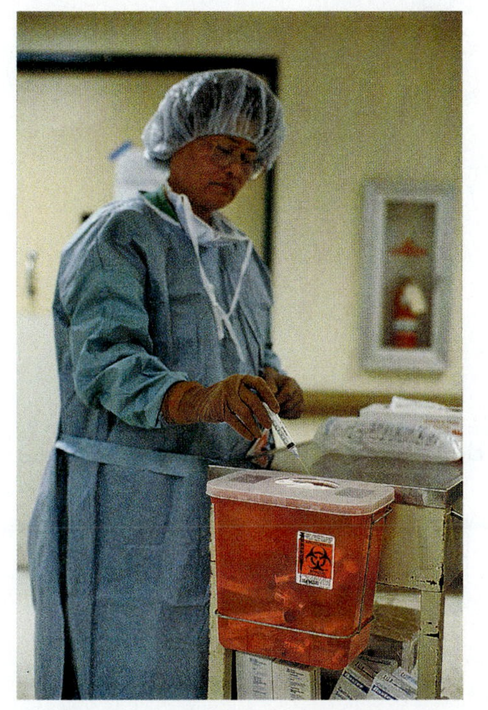

Figure 7.1 Puncture-resistant container for needles, syringes, and other "sharps."

SOURCE: Pearson Education, Inc.

Parts of a Syringe

A syringe consists of a barrel, a plunger, and a tip.

- **Barrel**: a hollow cylinder that holds the medication. It has calibrations (graduated markings) on the outer surface.
- **Plunger**: fits in the barrel and is moved back and forth. A rubber stopper attached to the plunger has two rings that fit snugly into the barrel. Pulling back on the plunger draws liquid or air into the syringe. Pushing in the plunger forces air or liquid out of the syringe.
- **Tip**: the end of the syringe that holds the needle. The needle slips onto the tip or can be twisted and locked in place (Luer-Lok™).

The inside of the barrel, plunger, and tip must always be sterile.

Needles

Needles are thin stainless steel tubes that come in various lengths and diameters. They are packaged with a protective cover that keeps them from being contaminated. The parts of a needle are the **hub**, which attaches to the syringe; the **shaft**, the long tube that is embedded in the hub; and the **bevel**, the slanted portion which makes the sharp point on the end of the needle. The **length** of the needle is the distance from the point to the hub. Needles most commonly used in medication administration range from $\frac{3}{8}$ *inch* to 2 *inches*. The **gauge** of the needle refers to the thickness of the needle and varies from 18 to 28 (the larger the gauge, the thinner the needle). The parts of a syringe and needle are shown in Figure 7.2.

NOTE

The two rings on the stopper are called "top" ring and "bottom" ring because when the syringe is held with the needle facing upward, the "top" ring is above the "bottom" ring.

Figure 7.2 Parts of a syringe and needle.

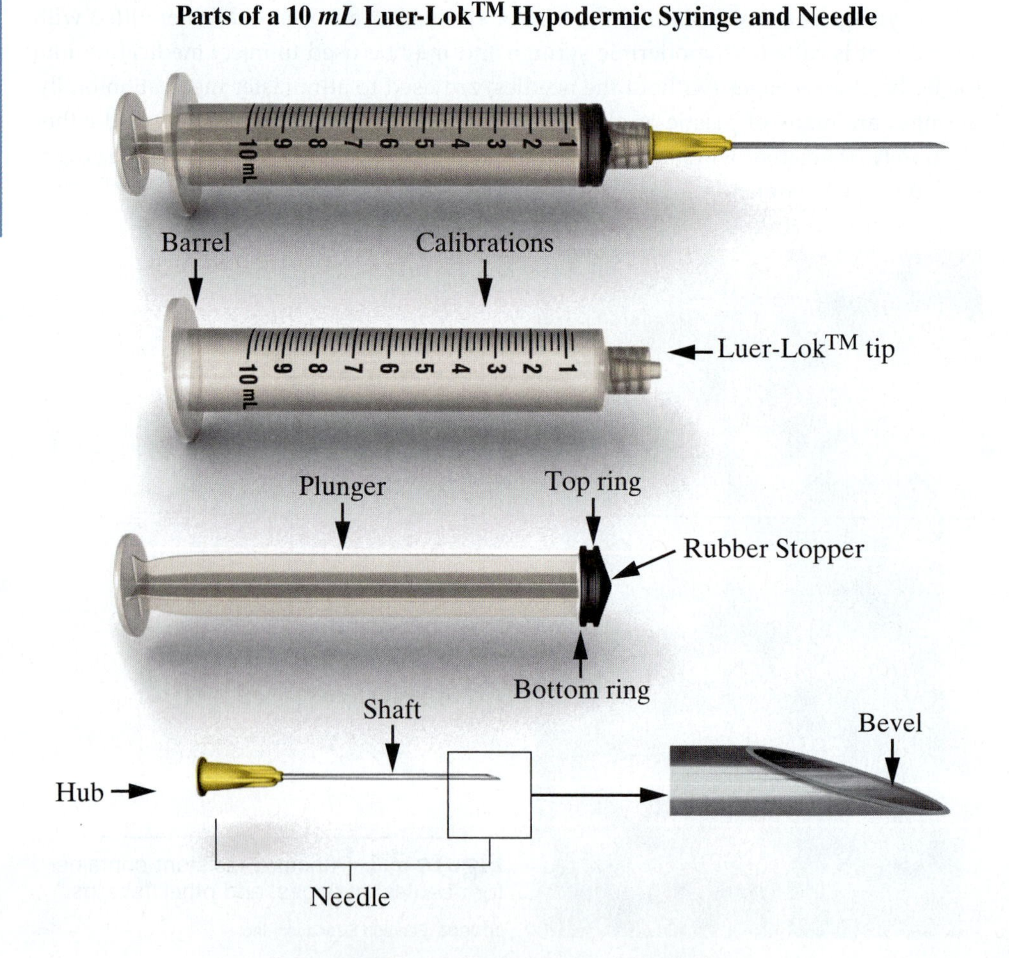

ALERT

The amount of fluid to be put in the syringe, the client's size, the type of tissue being injected, and the viscosity of the medication are factors that determine the size of the needle to be used. The inside of the barrel, the plunger, the tip of the syringe, and the needle should never come in contact with anything unsterile.

Commonly Used Sizes of Hypodermic Syringes

The two major types of syringes are hypodermic and oral. In 1853, doctors Charles Pravaz and Alexander Wood were the first to develop a syringe with a needle that was fine enough to pierce the skin. This is known as a **hypodermic syringe**. Use of oral syringes (without needles) are discussed in Chapter 12.

Hypodermic syringes are calibrated (marked) in *cubic centimeters* (cc), *milliliters* (*mL*), or units. Practitioners often refer to syringes by the volume they contain—for example, a 3-*cc* syringe. Although some syringes are still labeled in *cubic centimeters*, manufacturers are now phasing in syringes labeled in *milliliters*. In this text, we generally show *mL* instead of *cc* on the syringes.

The smaller-capacity syringes (0.5, 1, and 3 *mL*) are used most often for intradermal, subcutaneous, or intramuscular injections of medication. The larger sizes (5, 12, and 35 *mL*) are commonly used to draw blood or prepare medications for intravenous administration. A representative sample of commonly used syringes is shown in Figure 7.3.

Figure 7.3 A sample of commonly used hypodermic syringes (35 *mL*, 12 *mL*, 5 *mL*, 3 *mL*, 1 *mL*, and 0.5 *mL*).

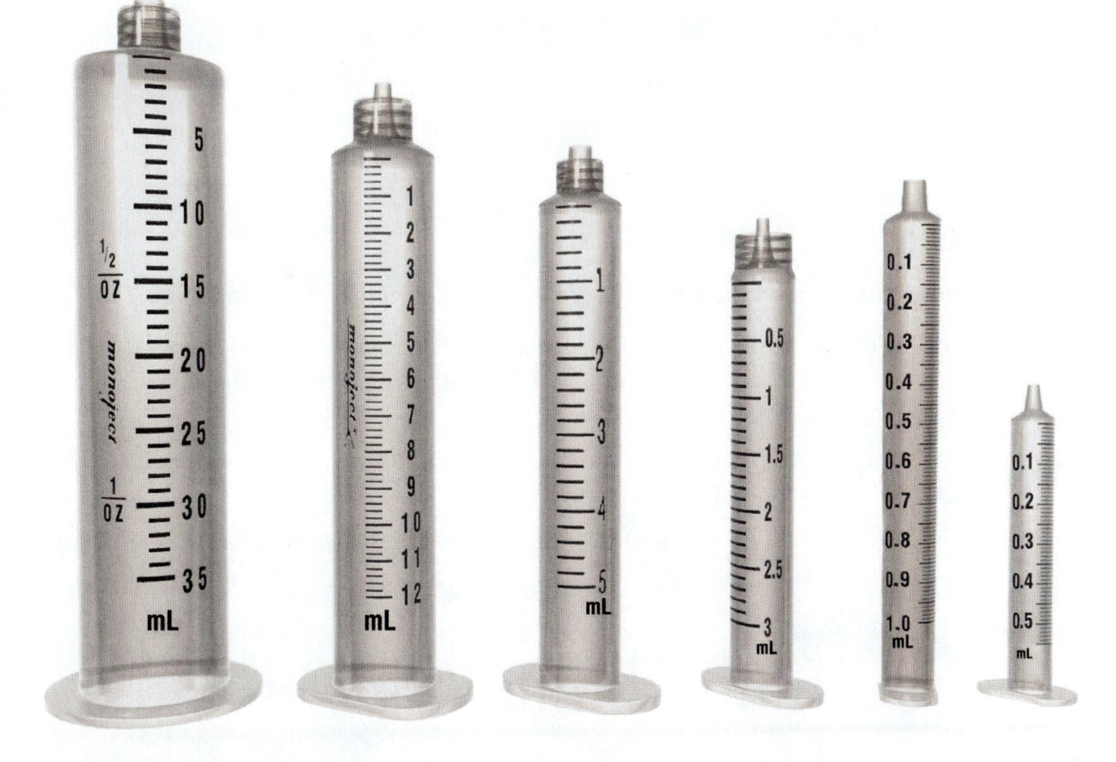

The space between two numbers on a syringe is broken up into either 2, 5, or 10 segments; this divides the space into halves, fifths, or tenths, respectively. For example, if the space between 2 *mL* and 3 *mL* on a syringe is divided into two equal segments, then each segment is $\frac{1}{2}$ or 0.5 *mL*. If the space between 2 *mL* and 3 *mL* is divided into five equal segments, then each segment is $\frac{1}{5}$ or 0.2 *mL*. If the space between 2 *mL* and 3 *mL* is divided into 10 equal segments, then each segment is $\frac{1}{10}$ or 0.1 *mL*.

A 35 *mL* syringe is shown in Figure 7.4. Each line on the barrel represents 1 *mL*, and the longer lines represent 5 *mL*.

Figure 7.4 A 35 *mL* syringe.

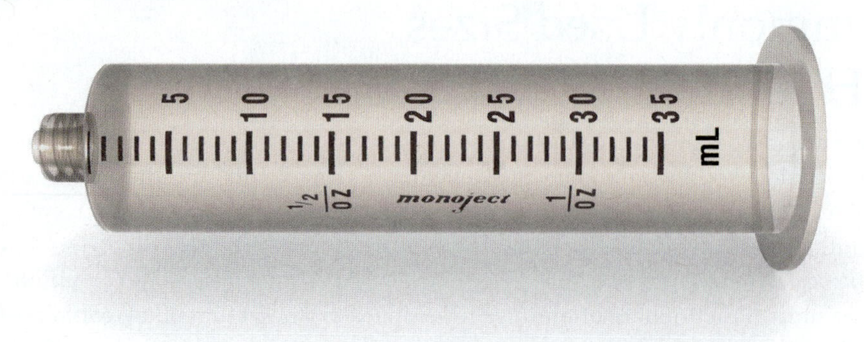

A 12 *mL* syringe is shown in Figure 7.5. Each line on the barrel represents 0.2 *mL*, and the longer lines represent 1 *mL*.

Figure 7.5 A 12 *mL* syringe.

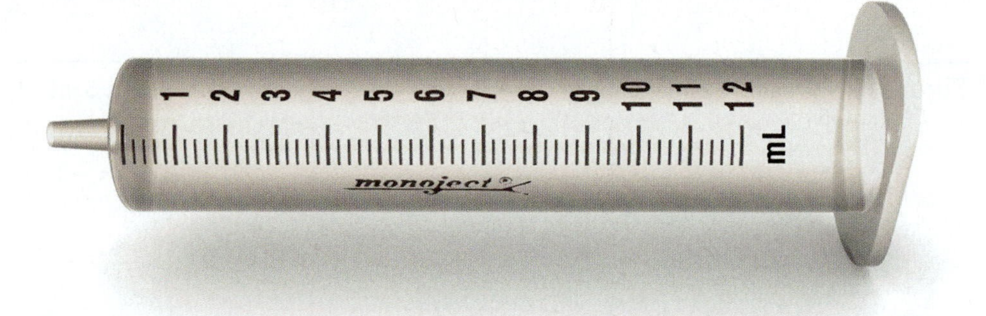

Example 7.1

How much liquid is in the partially filled 12 *mL* syringe shown in Figure 7.6?

The top ring of the plunger is at the second line after the 5 *mL* line. Because each line measures 0.2 *mL*, the second line measures 0.4 *mL*. Therefore, the amount in the syringe is 5.4 *mL*.

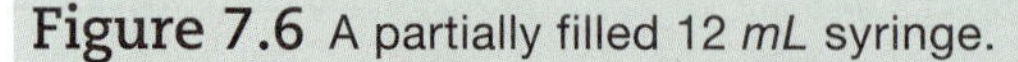

Figure 7.6 A partially filled 12 *mL* syringe.

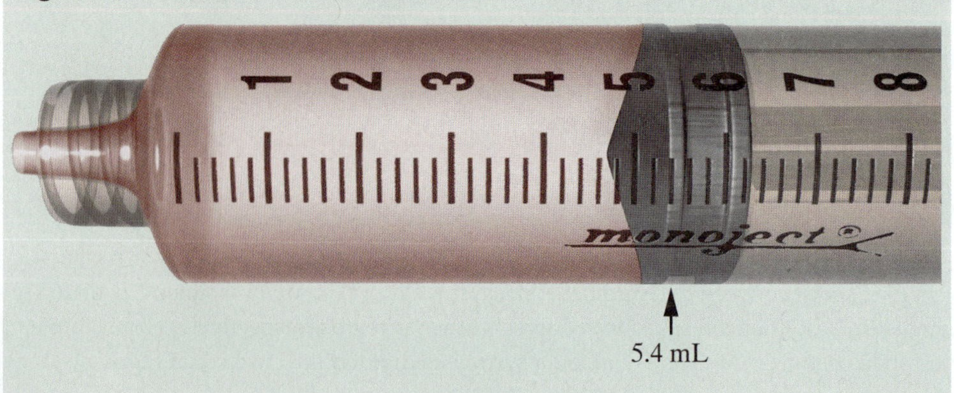

A 5 *mL* syringe is shown in Figure 7.7. Each line on the barrel represents 0.2 *mL*, and the longer lines represent 1 *mL*.

Figure 7.7 A 5 *mL* syringe.

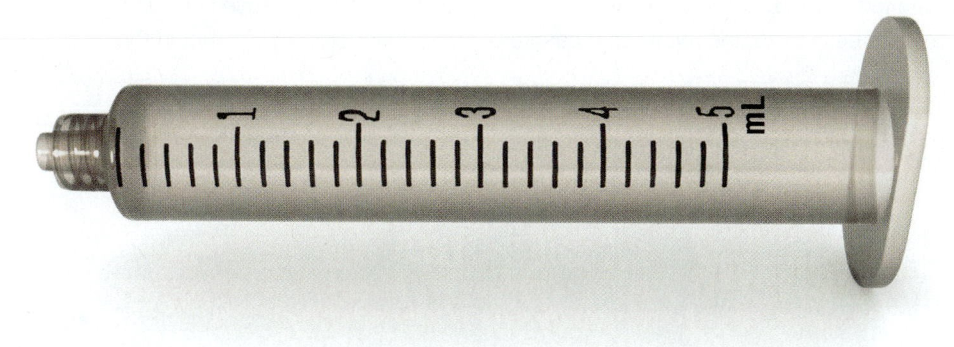

Example 7.2

How much liquid is in the 5 *mL* syringe shown in Figure 7.8?

The top ring of the plunger is at the third line after 4 *mL*. Because each line measures 0.2 *mL*, the third line measures 0.6 *mL*. Therefore, the amount of liquid in the syringe is 4.6 *mL*.

Figure 7.8 A partially filled 5 *mL* syringe.

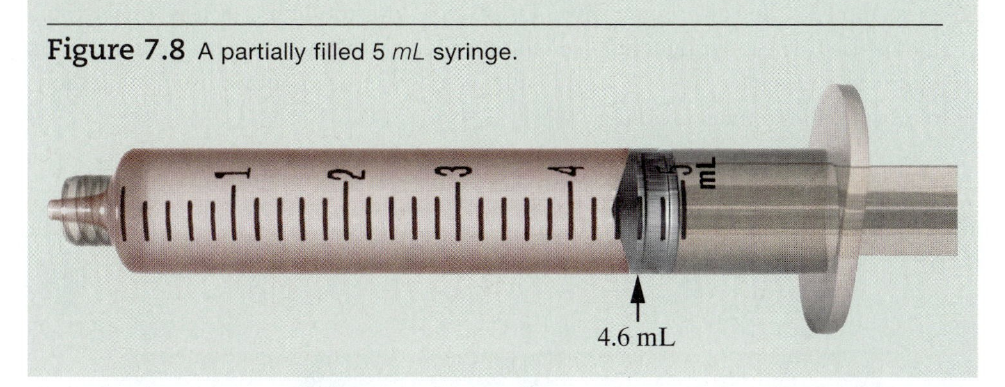

In Figure 7.9, a 3 *mL* syringe is shown. There are 10 spaces between the largest markings. This indicates that the syringe is measured in tenths of a milliliter. So, each of the lines is 0.1 *mL*. The longer lines indicate half and full milliliter measures. The liquid volume in a syringe is read from the *top ring*, **not** the bottom ring or the raised section in the middle of the plunger. Therefore, this syringe contains 0.9 *mL*.

Figure 7.9 A partially filled 3 *mL* syringe.

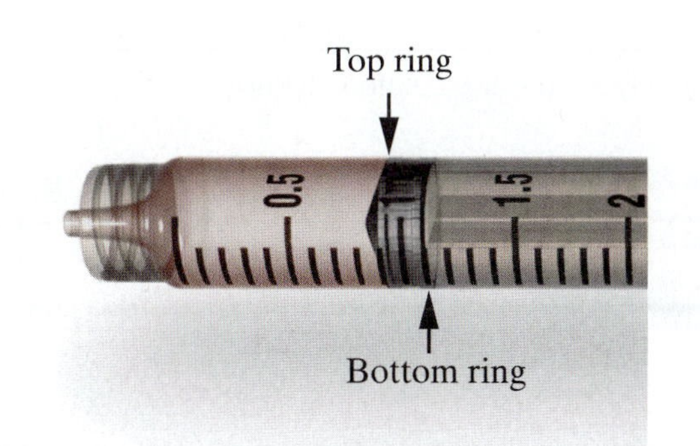

Example 7.3

How much liquid is in the 3 *mL* syringe shown in Figure 7.10?

The top ring of the plunger is at the second line after 1 *mL*. Because each line measures 0.1 *mL*, the two lines measure 0.2 *mL*. Therefore, the amount in the syringe is 1.2 *mL*.

Figure 7.10 A partially filled 3 *mL* syringe.

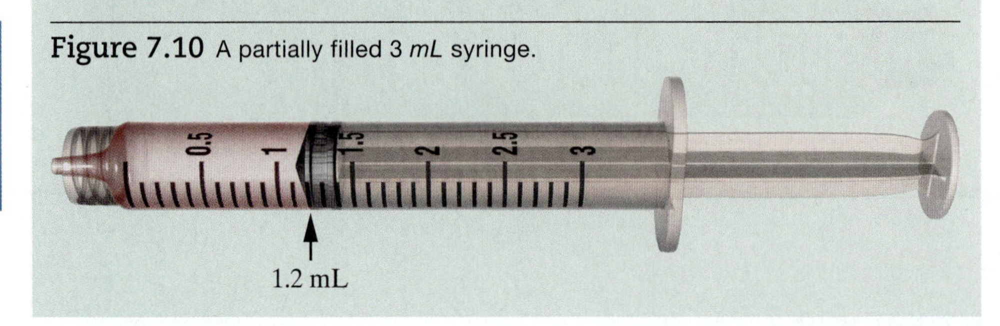

NOTE

When a volume of liquid must be administered, the smallest syringe that holds that volume would be the syringe of choice.

ALERT

The calibrations on the 1 *mL* syringe are very small and close together. Use caution when drawing up medication in this syringe.

When small volumes of 1 *milliliter* or less are required, a low-volume syringe provides the greatest accuracy. The 1 *mL* syringe, also called a tuberculin syringe, shown in Figure 7.11, is calibrated in hundredths of a *milliliter*. Because there are 100 lines on the syringe, each line represents 0.01 *mL*. The 0.5 *mL* syringe, shown in Figure 7.12, has 50 lines, and each line also represents 0.01 *mL*. For doses of 0.5 *mL* or less, this syringe should be used. These syringes are used for intradermal injection of very small amounts of substances in tests for tuberculosis and allergies, as well as for intramuscular injections of small quantities of medication.

Figure 7.11 A partially filled 1 *mL* safety tuberculin syringe.

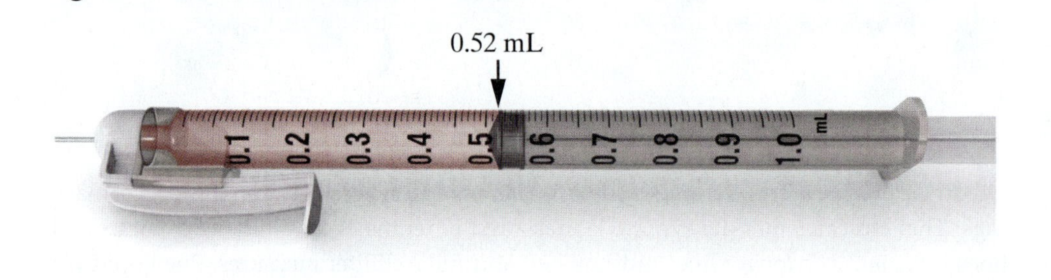

The top ring of the plunger in Figure 7.11 is at the second line after 0.5 *mL*. Therefore, the amount in the syringe is 0.52 *mL*.

Figure 7.12 A partially filled 0.5 *mL* safety syringe.

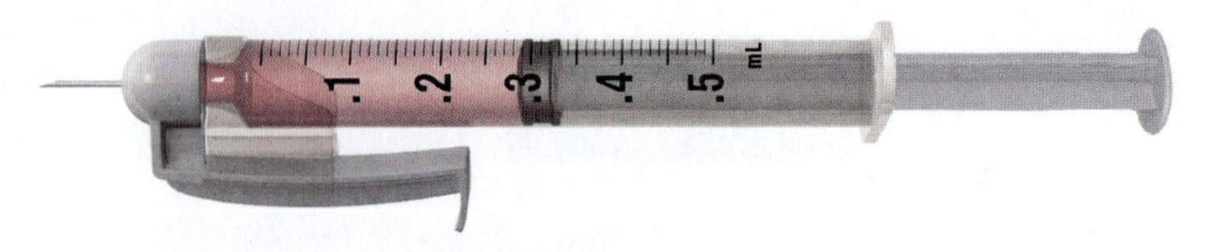

The top ring of the plunger in Figure 7.12 is at the first line before 0.3 *mL* (0.30 *mL*). Therefore, the syringe contains 0.29 *mL*.

Example 7.4

How much liquid is shown in the portion of the 1 *mL* tuberculin syringe shown in Figure 7.13?

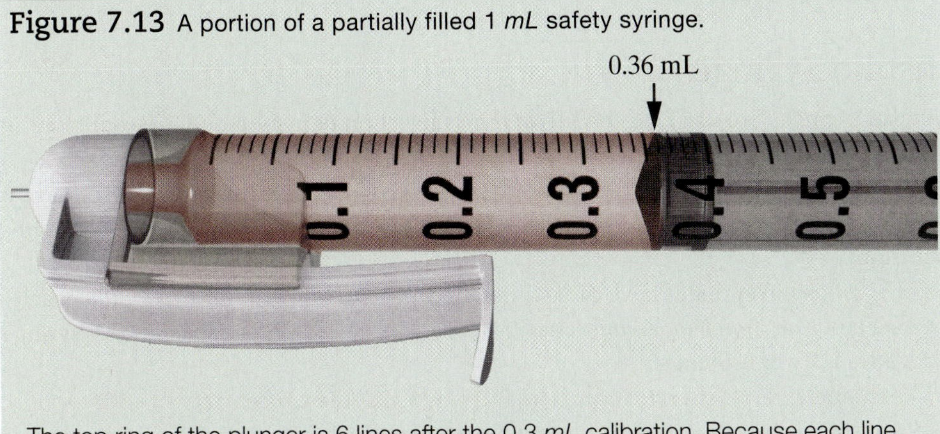

Figure 7.13 A portion of a partially filled 1 *mL* safety syringe.

The top ring of the plunger is 6 lines after the 0.3 *mL* calibration. Because each line represents 0.01 *mL*, the amount of liquid in the syringe is 0.36 *mL*.

Because 0.5 *mL* and 1 *mL* tuberculin syringes can accurately measure amounts to *hundredths* of a *milliliter*, the volume of fluid to be measured in these syringes is rounded to the nearest *hundredth*; for example, 0.358 *mL* is rounded off to 0.36 *mL*.

The 3 *mL* syringe can accurately measure amounts to *tenths* of a *milliliter*; therefore, the volume of fluid to be measured in this syringe is rounded to the nearest *tenth* of a *milliliter*. For example, 2.358 *mL* is rounded off to 2.4 *mL*. These rules are summarized in Table 7.1.

Table 7.1 Rules for Rounding Volumes in a Hypodermic Syringe.

Volume	Round to
Less than 1 *mL*	2 decimal places
More than 1 *mL*	1 decimal place

Insulin

Insulin is a hormone used to treat clients who have insulin-dependent diabetes mellitus (IDDM). Diabetes is fast becoming the epidemic of the 21st century.

Insulin is a high-risk medication. Therefore, a thorough understanding of the various types of insulins and insulin syringes is essential in preventing medication errors. Depending on its form, insulin can be administered via sub cutaneous injection, via intravenous route, via inhalation, or continuously via an insulin pump.

Insulin dosage is determined by the client's daily blood-glucose readings, frequently referred to as a "fingerstick." A blood-glucose monitor is small and can quickly analyze a drop of blood and display the amount of blood glucose measured in *milligrams per deciliter* (*mg/dL*). See Figure 7.14.

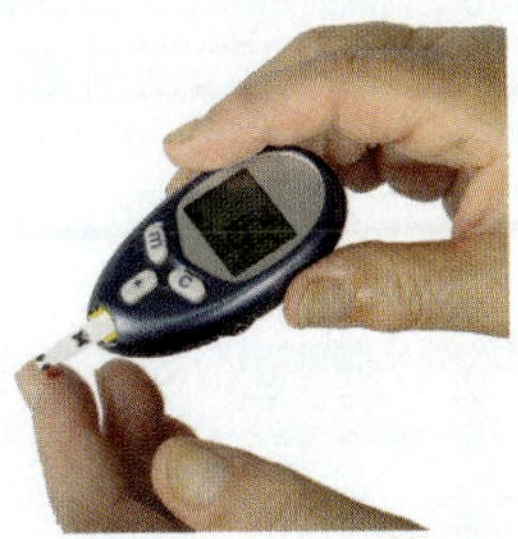

Figure 7.14 A blood-glucose monitor.

SOURCE: Dimitry/Fotolia

Insulin is supplied as a liquid measured in standardized units of potency rather than by weight or volume. These standardized units are called **USP** *units*, often shortened to *units*. The most commonly prepared concentration of insulin is 100 *units per milliliter*, which is referred to as *units 100 insulin* and abbreviated as U-100. Insulin in strengths of 200 units per *mL* (U-200), 300 units per *mL* (U-300), and 500 units per *mL* (U-500) are also available in the United States.

Insulin Syringes

Insulin syringes are used for the *subcutaneous* injection of insulin and are calibrated in *units* rather than *milliliters*.

Insulin syringes are calibrated for the administration of standard U-100 insulin only. Therefore, insulin syringes should not be used for administering nonstandard strengths of insulin.

U-100 insulin syringes have three different capacities: the standard 100-*unit* capacity and the **Lo-Dose** 50-*unit* or 30-*unit* capacities. There is a new FDA-approved U-500 syringe with a capacity of 250 units.

Extreme care must be taken when administering the concentrated U-500 insulin. U-500 insulin is five times the strength of U-100 insulin. To help avoid dosing errors, the new U-500 syringe MUST be used when administering U-500 insulin. This syringe has a volume of 0.5 *mL* with markings in 5-unit increments and allows for dosing up to 250 units. The syringe is color-coded green to align with the Humulin R U-500 insulin vial.

Figure 7.15 shows a *single-scale standard* 100-*unit* insulin syringe calibrated in 2-*unit* increments. Any odd number of units (e.g., 23, 35) is measured halfway between the even calibrations. These calibrations and spaces are very small, so this is not the syringe of choice for a person with impaired vision.

ALERT

Select the appropriate syringe and be very attentive to the calibrations when measuring insulin dosages. Both the single- and dual-scale standard 100-*unit* insulin syringes are calibrated in 2-*unit* increments. The Lo-Dose syringes are calibrated in 1-*unit* increments.

Figure 7.15 A single-scale standard 100-*unit* insulin syringe with 52 *units* of insulin.

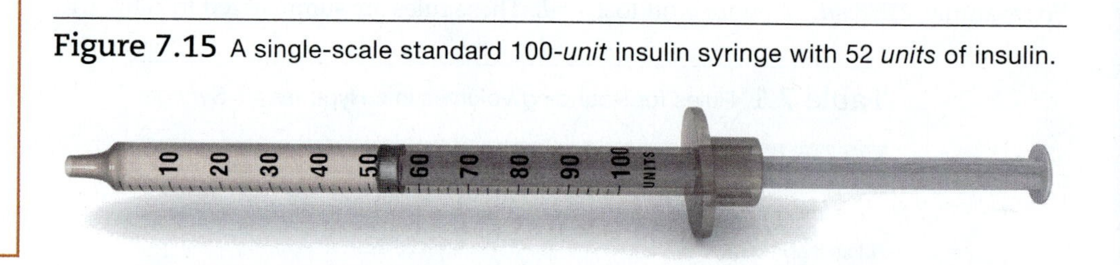

The dual-scale version of the 100-*unit* insulin syringe is easier to use. Figure 7.16 shows both sides of a *dual-scale* 100-*unit* insulin syringe, also calibrated in 2-*unit* increments. However, it has a scale with *even* numbers on one side and a scale with *odd* numbers on the opposite side. Both the even and odd sides are shown. Even-numbered doses

Figure 7.16 Two views of the same dual-scale standard 100-*unit* insulin safety syringe.

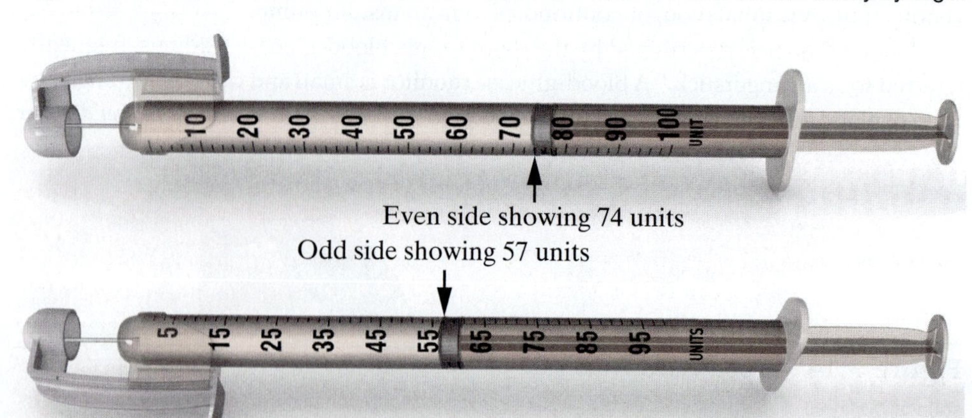

are measured using the "even" side of the syringe, whereas odd-numbered doses are measured using the "odd" side.

Each line on the barrel represents 2 *units*.

For small doses of insulin (50 *units* or fewer), Lo-Dose insulin syringes more accurately measure the doses and should be used. A 50-*unit* Lo-Dose insulin syringe, shown in Figure 7.17, is a single-scale syringe with 50 *units*. It is calibrated in 1-*unit* increments.

Figure 7.17 A 50-*unit* Lo-Dose insulin syringe with protective cap.

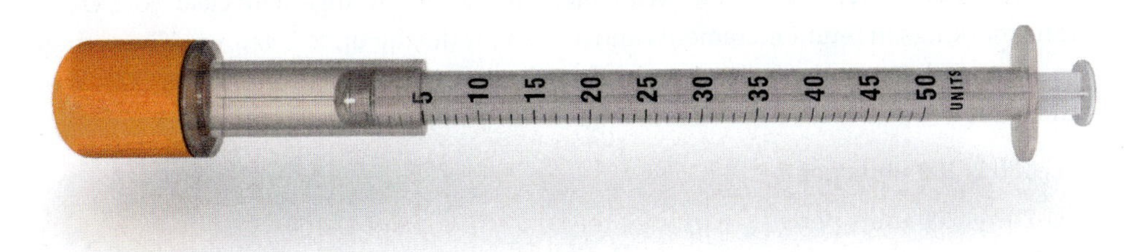

A 30-*unit* Lo-Dose insulin syringe, shown in Figure 7.18, is a syringe with a capacity of 30 *units*. It is calibrated in 1-*unit* increments and is used when the dose is less than 30 *units*.

Figure 7.18 A 30-*unit* Lo-Dose insulin syringe.

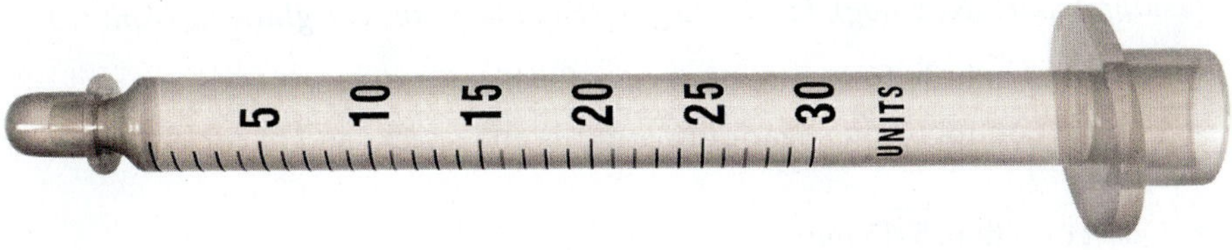

NOTE

Insulin is always ordered in *units*, the medication is supplied in 100 *units/mL*, and the syringes are calibrated for 100 *units/mL*. Therefore, no calculations are required to prepare insulin that is administered subcutaneously.

The insulin syringe is to be used in the measurement and administration of U-100 insulin **only**. *It must not be used to measure other medications that are also measured in units, such as heparin, Pitocin, or U-500 insulin.*

Types of Insulin

Human insulin has been replaced with synthetic insulins *(chemically altered DNA)*. These are called analogs of human insulin. An analog refers to something that is similar or analogous to something else. Insulin analogs are designed to mimic the body's natural pattern of insulin release. They have minor structural or amino acid changes that give them special desirable characteristics. Once absorbed by the body, they act on cells like human insulin, but they are absorbed from fatty tissue more predictably. The rapid-acting insulin analogs work more quickly, and the long-acting insulin analogs last longer and have a more even "peakless" effect.

In a vial or cartridge, human and animal insulins clump together. This clumping causes slow and unpredictable absorption from the subcutaneous tissue and a dose-dependent duration of action. The larger the dose, the longer the effect or duration.

Insulins are categorized by differences in: **Onset**: How quickly they act. **Peak**: How long it takes to achieve maximum effect. **Duration**: How long they last. **Concentration**: The most common concentration of insulin is 100 units per *mL* (U-100). In the United States, concentrations also now include 200 units per *mL* (U-200), 300 units per *mL* (U-300), and 500 units per *mL* (U-500). **Route of delivery**: Inhalation, subcutaneous, or intravenous.

Insulin Concentrations

- insulin lispro injection {rDNA} origin (Humalog) U-200 is available in a prefilled pen only (**Humalog Kwin Pen**)
- insulin glargine injection (Toujeo) U-300 is available in a prefilled pen only(**SoloStar**)
- insulin human injection {rDNA} origin (Humulin R) U-500 is available in a prefilled syringe (**Humulin R U-500 Kwik Pen**) and a 20 *mL* multiple-dose vial. The vial states that the insulin is concentrated and it includes a warning. In November 2016 the first **500-unit insulin syringe** became available. It is a 0.5 *mL* syringe with clear bold U-500 scale markings in 5-unit increments and allows for dosing up to 250 units. The syringe package and components are color-coded to align with the Humulin R U-500 label. Humulin R U-500 is used for clients who require more than 200 units per day.

ALERT

It is crucial that the nurse is very vigilant when reading the insulin label. There is potential to administer two, three, or five times the dose if the wrong insulin is selected. An overdose can result in irreversible insulin shock and death.

U-100 is 100 units per *mL*.

U-200 is 200 units per *mL*, two times the concentration of U-100.

U-300 is 300 units per *ml*, three times the concentration of U-100

U-500 is 500 units per *mL*, five times the concentration of U-100.

Types of Insulin

Fast-acting or Rapid-acting

insulin Aspart (Novolog), insulin Lispro (Humalog), insulin glulisine (Apidra)

- Absorbed quickly from fatty tissue into the bloodstream
- Used to control blood sugar during meals and snacks and to correct high blood sugars
- Onset of action: 5–15 minutes
- Peak effect: 1–2 hours
- Duration of action: 4–6 hours
- Clear in color
- Can be administered subcutaneously and intravenously
- Available in vials and pens

Intermediate-acting

NPH human insulin (Humulin N, Novolin N), premixed insulin (NPH with either regular human insulin or a rapid-acting insulin)

- Absorbed more slowly, lasts longer
- Used to control the blood sugar overnight, while fasting, and between meals.
- Onset: 1–2 hours
- Peak effect: 4–6 hours
- Duration: more than 12 hours

Long-acting

insulin glargine (Lantus) and insulin detemir (Levemir)

- Absorbed slowly, has a minimal peak effect and a stable plateau effect that lasts most of the day
- Used to control the blood sugar overnight, while fasting, and between meals
- Onset: $1-1\frac{1}{2}$ hours
- Effect: plateaus over next few hours
- Duration: 12–24 hours for insulin detemir and 24 hours for insulin glargine
- Clear in color

- Once daily dosing, any time of day, but same time every day
- Administered subcutaneously only
- Cannot be mixed with other insulins

Ultra-long-acting

insulin degludec (Tresiba)

- Onset: 30–90 minutes
- Peak: none due to slow release into systemic circulation
- Duration: more than 24 hours
- Clear in color
- Once daily dosing
- Available in **Unit-100 Flex-Touch** and **U-200 Flex-Touch pens**

Premixed combination

Humalog mix 50/50, Humalog 75/25, Humulin 50/50, Humulin 70/30, Novolog Mix 70/30, Novolin 70/30

- Combines fast-acting and intermediate-acting insulins
- Stimulates the varying levels of insulin within the body
- Decreases the need for client to mix insulins
- Decreases the number of injections required
- Available in vials and pens for administration

Inhaled

inhalation powder (Afrezza)

- Rapid-acting, inhaled at beginning of each meal
- Can be used for adults with type 1 or 2 diabetes
- Must be used in combination with injectable long-acting insulin
- Supplied in cartridges of 4 units, 8 units, and 12 units
- Onset: 12–15 minutes
- Peak effect: 30 minutes
- Duration: 180 minutes

New products

Glucagon-like peptide-1 (GLP-1) receptor agonist enhances glucose-dependent insulin secretion by the pancreatic beta-cell, suppresses inappropriately elevated glucagon secretion, and slows gastric emptying.

dulaglutide (Trulicity)

- Adjunct to diet and exercise to improve glycemic control in adults who have type 2 diabetes mellitus
- Administered subcutaneously once weekly any time of day
- Available as 0.75 *mg*/0.5 *mL* solution in a single-dose pen or prefilled syringe and 1.5 *mg*/0.5 *mL* solution in a single-dose pen or prefilled syringe

exenatide (Byetta)

- Used to treat people who have type 2 DM
- Adjunct to diet and exercise
- NOT a substitute for insulin
- Administer sub cut injection 60 *minutes* ac morning and evening meals (at least 6 *hours* or more apart)
- Available as 250 *mcg*/*mL* in 5 *mcg*/dose, 1.2 *mL* prefilled pen and 10 *mcg*/dose, 2.4 *mL* prefilled pen

> **ALERT**
>
> Insulin should be at room temperature when administered, and one source or brand of insulin should not be substituted for another without medical supervision.

Insulin glargine and lixisenatide (Soliqua® 100/33) 100 *units/mL* and 33 *mcg/mL*

- Contains Lantus and lixisenatide (a GLP-1 receptor agonist)
- Once daily injection subcut injection within the hour of first meal
- Available as 100-unit insulin glargine per *mL* and 33 *mcg* lixisenatide per *mL* in a prefilled 3 *mL* pen
- Available in U.S., January 2017

See Figure 7.19 for examples of drug labels for various types of insulin.

Figure 7.19 Drug labels for various types of insulin.

Intermediate-acting

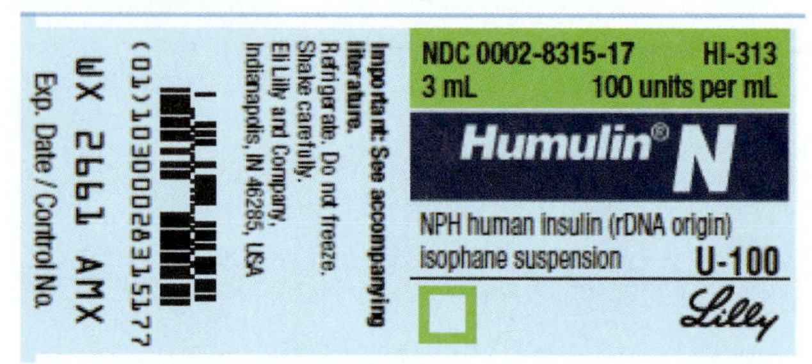

Intermediate-acting

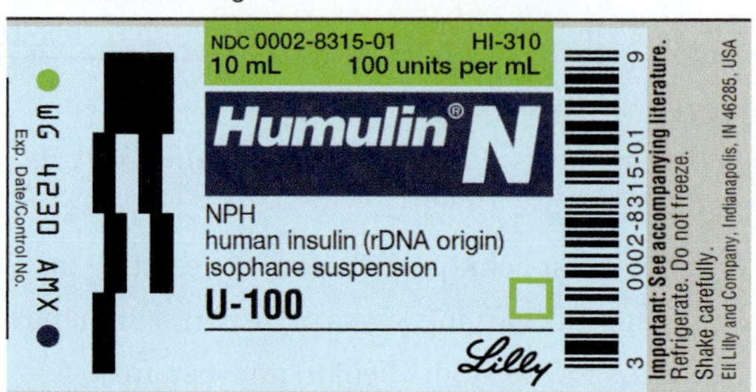

SOURCE: Courtesy of AbbVie

Short-acting

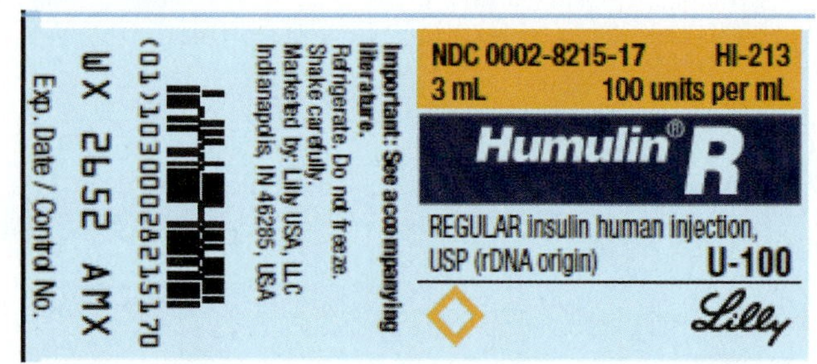

Short-acting

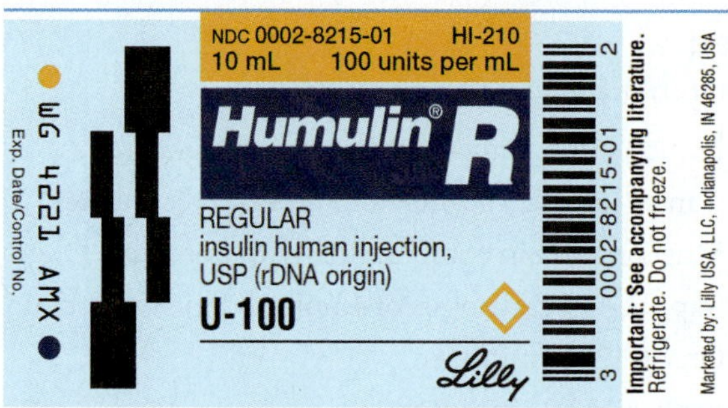

Rapid-acting

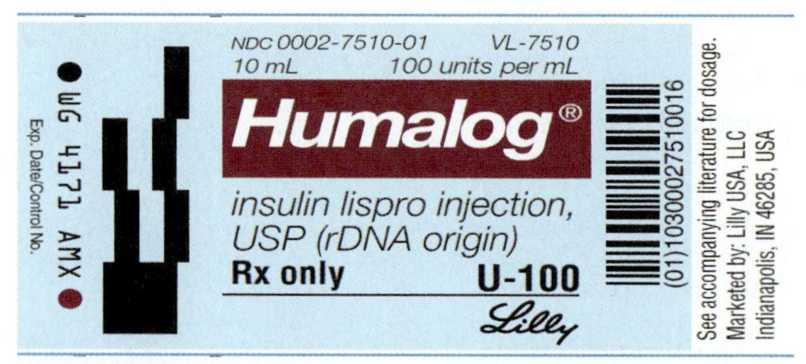

Rapid-acting

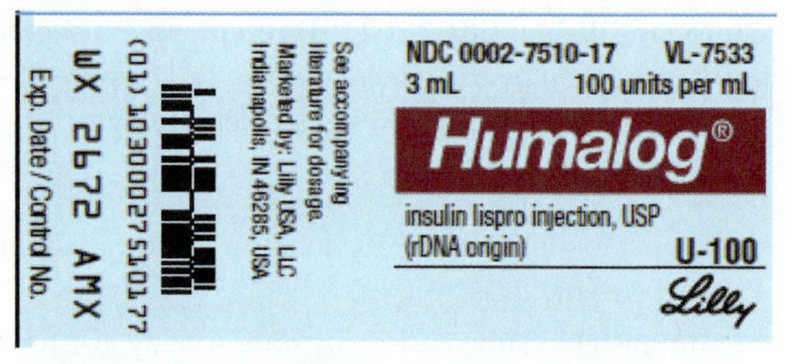

Combination 70% intermediate-acting and 30% short-acting

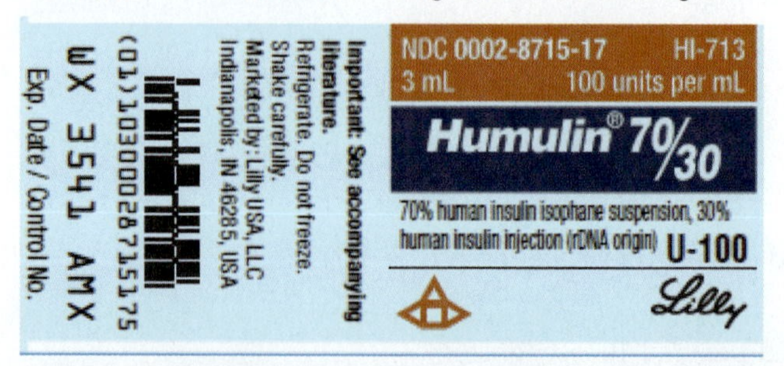

Combination 70% intermediate-acting and 30% short-acting

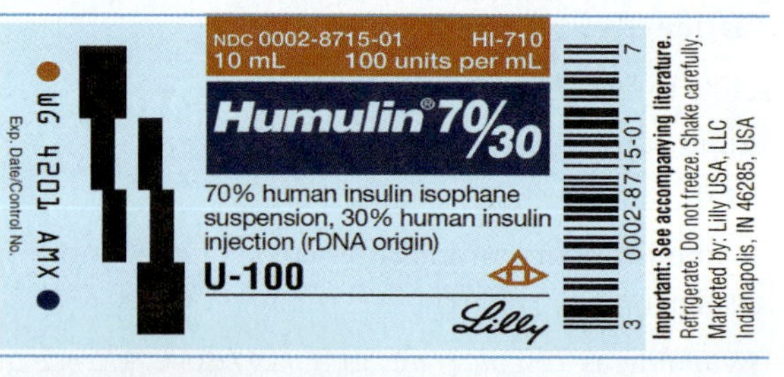

Figure 7.19 *(Continued)*

Combination 75% intermediate-acting and 25% rapid-acting

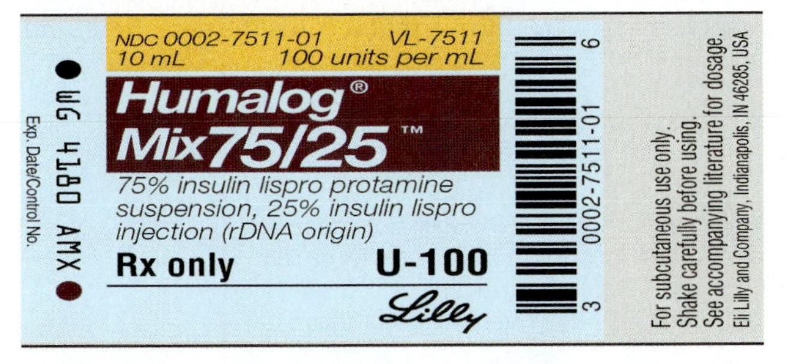

Combined 50% intermediate-acting and 50% rapid-acting

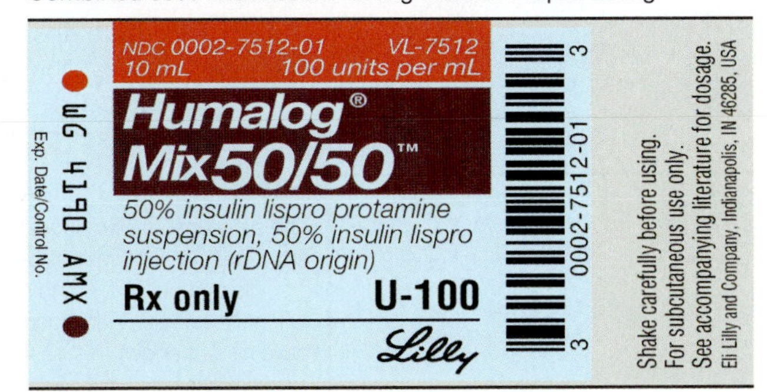

Rapid-acting 200 units per *mL*

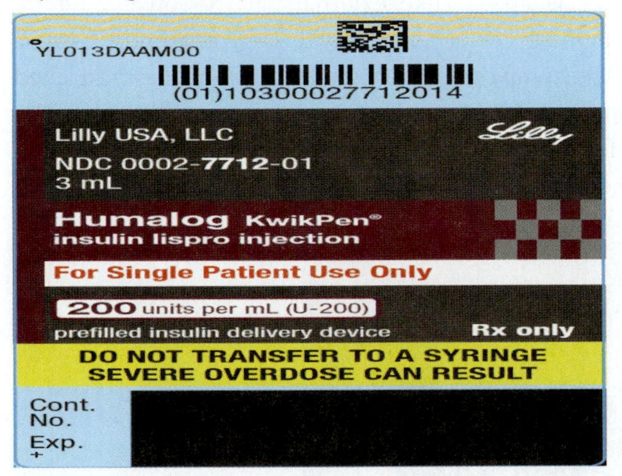

Short-acting 500 units per *mL*

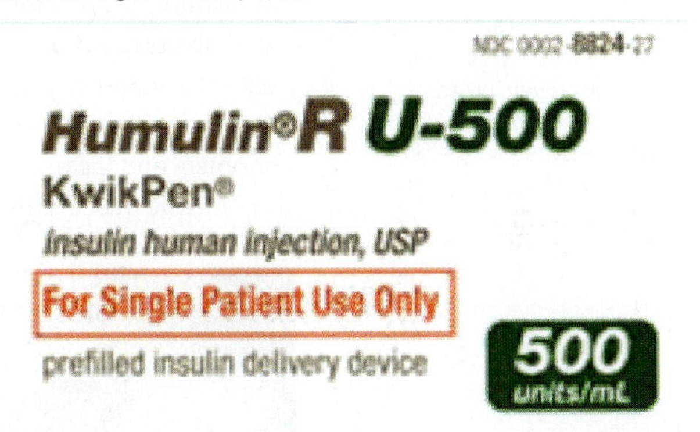

Insulin Pens

An insulin pen is an insulin delivery system that looks like a pen, uses an insulin cartridge, and has disposable needles. Compared to the traditional syringe and vial, a pen device is easier to use, provides greater dose accuracy, and is more acceptable to clients.

Some pens are disposed of after one use, whereas others have replaceable insulin cartridges. All pens use needles that minimize the discomfort of injection because they are extremely short and very thin.

The parts of an insulin pen are shown in Figure 7.20. The dose selector knob is used to "dial" the desired dose of insulin. Once the pen has been "primed" (cleared of any

Figure 7.20 An insulin pen.

See video demo of the FlexPen at http://www.levemir-us.com/about-levemir-FlexPen-demo.asp?WLac=LevemirFlexPen

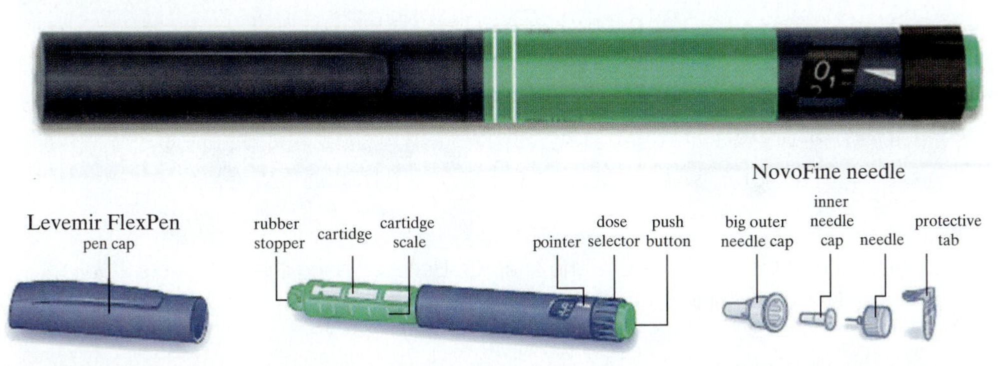

air in the cartridge) and the dose set, the insulin is injected by pressing on the injection button. Because preparing a dose with a pen involves dialing a mechanical device and not looking at the side of a syringe, insulin users with reduced visual acuity can be more assured of accurate dosing. Some pens have a "memory" that records the date, time, and amount of doses administered.

ALERT

The same insulin pen should not be used for multiple clients. The Joint Commission states that "insulin will not be borrowed or shared." Insulin pens are meant for use on a single person ONLY, and should NEVER be used for more than one person, even when the needle is changed (CDC 2012, FDA 2009). Therefore, each client should have his or her own insulin vial/pen.

ALERT

Insulin is a *high-alert medication*. Be sure to check your institution's policy regarding administration. For example, some agencies may require insulin doses to be checked by two nurses.

Insulin Pumps

An insulin pump, shown in Figure 7.21, is a beeperlike, external, battery-powered device that delivers rapid-acting insulin continuously for 24 *hours* a day through a **cannula** (a small, hollow tube) inserted under the skin. The pump contains an insulin cartridge that is attached to tubing with a cannula or needle on the end. The needle is inserted under the skin of the abdomen, and it can remain in place for two to three days. The insulin is delivered through this "infusion set." This eliminates the need for multiple daily injections of insulin.

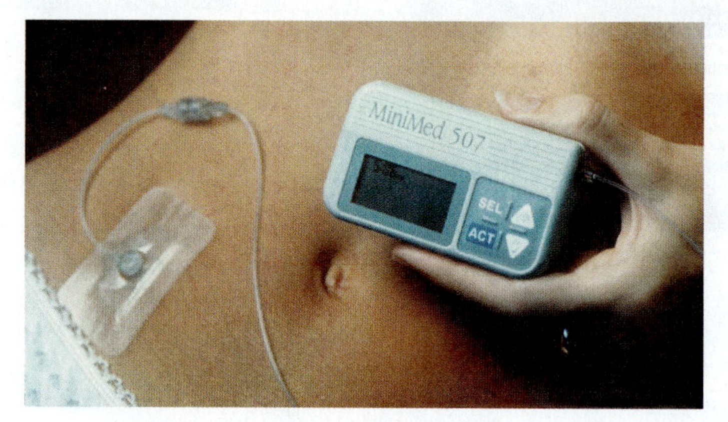

Figure 7.21
An insulin pump.

SOURCE: Ron May/Pearson Education, Inc.

The pump can be programmed to deliver a basal rate and/or a bolus dose. **Basal** insulin is delivered continuously over 24 *hours* to keep blood-glucose levels in range between meals and overnight. The basal rate can be programmed to deliver different rates at different times. **Bolus** doses can be delivered at mealtimes to provide control for additional food intake. The insulin pump currently on the market is the closest approximation to an artificial pancreas.

Example 7.5

What is the dose of insulin in the single-scale 100-*unit* insulin syringe shown in Figure 7.22?

Figure 7.22 A single-scale 100-*unit* insulin syringe.

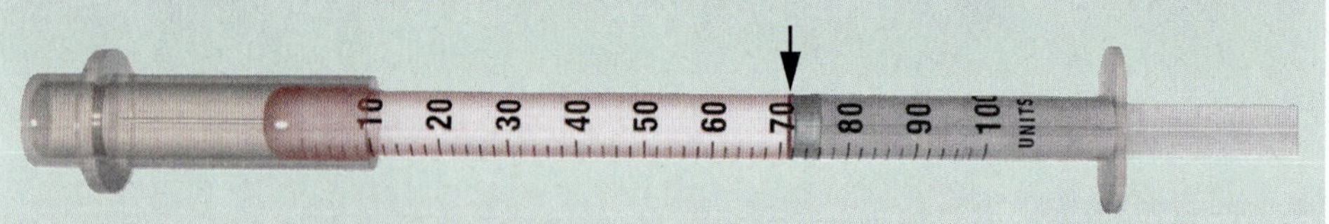

The top ring of the plunger is one line after 70. Because each line represents 2 *units*, the dose is 72 *units* of insulin.

Example 7.6

What is the dose of insulin in the dual-scale 100-*unit* insulin syringe shown in Figure 7.23?

Figure 7.23 Two views of a dual-scale insulin syringe.

100-unit dual-scale syringe

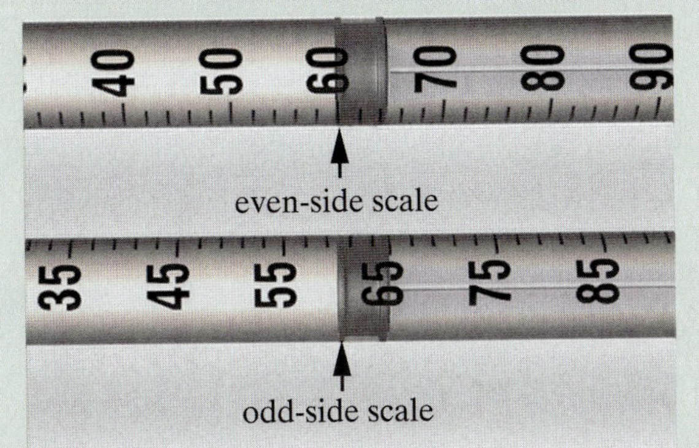

The top ring of the plunger is between calibrations and is slightly more than 2 lines after 55 on the odd-side scale. Notice how difficult it would be to determine where 60 *units* would measure using the odd-side scale of the syringe. However, on the even-side scale, the plunger falls exactly on the 60. So, the dose is 60 *units*.

Example 7.7

What is the dose of insulin in the 50-*unit* insulin syringe shown in Figure 7.24?

Figure 7.24 A 50-*unit* insulin syringe.

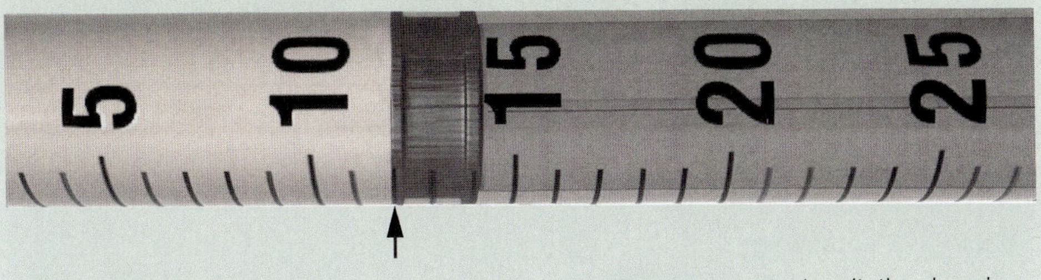

The top ring of the plunger is at 12. Because each line represents 1 *unit*, the dose is 12 *units*.

Example 7.8

What is the dose of insulin in the 30-*unit* insulin syringe shown in Figure 7.25?

Figure 7.25 A 30-*unit* Lo-Dose insulin syringe.

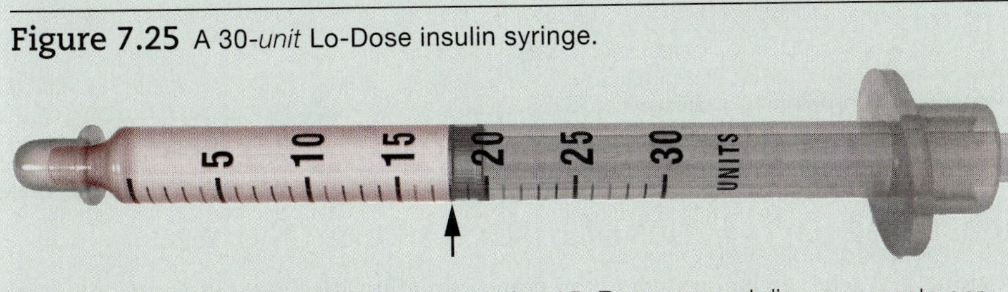

The top ring of the plunger is three lines after 15. Because each line represents one unit, the dose is 18 *units* of insulin.

Example 7.9

Order: *Humulin 70/30 (insulin human) 8 units subcut daily.*

(a) Choose the most appropriate of the three syringes shown in Figure 7.26, and place an arrow at the correct dosage level. See Figure 7.27 for the answer.
(b) How many 8-*unit* doses will a *10 mL* vial of *Humulin 70/30* contain?

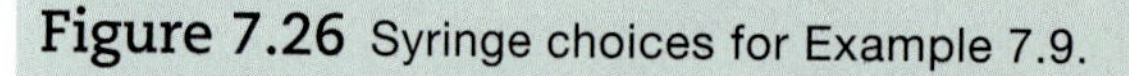

Figure 7.26 Syringe choices for Example 7.9.

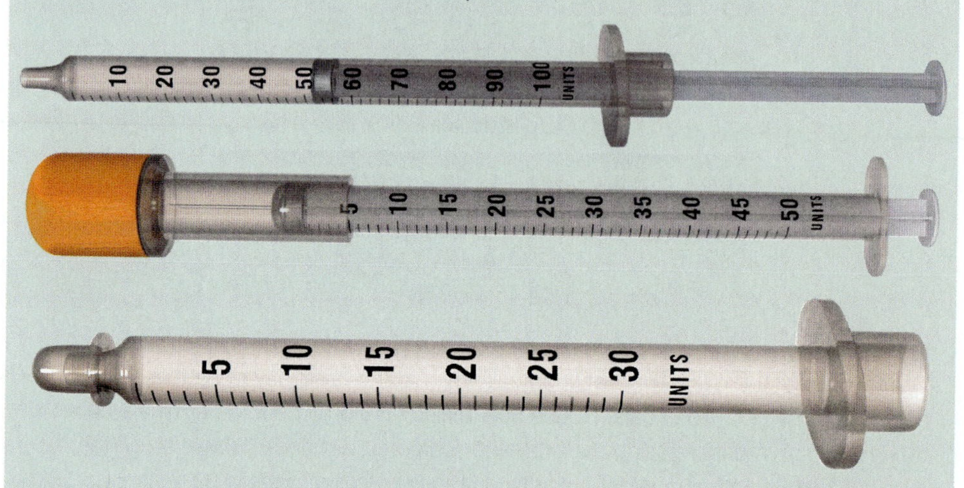

(a) The best choice would be the smallest syringe that contains the dose, that is, the 30 *mL* Lo-Dose insulin syringe.

Figure 7.27 Insulin syringe showing 8 *units* for Example 7.9.

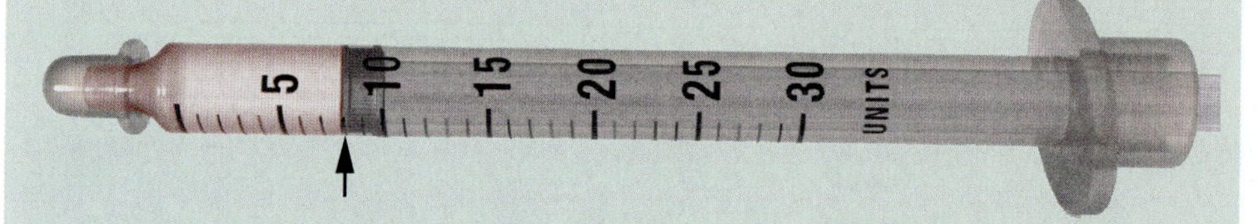

(b) You want to know how many doses would be contained in the vial. That is,

$$1\ vial = ?\ doses$$

You know the following:

- 1 *vial* contains a volume of 10 *mL*
- the standard strength of U-100 insulin is 100 *units/mL*
- 1 *dose* = 8 *units*

The above three items will provide the three unit fractions needed to do the problem as follows:

$$\frac{1\ \cancel{vial}}{1} \times \frac{10\ \cancel{mL}}{1\ \cancel{vial}} \times \frac{100\ \cancel{units}}{1\ \cancel{mL}} \times \frac{1\ dose}{8\ \cancel{units}} = 125\ doses$$

So, the vial contains 125 *doses*.

Measuring Two Types of Insulin in One Syringe

Individuals who have insulin-dependent diabetes mellitus (IDDM) often must have two different types of insulin administered at the same time. This combination is usually composed of a *rapid-acting* insulin with either an *intermediate-* or *long-acting* insulin; this can be accomplished by using an appropriate premixed combination drug. However, often the different insulin types are mixed in a single syringe just before administration, and the important points to remember in this process are:

- The *total volume* in the syringe is the *sum of the two insulin* amounts.
- The smallest-capacity syringe containing the dose should be used to measure the insulins because the enlarged scale is easier to read and therefore more accurate.
- The *amount of air equal to the amount of insulin to be withdrawn* from each vial must be injected into each vial.
- You must inject the air into the intermediate- or long-acting insulin before you inject the air into the regular insulin.
- The *regular* (rapid-acting) insulin is drawn up *first*; this prevents contamination of the regular insulin with the intermediate- or long-acting insulin.
- The intermediate- or long-acting insulins can precipitate; therefore, they must be well mixed before drawing up and administered without delay.
- Only insulins from the same source should be mixed together; for example, Humulin R and Humulin N are both human insulin and can be mixed.
- If you draw up too much of the intermediate- or long-acting insulin, you must discard the entire medication and start over.

The steps for preparing two types of insulin in one syringe are shown in **Example 7.10**.

ALERT

When injecting the air, do not touch the tip of the needle to the insulin in the vial.

NOTE

When you are mixing two types of insulin, think: "Clear, then Cloudy."

Example 7.10

The prescriber ordered 10 *units* Humulin R insulin and 30 *units* Humulin N insulin subcutaneously, 30 *minutes* before breakfast. Explain how you would prepare to administer this in one injection. Figures 7.28 and 7.29.

Figure 7.28 Mixing two types of insulin in one syringe.

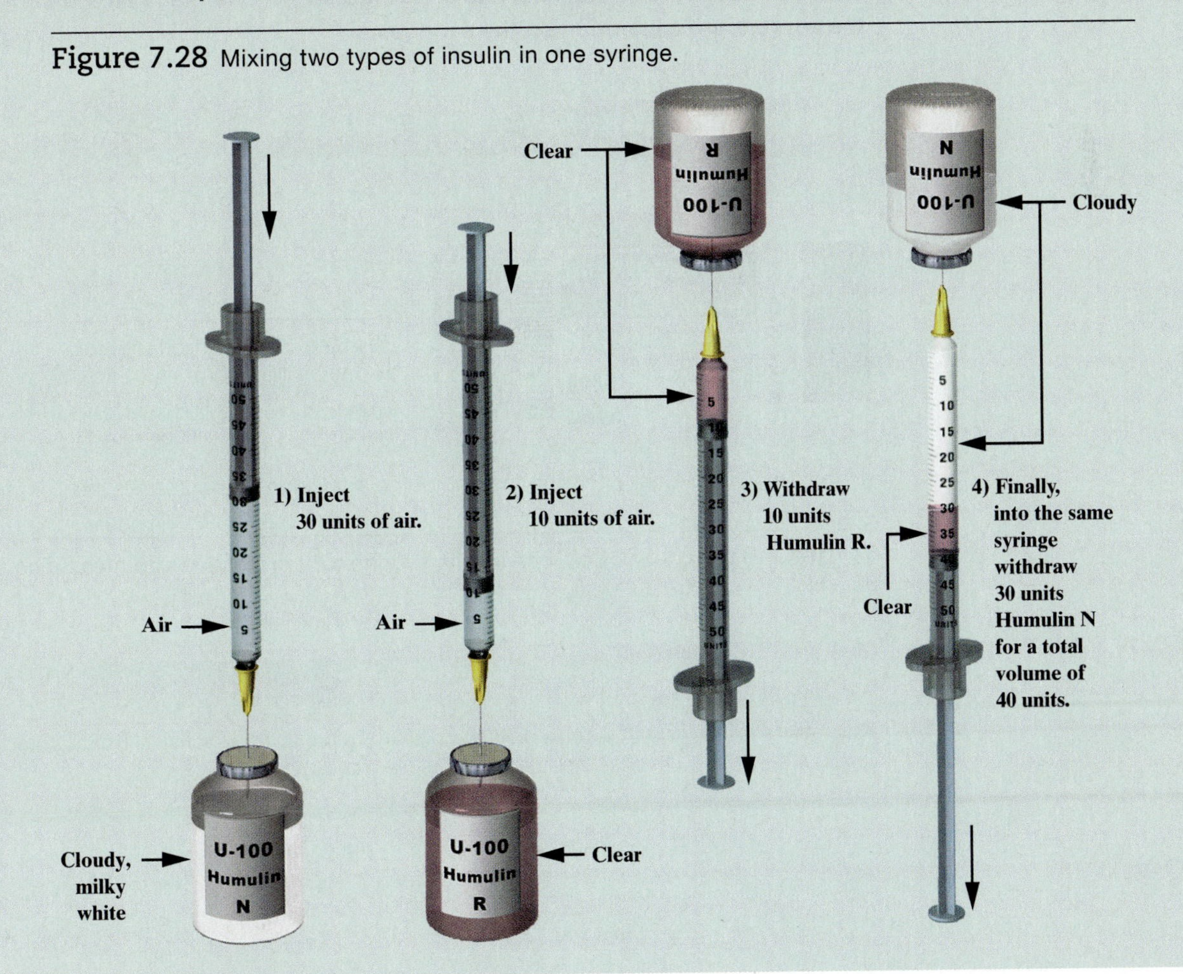

Figure 7.29 Combination of 30 *units* Humulin N and 10 *units* of Humulin R.

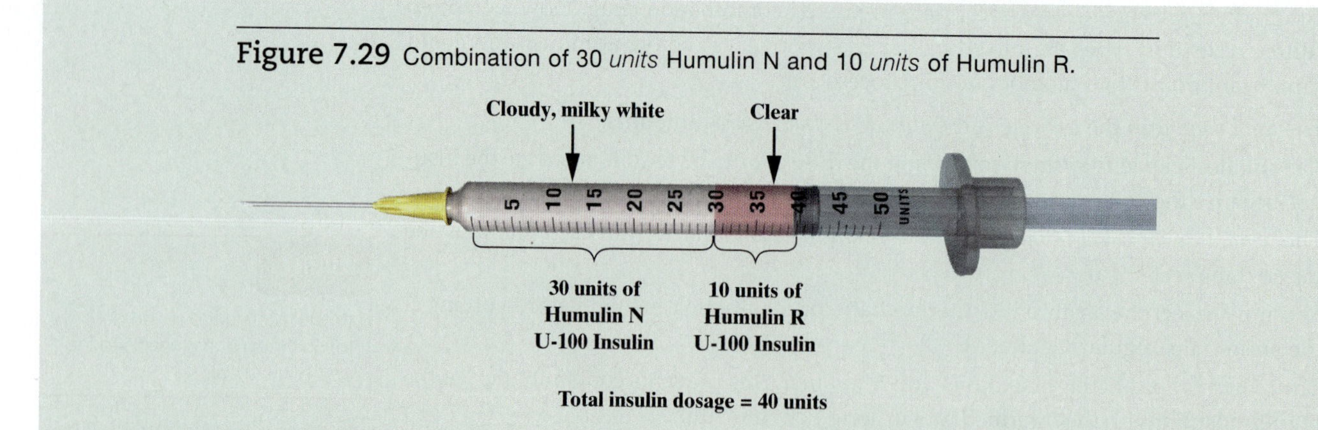

The total amount of insulin is 40 *units* (10 + 30). To administer this dose, use a 50-*unit* Lo-Dose syringe. Inject 30 *units* of air into the Humulin N vial and 10 *units* of air into the Humulin R vial. Withdraw 10 *units* of the Humulin R (rapid-acting) first and then withdraw 30 *units* of the Humulin N (intermediate-acting).

Premixed Insulin

Using premixed insulin eliminates errors that may occur when mixing two types of insulin in one syringe (Figure 7.28).

Example 7.11

Order: Give 35 *units* of Humalog Mix 50/50 insulin subcutaneously 30 *minutes* before breakfast. Use the label shown in Figure 7.30, and place an arrow at the appropriate calibration on the syringe.

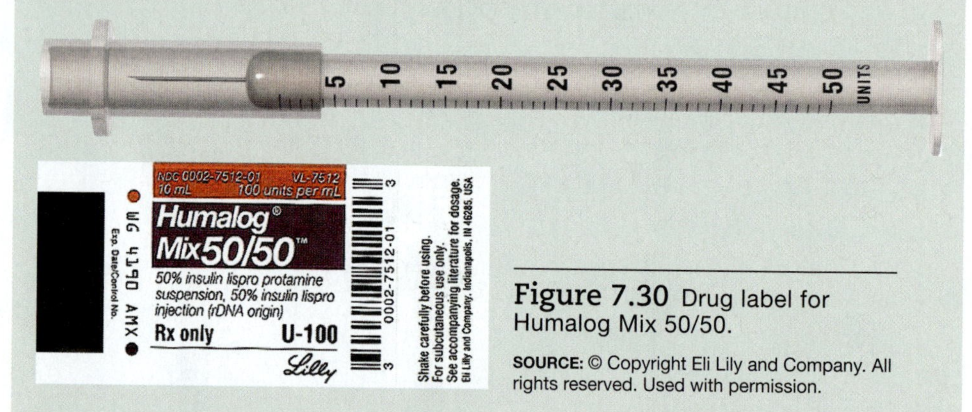

Figure 7.30 Drug label for Humalog Mix 50/50.

In the syringe in Figure 7.31, the top ring of the plunger is at the 35-*unit* line.

Figure 7.31 A 50-*unit* Lo-Dose insulin syringe with protective cap measuring 35 *units*.

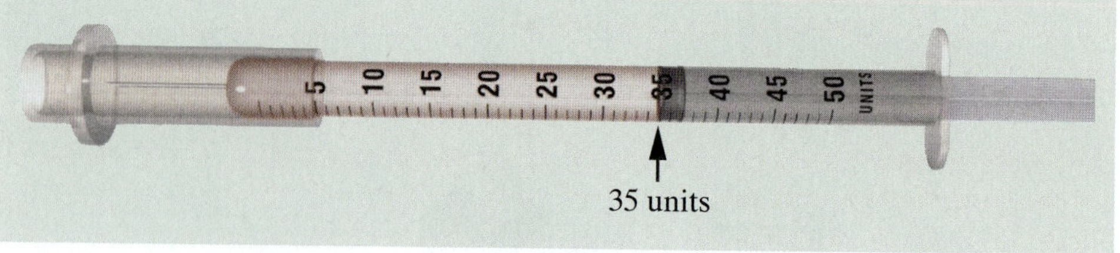

Insulin Coverage/Sliding-Scale Calculations

Regular insulin is sometimes ordered to lower ("cover") a client's blood-sugar level. The prescriber may order regular insulin to be given on a "sliding scale" schedule. The "sliding scale" recommends a dose based on blood-sugar level just before meals.

Example 7.12

Order: *fingersticks Q.I.D., at breakfast, lunch, and dinner and at bedtime. Give regular insulin as follows*:

glucose less than 150 mg/dL	*—no insulin*
glucose of 150–200 mg/dL	*—2 units*
glucose of 201–250 mg/dL	*—3 units*
glucose of 251–300 mg/dL	*—5 units*
glucose of more than 300 mg/dL	*—give 6 units and contact the prescriber stat*

Use the sliding scale to determine how much insulin you will give the client if the glucose level before lunchtime is:

(a) 125 *mg/dL*

(b) 278 *mg/dL*

(c) 350 *mg/dL*

(a) You need to compare the client's level with the information provided in the sliding scale. Because 125 *mg/dL* is less than 150 *mg/dL*, you would not administer any insulin.

(b) Because 278 *mg/dL* is between 251 and 300 *mg/dL*, you would administer 5 *units* of regular insulin immediately.

(c) Because 350 *mg/dL* is more than 300 *mg/dL*, you would give 6 units of regular insulin and contact the prescriber stat.

ALERT

More than 15 *units* of regular insulin for coverage is usually too much. Contact the physician.

NOTE

Currently, there is evidence that the routine use of the sliding scale should be discontinued because of an unacceptably high rate of hyper- and hypoglycemia and iatrogenic diabetic ketoacidosis in hospitalized clients with type 1 diabetes. Be sure to know your current hospital policies and protocols.

Prefilled Syringes

A prefilled, single-dose syringe contains the usual dose of a medication. Some prefilled glass cartridges are available for use with a special plunger called a Tubex or Carpuject syringe (Figure 7.32). If a medication order is for the exact amount of drug in the prefilled syringe, the possibility of measurement error by the person administering the drug is decreased.

Figure 7.32 Carpuject and Tubex prefilled cartridge holders.

SOURCE: Pearson Education, Inc.

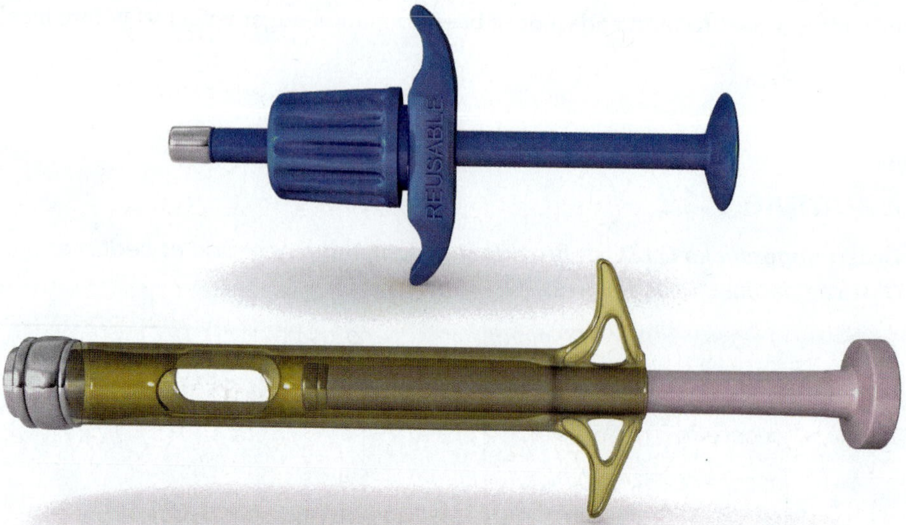

Example 7.13

The prefilled syringe cartridge shown in Figure 7.33 is calibrated so that each line measures 0.1 *mL*, and it has a capacity of 2.5 *mL*. How many *milliliters* are indicated by the arrow shown in Figure 7.33?

Figure 7.33 Prefilled cartridges.

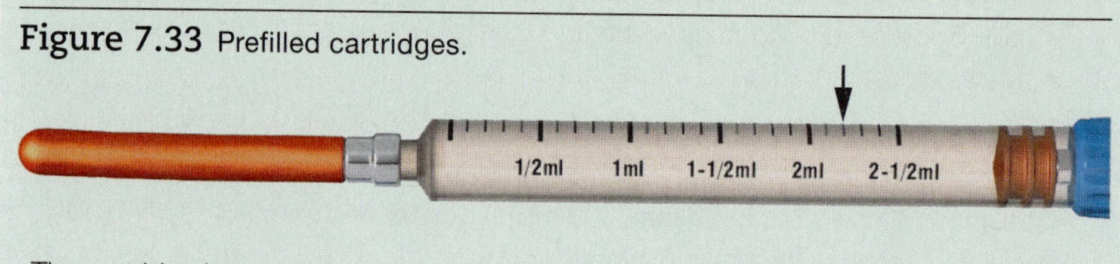

The cartridge has a total capacity of 2.5 *mL*, and the arrow is at 2.2 *mL*.

Example 7.14

How much medication is in the prepackaged cartridge shown in Figure 7.34?

Figure 7.34 Prefilled cartridge in holder.

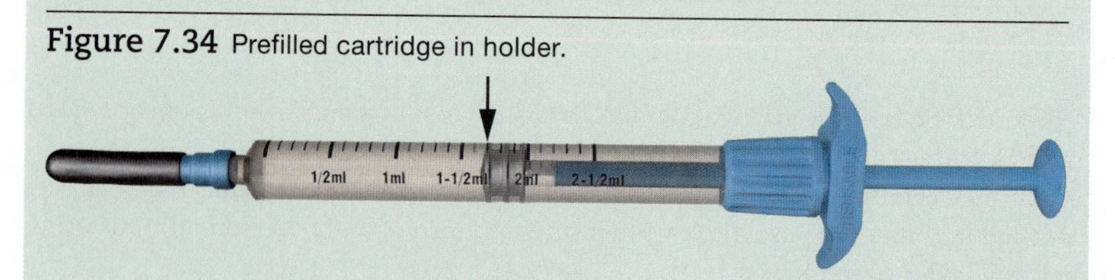

The top of the plunger is at two lines after the 1.5 *mL* line. Because each line measures 0.1 *mL*, the two lines measure 0.2 *mL*. Therefore, there are 1.7 *mL* of medication in this prefilled cartridge.

ALERT

To avoid errors when using Carpuject prefilled syringes, visually inspect the volume of solution in the cartridge to confirm that it contains the labeled fill volume. Cartridges with overfill should be returned to the pharmacy. Prefilled syringes should NOT be used as single- and multiple-dose vials, by withdrawing all or part of the medication in the cartridge into a syringe (ISMP Nurse Advisor ERR, Sept. 2012).

Safety Syringes

To prevent the transmission of blood-borne infections from contaminated needles, many syringes are now manufactured with various types of safety devices. For example, a syringe may contain a protective sheath (a) that can be used to protect the needle's sterility. This sheath is then pulled forward and locked into place to provide a permanent needle shield for disposal following injection. Others may have a needle that automatically retracts (b) into the barrel after injection. Each of these devices reduces the chance of needlestick injury. Figure 7.35 shows examples of safety syringes.

NOTE

To view an animation of the operation of a safety syringe, go to http://www.bd.com/hypodermic/products/integra/.

Figure 7.35 Safety syringes with (a) an active safety device and (b) a passive safety device.

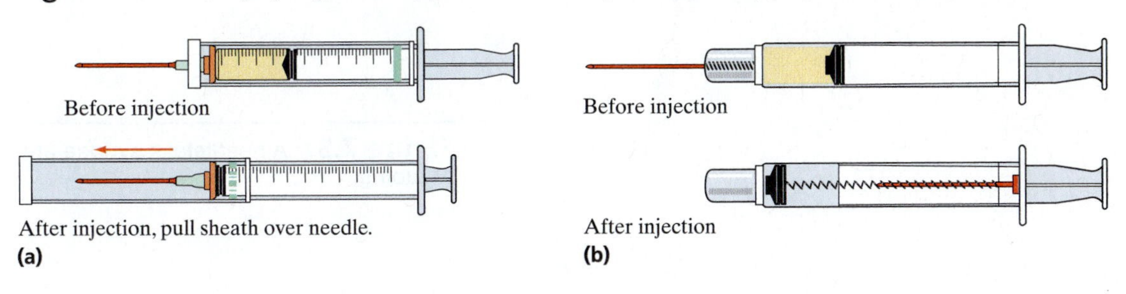

Needleless Syringes

A needleless syringe is a type of safety syringe designed to prevent needle punctures. It may be used to extract medication from a vial (see Figure 7.36), to add medication to intravenous (IV) tubing for medication administration (see Figure 7.37), or to administer medication by mouth (see Figure 7.38).

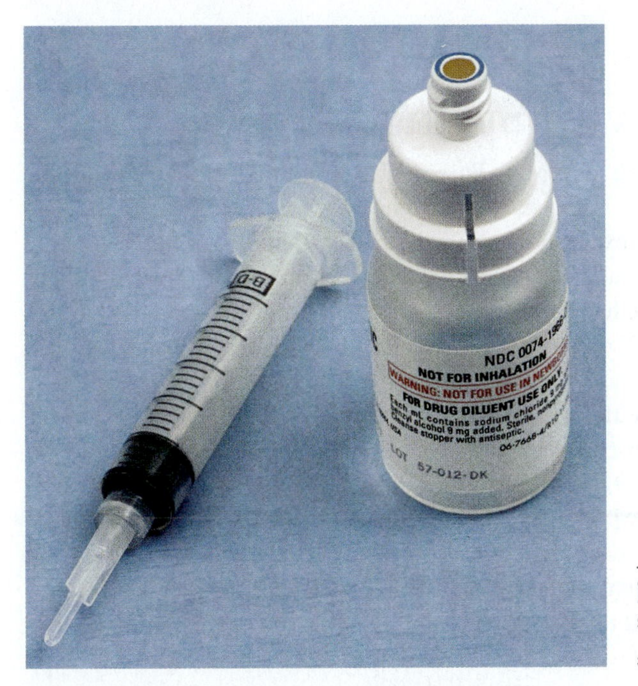

Figure 7.36 A needleless syringe and vial.

SOURCE: Al Dodge/Pearson Education, Inc.

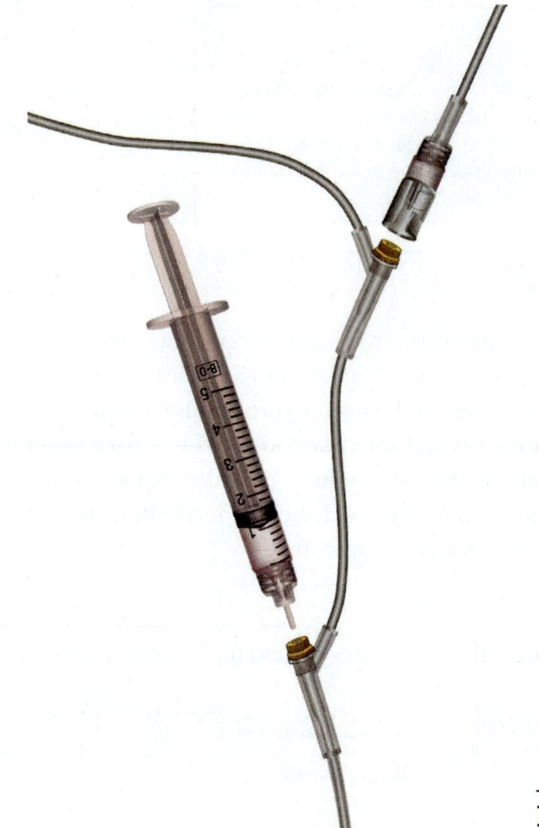

Figure 7.37 A needleless syringe and IV tubing.

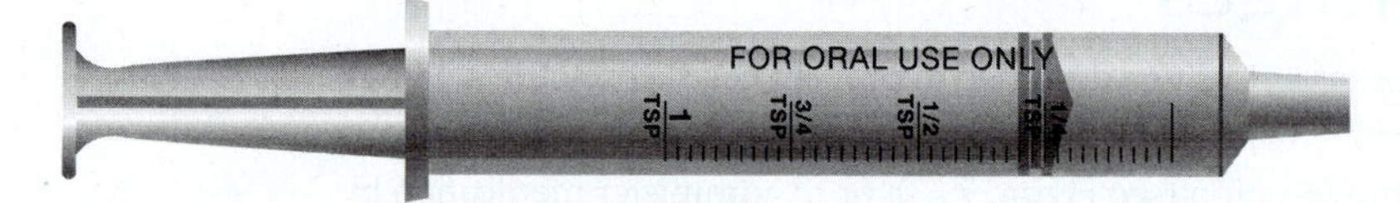

Figure 7.38 Oral syringe.

Dosing Errors with Syringes

Care must be taken when filling a syringe. Being off by even a small amount on the syringe scale can be critical. This is especially true when a syringe contains a relatively small portion of its capacity. For example, say a 3 *mL* syringe should correctly be filled to the prescribed 2.8 *mL* and by mistake it is filled to 2.9 *mL* (one extra tick on the scale). This results in about a 4% overdose [Change/Original = 0.1/2.8] On the other hand, if a 3 *mL* syringe should correctly be filled to 1 *mL* and by mistake it is filled to 1.1 *mL* (one extra tick), this results in a more serious, 10% overdose [Channge/Original = 0.1/1].

Rounding your final calculations also may lead to concerns. For example, say your computation yields a correct dose of 0.985 *mL*. If you correctly round off this result and administer 0.99 *mL*, you have increased the dose by about 0.5% [Change/Original = 0.005/0.985]. On the other hand, if your computation yields 0.025 *mL* and you correctly round off this result and administer 0.03 *mL*, then you have increased the dose by 20% [Change/Original = 0.005/0.025]. With pediatric and high-alert drugs, sometimes *rounding down* is used to avoid the possibility of overdose; consult the rounding protocols at your facility.

Summary

In this chapter, the various types of syringes were discussed. You learned how to measure the amount of liquid in various syringes. The types of insulin, how to measure a single dose, and how to mix two insulins in one syringe were explained. Prefilled, single-dose, and safety syringes were also presented.

- *Milliliters* (*mL*), rather than *cubic centimeters* (*cc*), are the preferred unit of measure for volume.
- All syringe calibrations must be read at the top ring of the plunger.
- Large-capacity hypodermic syringes (5, 12, 35 *mL*) are calibrated in increments from 0.2 *mL* to 1 *mL*.
- Small-capacity 3 *mL* hypodermic syringes are calibrated in tenths of a *milliter* (0.1 *mL*).
- The very small-capacity 0.5 *mL* and 1 *mL* hypodermic (tuberculin) syringes are calibrated in hundredths of a *milliliter*. They are the preferred syringes for use in measuring a dose of less than 1 *millimeter*.
- The calibrations on hypodermic syringes differ; therefore, be very careful when measuring medications in syringes.
- Amounts less than 1 *mL* are rounded to two decimal places.
- Amounts more than 1 *mL* are rounded to one decimal place.
- Standard insulin syringes are designed for measuring and administering U-100 insulin. They are calibrated for 100 *units* per *mL*.
- Lo-Dose insulin syringes are used for measuring small amounts of U-100 insulin. They have a capacity of 50 *units* or 30 *units*.
- Insulin is supplied in strengths of U-100, U-200, U-300, and U-500.
- For greater accuracy, use the smallest-capacity syringe possible to measure and administer doses. However, avoid filling a syringe to its capacity.
- When measuring two types of insulin in the same syringe, regular insulin is always drawn up in the syringe first. Think: *first clear, then cloudy*.
- The total volume when mixing insulins is the sum of the two insulin amounts.
- Insulin syringes are for measuring and administering insulin only. Tuberculin syringes are used to measure and administer other medications that are less than 1 *mL*. Confusion of the two types of syringes can cause a medication error.
- The prefilled single-dose syringe cartridge is to be used once and then discarded.
- Syringes intended for injections should not be used to measure or administer oral medications.
- Use safety syringes to prevent needlestick injuries.

Case Study 7.1

Read the Case Study and answer the questions. Answers can be found in Appendix A.

A 55-year-old male with a medical history of obesity, hypertension, hyperlipidemia, and diabetes mellitus comes to the emergency department complaining of constant abdominal pain, nausea and, vomiting, and constipation. He states that his pain is a 10 (on a 0–10 pain scale). His abdomen is distended, bowel sounds are hypoactive, and stool is positive for blood. Vital signs are B/P 154/94; T 101.4°F; P 110; and R 26. The diagnostic workup confirms a bowel obstruction, and he is admitted for a bowel resection.

Pre-op orders:

- NPO
- NG (nasogastric) tube to low suction
- V/S q 2h
- Morphine sulfate 2 *mg* subcut stat
- IV R/L @ 125 *mL/h*
- **Pre-op meds**: Demerol (meperidine hydrochloride) 75 *mg* and Phenergan (promethazine 25 *mg* IM 30 *minutes* before surgery;
- Cefoxitin 2 *g* IV 30 *minutes* before surgery

Post-op orders:

- NPO
- NG tube to low suction
- PCA as per pain management service
- V/S q2h
- IV D5RL@ 125 *mL/h*
- cefoxitin 1 *g* IVPB q8h for 3 *doses*, infuse in 100 *mL* D5W over 30 *min*
- ondansetron hydrochloride 4 *mg* IM stat
- heparin 2,000 units subcut q12h

(*continued*)

1. Read the morphine label and:
   (a) Draw a line indicating the dose on each of the following syringes.
   (b) Which syringe will most accurately measure the dose?

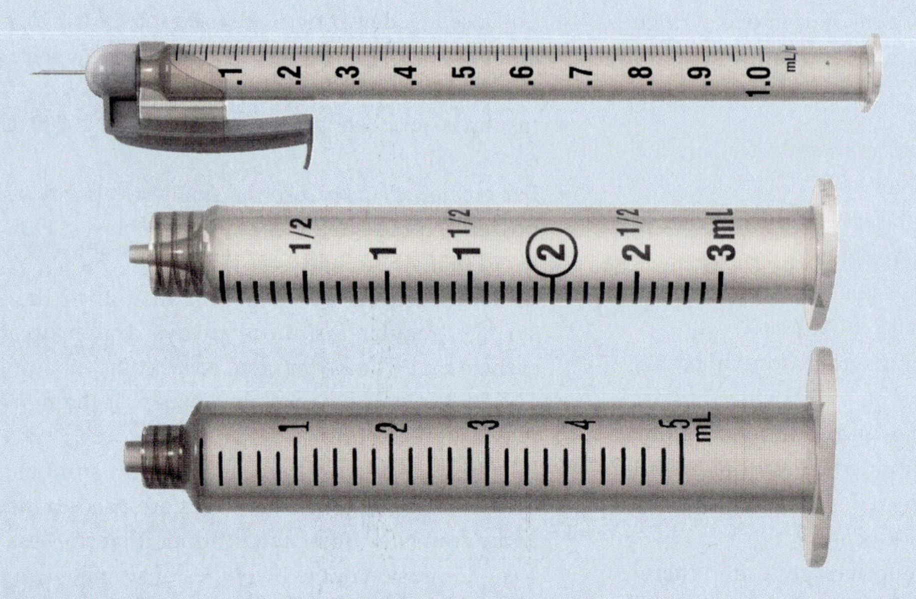

2. Calculate the pre-op dose of the Phenergan and Demerol to be administered 30 *minutes* before surgery. Phenergan is available in 25 *mg/mL* vials. Demerol is available in 2.5 *mL*–capacity prefilled syringes, each containing 1 *mL* of Demerol. The Demerol prefilled syringes have strengths of 10 *mg/mL*, 25 *mg/mL*, and 75 *mg/mL*.
   (a) How many *milliliters* of Phenergan will you prepare?
   (b) Which prepackaged syringe of Demerol will you use?
   (c) Indicate, on the appropriate syringe given, the dose of each of these drugs that you will administer.

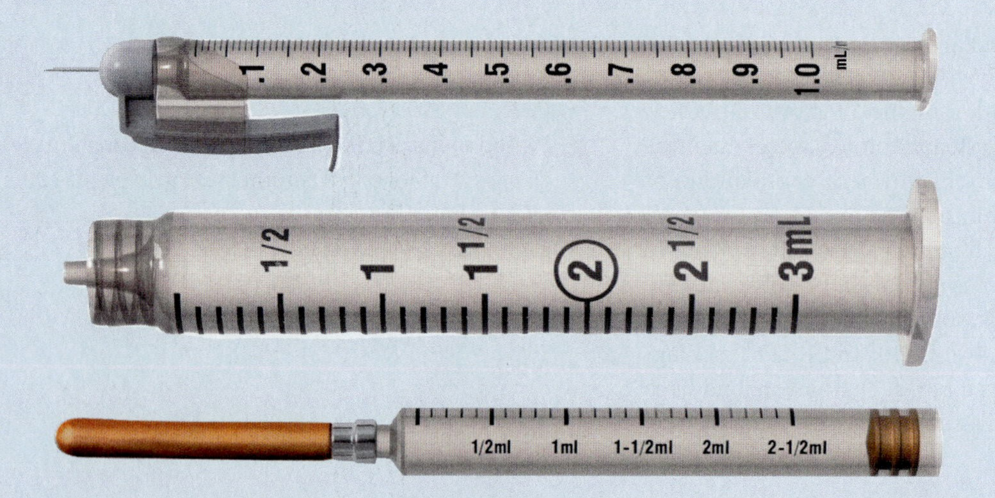

3. The label on the cefoxitin states: "add 10 *mL* of diluent to the 2 *g* vial." Draw a line on the appropriate syringe given, indicating the amount of diluent you will add to the vial.

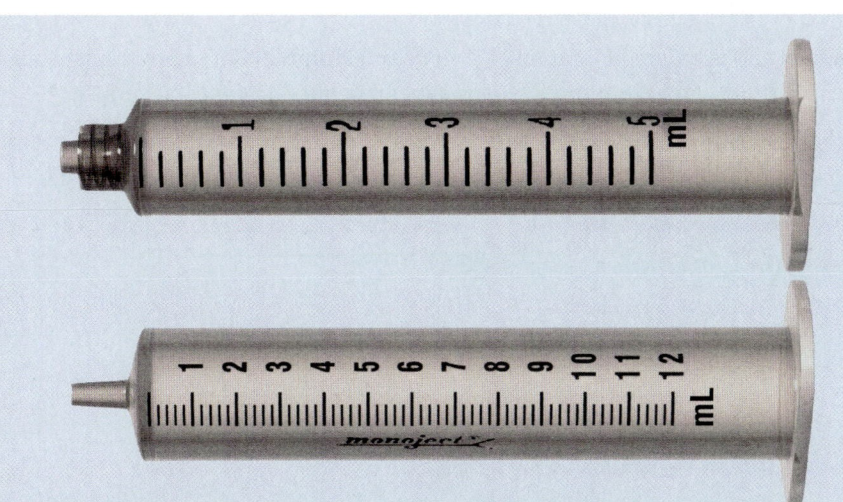

4. Read the ondansetron HCl label. Draw a line on the appropriate syringe, indicating the dose of ondansetron.

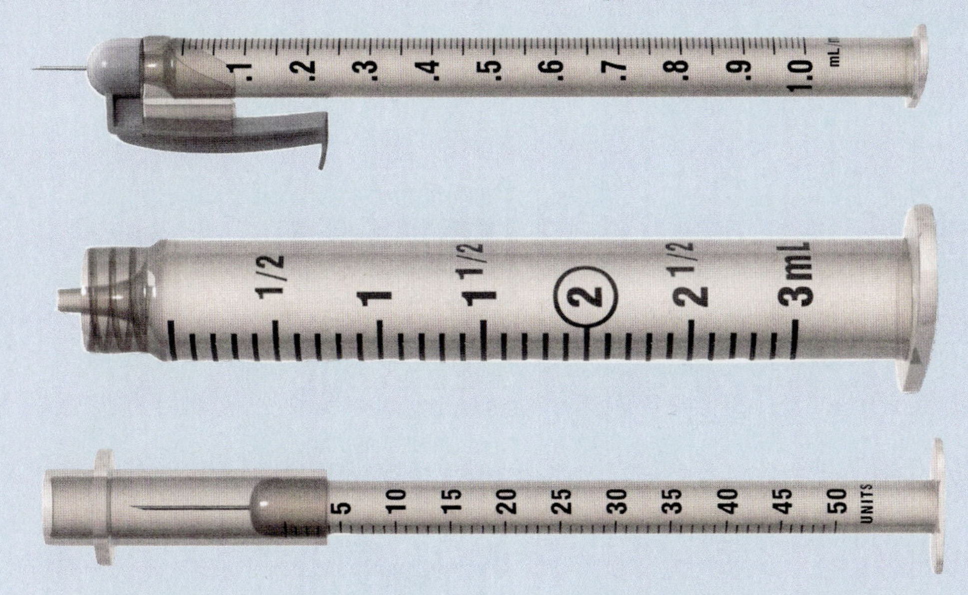

5. Read the heparin label and draw a line on the appropriate syringe, indicating the dose.

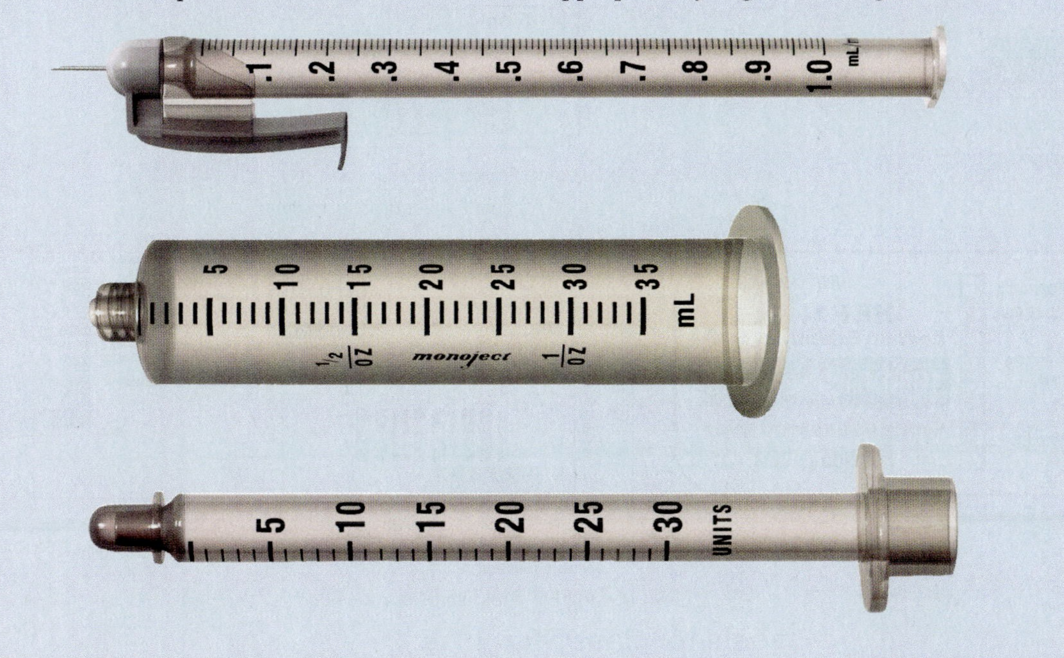

(continued)

6. The client has progressed to a regular diet and is ordered Humulin N 13 *units* and Humulin R 6 *units* subcutaneous 30 *minutes* ac breakfast, and Humulin N 5 *units* and Humulin R 5 *units* subcutaneous 30 *minutes* ac dinner.

   (a) How many units will the client receive before breakfast?

   (b) Indicate on the appropriate syringe given the number of units of each insulin required before breakfast.

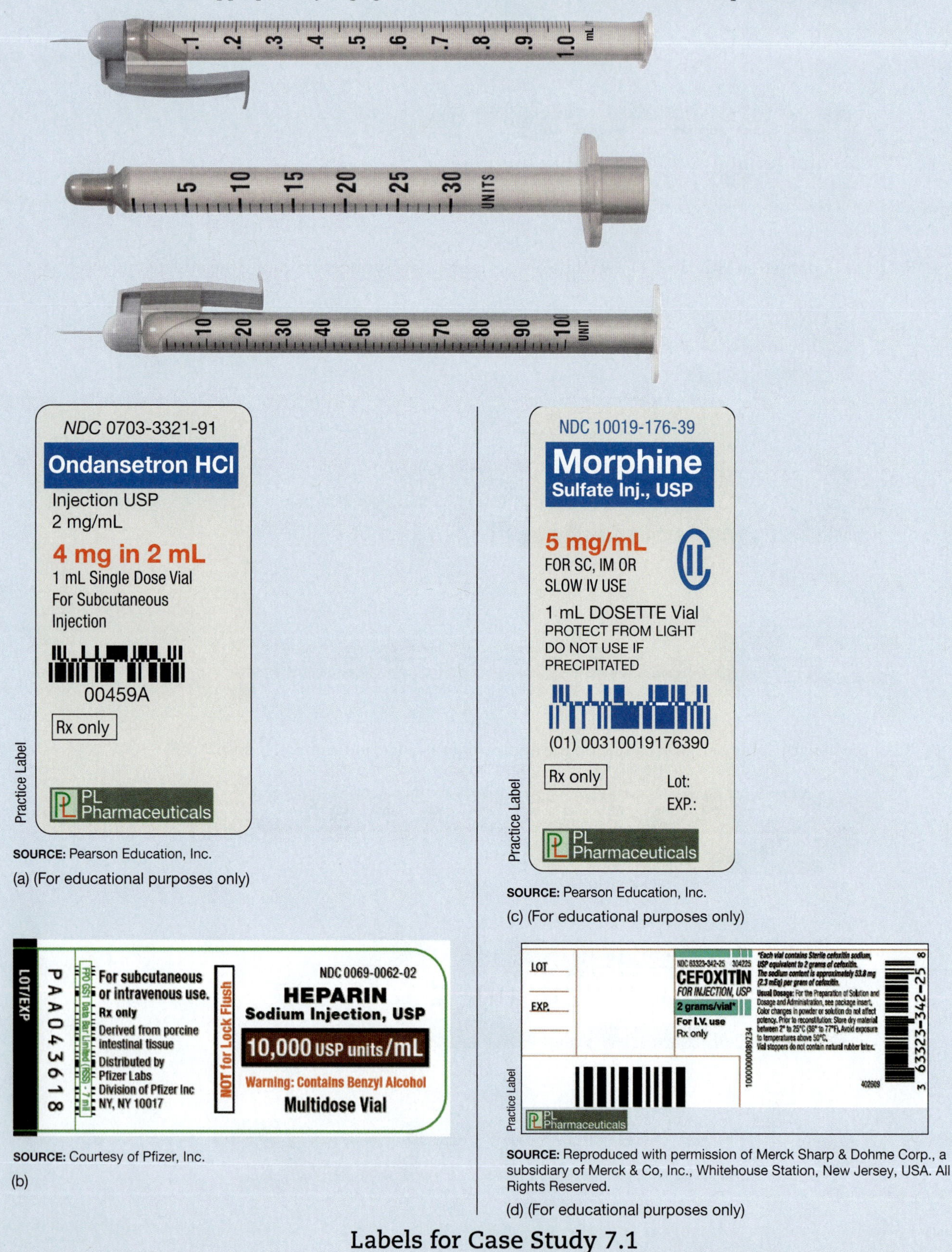

SOURCE: Pearson Education, Inc.

(a) (For educational purposes only)

SOURCE: Pearson Education, Inc.

(c) (For educational purposes only)

SOURCE: Courtesy of Pfizer, Inc.

(b)

SOURCE: Reproduced with permission of Merck Sharp & Dohme Corp., a subsidiary of Merck & Co, Inc., Whitehouse Station, New Jersey, USA. All Rights Reserved.

(d) (For educational purposes only)

Labels for Case Study 7.1

Practice Sets

The answers to *Try These for Practice, Exercises,* and *Cumulative Review Exercises* are found in Appendix A. Ask your instructor for the answers to the *Additional Exercises.*

Try These for Practice

Test your comprehension after reading the chapter.

In problems 1 through 4, identify the type of syringe shown in the figure. Place an arrow at the appropriate level of measurement on the syringe for the volume given.

1. ______________ syringe; 0.68 *mL*

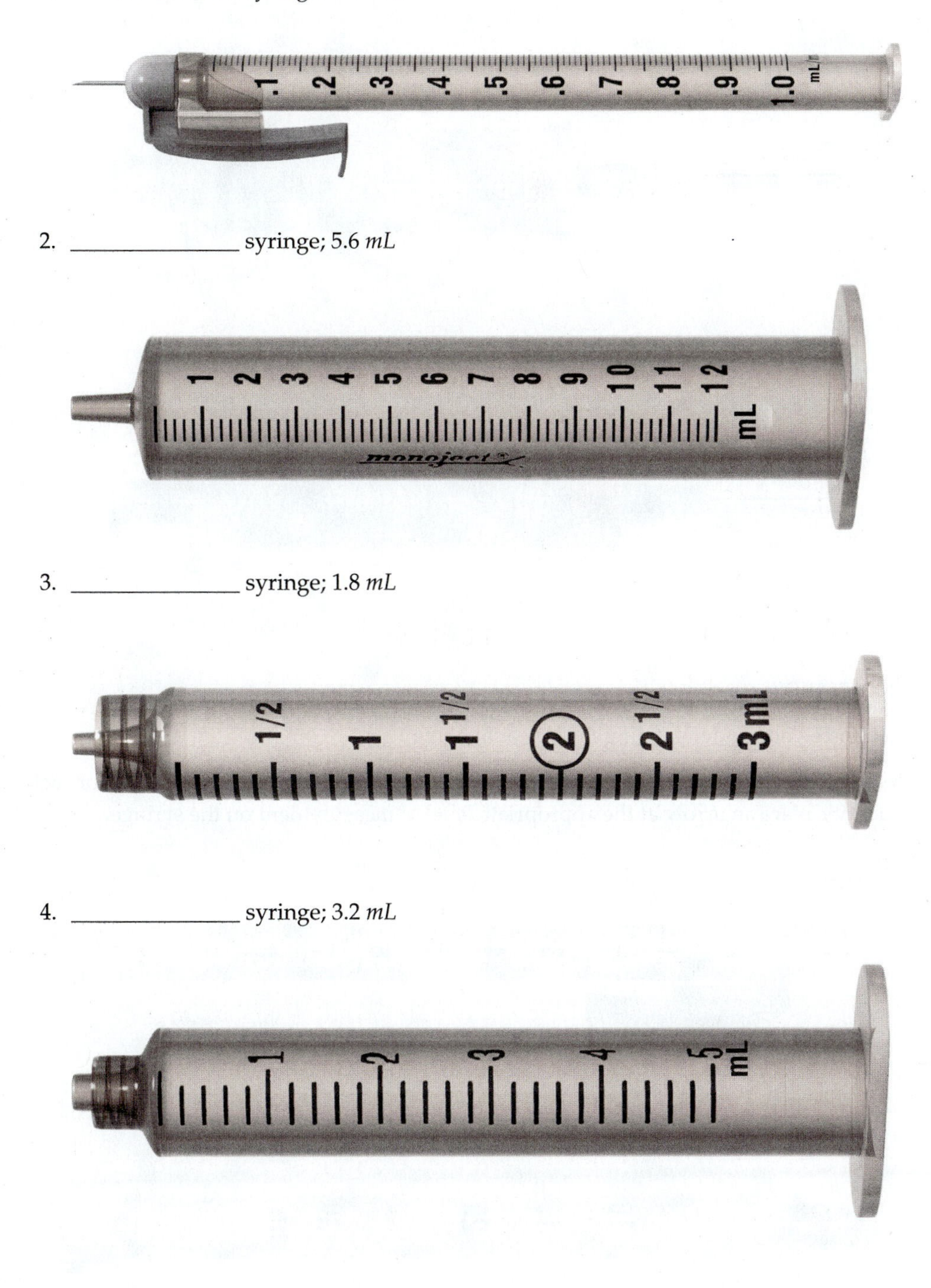

2. ______________ syringe; 5.6 *mL*

3. ______________ syringe; 1.8 *mL*

4. ______________ syringe; 3.2 *mL*

5. Order: *methylprednisolone acetate (Depo Medrol) 80 mg IM every other week.*

   The strength on the label is 40 *mg/mL*. Draw an arrow on the most appropriate syringe indicating the number of *milliliters* you will administer.

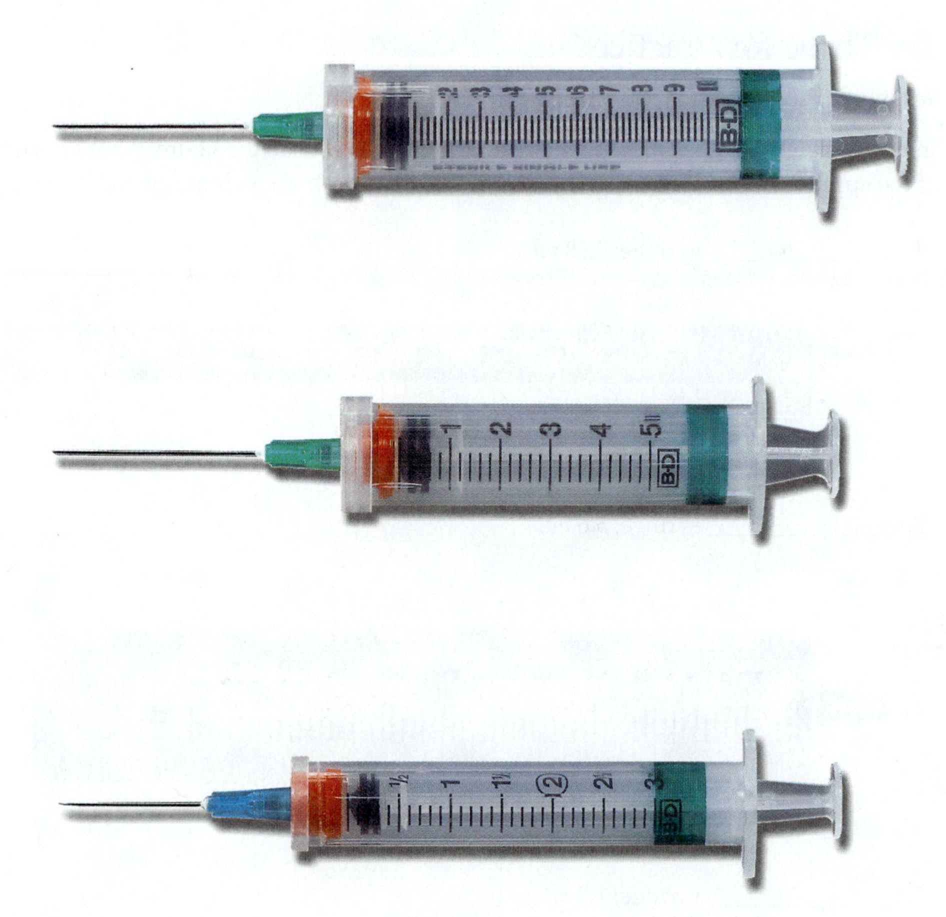

Exercises

Reinforce your understanding in class or at home.

In problems 1 through 14, identify the type of syringe shown in the figure. Then, for each quantity, place an arrow at the appropriate level of measurement on the syringe.

1. _______________ syringe; 0.45 *mL*

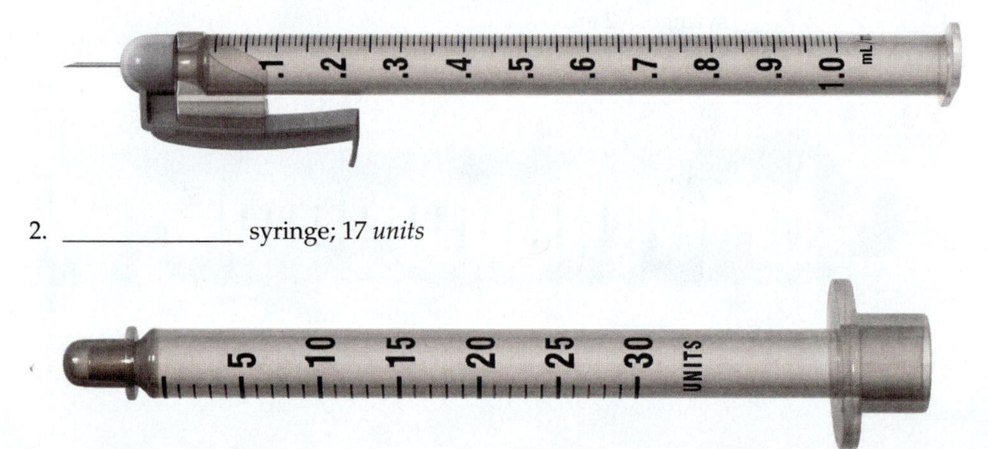

2. _______________ syringe; 17 *units*

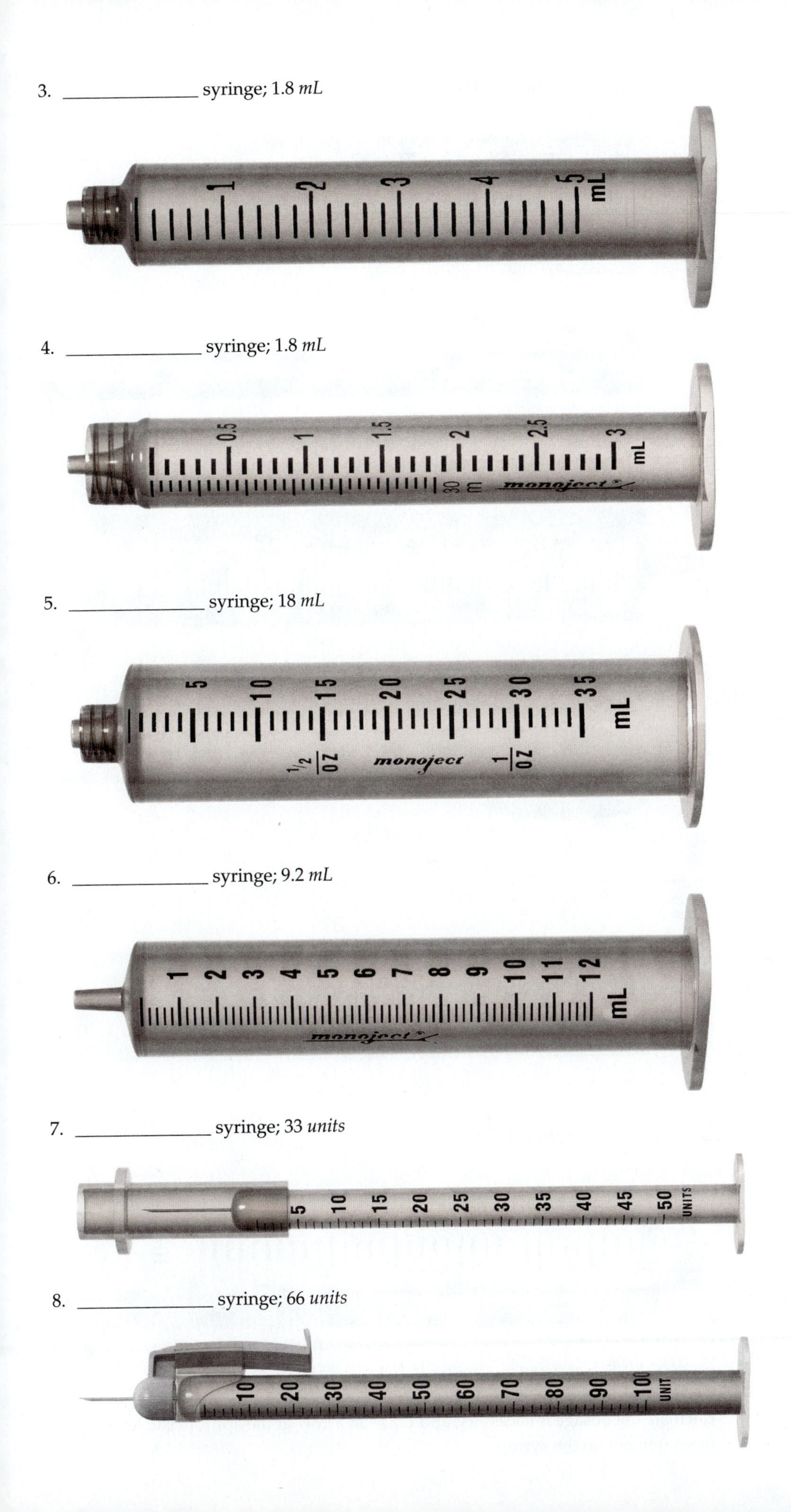
3. _______________ syringe; 1.8 *mL*
1 2 3 4 5 mL
4. _______________ syringe; 1.8 *mL*
0.5 1 1.5 2 2.5 3 mL
30 m
monoject
5. _______________ syringe; 18 *mL*
5 10 15 20 25 30 35 mL
1/2 OZ
monoject
1 OZ
6. _______________ syringe; 9.2 *mL*
1 2 3 4 5 6 7 8 9 10 11 12 mL
monoject
7. _______________ syringe; 33 *units*
5 10 15 20 25 30 35 40 45 50 UNITS
8. _______________ syringe; 66 *units*
10 20 30 40 50 60 70 80 90 100 UNIT

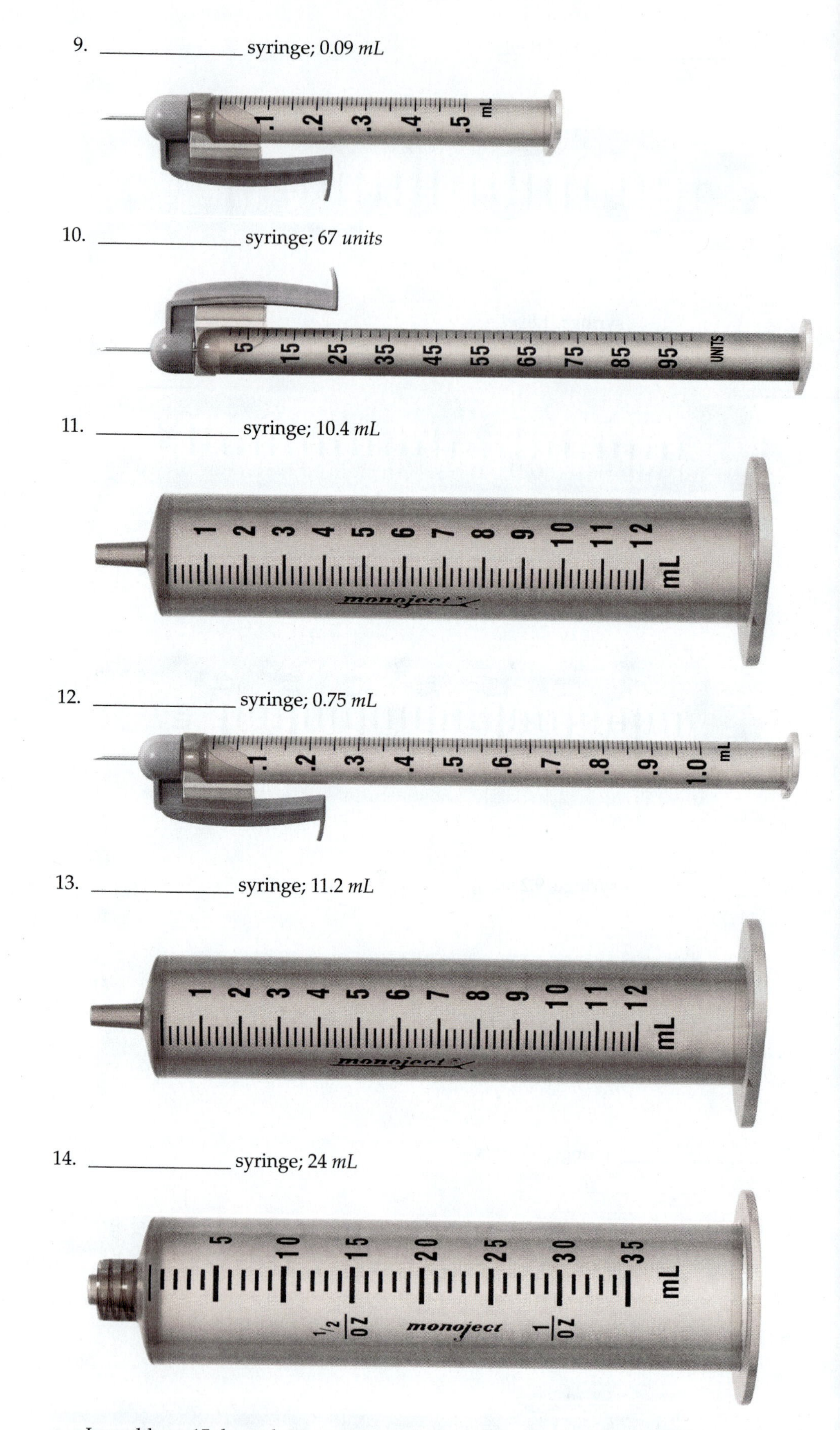

9. ______________ syringe; 0.09 *mL*

10. ______________ syringe; 67 *units*

11. ______________ syringe; 10.4 *mL*

12. ______________ syringe; 0.75 *mL*

13. ______________ syringe; 11.2 *mL*

14. ______________ syringe; 24 *mL*

In problems 15 through 20, read the order, use the appropriate label in Figure 7.39, calculate the dosage if necessary, and place an arrow at the appropriate level of measurement on the syringe.

Figure 7.39 Drug labels and drug guide information for Exercises 15–20.

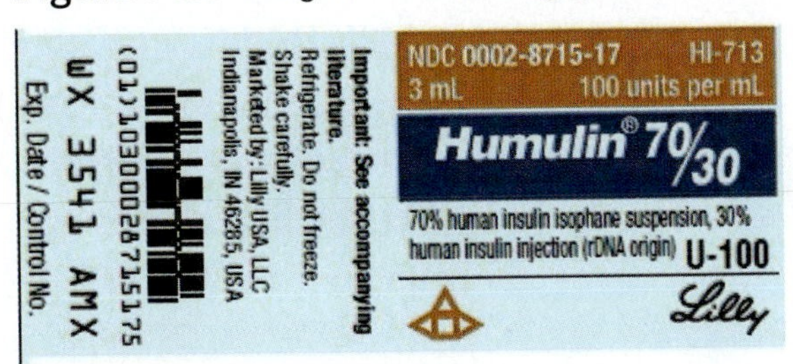

SOURCE: © Copyright Eli Lily and Company. All rights reserved. Used with permission.

(a)

SOURCE: Endo Pharmaceuticals Inc.

(b)

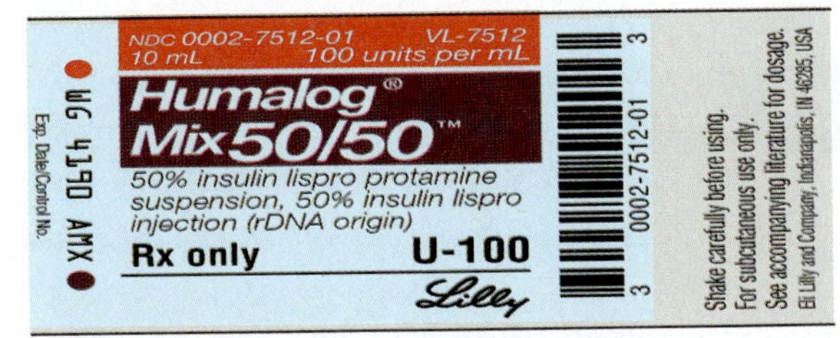

SOURCE: © Copyright Eli Lily and Company. All rights reserved. Used with permission.

(c)

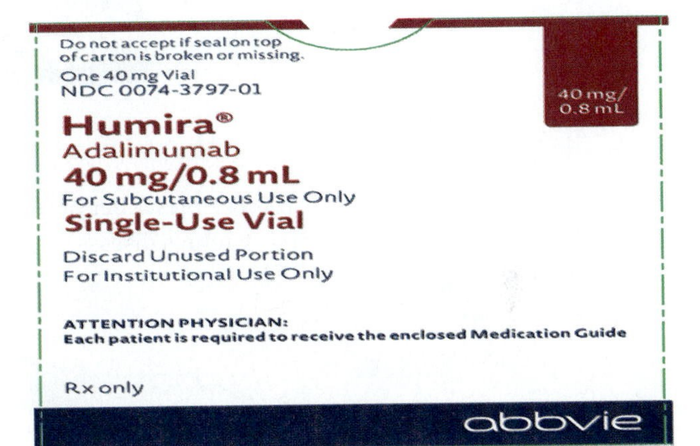

SOURCE: Courtesy of AbbVie

(d)

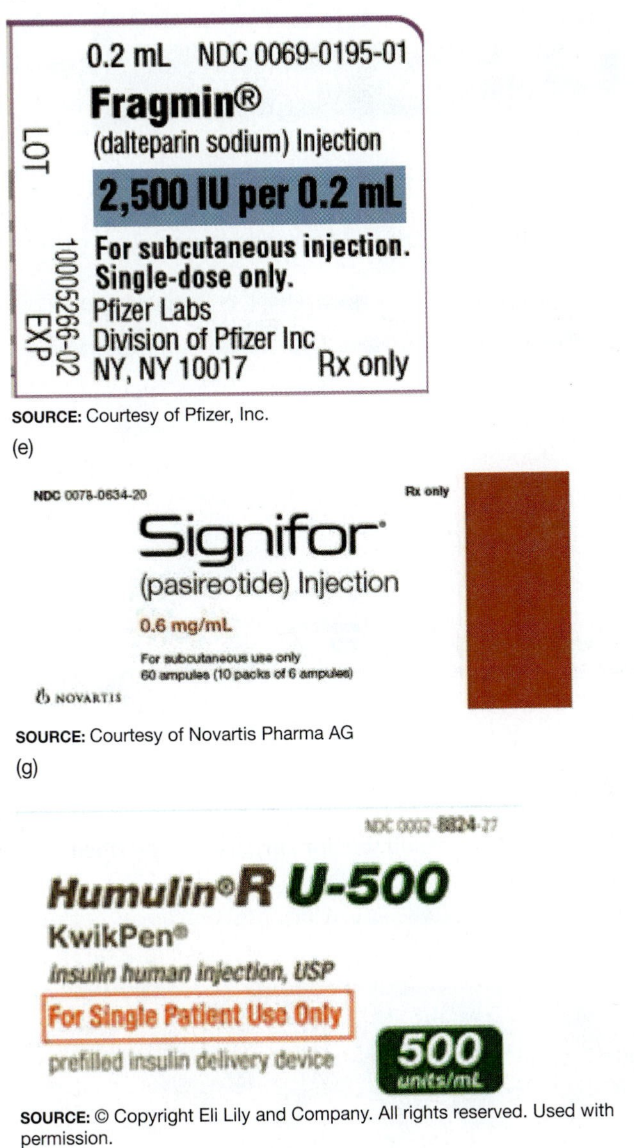

SOURCE: Courtesy of Pfizer, Inc.

(e)

SOURCE: Courtesy of Novartis Pharma AG

(g)

SOURCE: © Copyright Eli Lily and Company. All rights reserved. Used with permission.

(h)

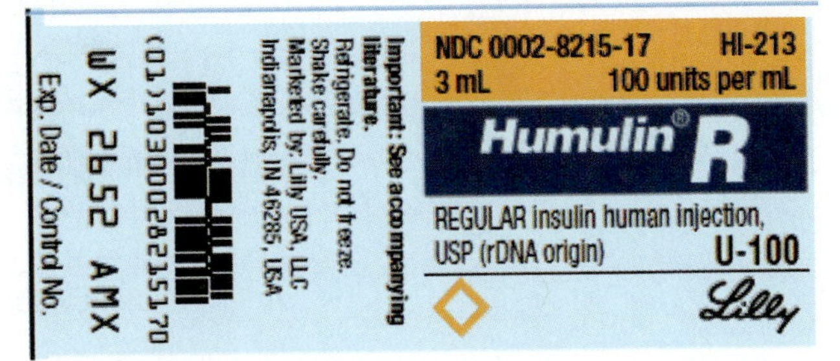

SOURCE: © Copyright Eli Lily and Company. All rights reserved. Used with permission.

(f)

SOURCE: Courtesy of Pfizer, Inc.

(i)

15. Order: *testosterone undecanoate (Aveed) injection 600 mg IM stat.*

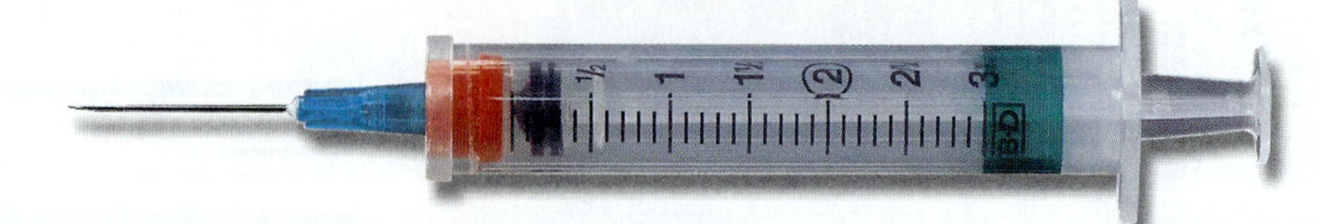

16. Order: *Humalog 70/30 22 units subcut 30 minutes before breakfast.*

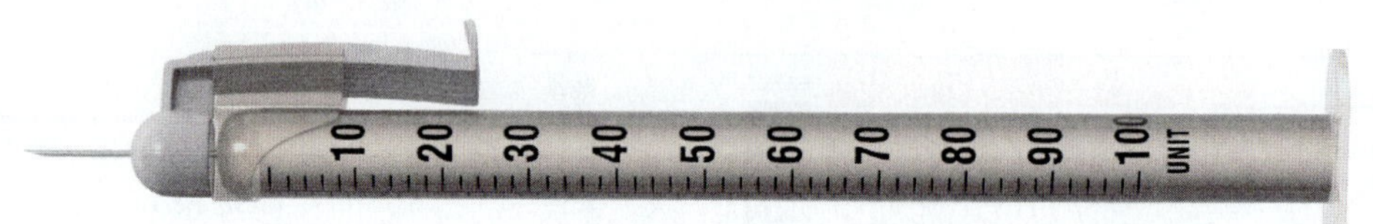

17. The prescriber ordered *adalimumab (Humira) 80 mg subcut stat* for a client who has Crohn's disease.

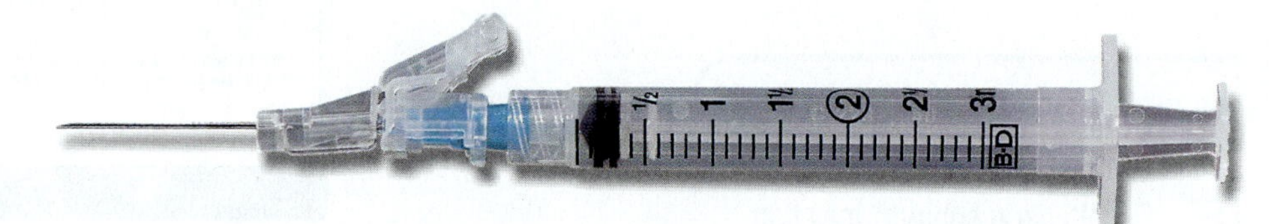

18. Order: *dalteparin sodium (Fragmin) 5,000 units subcut 1 hour prior to surgery*

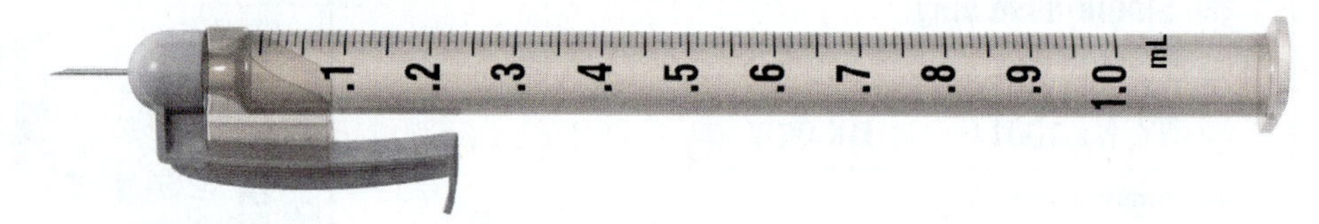

19. Order: *Humulin R 4 units subcut stat*

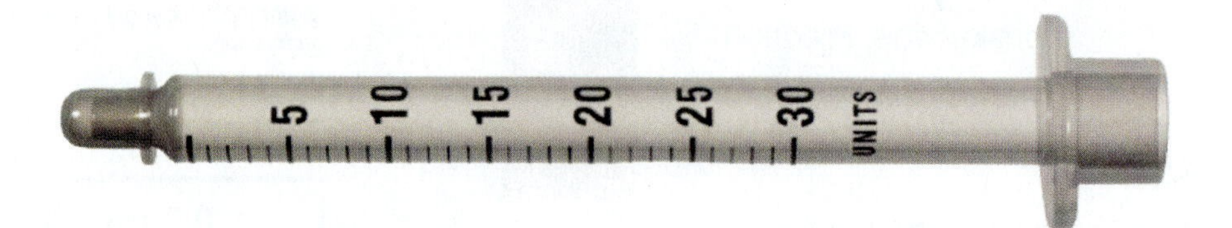

20. A client who has Cushing's disease and is not suitable for surgery is prescribed pasireotide (Signifor) 0.9 *mg* subcut B.I.D.

Additional Exercises

Now, test yourself!

In problems 1 through 15, identify the type of syringe shown in the figure. Then, for each quantity, place an arrow at the appropriate level of measurement on the syringe.

1. ______________ syringe; 66 *units*

2. ______________ syringe; 21 *units*

3. ______________ syringe; 1.4 *mL*

4. ______________ syringe; 1.4 *mL*

5. ______________ syringe; 8.3 *mL*

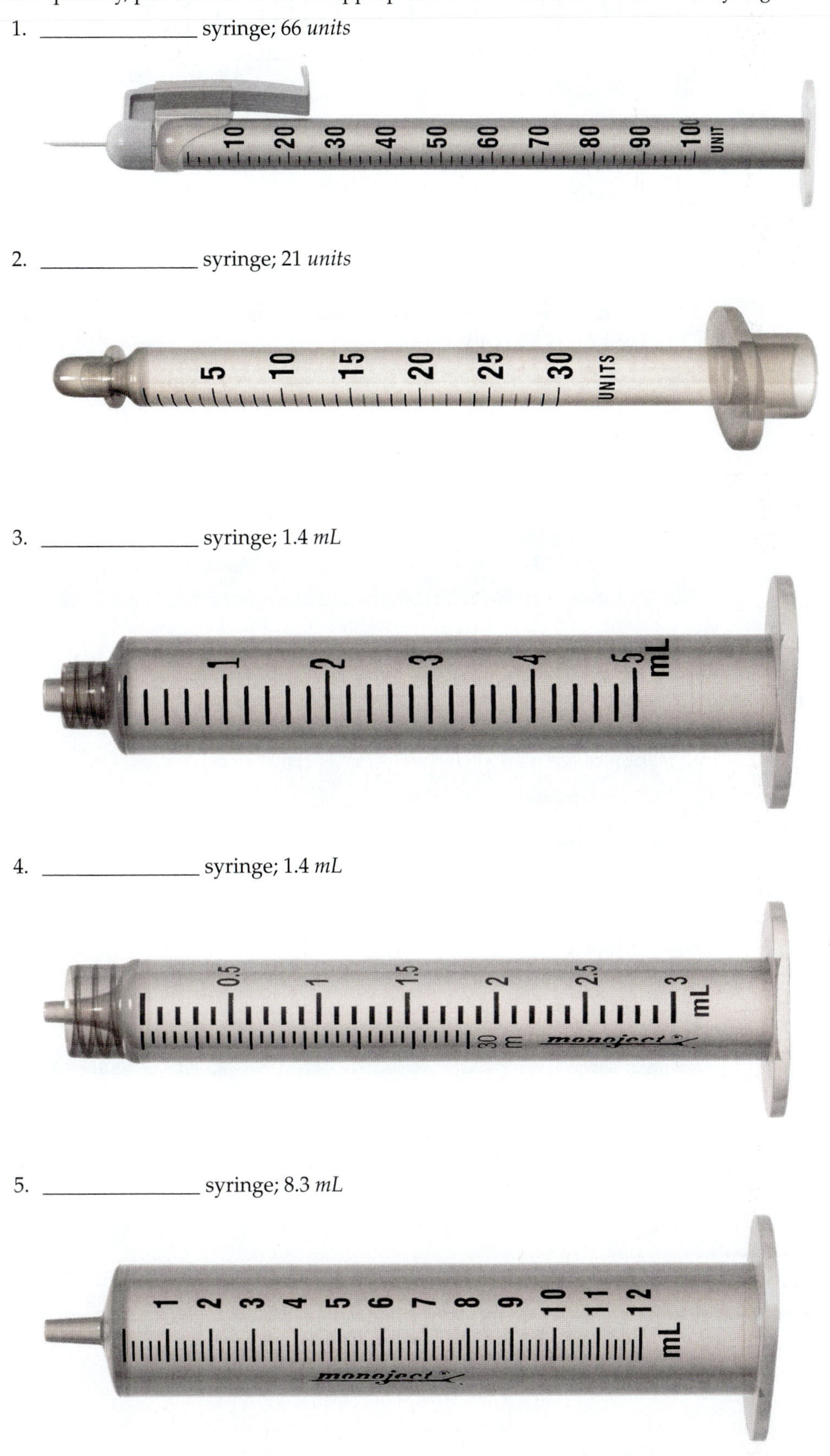

6. ______________ syringe; 14 *mL*

7. ______________ syringe; 29 *units*

8. ______________ syringe; 78 *units*

9. ______________ syringe; 0.43 *mL*

10. ______________ syringe; 81 *units*

11. ______________ syringe; 8.6 *mL*

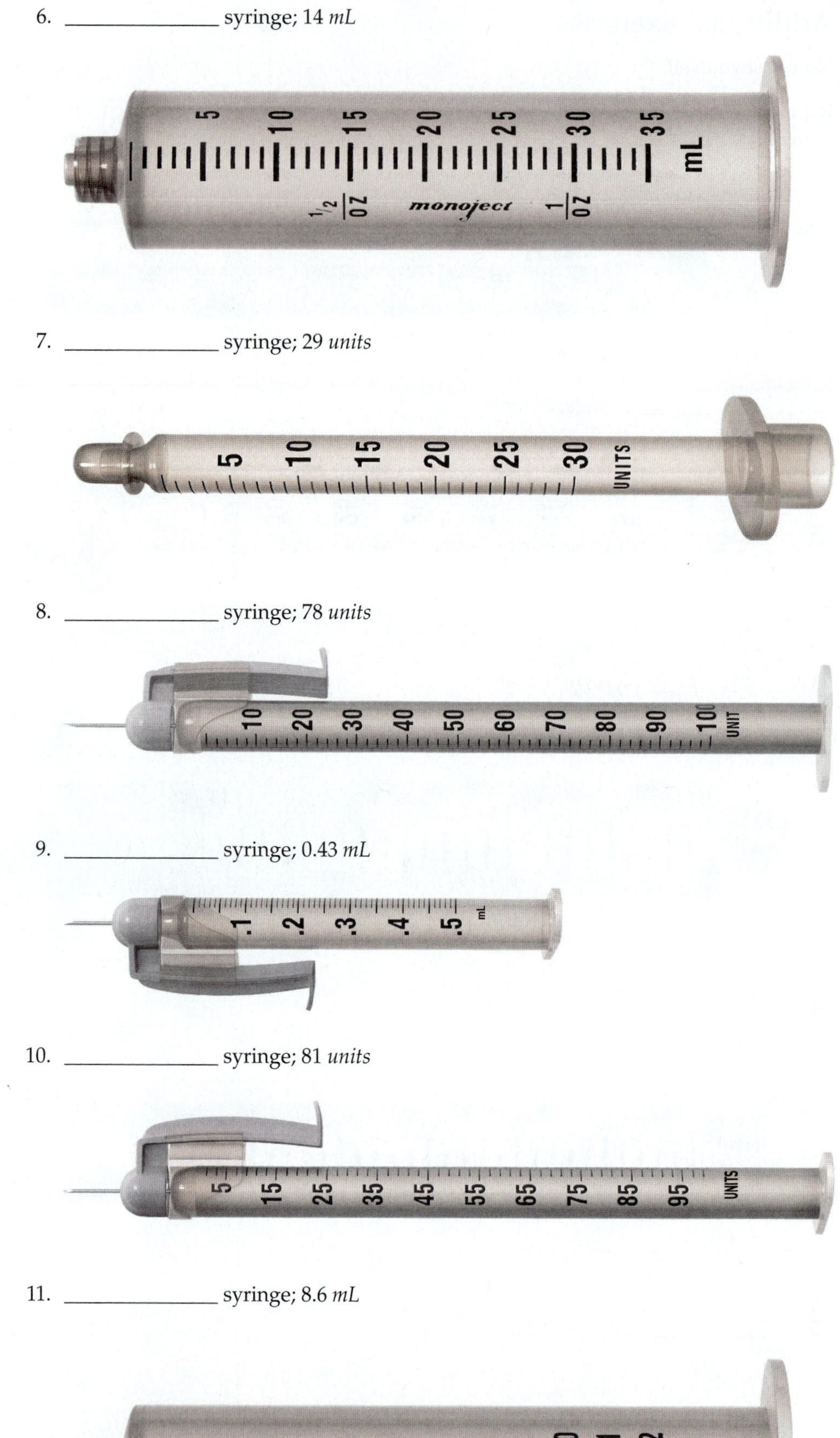

12. ______________ syringe; 0.56 *mL*

13. ______________ syringe; 9.2 *mL*

14. ______________ syringe; 33 *mL*

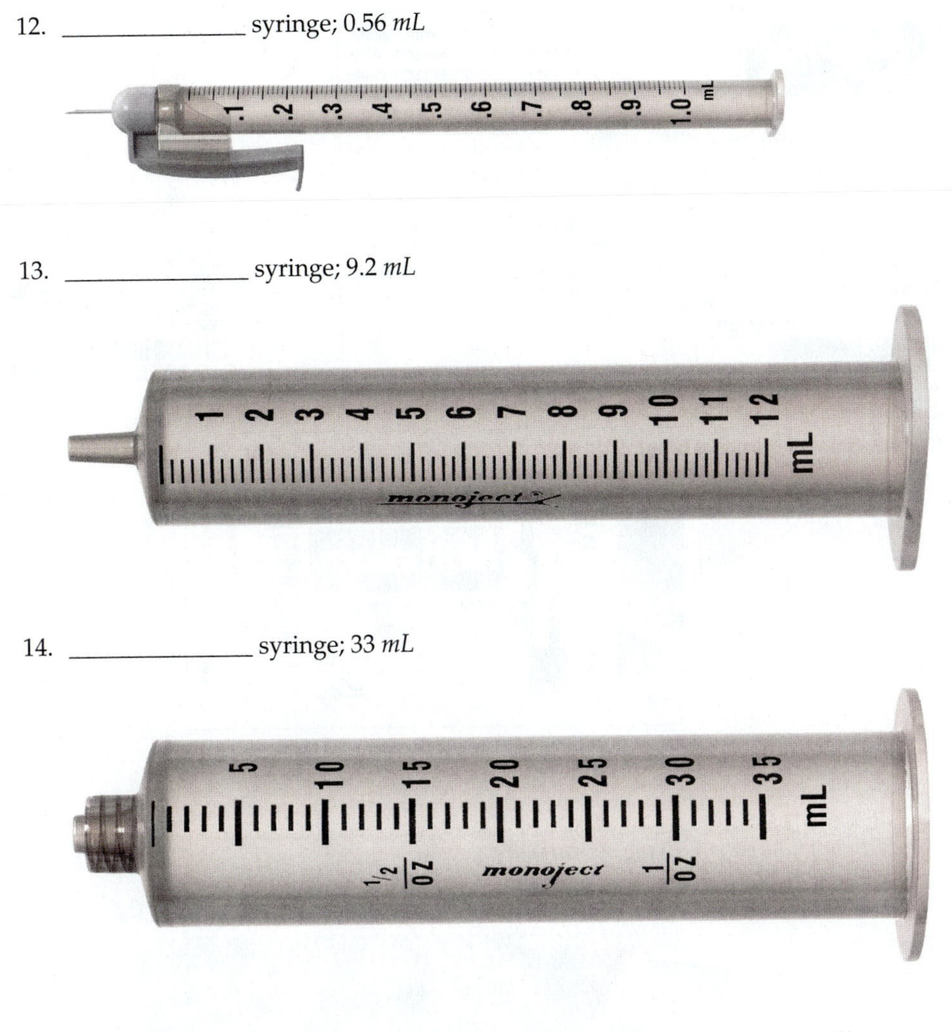

In problems 15 through 20, consult the labels in Figure 7.40 to answer the questions, and then place arrows at the appropriate level of measurement on the syringes.

Figure 7.40 Drug labels for Additional Exercises 15–20.

(a)

2.5 mL
Streptomycin Sulfate Injection, USP
1 g/2.5 mL
(400 mg/mL)
(of streptomycin)
*For **IM** use only*
Store under refrigeration at 36° to 46°F (2° to 8°C)
CAUTION: Federal law prohibits dispensing without prescription.
LOT 8E31A
EXP
Pfizer Roerig
Division of Pfizer Inc, NY, NY 10017

SOURCE: Courtesy of Pfizer, Inc.

(b)

NAFCILLIN SODIUM
(naf-sill'in)
Classifications: BETA-LACTAM ANTIBIOTIC; PENICILLIN
Therapeutic: ANTISTAPHYLOCOCCAL PENICILLIN

Staphylococcal Infections
Adult: **IV** 500 mg–1 g q4h (max: 12 g/day) **IM** 500 mg q4–6h
Child: **IV** 50–200 mg/kg/day divided q4–6h (max: 12 g/day) **IM** *Weight greater than 40 kg,* 500 mg q4–6h; *weight less than 40 kg,* 25 mg/kg b.i.d.
Neonate: **IV** 50–100 mg/kg/day divided q6–12h **IM** 25–50 mg/kg b.i.d.

(c)

NALBUPHINE HYDROCHLORIDE
(nal'byoo-feen)
Nubain
Classifications: ANALGESIC; NARCOTIC (OPIATE) AGONIST-ANTAGONIST
Therapeutic: NARCOTIC ANALGESIC

Moderate to Severe Pain
Adult: **IV/IM/Subcutaneous** 10 mg/70 kg q3–6h prn (max: 160 mg/day)

Surgery Anesthesia Supplement
Adult: **IV** 0.3–3 mg/kg, then 0.25–0.5 mg/kg as required

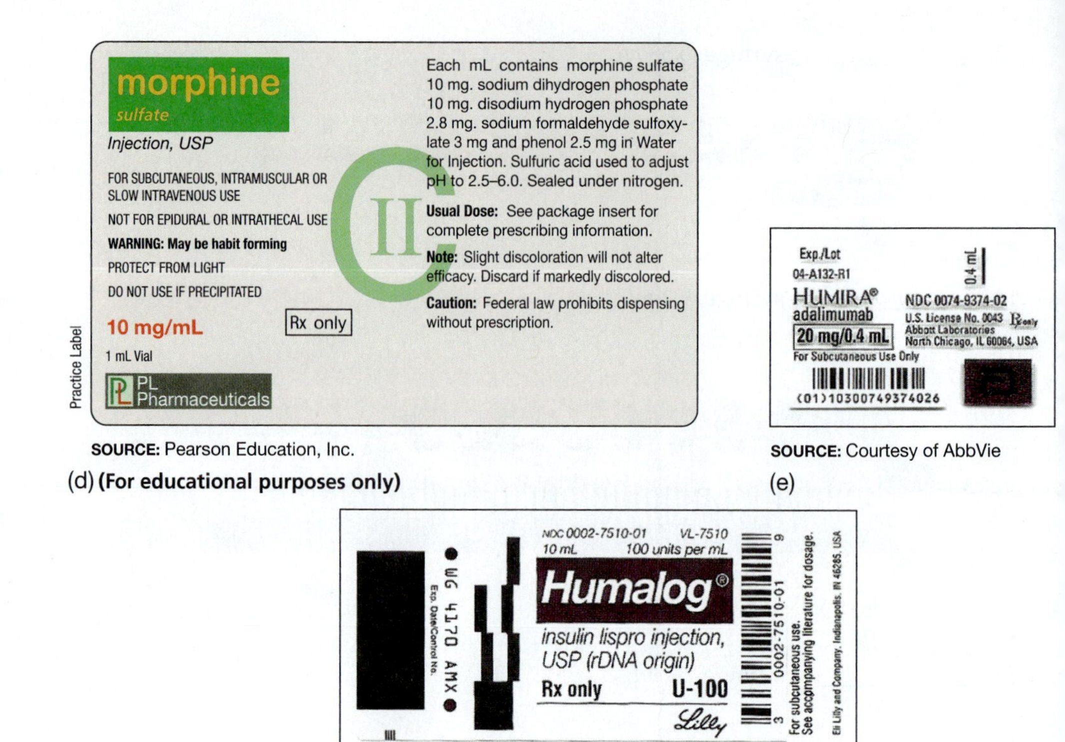

SOURCE: Pearson Education, Inc.

(d) **(For educational purposes only)**

SOURCE: Courtesy of AbbVie

(e)

SOURCE: © Copyright Eli Lily and Company. All rights reserved. Used with permission.

(f)

15. Order: *morphine sulfate 15 mg subcut q4h prn pain.*

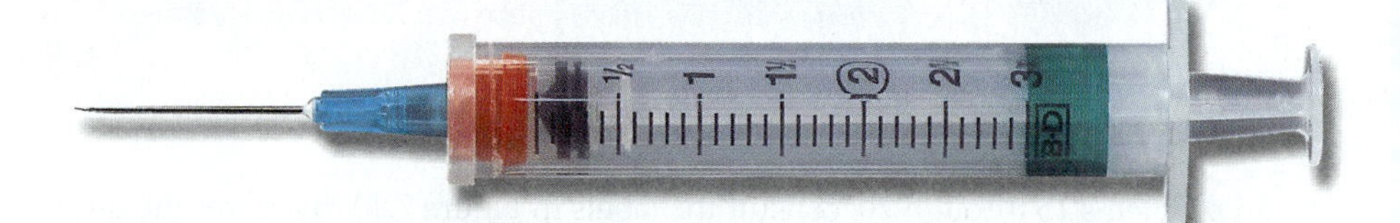

16. The client weighs 220 *pounds*. The order is *insulin lispro 0.5 units/kg subcut daily 10 min ac.*

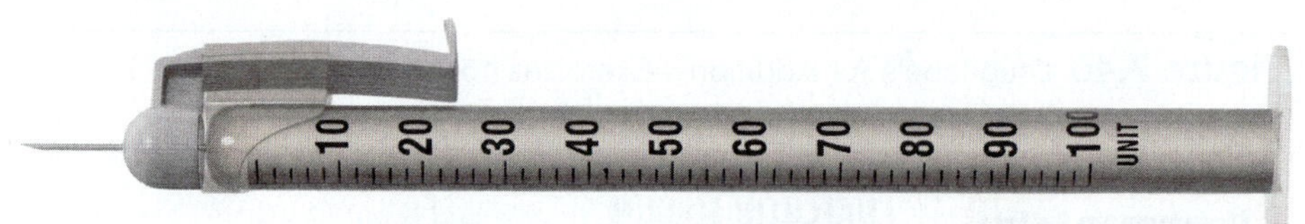

17. Order: *Streptomycin 800 mg IM daily.*

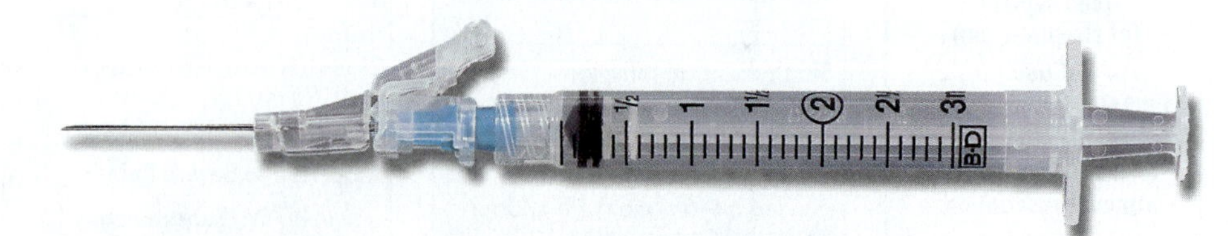

18. Order: *Humira 20 mg subcut stat.*

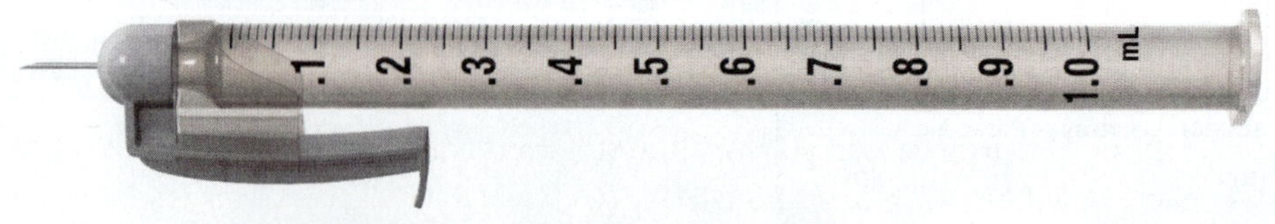

19. Nafcillin sodium is ordered IM for an adult client. The strength of the nafcillin sodium on hand is 250 *mg/mL*. Is the amount shown by the arrow on the syringe the correct dose to administer?

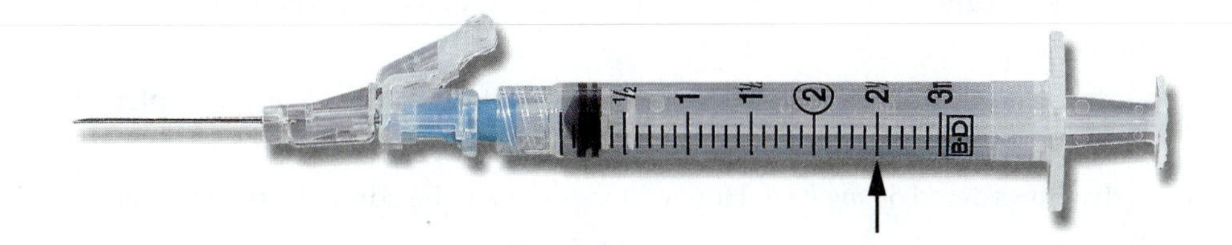

20. Indicate, by placing an arrow on the syringe, the dose of nalbuphine HCl to be administered IM for severe pain. The strength available is 10 *mg/mL*, and the adult client weighs 105 *kg*.

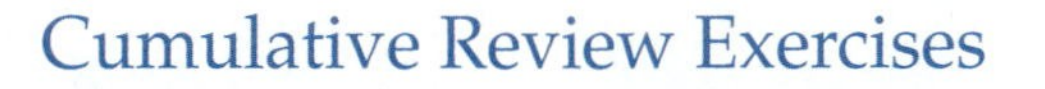

Cumulative Review Exercises

Review your mastery of previous chapters.

1. Prescriber's order: *Administer Humulin R (regular insulin [rDNA origin]) subcutaneously as per the following blood-glucose results:*

For glucose less than 160 mg/dL	*—no insulin*
glucose 160 mg/dL–220 mg/dL	*—give 2 units*
glucose 221 mg/dL–280 mg/dL	*—give 4 units*
glucose 281 mg/dL–340 mg/dL	*—give 6 units*
glucose 341 mg/dL–400 mg/dL	*—give 8 units*
glucose greater than 400 mg/dL	*—notify MD stat*

   How many units will you administer if the client's glucose level at lunchtime is
   (a) *140 mg/dL?*
   (b) *200 mg/dL?*
   (c) *450 mg/dL?*

2. If *40 mg* of a drug is ordered *po daily* and the strength of the drug is *10 mg/mL*, how many *milliliters* will you administer?
3. If *40 mg* of a drug is ordered *po b.i.d.* and the strength of the drug is *10 mg/mL*, how many *milliliters* will you administer?
4. If *40 mg* of a drug is ordered *po daily in two divided doses* and the strength of the drug is *10 mg/mL*, how many *milliliters* will you administer?
5. If *40 mg* of a drug is ordered *po q12h* and the strength of the drug is *10 mg/mL*, how many *milliliters* will you administer?

6. Order: *Dilantin (phenytoin) 250 mg po stat*. The concentration of the Dilantin is 125 *mg*/5 *mL*. How many teaspoons will you administer?
7. Order: *Camptosar (irinotecan)* 350 *mg*/m^2 *IV over 90 minutes on day 1 every 3 weeks*. How many *g* will be administered to a client who has a BSA of 1.95 m^2?
8. Find the weight, to the nearest tenth of a *kilogram*, of a client who weighs 200 *pounds*.
9. Order: *Glucotrol (glipizide) 15 mg po daily*. Available tablets are 5 *mg* per tablet. How many tablets will you administer?
10. A drug is ordered *50 mg b.i.d.* How many *grams* will be administered in 10 days?
11. Order: *methylprednisolone acetate (Depo Medrol) 10 mg IM every other week*. The strength on the label is 20 *mg*/*mL*. How many milliliters will you administer and what size syringe will you use?
12. Using the formula, find the BSA of a client who is 5 *feet* 3 *inches* tall and weighs 195 *pounds*.
13. Order: Novolin R U-100 8 units subcut and Novolin N U-100 15 units subcut ac breakfast. What size syringe will you use and how many units will the client receive?
14. Order: *ampicillin 375 mg IM q6h*. The strength on the label is 250 *mg*/*mL*. How many *milliliters* will you administer and what size syringe will you use?
15. Order: *fentanyl citrate injection 50 mcg IM q 1-2 h prn postoperative pain*. The strength on the label is 250 *mcg*/5 *mL*. How many *milliliters* will you administer and what size syringe will you use?

Chapter 8

Solutions

Learning Outcomes

After completing this chapter, you will be able to

8.1 Find the strength of a solution as a ratio, as a fraction, and as a percent.

8.2 Determine the amount of solute in a given amount of solution.

8.3 Determine the amount of solution that would contain a given amount of solute.

8.4 Do the calculations necessary to prepare solutions from pure drugs.

8.5 Do the calculations necessary to prepare solutions for irrigations, soaks, and nutritional feedings.

In this chapter you learn about solutions. Although medicinal solutions are generally prepared by the pharmacist, others may be required to prepare solutions for irrigations, soaks, and nutritional feedings.

Drugs are manufactured in both pure and diluted forms. A pure drug contains only the drug and nothing else. A pure drug can be diluted by dissolving a quantity of the pure drug in a liquid to form a **solution**. The pure drug (either dry or liquid) is called the **solute**. The liquid added to the pure drug to form the solution is called the **solvent** or **diluent**.

Introduction

To make a cup of coffee, you might dissolve 2 *teaspoons* of instant coffee granules in a cup of hot water. The instant coffee granules (*solute*) are added to the hot water (*solvent*) to form the cup of coffee (*solution*). If instead of 2 teaspoons of instant coffee granules, you add either 1 or 3 teaspoons of instant coffee granules to the cup of hot water, the coffee solution will taste quite different. The **strength** or **concentration** of the coffee could be described in terms of *teaspoons per cup* (*t/cup*). Thus, a coffee solution with a strength of *1 t/cup* is a *"weaker"* solution than a coffee solution with a strength of 2 *t/cup*, and a strength of *3 t/cup* is *"stronger"* than a strength of 2 *t/cup*.

Important terms for the elements of a solution:

- The **solute** is the solid or liquid to be dissolved or diluted. Some solutes are powdered drugs, chemical salts, and liquid nutritional supplements.
- The **solvent** (**diluent**) is the liquid that dissolves the solid solute or dilutes the liquid solute. Two commonly used solvents are sterile water and normal saline.
- The **solution** is the liquid resulting from the combination of the solute and the solvent.

Strengths of Solutions Using Explicit Units of Measurement

The strength of a drug is stated on the label. Liquid drugs are solutions. The strength of these solutions compares the *amount of drug (solute)* in the solution to the *volume of solution*. Some examples of drug strengths or concentrations are *Lanoxin 500 mcg/2 mL, KCl 2 mEq/mL, Garamycin 80 mg/2 mL*, and *heparin 10,000 units/mL*.

Suppose a vial is labeled *furosemide 5 mg/mL*. This means that there are 5 *milligrams* of furosemide in each *milliliter* of the solution. If a second vial is labeled *furosemide 10 mg/mL*, then this second solution is "stronger" than the first because there are 10 *mg* of furosemide in each *milliliter* of the solution. If an order is *furosemide 10 mg po stat*, then to receive 10 *mg* of the drug, the client would receive either 2 *mL* of the "weaker" first solution or 1 *mL* of the "stronger" second solution.

NOTE

This textbook does not make a distinction between the words *strength* and *concentration*. Some references call *5 g/100 mL* a "concentration" because it contains units of measurement, and *5%* a "strength" because it contains no units of measurement.

Strengths of Solutions as Ratios, Fractions, and Percents

Sometimes the strength of a solution is specified *without using explicit units of measurement such as milligrams* or *milliliters* but by comparing the number of parts of *solute* to the number of parts of *solution*. This method of stating strength is generally expressed by using either *ratios, fractions*, or *percents*. Some examples of these strengths are *epinephrine 1:1,000 (ratio), Enfamil $\frac{1}{2}$ strength (fraction)*, and *0.9% NaCl (percent)*. In fractional form, the strength of a solution equals the amount of solute (drug) over the amount of solution.

$$\text{STRENGTH} = \frac{\text{SOLUTE}}{\text{SOLUTION}}$$

If a solution contains *1 part solute* in *2 parts of solution*, the strength could be expressed in the form of the *ratio 1:2* (read "1 to 2"), the *fraction $\frac{1}{2}$ strength*, or (because $\frac{1}{2} = 50\%$) the *percentage 50%*. See Figure 8.1.

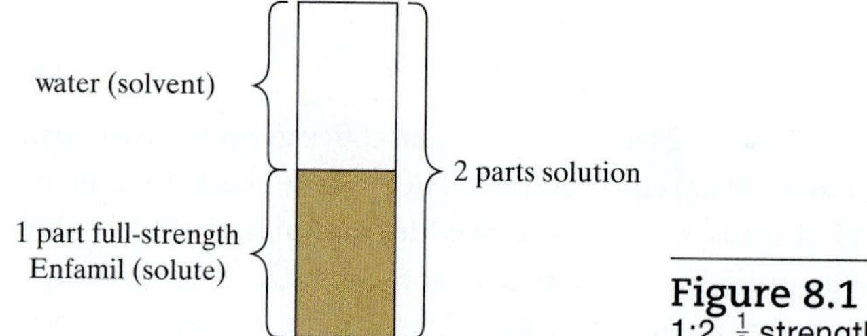

Figure 8.1 A model of the structure of a 1:2, $\frac{1}{2}$ strength, or 50% Enfamil solution.

The ratio *1:5* means that there is 1 part *solute* in 5 parts *solution*. This solution is also referred to as a $\frac{1}{5}$ strength solution or as a *20%* solution. See Figure 8.2.

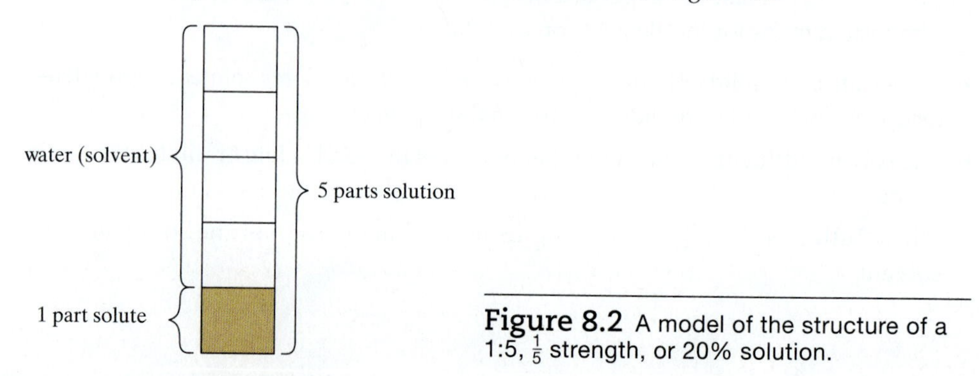

Figure 8.2 A model of the structure of a 1:5, $\frac{1}{5}$ strength, or 20% solution.

A $\frac{1}{3}$ strength solution can be expressed as a *1:3* solution. This has 1 part *solute* for 3 parts *solution*. Because $\frac{1}{3} = 33\frac{1}{3}\%$, this is a $33\frac{1}{3}\%$ solution. See Figure 8.3.

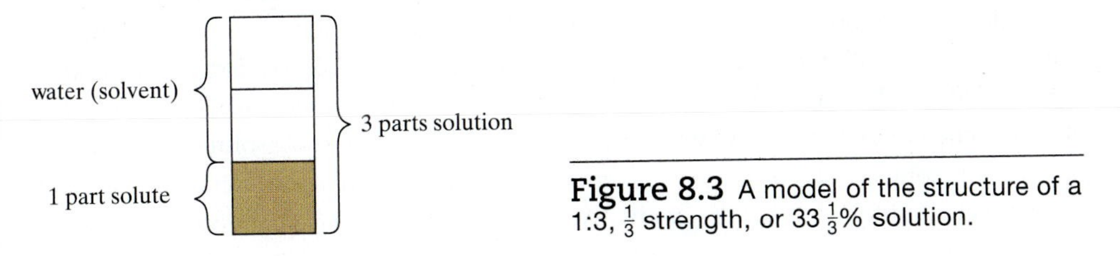

Figure 8.3 A model of the structure of a 1:3, $\frac{1}{3}$ strength, or $33\frac{1}{3}\%$ solution.

A *60%* solution can be referred to (in fractional form) as a 60/100 solution and, after reducing, this fraction becomes $\frac{3}{5}$. In ratio form this strength would be *3:5*. This solution has 3 parts *solute* for 5 parts *solution*. See Figure 8.4.

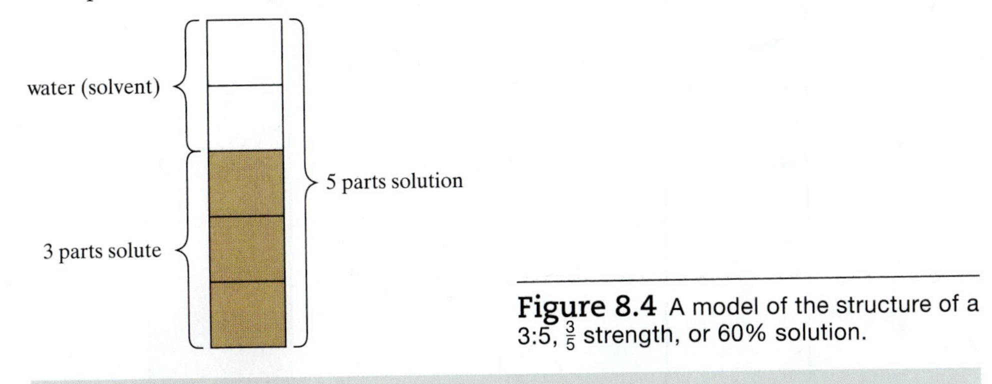

Figure 8.4 A model of the structure of a 3:5, $\frac{3}{5}$ strength, or 60% solution.

Example 8.1

Fill in the missing items in each line by following the pattern of the first line.

The solution contains:	The strength of the solution is		
	ratio	**fraction**	**percent**
1 part solute in 2 parts solution	1:2	$\frac{1}{2}$	50%
	1:4		
		$\frac{1}{5}$	
			3%
			5%
		$\frac{2}{5}$	
1 part solute in 1,000 parts solution			

Here are the answers.

The solution contains:	The strength of the solution is		
	ratio	**fraction**	**percent**
1 part solute in 2 parts solution	1:2	$\frac{1}{2}$	50%
1 part solute in 4 parts solution	1:4	$\frac{1}{4}$	25%
1 part solute in 5 parts solution	1:5	$\frac{1}{5}$	20%
3 parts solute in 100 parts solution	3:100	$\frac{3}{100}$	3%
1 part solute in 20 parts solution	1:20	$\frac{1}{20}$	5%
2 parts solute in 5 parts solution	2:5	$\frac{2}{5}$	40%
1 part solute in 1,000 parts solution	1:1,000	$\frac{1}{1,000}$	0.1%

In 2016 the USP no longer allows the use of ratio expressions on single-entity drug products. For example, the strength of EPINEPHrine 1:1,000 will only be displayed as 1 *mg/mL*, However, combination drugs such as lidocaine 1% and EPINEPHrine 1:100,000 will retain ratio expressions.

Liquid Solutes

For a solute that is in liquid form, the ratio *1:40* means there is 1 part of solute in every 40 parts of solution. This could be 1 ounce of solute in every 40 ounces of solution, 1 *cup* of solute in every 40 *cups* of solution, or 1 *milliliter* of solute in every 40 *milliliters* of solution. For most solutions, *milliliters* will be used. So 40 *milliliters* of a *1:40* acetic acid solution means that 1 *milliliter* of pure acetic acid is diluted with water to make a total of 40 *milliliters* of solution. You would prepare this solution by placing 1 *milliliter* of pure acetic acid in a graduated cylinder and adding water until the level in the graduated cylinder reaches 40 *milliliters*. See Figure 8.5.

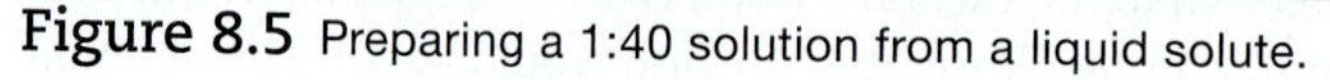

Figure 8.5 Preparing a 1:40 solution from a liquid solute.

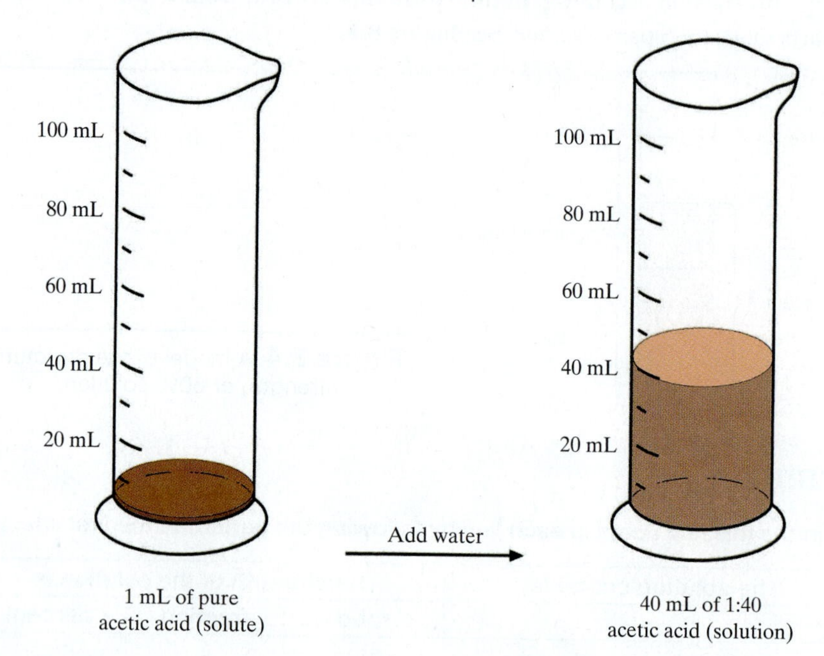

A 1% solution means that there is 1 part of the solute in 100 parts of solution. So you would prepare 100 *mL* of a 1% creosol solution by placing 1 *milliliter* of pure creosol in a graduated cylinder and adding water until the level in the graduated cylinder reaches 100 *mL*. See Figure 8.6.

Figure 8.6 Preparing a 1% solution from a liquid solute.

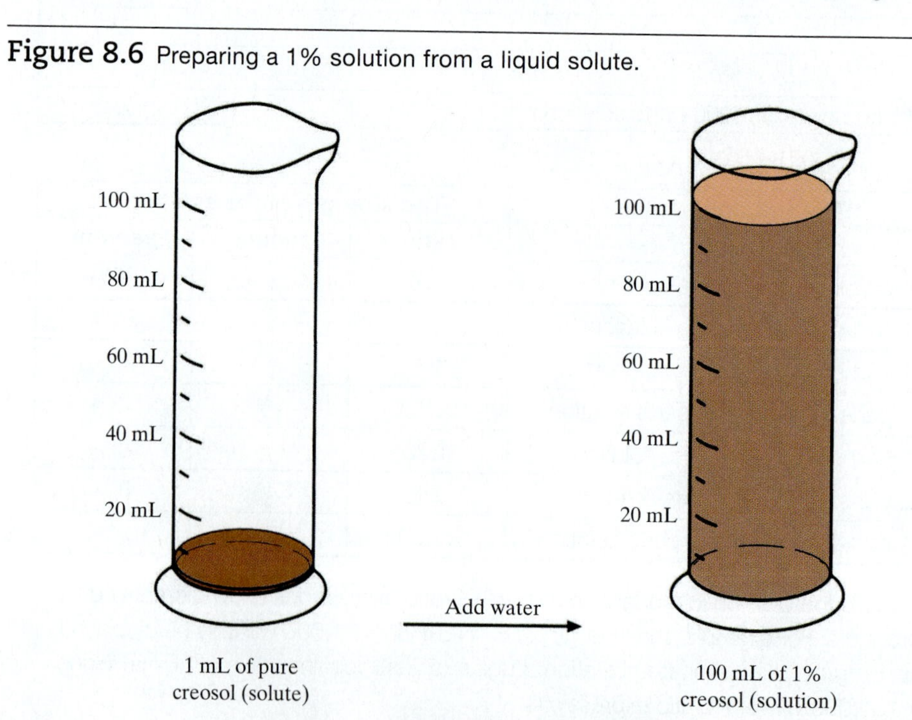

Example 8.2

Suppose 40 *mL* of an iodine solution contains 10 *mL* of (solute) pure iodine. Express the strength of this solution as a ratio, a fraction, and a percentage.

The strength of a solution may be expressed as the ratio of the *amount of pure drug in the solution to the total amount of the solution*. The amount of the solution is always expressed in *milliliters*, and because iodine is a liquid in pure form, the amount of iodine is also expressed in *milliliters*.

There are 10 *mL* of iodine (*solute*) in 40 *mL* of *solution*.

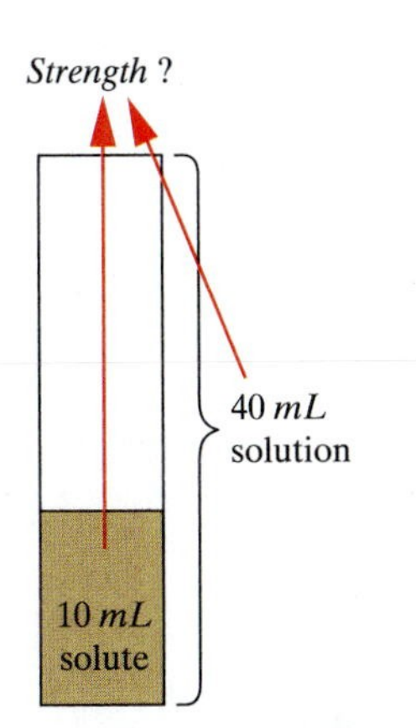

$$\text{Strength} = \frac{\text{Solute}}{\text{Solution}}$$

$$\text{Strength} = \frac{10\ mL}{40\ mL}$$

$$\text{Strength} = \frac{10\ \cancel{mL}}{40\ \cancel{mL}} = \frac{1}{4}$$

There are 10 *mL* of pure iodine in 40 *mL* of the solution, so the strength of this iodine solution may be expressed as the ratio *1:4*, as the fraction $\frac{1}{4}$ *strength*, and as the percentage *25%*.

Dry Solutes

The ratio *1:20* means 1 part of the solute in 20 parts of solution, or 2 parts of the solute in 40 parts of solution, or 3 parts in 60, or 4 parts in 80, or 5 parts in 100, and so on. When a drug is in *dry* form, the ratio *1:20* means 1 *g* of drug in every 20 *mL* of solution. So 100 *mL* of a *1:20* potassium permanganate solution means 5 *g* of potassium permanganate dissolved in water to make a total of 100 *mL* of the solution. A *1:20* solution is the same as a 5% solution. If each tablet is 5 *g*, then you would prepare this solution by placing 1 tablet of potassium permanganate in a graduated cylinder and adding some water to dissolve the tablet; then add more water until the level in the graduated cylinder reaches 100 *mL*.

Because a 5% potassium permanganate solution means 5 *g* of potassium permanganate in 100 *mL* of solution, the strength is also written as $\frac{5\ g}{100\ mL}$ or $\frac{1\ g}{20\ mL}$. See Figure 8.7.

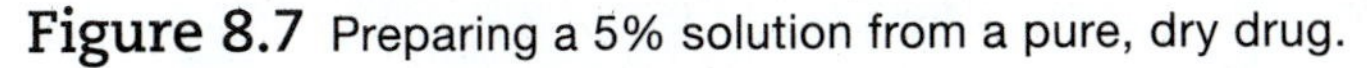

Figure 8.7 Preparing a 5% solution from a pure, dry drug.

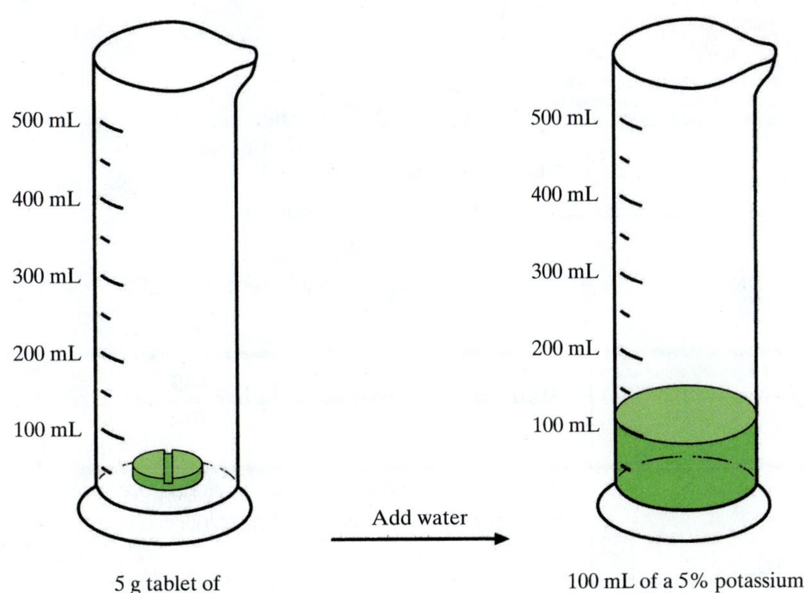

For solutions with dry solutes, remember that 1 *mL* of water weighs *1 gram*. So, with such solutions you can think of *grams* and *milliliters* as "equivalent," and therefore *grams* and *milliliters* may be "cancelled." So, the strength of the above solution can be calculated as follows:

$$\frac{1\,g}{20\,mL} = \frac{1\,\cancel{g}}{20\,\cancel{mL}} = \frac{1}{20}\,strength$$

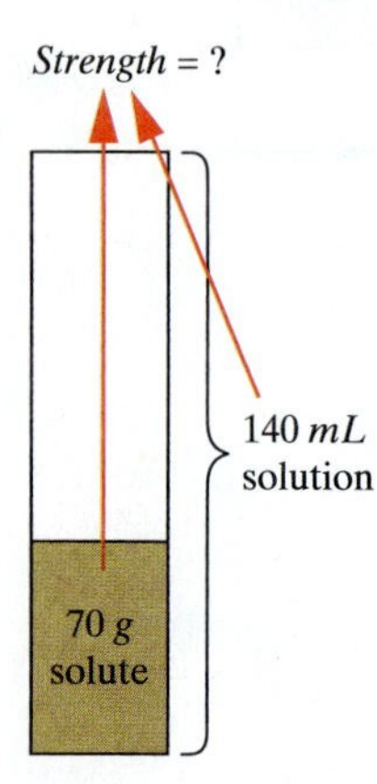

Example 8.3

There are 70 *grams* of a drug dissolved in 140 *milliliters* of a solution. What is the strength of this solution expressed as a fraction, a ratio, and a percent?

$$Strength = \frac{\text{Solute}}{\text{Solution}}$$

There are 70 *g* of *solute* in 140 *mL* of *solution*.

$$\text{Strength} = \frac{70\,g}{140\,mL}$$

Because 1 *milliliter* of water weighs 1 *gram*, you may cancel *grams* with *milliliters* and reduce the fraction.

$$\text{Strength} = \frac{70\,\cancel{g}}{140\,\cancel{mL}} = \frac{7\cancel{0}}{14\cancel{0}} = \frac{1}{2}$$

So, the strength of this solution can be expressed as $\frac{1}{2}$ strength, as 1:2, or as 50%.

Example 8.4 illustrates how to compare two strengths, one expressed *with* and another expressed *without* using explicit units of measurement.

Example 8.4

Read the label in Figure 8.8 and verify that the two strengths stated on the label are equivalent.

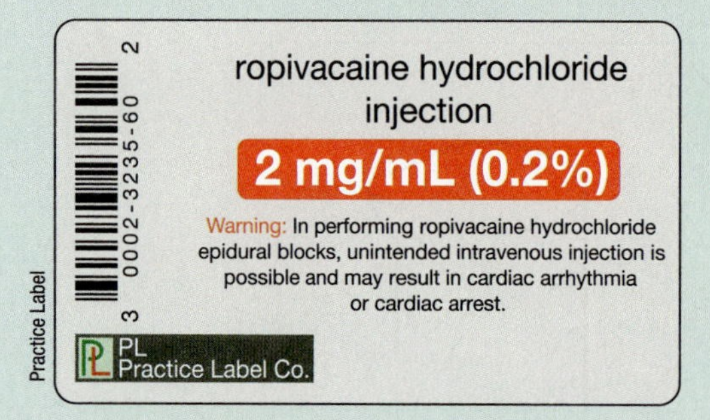

Figure 8.8 Practice label for ropivacaine HCl. (For educational purposes only)

SOURCE: Pearson Education, Inc.

The two strengths stated on this label are *2 mg/mL* and *0.2%*. To show that they are equivalent, take either one of these strengths and show how to change it to the other.

Method 1: Change $\frac{2\,mg}{mL}$ = ?%

Change 2 *mg* to *grams* by moving the decimal point 3 places to the left.

$$2\,mg = 2.\,mg = .0\,0\,2\,g = 0.002\,g$$

Method 2: Change 0.2% *to*? $\frac{mg}{mL}$

A solution whose strength is 0.2% has 0.2 *g* of solute (ropivacaine HCl) in 100 *mL* of solution. As a fraction, this is 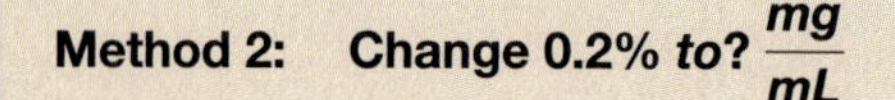 $\frac{0.2\,g}{100\,mL}$.

So, 2 *mg/mL* equals *0.002g/mL*. Now cancel the *grams* and *milliliters* and write the resulting number as a percent.

$$\frac{2\ mg}{1\ mL} = \frac{0.002\ g}{1\ mL} = \frac{0.002}{1} = 0.002 = 0.2\%$$

You need to change this fraction to *mg/mL*. That is,

$$\frac{0.2\ g}{100\ mL} = \frac{?\ mg}{mL}$$

One way to change $\frac{0.2\ g}{100\ mL}$ to $\frac{?\ mg}{mL}$ is to convert 0.2 *g* to *mg* by moving the decimal point three places to the right as follows:

$$0.2\ g = 0.200\ g = 0200.\ mg = 200\ mg$$

Therefore,

$$\frac{0.2\ g}{100\ mL} = \frac{200\ mg}{100\ mL} = \frac{200\ mg}{100\ mL} = \frac{2\ mg}{1\ mL}$$

So, the two strengths (0.2% and 2 *mg/mL*) on the label are equivalent.

Determining the Amount of Solute in a Given Amount of Solution

Either the dimensional analysis or ratio & proportion method can be used to determine the amount of solute in a given amount of a solution of known strength.

The units of measurement for the amount of solution (volume), strength of the solution, and amount of solute are listed as follows:

Amount of solution: Use *milliliters*.

Strength: Always write as a fraction for calculations.

For liquid solutes:

1:40 acetic acid solution is written as $\frac{1\ mL}{40\ mL}$

5% acetic acid solution is written as $\frac{5\ mL}{100\ mL}$

For dry or powder solutes:

1:20 potassium permanganate solution is written as $\frac{1\ g}{20\ mL}$

12% potassium permanganate solution is written as $\frac{12\ g}{100\ mL}$

Amount of solute: Use *milliliters* for liquids.

Use *grams* for tablets or powders.

To prepare a given amount of a solution of a given strength, you must first determine the amount of solute that will be in that solution. Examples 8.5 through 8.7 illustrate how this is done for dry solutes, and examples 8.8 and 8.9 have liquid solutes.

Example 8.5

A solute is supplied in powdered form. How many *grams* of this solute would be needed to prepare *500 mL* of a *3/4 strength* solution?

Given:	Amount of Solution:	500 *mL*
	Strength:	3/4 strength
Find:	Amount of Solute:	? *grams*

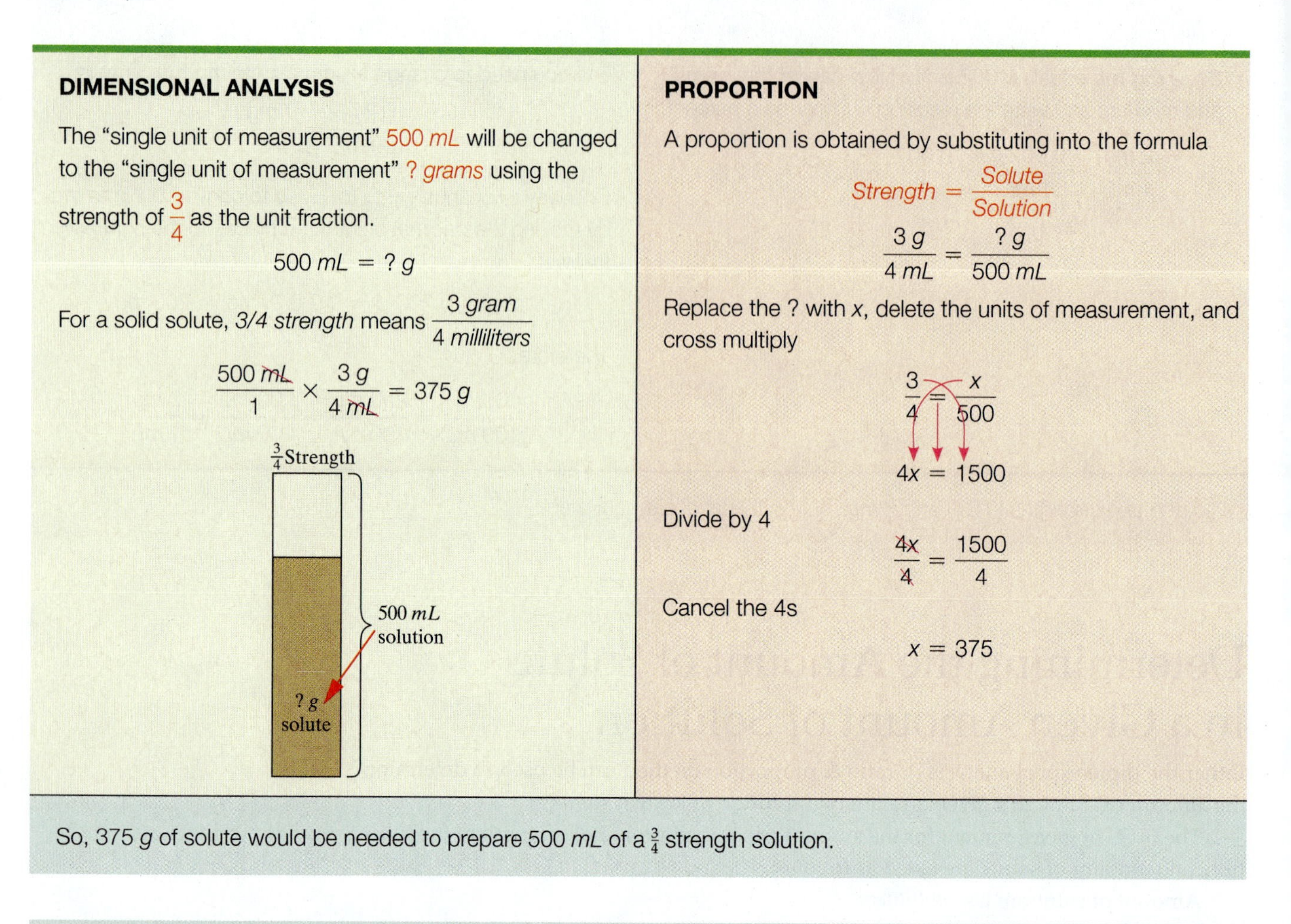

DIMENSIONAL ANALYSIS

The "single unit of measurement" 500 *mL* will be changed to the "single unit of measurement" ? *grams* using the strength of $\frac{3}{4}$ as the unit fraction.

$$500\ mL = ?\ g$$

For a solid solute, *3/4 strength* means $\frac{3\ gram}{4\ milliliters}$

$$\frac{500\ \cancel{mL}}{1} \times \frac{3\ g}{4\ \cancel{mL}} = 375\ g$$

PROPORTION

A proportion is obtained by substituting into the formula

$$Strength = \frac{Solute}{Solution}$$

$$\frac{3\ g}{4\ mL} = \frac{?\ g}{500\ mL}$$

Replace the ? with *x*, delete the units of measurement, and cross multiply

$$\frac{3}{4} = \frac{x}{500}$$

$$4x = 1500$$

Divide by 4

$$\frac{\cancel{4}x}{\cancel{4}} = \frac{1500}{4}$$

Cancel the 4s

$$x = 375$$

So, 375 *g* of solute would be needed to prepare 500 *mL* of a $\frac{3}{4}$ strength solution.

Example 8.6

Read the label in Figure 8.9. How many *grams* of dextrose are contained in 30 *mL* of this solution?

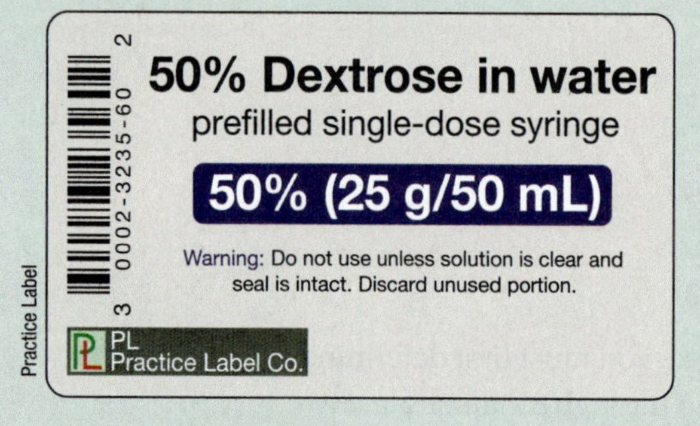

Figure 8.9 Practice label for 50% Dextrose. (For educational purposes only)

SOURCE: Pearson Education, Inc.

DIMENSIONAL ANALYSIS

Given: Amount of solution: 30 *mL*

Strength: 50% or $\frac{50\ g}{100\ mL}$

Find: Amount of solute: g

$$30\ mL = ?\ g$$

$$30\ mL \times \frac{50\ g}{100\ mL} = ?\ g$$

$$3\cancel{0}\ \cancel{mL} \times \frac{5\cancel{0}\ g}{10\cancel{0}\ \cancel{mL}} = 15\ g$$

RATIO & PROPORTION

A proportion is obtained by substituting into the formula

$$Strength = \frac{Solute}{Solution}$$

Substituting, you get

$$\frac{50\ g}{100\ mL} = \frac{x\ g}{30\ mL}$$

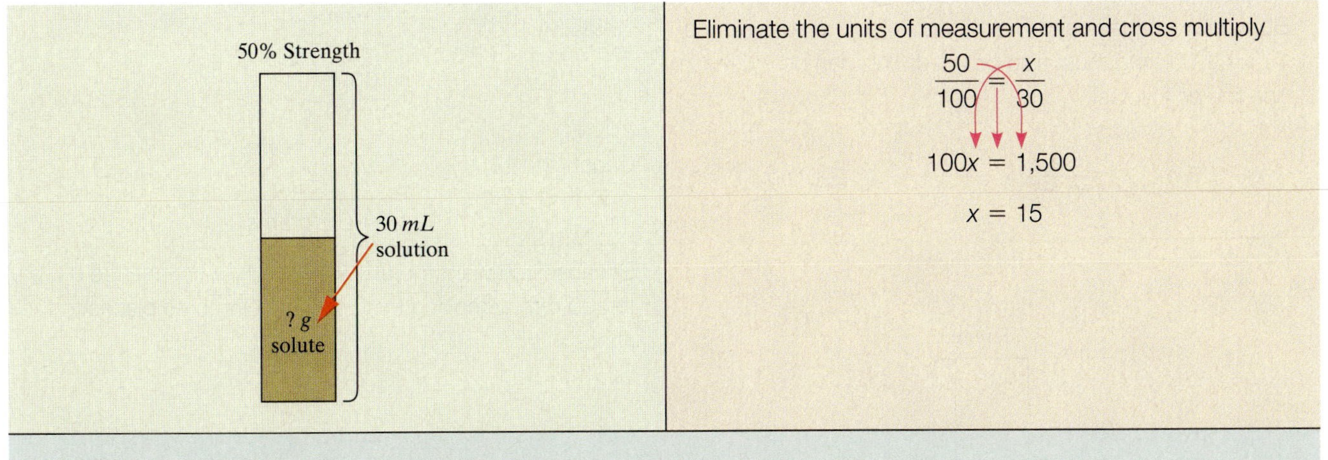

Eliminate the units of measurement and cross multiply

$$\frac{50}{100} = \frac{x}{30}$$

$$100x = 1{,}500$$

$$x = 15$$

So, 15 *g* of dextrose are contained in 30 *mL* of a 50% dextrose solution.

Example 8.7

Read the label in Figure 8.10 and determine the number of *milligrams* of lidocaine that are contained in 5 *mL* of this lidocaine solution.

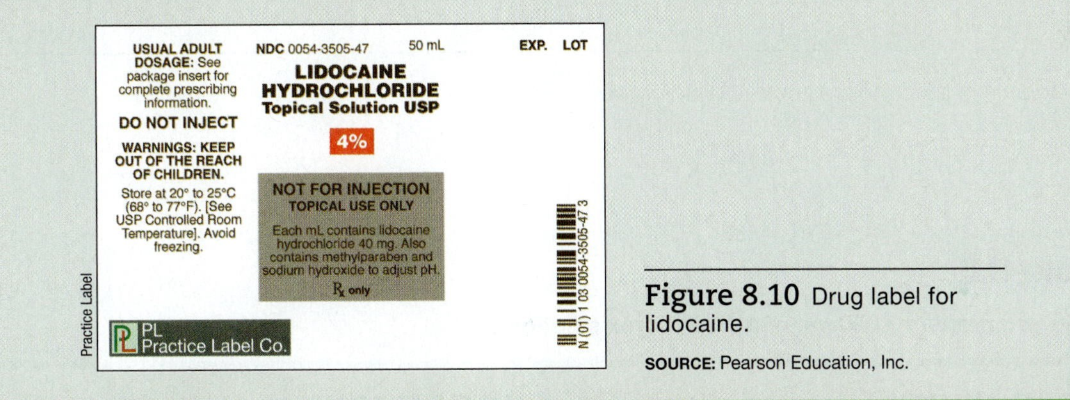

Figure 8.10 Drug label for lidocaine.

SOURCE: Pearson Education, Inc.

DIMENSIONAL ANALYSIS

Given: Amount of solution: 5 *mL*
Strength: 4%
Find: Amount of solute: ? *mg*

You want to convert the amount of the solution (5 *mL*) to the amount of the solute (? *mg*).

$$5\ mL = ?\ mg$$

Note that lidocaine is a powder in pure form, so the strength of the 4% solution is expressed in fraction form as $\frac{4\ g}{100\ mL}$.

This strength can be used to find the amount of lidocaine in *grams*.

$$5\ \cancel{mL} \times \frac{4\ g}{100\ \cancel{mL}} = ?\ mg$$

RATIO & PROPORTION

Because lidocaine is a solid in its pure form, it is measured in *grams*. So, 4% strength means 4 *g* of lidocaine in each 100 *mL* of the solution. You need to determine the number of *mg* of lidocaine that are in 5 *mL* of this solution.

A proportion is obtained by substituting into the formula

$$Strength = \frac{Solute}{Solution}$$

$$\frac{4\ g}{100\ mL} = \frac{?\ g}{5\ mL}$$

Replace the ? with *x*, and delete the units of measurement and cross multiply

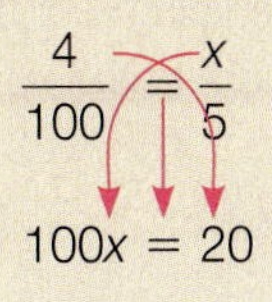

$$\frac{4}{100} = \frac{x}{5}$$

$$100x = 20$$

(Continued)

But you want the answer in *milligrams*, so the equivalence $1\ g = 1{,}000\ mg$ must also be used. This can be written in one line as follows:

$$5\ mL \times \frac{4\ g}{100\ mL} \times \frac{1{,}000\ mg}{g} = 200\ mg$$

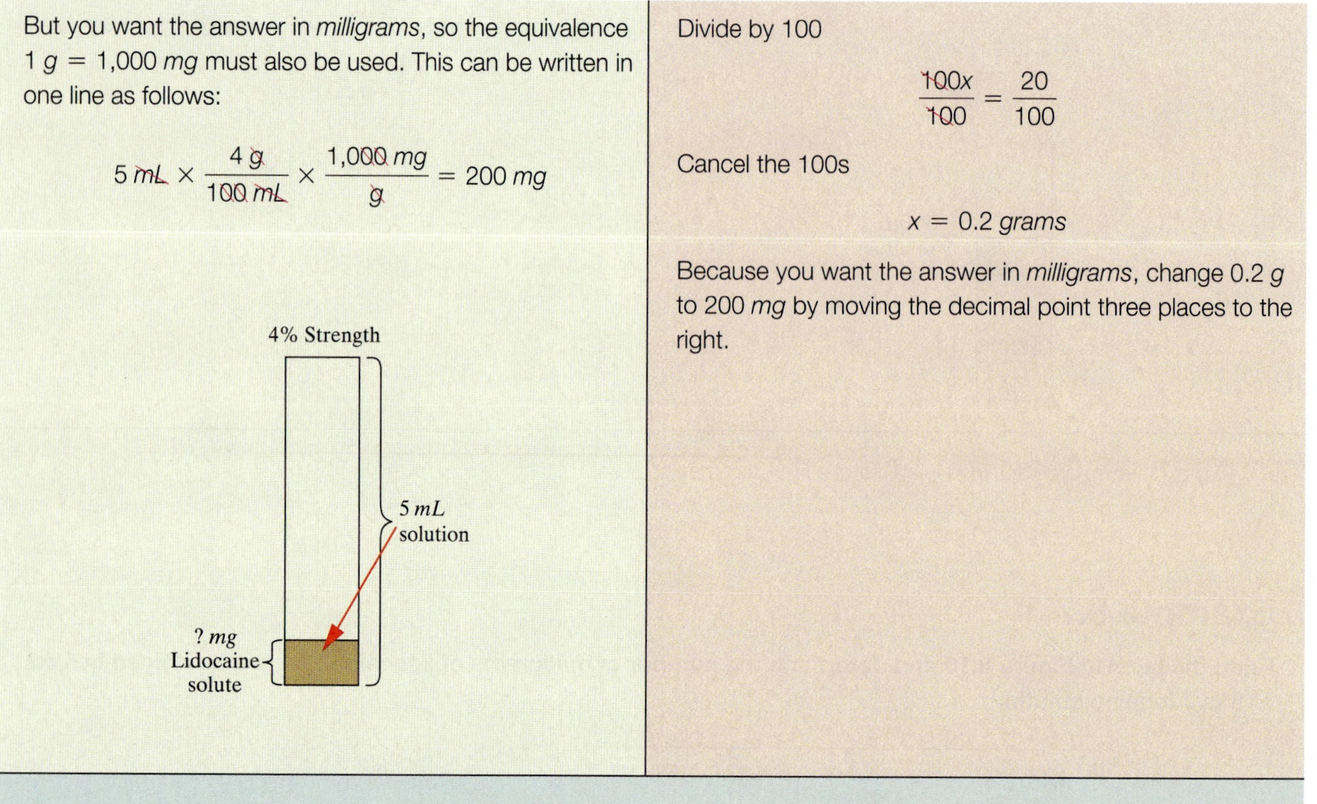

Divide by 100

$$\frac{100x}{100} = \frac{20}{100}$$

Cancel the 100s

$$x = 0.2\ grams$$

Because you want the answer in *milligrams*, change 0.2 *g* to 200 *mg* by moving the decimal point three places to the right.

So, 200 *milligrams* of lidocaine are contained in 5 *milliliters* of a 4% lidocaine solution.

Example 8.8

How would you prepare 2,000 *mL* of a *1:10* Clorox solution?

DIMENSIONAL ANALYSIS

Given: Amount of solution: 2,000 *mL*

Strength: 1:10 or $\frac{1}{10}$

Find: Amount of solute: ? *mL*

Because Clorox is a liquid in its pure form, it is measured in *milliliters*. So, a *1:10* strength means that 1 *mL* of Clorox is in each 10 *mL* of the solution.

You want to convert the amount of the solution (2,000 *mL*) to the amount of the solute Clorox.

$$2{,}000\ mL = ?\ mL$$

The preceding expression contains *mL* on both sides. This can be confusing! To make it clearer, note that on the left side "*mL*" refers to the volume of the solution, whereas on the right side "*mL*" refers to the volume of the full-strength Clorox.

So, you have the following:

$$2{,}000\ mL\ \text{(solution)} = ?\ mL\ \text{(Clorox)}$$

RATIO & PROPORTION

Because Clorox is a liquid in its pure form, it is measured in *milliliters*. So, *1:10* strength means 1 *mL* of Clorox in each 10 *mL* of the solution.

A proportion is obtained by substituting into the formula

$$\text{Strength} = \frac{\text{Solute}}{\text{Solution}}$$

Substituting, you get

$$\frac{1\ mL\ \text{(Clorox)}}{10\ mL\ \text{(solution)}} = \frac{x\ mL\ \text{(Clorox)}}{2{,}000\ mL\ \text{(solution)}}$$

Eliminate the units of measurement and cross multiply

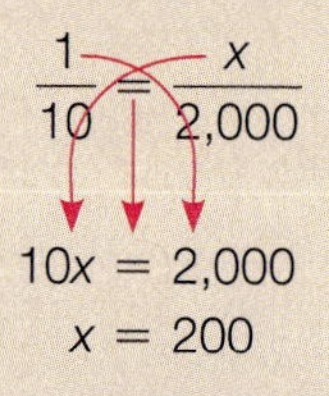

$$\frac{1}{10} = \frac{x}{2{,}000}$$

$$10x = 2{,}000$$

$$x = 200$$

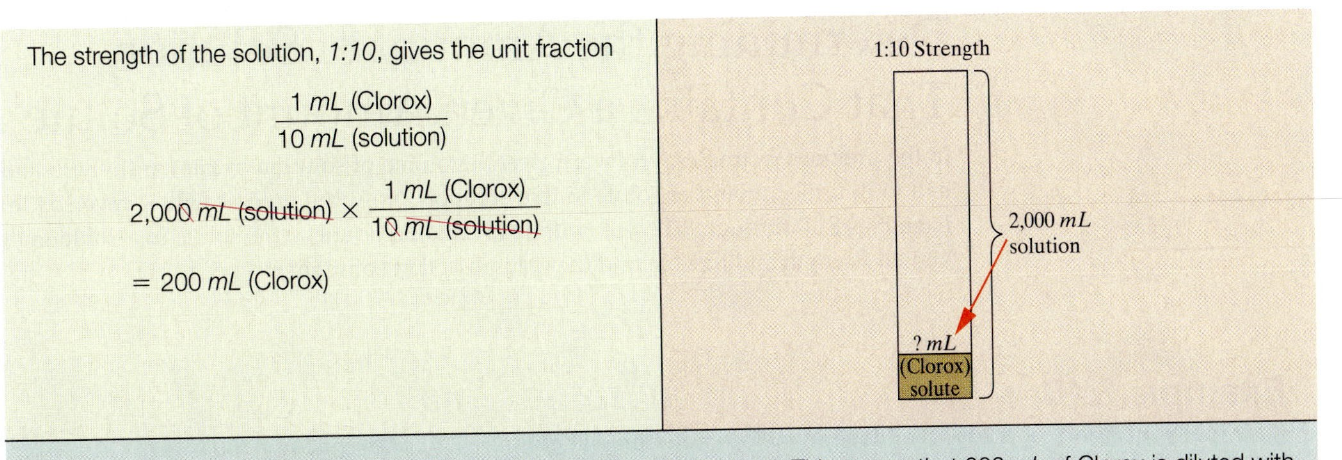

The strength of the solution, *1:10*, gives the unit fraction

$$\frac{1\ mL\ (\text{Clorox})}{10\ mL\ (\text{solution})}$$

$$2{,}000\ \cancel{mL\ (\text{solution})} \times \frac{1\ mL\ (\text{Clorox})}{10\ \cancel{mL\ (\text{solution})}}$$

$$= 200\ mL\ (\text{Clorox})$$

So, you need 200 *mL* of Clorox to prepare 2,000 *mL* of a *1:10* solution. This means that 200 *mL* of Clorox is diluted with water to 2,000 *mL* of solution.

Example 8.9

How would you prepare 250 *mL* of a $\frac{1}{2}$% Lysol solution?

DIMENSIONAL ANALYSIS

Given: Amount of solution: 250 *mL*

Strength: $\frac{1}{2}\%$

Find: Amount of pure Lysol: ? *mL*

Because Lysol is a liquid in undiluted form, the amount of Lysol to be found is measured in *milliliters*.

$\frac{1}{2}$% can be written as 0.5% or as

$$\frac{0.5\ mL\ (\text{Lysol})}{100\ mL\ (\text{solution})}$$

Convert the amount of the solution (250 *mL*) to the amount of Lysol.

$$250\ mL\ (\text{solution}) = ?\ mL\ (\text{Lysol})$$

Use the strength of the solution

$$\frac{0.5\ mL\ (\text{Lysol})}{100\ mL\ (\text{solution})}$$ as the unit fraction.

$$250\ \cancel{mL\ (\text{solution})} \times \frac{0.5\ mL\ (\text{Lysol})}{100\ \cancel{mL\ (\text{solution})}}$$

$$= 1.25\ mL\ (\text{Lysol})$$

RATIO & PROPORTION

Because Lysol is a liquid in its pure form, it is measured in *milliliters*. So, $\frac{1}{2}$% (0.5%) strength means 0.5 *mL* of Lysol is contained in each 100 *mL* of the solution.

A proportion is obtained by substituting into the formula

$$\text{Strength} = \frac{\text{Solute}}{\text{Solution}}$$

Substituting, you get

$$\frac{0.5\ mL(\text{Lysol})}{100\ mL(\text{solution})} = \frac{x\ mL(\text{Lysol})}{250\ mL(\text{solution})}$$

Eliminate the units of measurement and cross multiply

$$\frac{0.5}{100} = \frac{x}{250}$$

$$100x = 125$$

$$x = 1.25$$

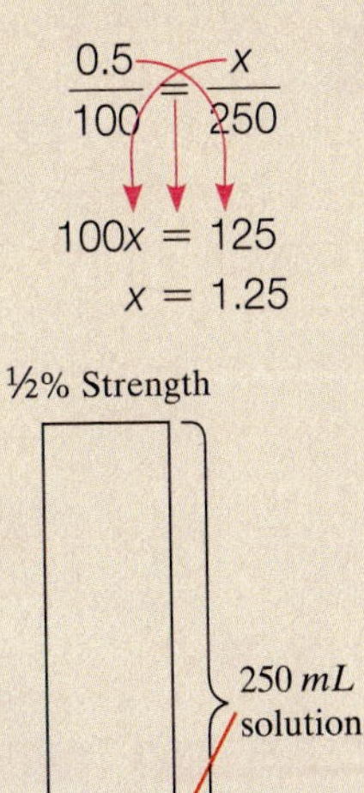

So, you need 1.25 *mL* of Lysol to prepare 250 *mL* of a $\frac{1}{2}$% Lysol solution. This means that 1.25 *mL* of Lysol is diluted with water to 250 *mL* of solution.

Determining the Amount of Solution That Contains a Given Amount of Solute

In the previous examples, you were given a volume of solution of known strength and had to find the amount of solute in that solution. Now, the process will be reversed. In Examples 8.10 through 8.12, you will be given an amount of the solute in a solution of known strength and have to find the volume of that solution.

Example 8.10

How many *milliliters* of a 20% magnesium sulfate solution will contain 40 *g* of magnesium sulfate?

DIMENSIONAL ANALYSIS

You need to determine the number of *milliliters* of this solution that contains 40 *g* of magnesium sulfate.

Given: Amount of solute: 40 *g*

Strength: 20%

Find: Amount of solution: ? *mL*

You want to convert the 40 *g* of solute to *milliliters* of solution.

$$40\ g = ?\ mL$$

You want to cancel the *grams* and obtain the equivalent amount in *milliliters*.

$$40\ g \times \frac{?\ mL}{?\ g} = ?\ mL$$

In a 20% solution there are 20 *g* of magnesium sulfate per 100 *mL* of solution. So, the unit fraction is

$$\frac{100\ mL}{20\ g}$$

$$\overset{2}{\cancel{40}}\ \cancel{g} \times \frac{100\ mL}{\underset{1}{\cancel{20}}\ \cancel{g}} = 200\ mL$$

RATIO & PROPORTION

The 20% strength means that there is 20 *g* of magnesium sulfate in every 100 *mL* of this solution.

A proportion is obtained by substituting into the formula

$$Strength = \frac{Solute}{Solution}$$

Substituting, you get

$$\frac{20\ g}{100\ mL} = \frac{40\ g}{x\ mL}$$

Eliminate the units of measurement and cross multiply

$$\frac{20}{100} = \frac{40}{x}$$

$$4{,}000 = 20x$$

$$200 = x$$

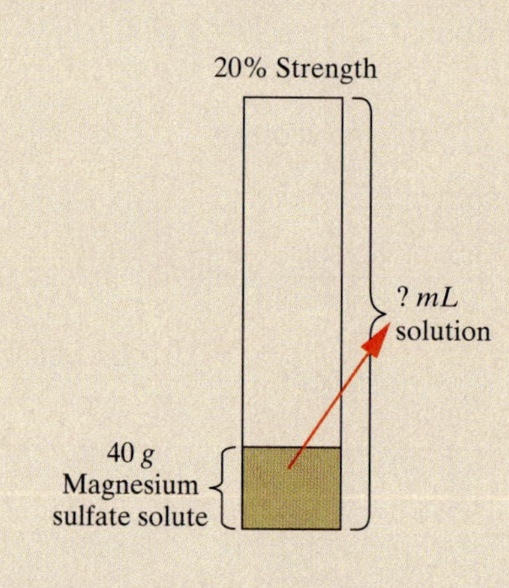

So, 200 *mL* of a 20% magnesium sulfate solution contains 40 *g* of magnesium sulfate.

Example 8.11

How many *milliliters* of the zoledronic acid solution (Figure 8.11) contain 10 *mg* of the drug?

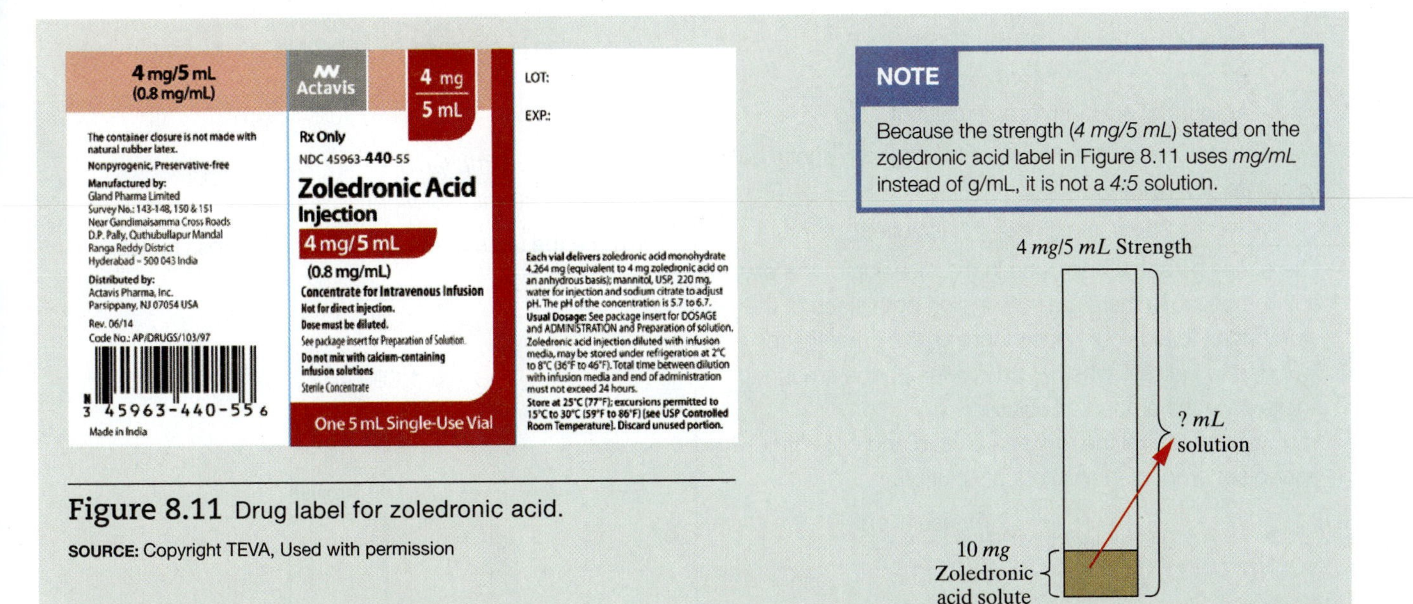

Figure 8.11 Drug label for zoledronic acid.

SOURCE: Copyright TEVA, Used with permission

NOTE

Because the strength (*4 mg/5 mL*) stated on the zoledronic acid label in Figure 8.11 uses *mg/mL* instead of g/mL, it is not a *4:5* solution.

DIMENSIONAL ANALYSIS

You need to determine the number of *milliliters* of the solution that contains 10 *mg* of the solute.

Given: Amount of solute: 10 *mg*

Strength: 4 *mg*/5 *mL*

Find: Amount of solution: ? *mL*

You want to convert the amount of the solute (10 *mg*) to the amount of the solution (? *mL*).

$$10\ mg = ?\ mL$$

Use the strength of the solution $\frac{4\ mg}{5\ mL}$ as the unit fraction.

In this case, the *milligrams* need to cancel. So, the fraction must be inverted to have *mg* in the denominator

$$10\ \cancel{mg} \times \frac{5\ mL}{4\ \cancel{mg}} = 12.5\ mL$$

RATIO & PROPORTION

The *4 mg/5 mL* strength means that there is 4 *mg* of the drug (zoledronic acid) in every 5 *mL* of this solution. You need to determine the number of *milliliters* of this solution that contain 10 *mg* of the drug.

A proportion is obtained by substituting into the formula

$$Strength = \frac{Solute}{Solution}$$

Substituting, you get

$$\frac{4\ mg}{5\ mL} = \frac{10\ mg}{x\ mL}$$

Eliminate the units of measurement and cross multiply

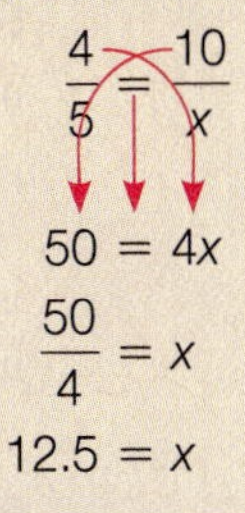

$$\frac{4}{5} = \frac{10}{x}$$

$$50 = 4x$$

$$\frac{50}{4} = x$$

$$12.5 = x$$

So, 12.5 *mL* of the zoledronic acid solution contain 10 *mg* of zoledronic acid.

Example 8.12

How many *milliliters* of a *1:40* acetic acid solution will contain 25 *mL* of acetic acid?

DIMENSIONAL ANALYSIS

You need to determine the number of *milliliters* of this solution that contain 25 *mL* of acetic acid.

RATIO & PROPORTION

The *1:40* strength means that there is 1 *mL* of acetic acid in every 40 *mL* of this solution. You need to determine the number of *milliliters* of this solution that contain 25 *mL* of the pure acetic acid.

(Continued)

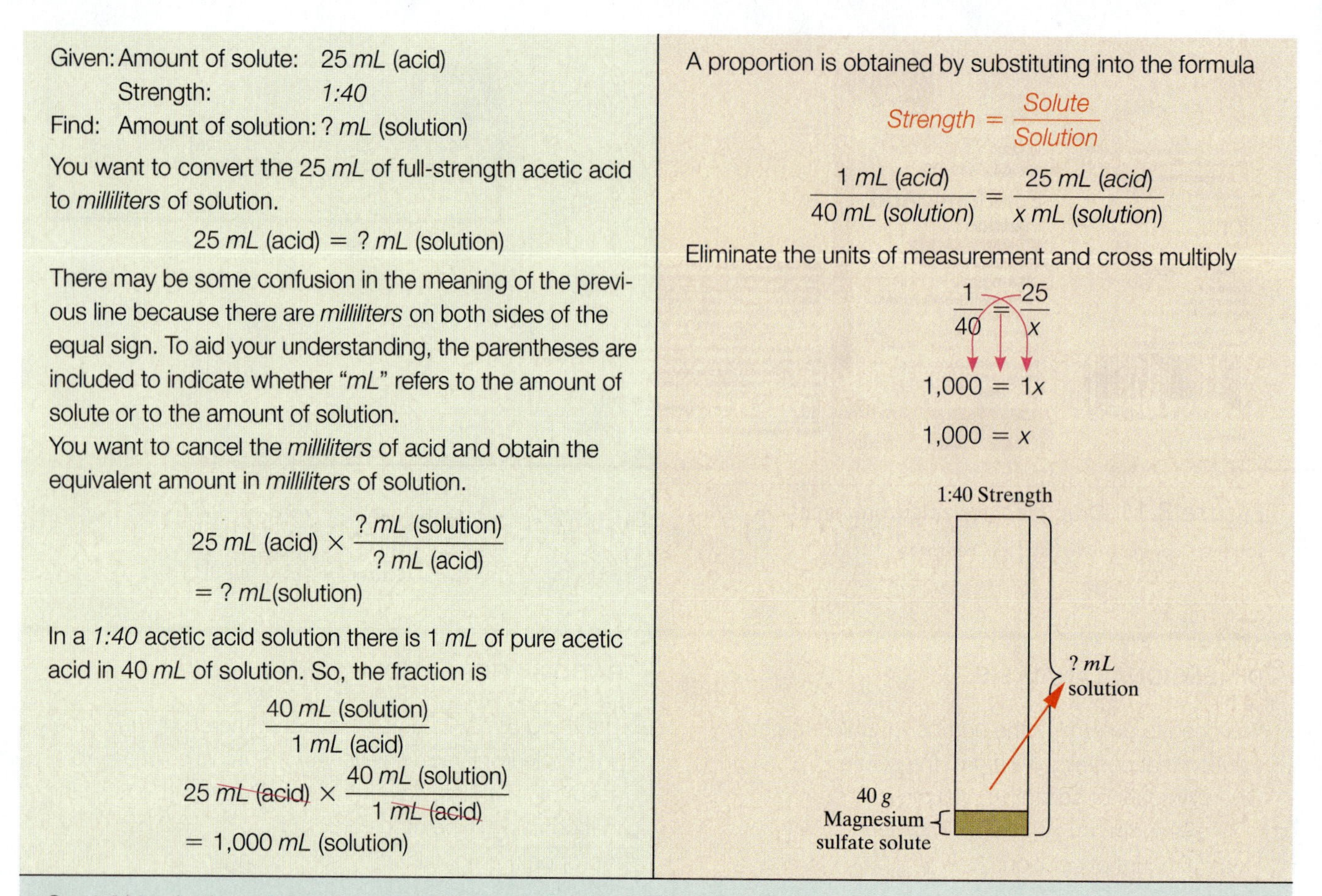

Given: Amount of solute: 25 *mL* (acid)
Strength: *1:40*
Find: Amount of solution: ? *mL* (solution)

You want to convert the 25 *mL* of full-strength acetic acid to *milliliters* of solution.

$$25\ mL\ (\text{acid}) = ?\ mL\ (\text{solution})$$

There may be some confusion in the meaning of the previous line because there are *milliliters* on both sides of the equal sign. To aid your understanding, the parentheses are included to indicate whether "*mL*" refers to the amount of solute or to the amount of solution.

You want to cancel the *milliliters* of acid and obtain the equivalent amount in *milliliters* of solution.

$$25\ mL\ (\text{acid}) \times \frac{?\ mL\ (\text{solution})}{?\ mL\ (\text{acid})} = ?\ mL(\text{solution})$$

In a *1:40* acetic acid solution there is 1 *mL* of pure acetic acid in 40 *mL* of solution. So, the fraction is

$$\frac{40\ mL\ (\text{solution})}{1\ mL\ (\text{acid})}$$

$$25\ \cancel{mL\ (\text{acid})} \times \frac{40\ mL\ (\text{solution})}{1\ \cancel{mL\ (\text{acid})}} = 1{,}000\ mL\ (\text{solution})$$

A proportion is obtained by substituting into the formula

$$\text{Strength} = \frac{\text{Solute}}{\text{Solution}}$$

$$\frac{1\ mL\ (\text{acid})}{40\ mL\ (\text{solution})} = \frac{25\ mL\ (\text{acid})}{x\ mL\ (\text{solution})}$$

Eliminate the units of measurement and cross multiply

$$\frac{1}{40} = \frac{25}{x}$$

$$1{,}000 = 1x$$

$$1{,}000 = x$$

So, 1,000 *mL* of a *1:40* acetic acid solution contain 25 *mL* of acetic acid.

Irrigating Solutions, Soaks, and Oral Feedings

Sometimes healthcare professionals are required to prepare irrigating solutions, soaks, and nutritional feedings. These may be supplied in ready-to-use form, or they can be prepared from dry powders or from liquid concentrates.

Irrigating solutions and soaks are used for sterile irrigation of body cavities, wounds, indwelling catheters; washing and rinsing purposes; or for soaking of surgical dressings, instruments, and laboratory specimens.

Enteral feedings are nutritional solutions that can be supplied in ready-to-use form or they may be reconstituted from powders or from liquid concentrates. The nutritional solutions may be administered either orally or parenterally.

ALERT

Full-strength (ready-to-use) hydrogen peroxide is generally supplied as a 3% solution. This stock solution may be diluted to form weaker solutions depending on the application. These dilutions must be performed using aseptic techniques.

Example 8.13

Using a full-strength hydrogen peroxide solution, how would you prepare 300 *mL* of $\frac{2}{3}$ strength hydrogen peroxide solution for a wound irrigation, using normal saline as the diluent?

The $\frac{2}{3}$ strength means that there are 2 *mL* of full-strength hydrogen peroxide solute in every 3 *mL* of the $\frac{2}{3}$ strength solution. You need to determine the number of *milliliters* of full-strength hydrogen peroxide solute that are contained in 300 *mL* of the $\frac{2}{3}$ strength solution.

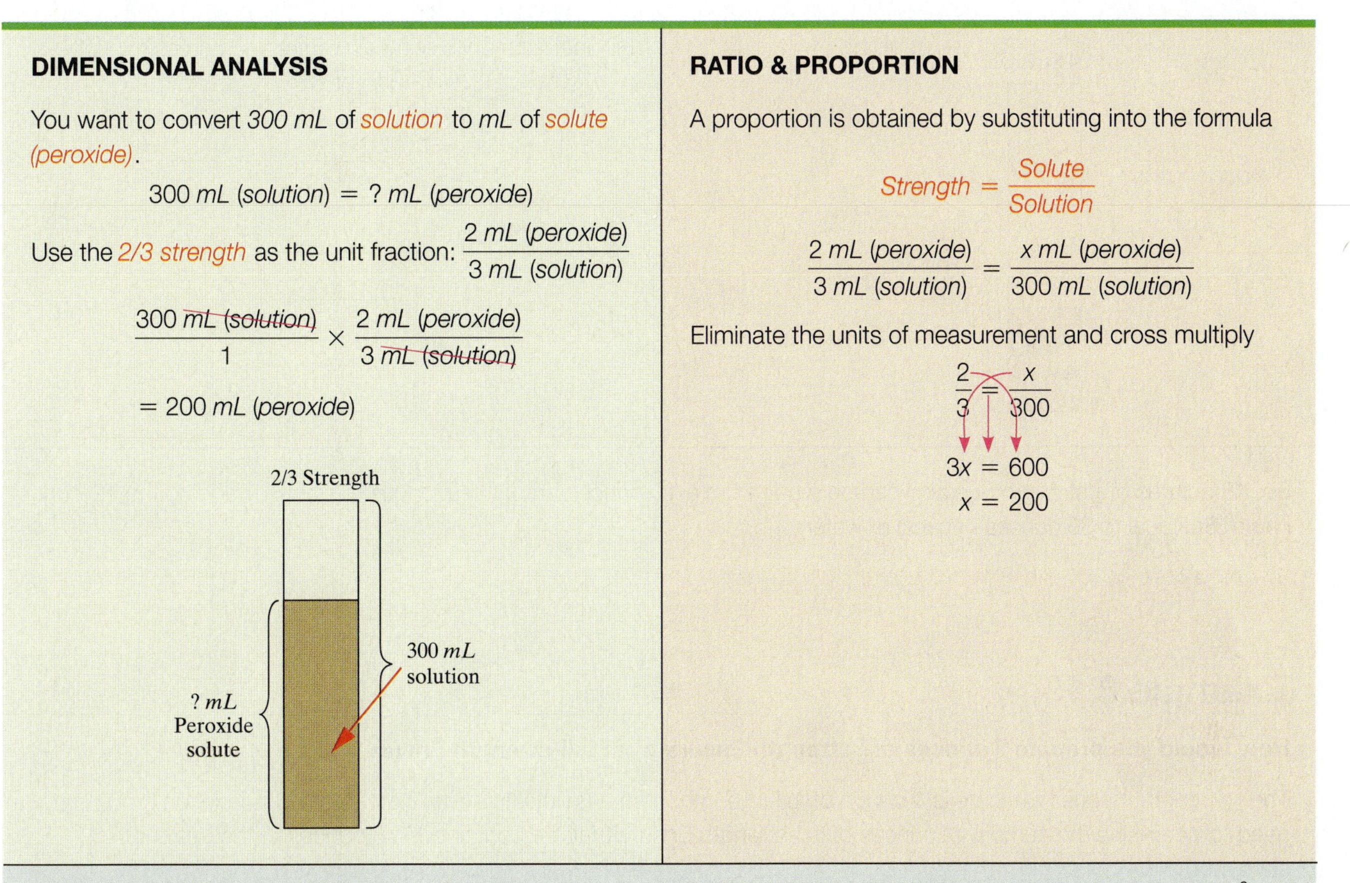

DIMENSIONAL ANALYSIS

You want to convert *300 mL* of *solution* to *mL* of *solute (peroxide)*.

$$300\ mL\ (solution) = ?\ mL\ (peroxide)$$

Use the *2/3 strength* as the unit fraction: $\frac{2\ mL\ (peroxide)}{3\ mL\ (solution)}$

$$\frac{300\ \cancel{mL\ (solution)}}{1} \times \frac{2\ mL\ (peroxide)}{3\ \cancel{mL\ (solution)}}$$

$$= 200\ mL\ (peroxide)$$

RATIO & PROPORTION

A proportion is obtained by substituting into the formula

$$Strength = \frac{Solute}{Solution}$$

$$\frac{2\ mL\ (peroxide)}{3\ mL\ (solution)} = \frac{x\ mL\ (peroxide)}{300\ mL\ (solution)}$$

Eliminate the units of measurement and cross multiply

$$\frac{2}{3} = \frac{x}{300}$$

$$3x = 600$$

$$x = 200$$

So, 200 *mL* of full-strength hydrogen peroxide would be diluted with 100 *mL* of normal saline to make 300 *mL* of a $\frac{2}{3}$ strength solution.

Example 8.14

How many ounces of $\frac{1}{4}$ strength Sustacal can be made from a 12-*ounce* can of full-strength Sustacal?

The $\frac{1}{4}$ strength means that there is 1 *ounce* of full-strength Sustacal (solute) in every 4 *ounces* of this solution. You need to determine the number of ounces of $\frac{1}{4}$ strength Sustacal that can be made from 12 *oz* of full-strength Sustacal.

DIMENSIONAL ANALYSIS

You want to convert *12 oz* of *Sustacal (solute)* to *oz* of *solution*.

$$12\ oz\ (Sustacal) = ?\ oz\ (solution)$$

Use the *1/4 strength* as the unit fraction: $\frac{4\ oz\ (solution)}{1\ oz\ (Sustacal)}$

$$\frac{12\ \cancel{oz\ (Sustacal)}}{1} \times \frac{4\ oz\ (solution)}{1\ \cancel{oz\ (Sustacal)}}$$

$$= 48\ oz\ (solution)$$

RATIO & PROPORTION

A proportion is obtained by substituting into the formula

$$Strength = \frac{Solute}{Solution}$$

$$\frac{1\ oz\ (Sustacal)}{4\ oz\ (solution)} = \frac{12\ oz\ (Sustacal)}{x\ oz\ (solution)}$$

(Continued)

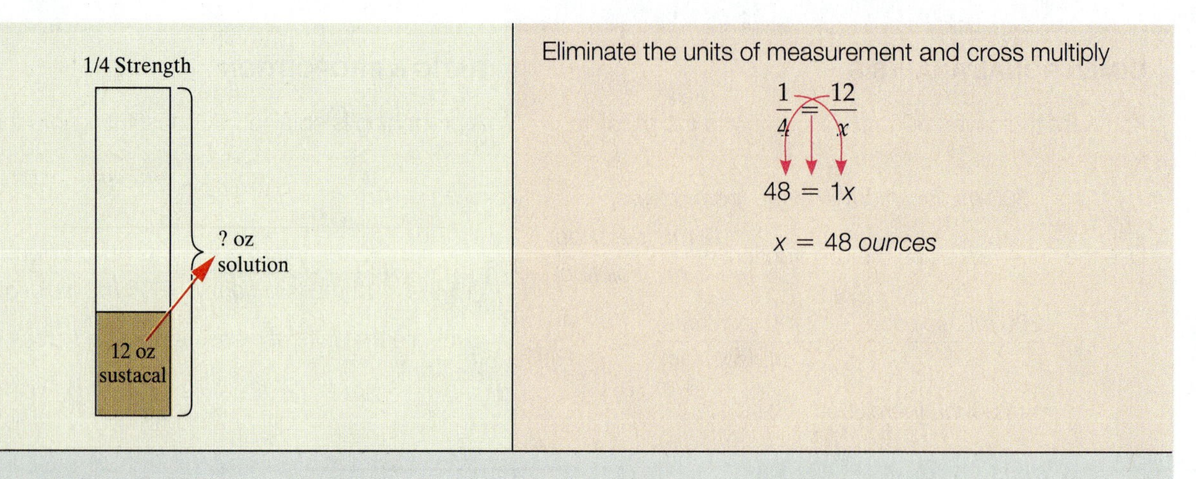

Eliminate the units of measurement and cross multiply

$$\frac{1}{4} = \frac{12}{x}$$

$$48 = 1x$$

$$x = 48 \text{ ounces}$$

So, 48 ounces of $\frac{1}{4}$ strength Sustacal can be made from a 12-*ounce* can of full-strength Sustacal by adding the 12-*ounce* can of Sustacal to 36 *ounces* (3 cans) of water.

Example 8.15

How would you prepare 8 *ounces* of $\frac{1}{2}$ strength Ensure from full-strength Ensure?

The $\frac{1}{2}$ strength means that there is 1 *ounce* of full-strength Ensure (solute) in every 2 *ounces* of this solution. You need to determine the number of ounces of full-strength Ensure that are contained in 8 *ounces* of the $\frac{1}{2}$ strength solution.

DIMENSIONAL ANALYSIS

You want to convert *8 oz* of *(solution)* to ? *oz* of *Ensure (solute).*

$$8 \text{ oz (solution)} = ? \text{ oz (Ensure)}$$

Use the *1/2 strength* as the unit fraction: $\frac{1 \text{ oz (Ensure)}}{2 \text{ oz (Solution)}}$

$$\frac{8 \text{ oz (solution)}}{1} \times \frac{1 \text{ oz (Ensure)}}{2 \text{ oz (solution)}}$$

$$= 4 \text{ oz (Ensure)}$$

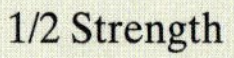

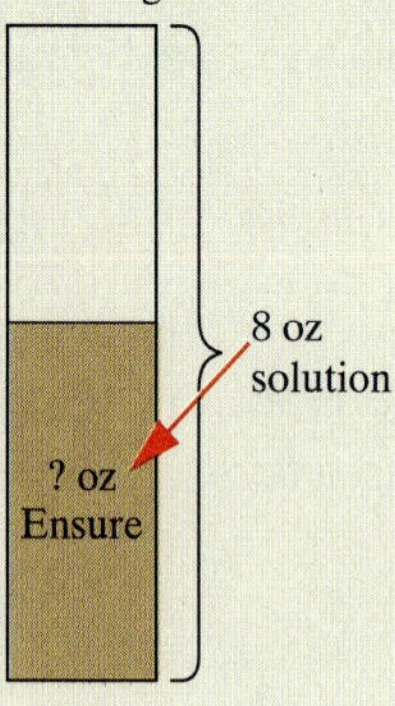

RATIO & PROPORTION

A proportion is obtained by substituting into the formula

$$\text{Strength} = \frac{\text{Solute}}{\text{Solution}}$$

$$\frac{1 \text{ oz (Ensure)}}{2 \text{ oz (solution)}} = \frac{x \text{ oz (Ensure)}}{8 \text{ oz (solution)}}$$

Eliminate the units of measurement and cross multiply

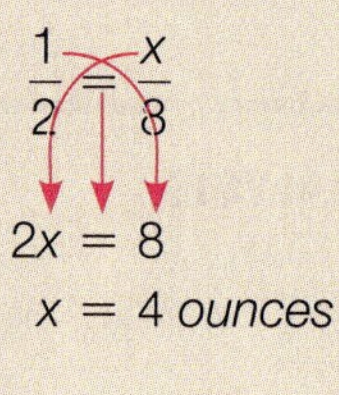

$$\frac{1}{2} = \frac{x}{8}$$

$$2x = 8$$

$$x = 4 \text{ ounces}$$

So, 4 *oz* of full-strength Ensure are contained in 8 *ounces* of $\frac{1}{2}$ strength Ensure. To prepare the solution, add 4 *ounces* of water to 4 *ounces* of full-strength Ensure to make 8 *ounces* of the $\frac{1}{2}$-strength solution.

Summary

In this chapter, you learned that there are three important quantities associated with a solution: the *strength* of the solution, the *amount of solute* dissolved in the solution, and the total *volume of the solution*. If any two of these three quantities are known, the remaining quantity can be found.

- The *strength* of a solution is the ratio of the *amount of solute* dissolved in the solution to the total *volume of the solution*.
- The strength of a solution may be expressed in the form of a *ratio*, *fraction*, or *percentage*.
- A $\frac{1}{2}$ *strength* solution is a *1:2* or a *50%* solution and should not be confused with a $\frac{1}{2}$% solution.
- The amount of solute dissolved in the solution should be expressed in *milliliters* if the solute is a *liquid*.
- The amount of solute dissolved in the solution should be expressed in *grams* if the solute is a *solid* or *powder*.
- The *volume of a solution* should be expressed in *milliliters*.
- $\text{Strength} = \dfrac{\text{Solute}}{\text{Solution}}$
- To determine the amount of solute contained in a given amount of a solution of known strength, use the strength as the known equivalence.
- To determine the amount of a solution of known strength containing a given amount of solute, use the strength as the known equivalence.
- Use aseptic technique when diluting stock solutions for irrigations, soak, and nutritional liquids.
- The strength of a particular solution may be written in many different forms. The following strengths are all equivalent:

With Stated Units of Measurement

$$\textit{Rates} \begin{cases} 500\ mg/mL \\ 500\ mg \text{ per } mL \\ \dfrac{500\ mg}{1\ mL} \end{cases}$$

Equivalence $500\ mg = 1\ mL$

Without Stated Units of Measurement

Fraction	$\frac{1}{2}$ strength
Ratio	1:2
Precentage	50%

Case Study 8.1

Read the Case Study and answer the questions. Answers can be found in Appendix A.

A 65-year-old male is admitted to a rehab facility, status post right-sided cerebral vascular accident (CVA). He has a past medical history of hypertension, hyperlipidemia, atrial fibrillation, osteoarthritis, and insulin-dependent diabetes mellitus. He is alert and oriented to person, place, time, and recent memory. He has left-sided weakness, needs assistance with activities of daily living (ADL), and has a 3 *cm* wound on his left heel. He rates his pain level as 8 on a scale of 0–10. Vital signs are T 98.7° F; P 88 R 24; B/P 134/82.
His orders are as follows:

- diltiazem LA 120 *mg* po daily
- nabumetone 1,000 *mg* po at bedtime
- warfarin 2.5 *mg* po daily
- simvastatin 40 *mg* po at bedtime
- Sustacal 2 *oz* po with each oral medication administration
- Humulin R insulin 10 *units* and Humulin N insulin 34 *units* subcut 30 *minutes* ac breakfast
- Humulin R insulin 10 *units* and Humulin N insulin 28 *units* subcut 30 *minutes* ac dinner
- Pneumovax 0.5 *mL* IM stat for 1 dose
- Cleanse left heel with NS solution (0.9% Na Cl) and apply DSD daily

Refer to the labels below when necessary to answer the following questions.

1. Select the correct label for the diltiazem dose. How many tablets will you administer?
2. Select the correct label for the warfarin dose. How many tablets will you administer?
3. How many tablets of simvastatin will you administer?
4. How many tablets of nabumetone will you administer?
5. How many *mL* of Sustacal will the client receive daily?

(continued)

6. The pneumovax vial contains 2.5 *mL*. Choose the appropriate syringe below and place an arrow at the dose.

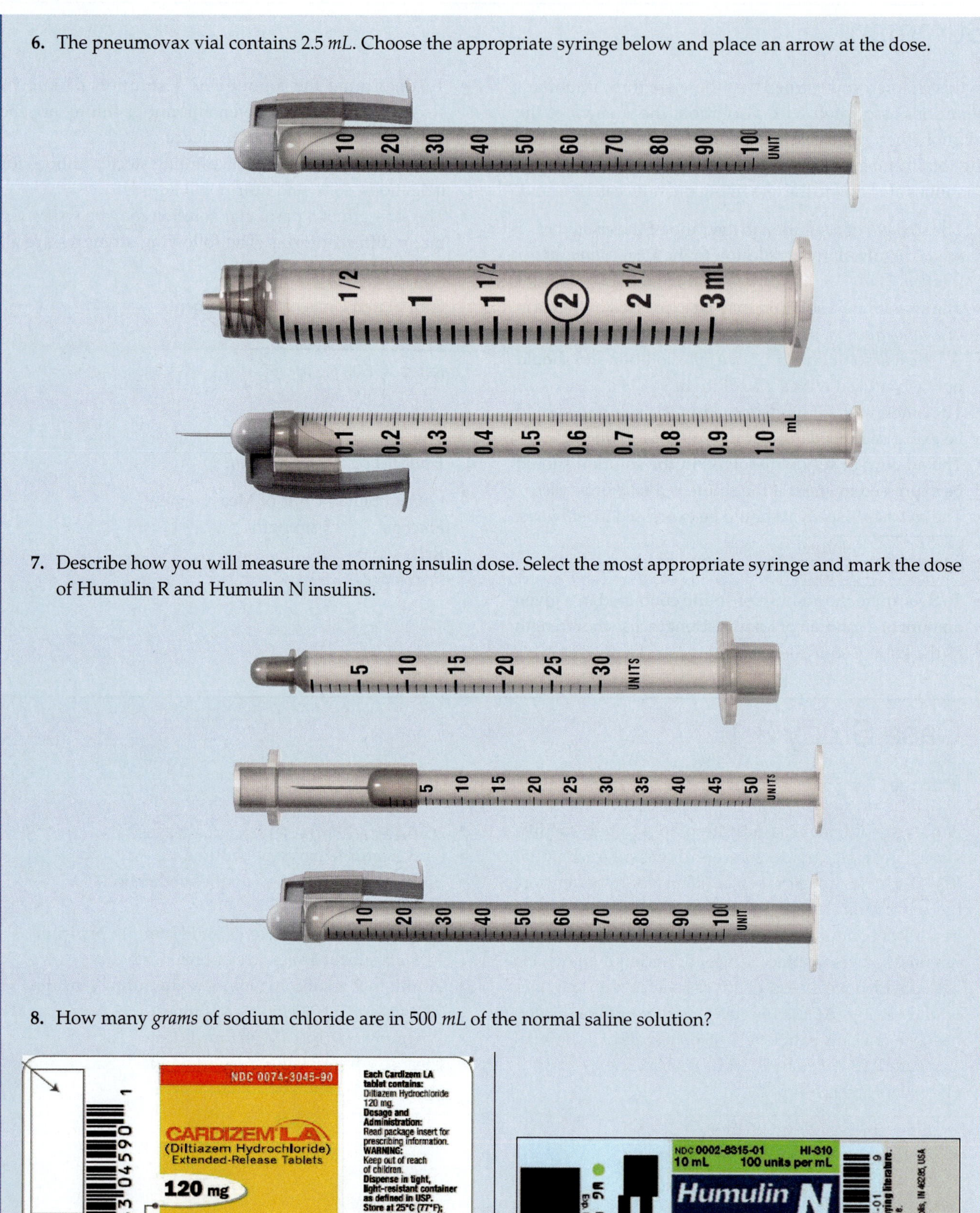

7. Describe how you will measure the morning insulin dose. Select the most appropriate syringe and mark the dose of Humulin R and Humulin N insulins.

8. How many *grams* of sodium chloride are in 500 *mL* of the normal saline solution?

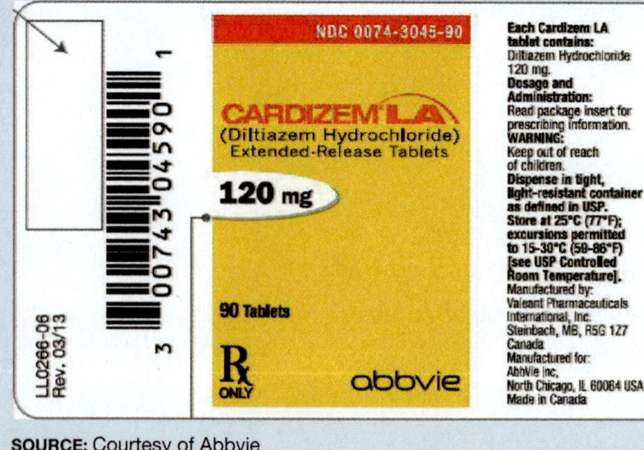

SOURCE: Courtesy of Abbvie

(a) (For educational purposes only)

NDC 0002-8315-01 HI-310
10 mL 100 units per mL
Humulin N
NPH
human insulin (rDNA origin)
isophane suspension
U-100
Lilly
Important: See accompanying literature.
Refrigerate. Do not freeze.
Shake carefully.
Eli Lilly and Company, Indianapolis, IN 46285, USA

SOURCE: © Copyright Eli Lily and Company. All rights reserved. Used with permission.

(b)

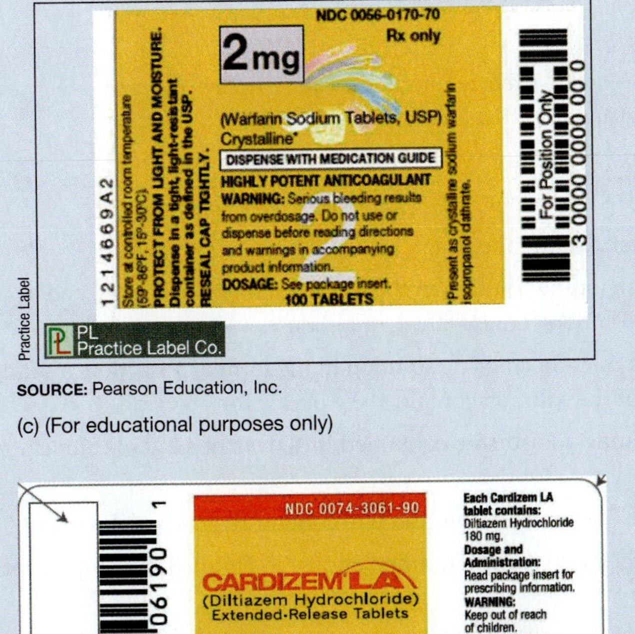

SOURCE: Pearson Education, Inc.

(c) (For educational purposes only)

NDC 0074-3061-90

CARDIZEM LA

(Diltiazem Hydrochloride) Extended-Release Tablets

180 mg

90 Tablets

Rx ONLY

abbvie

Each Cardizem LA tablet contains: Diltiazem Hydrochloride 180 mg.
Dosage and Administration: Read package insert for prescribing information.
WARNING: Keep out of reach of children.
Dispense in tight, light-resistant container as defined in USP.
Store at 25°C (77°F); excursions permitted to 15-30°C (59-86°F) [see USP Controlled Room Temperature].
Manufactured by: Valeant Pharmaceuticals International, Inc., Steinbach, MB, R5G 1Z7 Canada
Manufactured for: AbbVie Inc., North Chicago, IL 60064 USA
Made in Canada

3 00743 06190 1

LL0269-06 Rev. 03/13

SOURCE: Courtesy of Abbvie

(d) (For educational purposes only)

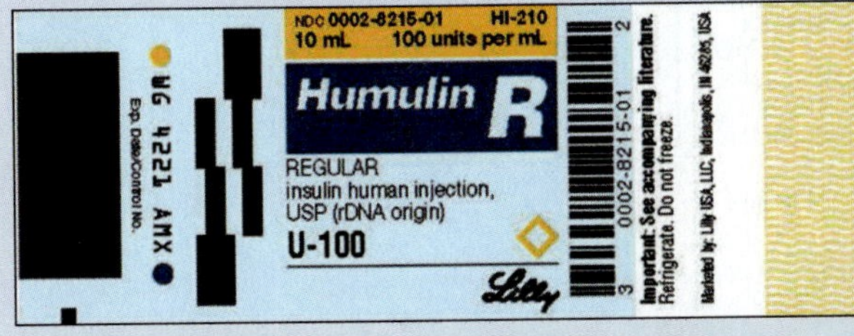

SOURCE: © Copyright Eli Lily and Company. All rights reserved. Used with permission.

(e)

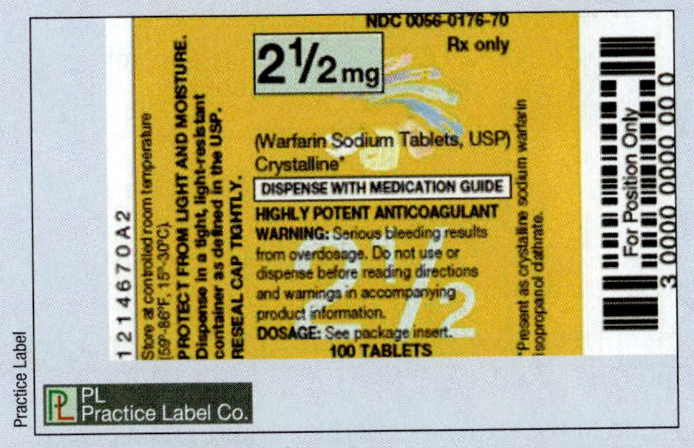

SOURCE: Pearson Education, Inc.

(f) (For educational purposes only)

NDC 0093-1015-10

NABUMETONE Tablets USP 500 mg

Each tablet contains: nabumetone, USP 500 mg

ATTENTION PHARMACIST: Each patient is required to receive a Medication Guide.

Rx only

1000 TABLETS

TEVA

Usual Dosage: See package insert for full prescribing information.
Store at 20° to 25°C (68° to 77°F) [See USP Controlled Room Temperature].
Dispense in a tight, light-resistant container as defined in the USP, with a child-resistant closure (as required).
KEEP THIS AND ALL MEDICATIONS OUT OF THE REACH OF CHILDREN.
Manufactured In Israel By: TEVA PHARMACEUTICAL IND. LTD. Jerusalem, 91010, Israel
Manufactured For: TEVA PHARMACEUTICALS USA Sellersville, PA 18960
323K25201070S
Rev. D 6/2005
N 3 0093-1015-10 5

SOURCE: Copyright TEVA, Used with permission

(g)

Zocor® 40 mg
(Simvastatin)

Manuf. for: MERCK & CO., INC. Whitehouse Station, NJ 08889, USA
By: MERCK SHARP & DOHME LTD. Cramlington, Northumberland, UK NE23 3JU
Formulated in UK

Each tablet contains 40 mg of simvastatin.

90 Tablets

MSD 749

Lot

NDC 0006-0749-54

USUAL ADULT DOSAGE: See accompanying circular.
Store between 5-30°C (41-86°F).
Rx only

9782900 90| No.8148

N 3 0006-0749-54 4

SOURCE: Reproduced with permission of Merck Sharp & Dohme Corp., a subsidiary of Merck & Co, Inc., Whitehouse Station, New Jersey, USA. All Rights Reserved.

(h) (For educational purposes only)

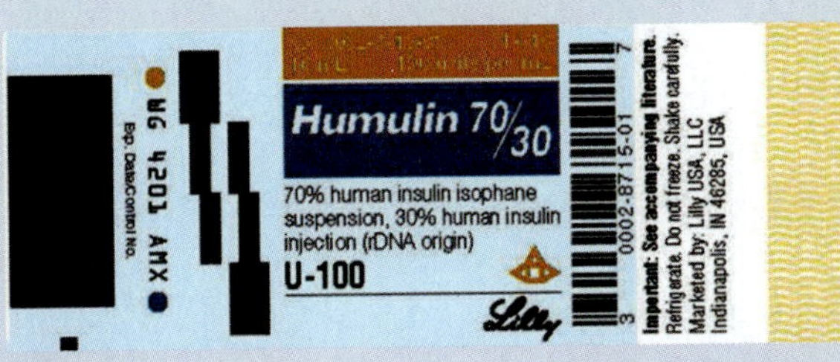

SOURCE: © Copyright Eli Lily and Company. All rights reserved. Used with permission.

(i)

Drugs Labels for Case Study 8.1

Practice Sets

The answers to *Try These for Practice, Exercises,* and *Cumulative Review Exercises* are found in Appendix A. Ask your instructor for the answers to the *Additional Exercises.*

Try These for Practice

Test your comprehension after reading the chapter.

1. Express the strength of an iodine solution in the form of a fraction, a ratio, and a percent if 400 *mL* of the solution contain 80 *mL* of iodine.
2. Express the strength of a calcium chloride solution in the form of a fraction, a ratio, and a percent if 250 *mL* of the solution contain 100 *g* of calcium chloride.
3. How many *grams* of sodium chloride are contained in 400 *mL* of a 2% sodium chloride solution?
4. How many *milliliters* of a 5% dextrose solution will contain 10 *grams* of dextrose?
5. Express the strength of the cyclosporine solution shown in Figure 8.12 as a percent.

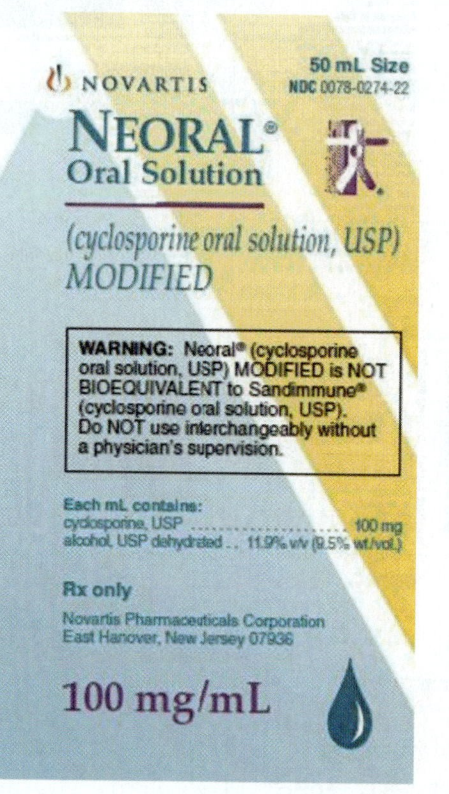

Figure 8.12 Drug label for cyclosporine oral solution.

SOURCE: Courtesy of Novartis Pharma AG

Exercises

Reinforce your understanding in class or at home.

1. Express the strength of a solution in the form of a fraction, a ratio, and a percent if *200 mL* of the solution contain *50 mL* of a drug.
2. Express the strength of a solution in the form of a fraction, a ratio, and a percent if *8 mL* of the solution contain *3 g* of a drug.
3. Express the strength of a solution in the form of a fraction, a ratio, and a percent if *1 L* of the solution contains *60,000 mg* of a drug.
4. Express the strength of a solution of Isocal in the form of a fraction, a ratio, and a percent if *240 ounces* of the solution contain *80 ounces* of full-strength Isocal.

5. A vial of lidocaine solution has a strength of *0.5%*. A different vial of lidocaine solution has a strength of *40 mg/mL*. Which solution is stronger?
6. Which of the following could not be a solution strength?

   0.04%   2:7   6 *mL*   4 *g/mL*   *half-strength*

7. Fill in the following chart of equivalent strengths.

Ratio	Fraction	Percent
1:5		
	$\frac{1}{4}$	
		10%
1:200		
	$\frac{9}{1{,}000}$	

8. Calculate the number of *grams* of dextrose in 500 *mL* of a 5% dextrose solution.
9. How many *liters* of a normal saline (0.9% NaCl) solution will contain 18 *grams* of NaCl?
10. What is the strength of an Isocal solution made by adding 1 can of Isocal to 3 cans of water? Express as a fraction.
11. How many *milligrams* of sodium chloride are contained in 1 *liter* of 0.9% sodium chloride solution?
12. How many ounces of Sustacal are contained in 60 *ounces* of a 2/3 strength Sustacal solution?
13. How many *milliliters* of a 0.5% solution contain 4 *grams* of a drug?
14. How many *grams* of sodium chloride are contained in 2 *L* of a 4% sodium chloride solution?
15. How would 200 *mL* of a 10% solution be prepared using tablets that each contain 10 *grams* of the drug?
16. How many *mg* of NaCl are contained in 500 *mL* of a 0.45% NaCl solution?
17. See the label in Figure 8.13. How many *mg* of cromolyn sodium are contained in 3 *mL* of this solution?

Figure 8.13 Drug label for cromolyn sodium.

SOURCE: Meda Pharmaceuticals Inc.

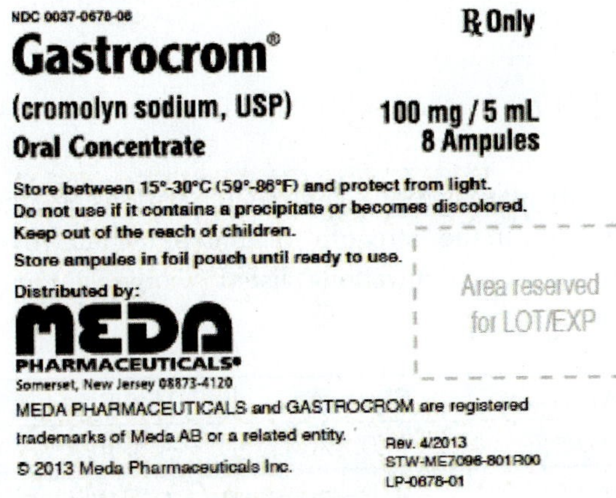

18. The strengths of two solutions are $\frac{1}{2}$ strength and 50%. Which is stronger?
19. An IV bag contains 200 *mL* of a 5% mannitol solution. How many *grams* of mannitol are in the IV bag?
20. How many *milliliters* of a 15% magnesium sulfate solution will contain 60 *grams* of magnesium sulfate?

Additional Exercises

Now, test yourself!

1. Express the strength of a solution both as a ratio and as a percentage if 500 *mL* of the solution contain 25 *mL* of solute.
2. Express the strength of a solution both as a ratio and as a percentage if 200 *mL* of the solution contain 40 *g* of solute.
3. Express the strength of a solution both as a ratio and as a percentage if 2 *L* of the solution contain 400 *mg* of solute.
4. Betadine solution is a 10% povidone-iodine solution. Express this strength both as a fraction and as a ratio.
5. Thorazine is available in a strength of 25 *mg/mL*. Express this strength as a percent.
6. Which of the following could be solution strengths?

   1:10,000 0.5% 25 *mL* $\frac{1}{3}$ 2 *mg/mL* 100 *g*

7. Read the label in Figure 8.14 and determine the number of *milligrams* of hydroxyzine pamoate that are contained in the vial of Vistaril.

Figure 8.14 Drug label for Vistaril.

SOURCE: Courtesy of Pfizer, Inc.

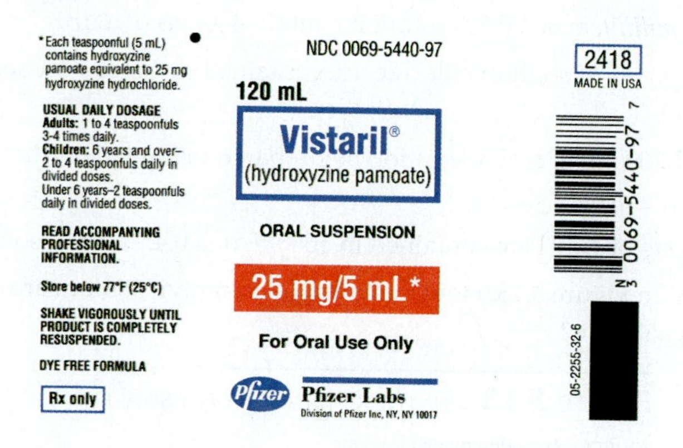

8. How many *mL* of a 10% magnesium sulfate solution will contain 14 *grams* of magnesium sulfate?
9. A pharmaceutical company sells ropivacaine HCl in various strengths as listed in the chart. Find the error in the "strength" column of the table by trying to verify that each of the four "concentrations" listed is equivalent to each of the corresponding "strengths."

Concentration	Strength	Vial Size
2 *mg/mL*	0.2%	100 *mL*
5 *mg/mL*	0.4%	30 *mL*
7.5 *mg/mL*	0.75%	20 *mL*
10 *mg/mL*	1%	20 *mL*

10. How many *mL* of the lidocaine viscous solution shown in Figure 8.15 will contain 10 *mg* of lidocaine?

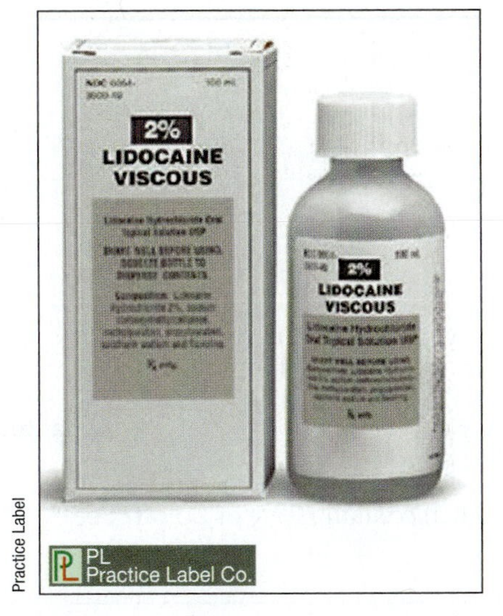

Figure 8.15 Drug packaging for 2% lidocaine viscous. (For educational purposes only)

SOURCE: Pearson Education, Inc.

11. How many *mg* of fluconazole are contained in 200 *mL* of a 0.2% solution?
12. Express as a percent the strength of the pneumococcal vaccine whose label is in Figure 8.16.

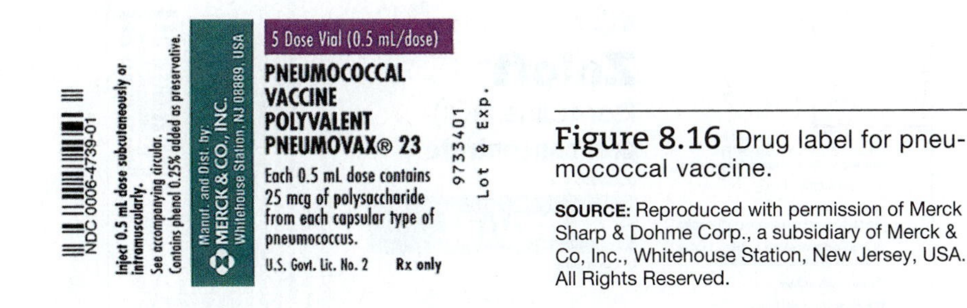

Figure 8.16 Drug label for pneumococcal vaccine.

SOURCE: Reproduced with permission of Merck Sharp & Dohme Corp., a subsidiary of Merck & Co, Inc., Whitehouse Station, New Jersey, USA. All Rights Reserved.

13. The nutritional formula Sustacal is supplied in 10-*ounce* cans. How would you prepare 40 *ounces* of a half-strength Sustacal solution?
14. How would you prepare 1 *liter* of a 25% boric acid solution from boric acid crystals?
15. How would 400 *mL* of a 20% solution be prepared using tablets that each contain 10 *grams* of the drug?
16. How many *mg* of NaCl are contained in 250 *mL* of a 0.45% NaCl solution?
17. The label on the vial of metoprolol tartrate indicates a strength of 5 *mg*/5 *mL*. How many *mg* of metoprolol tartrate are contained in 87 *mL* of this solution?
18. Are the following two strengths equivalent: 2% and 20 *mg*/*mL*?
19. The label on a 20 *mL* aminophylline vial indicates a strength of 500 *mg*/20 *mL*.
    (a) How many *mL* of aminophylline would contain 200 *mg* of this drug?
    (b) How many *mg* of aminophylline would be contained in 1 *mL* of this solution?
20. How many *milliliters* are in one spray of the ipratropium bromide solution shown in Figure 8.17?

Figure 8.17 Container and packaging for ipratropium bromide. (For educational purposes only)

SOURCE: Pearson Education, Inc.

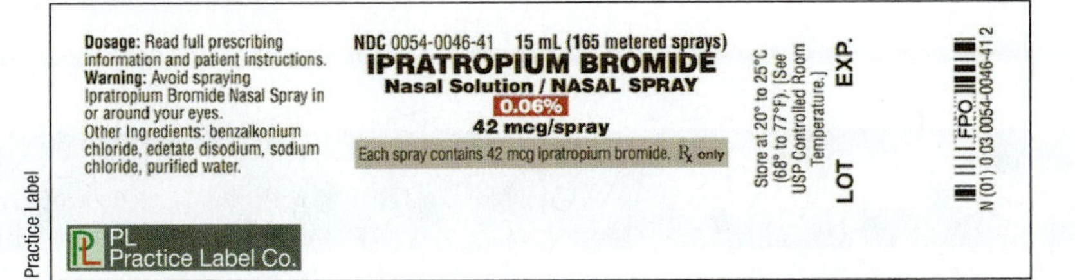

Cumulative Review Exercises

Review your mastery of previous chapters.

1. 0.6 *g* = __________ *mg*
2. 3 T = __________ *oz*
3. 110 *lb* = __________ *kg*
4. 45 *mm* = __________ *cm*
5. 1 *pt* = __________ *oz*
6. 8 *oz/day* = __________ *lb/wk*
7. A client enters the ICU at 2230 *h* on Tuesday and leaves 10 *hours* later. At what time (and day) does the client leave the ICU?
8. How many *milliliters* of Zoloft (sertraline HCl) contain 70 *mg* of Zoloft? See Figure 8.18.

Figure 8.18 Drug label for Zoloft.

SOURCE: Courtesy of Pfizer, Inc.

11015101
LOT
EXP

Store at 25°C (77°F); excursions permitted to 15-30°C (59-86°F) [see USP Controlled Room Temperature].

STORE UPRIGHT.

DOSAGE AND USE
See accompanying prescribing information.

*Each mL contains sertraline hydrochloride equivalent to 20 mg of sertraline.

Contains 12% alcohol.

THE PACKAGING OF THIS PRODUCT CONTAINS DRY NATURAL RUBBER.

ALWAYS DISPENSE WITH MEDICATION GUIDE

Pfizer

Rx only

Zoloft®
(sertraline HCl)
oral concentrate
equivalent to
20 mg/mL*
of sertraline

60 mL

ZOLOFT ORAL CONCENTRATE MUST BE DILUTED BEFORE USE.

MIXING INSTRUCTIONS
Just before taking, use the dropper provided to remove the required amount of ZOLOFT Oral Concentrate and mix with 4 oz (1/2 cup) of water, ginger ale, lemon/lime soda, lemonade or orange juice ONLY. Do not mix ZOLOFT Oral Concentrate with anything other than the liquids listed. At times, a slight haze may appear after mixing; this is normal. The medicine should be given immediately after mixing.
DO NOT MIX IN ADVANCE.

Distributed by
Roerig
Division of Pfizer Inc
NY, NY 10017

N 1 03 0049-4940-23-1

FPO - RSS 12 mil Limited

9. How many *milligrams* of a drug should be administered to the client if the order specifies 80 *mg* daily in 2 divided doses?
10. A 0.5 *mL* prefilled syringe contains 30 *mcg* of Avonex. How many *mcg* are contained in 0.25 *mL*?
11. Write 3:25 P.M. in military time.
12. Convert the rate of 2 *pt/day* to a rate measured in *mL/h*.
13. Order: *prednisone 30 mg po in three divided doses per day*. If the recommended safe dose range is 5–60 *mg/day*, is the order safe?
14. Order: *primaquine phosphate 0.3 mg/kg PO daily for 2 wk*. How many *mg* will be given to a 40-*kg* child?
15. Find the BSA of a person who weighs 150 *lb* and is 6 *ft* tall.

Pearson Nursing Student Resources Find additional review materials at: **nursing.pearsonhighered.com**

Chapter 9

Parenteral Medications

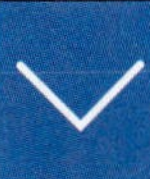

Learning Outcomes

After completing this chapter, you will be able to

9.1 Calculate doses for parenteral medications in liquid form.

9.2 Interpret the directions on drug labels and package inserts for reconstituting medications supplied in powdered form.

9.3 Label reconstituted multi-dose medication containers with the necessary information.

9.4 Choose the most appropriate diluent volume when reconstituting a multiple-strength medication.

9.5 Calculate doses of parenteral medications measured in units.

9.6 Calculate doses for subcutaneous heparin.

This chapter introduces the calculations you will use to prepare and administer parenteral medications safely. Chapter 2 discussed the most common parenteral sites: intramuscular (IM), subcutaneous (subcut), and intravenous (IV). This chapter focuses on calculations for administering medications via the subcutaneous and intramuscular routes.

Parenteral Medications

Parenteral medications are those that are injected into the body by various routes. Drugs for parenteral medications may be packaged in a variety of forms, including ampules, vials, and prefilled cartridges or syringes. Prefilled cartridges and syringes were discussed in Chapter 7.

An **ampule** is a glass container that holds a single dose of medication. It has a narrow neck that is designed to snap open. The medication is aspirated into a syringe by gently pulling back on the plunger, which creates a negative pressure and allows the liquid to be pulled into the syringe (Figure 9.1).

Figure 9.1 Ampules.

SOURCE: Pearson Education, Inc.

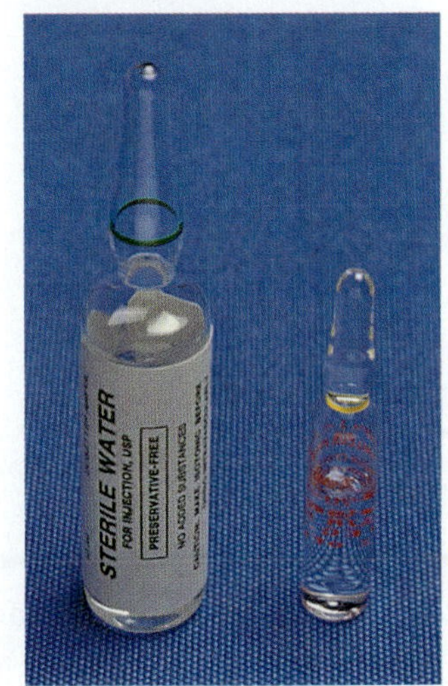

A **vial** is a glass or plastic container that has a rubber membrane on the top. This membrane is covered with a lid that maintains the sterility of the membrane until the vial is used for the first time. Multi-dose vials contain more than one dose of a medication. Single-dose vials contain one dose of medication, and many drugs are now prepared in single-dose format to reduce the chance of error. The medication in a vial may be supplied in liquid or powder form (Figure 9.2).

The CDC's guidelines state that medications labeled "single dose" or "single use" are to be used only once. Because single-dose vials (SDVs) typically lack antimicrobial preservatives, this practice protects clients from life-threatening infections that occur when medications get contaminated from unsafe use.

NOTE

Be sure to use a plastic ampule opener to safely break the ampule and a filter needle to withdraw the contents from the ampule. *Do not* use the filter needle to administer the medication. Dispose safely according to the facility policy.

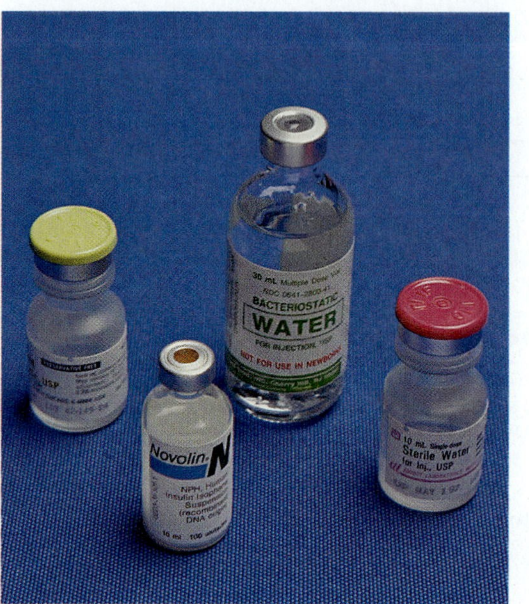

Figure 9.2 Vials.

SOURCE: Pearson Education, Inc.

NOTE

Single-dose ampules and vials may contain a little more drug than indicated on the label. Therefore, if the order is for the exact amount of medication stated on the label, it is important to carefully measure the amount of medication to be withdrawn. Before a fluid can be extracted from a vial, that same volume of air must be injected into the vial, in order to prevent a vacuum from being created.

Parenteral Medications Supplied as Liquids

When parenteral medications are in liquid form, you must calculate the volume of the solution that contains the prescribed amount of the medication. To perform this calculation, you also need to know the strength of the solution. You use Dimensional Analysis to calculate the volume that will be administered.

The following rough guidelines for the volumes generally administered subcutaneously or intramuscularly can be used to test the reasonableness of your calculated dosages.

Subcut:	Infant:	less than 0.1 *mL*
	Child:	less than 0.5 *mL*
	Adult:	from 0.5 *mL* to 1 *mL*
IM:	Infant:	less than 1 *mL*
	Child:	less than 2 *mL*
	Adult:	less than 3 *mL* (in the deltoid less than 2 *mL*)

Example 9.1

The prescriber ordered *Sandostatin (octreotide acetate) 50 mcg subcut q8h*. Read the label in Figure 9.3a and determine how many *milliliters* of this hormone suppressant you will administer. Indicate the dose on the syringe shown in Figure 9.3b.

Figure 9.3a Drug label for Sandostatin.

SOURCE: Courtesy of Novartis Pharma AG

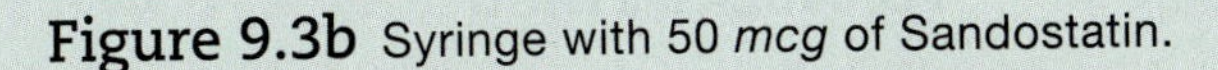

Figure 9.3b Syringe with 50 *mcg* of Sandostatin.

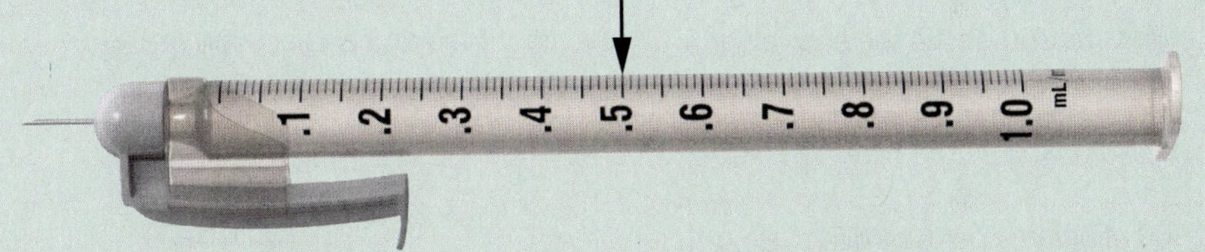

Begin by determining how many *milliliters* contain the prescribed quantity of the medication. That is, you want to convert 50 *mcg* to an equivalent in *milliliters*.

DIMENSIONAL ANALYSIS

$$50\ mcg = ?\ mL$$

You cancel the micrograms and obtain the equivalent quantity in *milliliters*.

$$50\ mcg \times \frac{?\ ml}{?\ mcg} = ?\ mL$$

The label reads "100 *micrograms* per 1 *milliliter*." Therefore, the unit fraction is $\frac{1\ mL}{50\ mcg}$

$$50\ \cancel{mcg} \times \frac{1\ mL}{100\ \cancel{mcg}} = 0.5\ mL$$

FORMULA METHOD

D (desired dose) = 50 *mcg*
H (dose on hand) = 100 *mcg*
Q (dosage unit) = 1 *mL*
X (unknown) = ? *mL*

Fill in the formula $\frac{D}{H} \times Q = X$

$$\frac{50\ mcg}{100\ mcg} \times 1\ mL = ?\ mL$$

Cancel and multiply $\frac{50\ \cancel{mcg}}{100\ \cancel{mcg}} \times 1\ mL = \frac{1}{2}\ mL$

So, you would administer 0.5 *mL* of Sandostatin.

ALERT

In Example 9.1, the strength indicates that 100 *mcg* = 1 *mL*. Because the order (50 *mcg*) is less than 100 *mcg*, you would administer less than 1 *mL*. Always check to see whether the amount of drug prescribed is smaller (or larger) than the amount of drug stated in the strength available.

Example 9.2

The prescriber ordered *Cleocin (clindamycin)* 600 *mg IM q12h*. Read the label in Figure 9.4 and calculate how many *milliliters* of this lincosamide antibiotic you will administer.

(Continued)

Figure 9.4 Drug label for Cleocin.

SOURCE: Pearson Education, Inc.

6 mL Vial NDC 0009-0902-11
Cleocin Phosphate®
clindamycin injection, USP
900 mg/6 mL*
(150 mg/mL)
For intramuscular or intravenous use
Rx only
Single Dose Container
Store at controlled room temperature 20° to 25°C (68° to 77°F) [see USP].
Do not refrigerate.
DOSAGE AND USE:
See accompanying prescribing information.
*Each 6 mL contains clindamycin phosphate equivalent to 900 mg of clindamycin.
Distributed by Pharmacia & Upjohn Co Division of Pfizer Inc, NY, NY 10017
LOT/EXP

Begin by determining how many *milliliters* contain the prescribed quantity of the medication (600 *mg*). That is, you want to convert 600 *mg* to an equivalent in *milliliters*.

DIMENSIONAL ANALYSIS

$$600\ mg = ?\ mL$$

You cancel the *milligrams* and obtain the equivalent quantity in *milliliters*.

$$600\ mg \times \frac{?\ ml}{?\ mg} = ?\ mL$$

The label reads 900 *milligrams* per 6 *milliliters*. So, the unit fraction is $\frac{6\ mL}{900\ mg}$

$$6\cancel{00}\ \cancel{mg} \times \frac{6\ mL}{9\cancel{00}\ \cancel{mg}} = 4\ mL$$

FORMULA METHOD

D (desired dose) $= 600\ mg$
H (dose on hand) $= 900\ mg$
Q (dosage unit) $= 6\ mL$
X (unknown) $= ?\ mL$

Fill in the formula $\frac{D}{H} \times Q = X$

$$\frac{600\ mg}{900\ mg} \times 6\ mL = ?\ mL$$

Cancel and multiply $\frac{600\ \cancel{mg}}{900\ \cancel{mg}} \times 6\ mL = 4\ mL$

So, you would administer 4 *mL* of Cleocin.

Example 9.3

The prescriber ordered *deferoxamine mesylate (Desferal) 500 mg IM q4h for two doses* for an adult client who has acute iron intoxication. Read the label and reconstitution chart in Figure 9.5.

(a) How many *milliliters* will you use to reconstitute the drug?

(b) How many *milliliters* of this chelating agent will you administer?

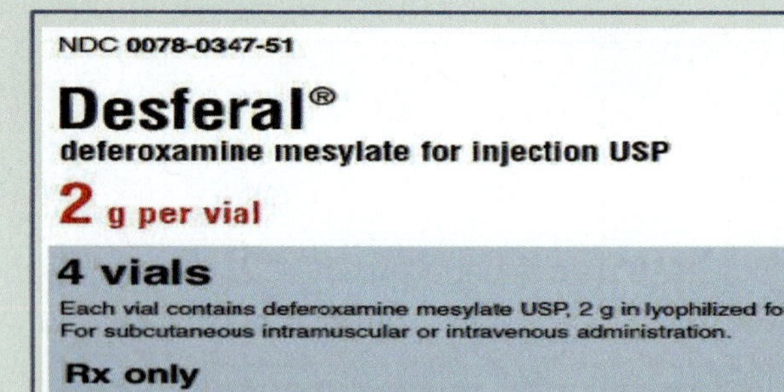

Figure 9.5 Drug label and portion of package insert for deferoxamine mesylate.

SOURCE: Courtesy of Novartis Pharma AG

Reconstitution and Preparation for Intramuscular Administration

Vial Size	Amount of Sterile Water for Injection Required for Reconstitution	Total Drug Content after Reconstitution	Final Concentration per *mL* after Reconstitution
500 *mg*	2 *mL*	500 *mg*/2.35 *mL*	213 *mg/mL*
2 *grams*	8 *mL*	2 *grams*/9.4 *mL*	213 *mg/mL*

(a) First read the information in the chart, and you will see that the 500 *mg* vial should be reconstituted with 2 *mL* of sterile water for injection.

(b) Following reconstitution the strength of the solution is 213 *mg* per *mL*.

DIMENSIONAL ANALYSIS

$$500\ mg = ?\ mL$$

Use the strength to obtain the unit fraction $\frac{1\ mL}{213\ mg}$ to change the *mg* to *mL*.

$$\frac{500\ \cancel{mg}}{1} \times \frac{1\ mL}{213\ \cancel{mg}} = 2.347\ mL$$

PROPORTION

Think: $213\ mg = 1\ mL$
$500\ mg = ?\ mL$

Make a proportion $\frac{213\ mg}{1\ mL} = \frac{500\ mg}{x\ mL}$

Cross multiply $213x = 500$
$x = 2.347\ mL$

So, you would administer 2.3 *mL* to the client.

Example 9.4

The prescriber ordered *haloperidol* 3 *mg IM q4h prn*. Figure 9.6 and determine how many *milliliters* of this antipsychotic drug you will prepare. Indicate the dose on the syringe below.

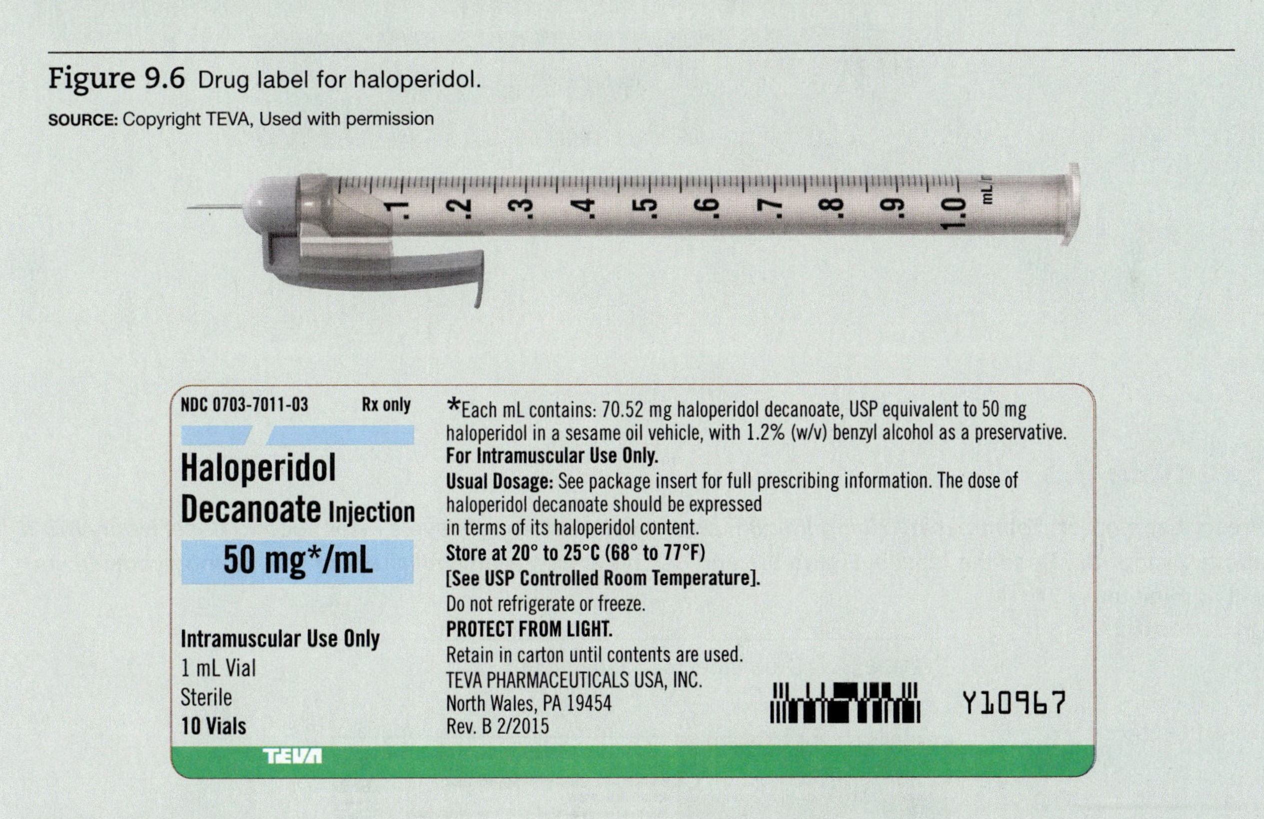

Figure 9.6 Drug label for haloperidol.

SOURCE: Copyright TEVA, Used with permission

You have a 5 *mL* multiple-dose vial, and the label indicates the strength is 50 *mg/mL*. Begin by determining how many *milliliters* of the solution in the vial contain the prescribed quantity of the medication. That is, you want to convert 3 *mg* to an equivalent in *milliliters*.

(Continued)

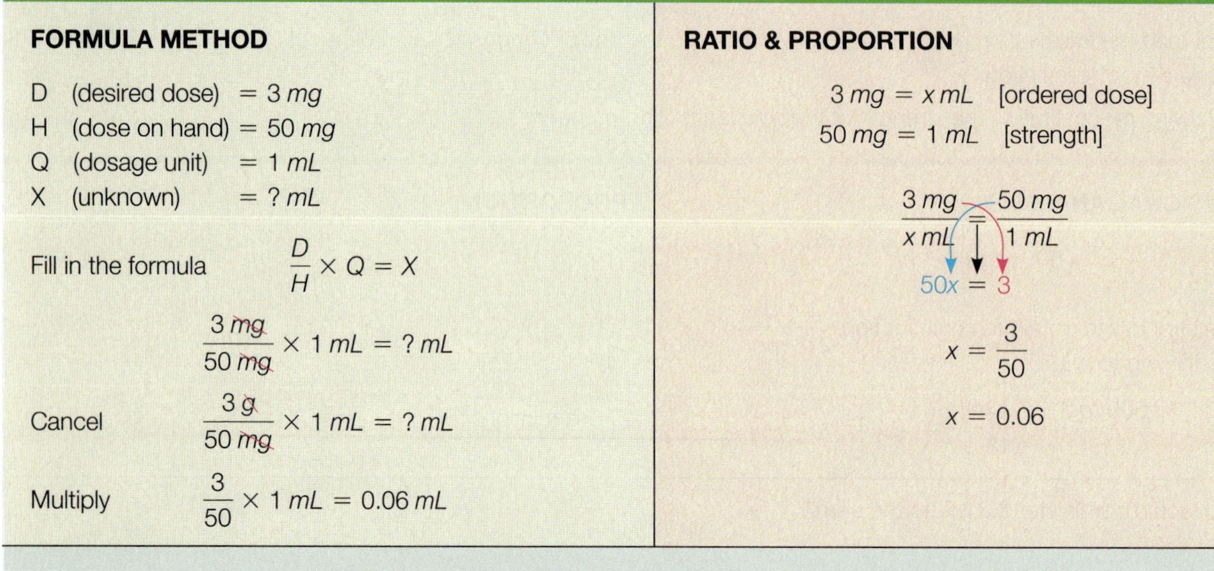

FORMULA METHOD	RATIO & PROPORTION
D (desired dose) = 3 *mg* H (dose on hand) = 50 *mg* Q (dosage unit) = 1 *mL* X (unknown) = ? *mL*	$3\ mg = x\ mL$ [ordered dose] $50\ mg = 1\ mL$ [strength]
Fill in the formula $\frac{D}{H} \times Q = X$	$\frac{3\ mg}{x\ mL} = \frac{50\ mg}{1\ mL}$
$\frac{3\ \cancel{mg}}{50\ \cancel{mg}} \times 1\ mL = ?\ mL$	$50x = 3$
Cancel $\frac{3\ \cancel{g}}{50\ \cancel{mg}} \times 1\ mL = ?\ mL$	$x = \frac{3}{50}$
Multiply $\frac{3}{50} \times 1\ mL = 0.06\ mL$	$x = 0.06$

So, you would use a 1*mL* syringe and give the client 0.06 *mL*.

Figure 9.6(b) Syringe with 3 *mg* of haloperidol (0.06 *mL*).

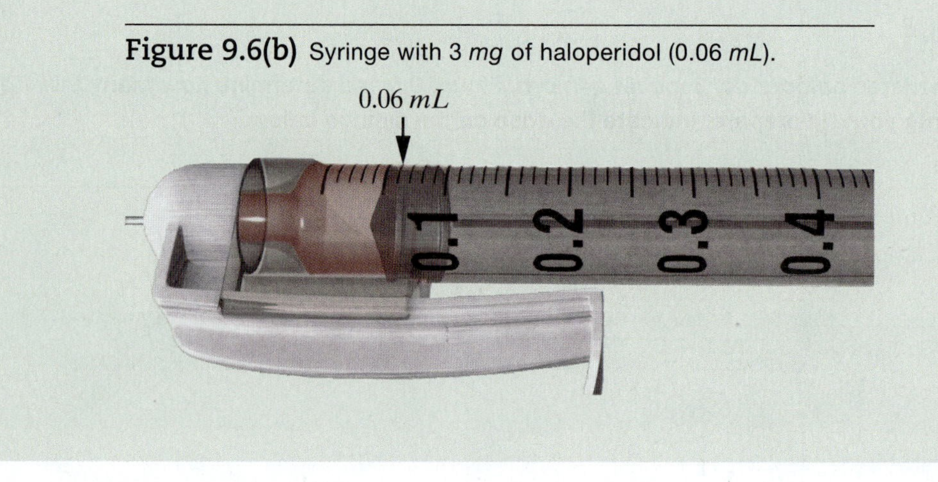

Example 9.5

Prescriber's order: *Tobramycin* 120 *mg IM q8h, draw peak and trough levels after second dose. Notify MD if above 2 mcg/mL*. Read the label in Figure 9.7 and calculate how many *milliliters* of this aminoglycoside you will administer.

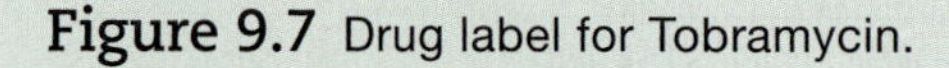

Figure 9.7 Drug label for Tobramycin.

SOURCE: Courtesy of Pfizer, Inc.

Determine how many milliliters of the solution in the vial contain the prescribed quantity of the medication. That is, you want to convert 120 *mg* to an equivalent in milliliters.

DIMENSIONAL ANALYSIS

$$120\ mg = ?\ mL$$

You cancel the *milligrams* and obtain the equivalent quantity in *milliliters*.

$$120\ mg \times \frac{?\ mL}{?\ mg} = ?\ mL$$

The label indicates that the strength is 40 *mg* per *milliliter*.

Therefore, the unit fraction is $\frac{1\ mL}{40\ mg}$

$$120\ \cancel{mg} \times \frac{1\ mL}{40\ \cancel{mg}} = 3\ mL$$

PROPORTION

Think:

$$40\ mg = 1\ mL$$
$$120\ mg = ?\ mL$$

Make a proportion $\frac{40\ mg}{1\ mL} = \frac{120\ mg}{x\ mL}$

Cross multiply $40x = 120$

$$x = 3\ mL$$

So, you would administer 3 *mL* of Tobramycin to the client.

Example 9.6

The order for an adult who has adrenal insufficiency is *dexamethasone sodium phosphate* 5 *mg IM q12h*. The client weighs 100 *kg*. Read the label in Figure 9.8.

Figure 9.8 Label for dexamethasone sodium phosphate.

Source: Courtesy of Pfizer, Inc.

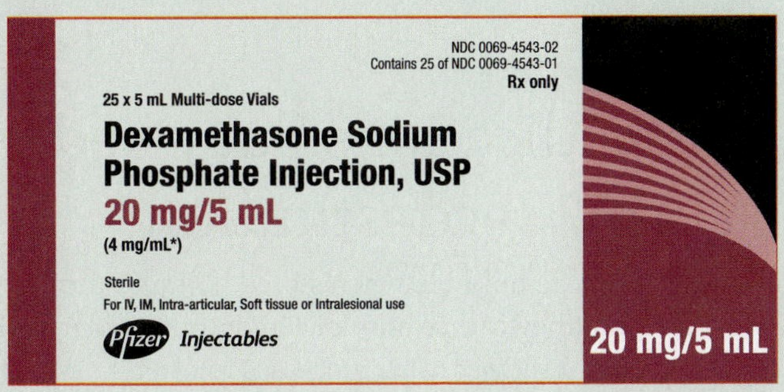

(a) If the recommended daily dosage is 0.03–0.15 *mg/kg*, is the prescribed dosage safe?

(b) How many *milliliters* will you administer?

(a) Using the recommended daily dosage, calculate the minimum and maximum number of *milligrams* the client could receive each day. Notice that the strength of the dexamethasone is 20 *mg*/5 *mL* or, equivalently, 4 *mg/mL*.

Minimum Daily Dosage

Because the *minimum* recommended daily dosage (0.03 *mg/kg*) is based on the size of the client (100 *kg*), multiply these as follows:

$$100\ \cancel{kg} \times \frac{0.03\ mg}{\cancel{kg}} = 3\ mg$$

Maximum Daily Dosage

Because the *maximum* recommended daily dosage (0.15 *mg/kg*) is based on the size of the client (100 *kg*), multiply these as follows:

$$100\ \cancel{kg} \times \frac{0.15\ mg}{\cancel{kg}} = 15\ mg$$

So, the safe dose range for this client is 3–15 *mg* daily.

The prescribed dosage is safe because the prescribed dosage of 5 *mg* q12h means the client would receive 10 *mg* per day, which is in the safe dose range of 3–15 *mg* per day.

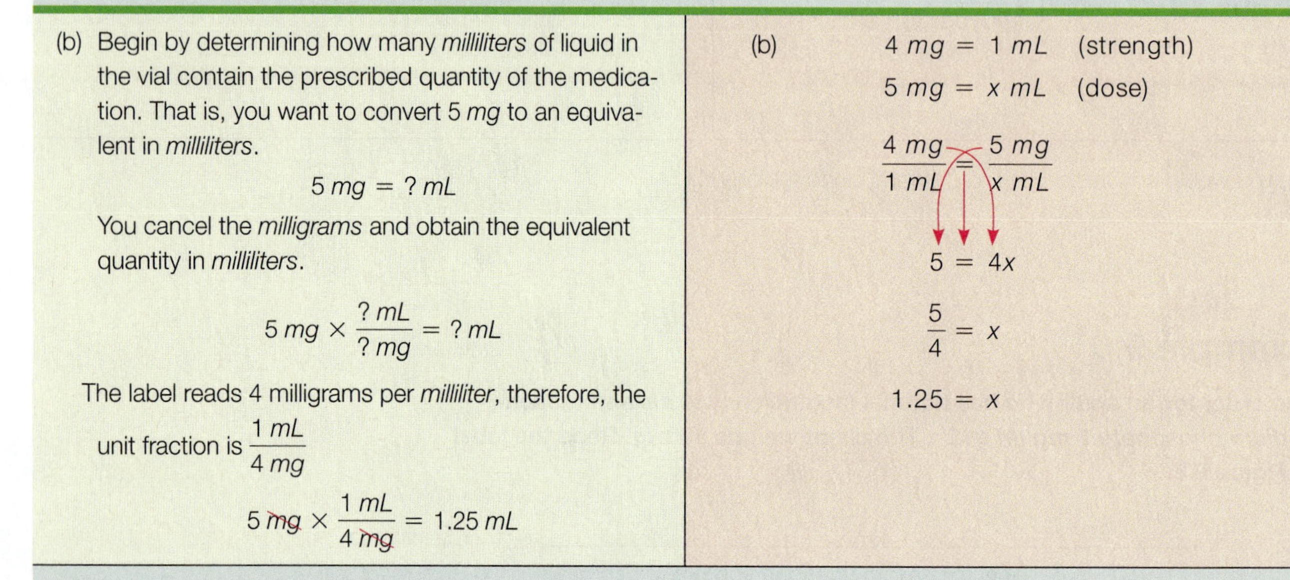

(b) Begin by determining how many *milliliters* of liquid in the vial contain the prescribed quantity of the medication. That is, you want to convert 5 *mg* to an equivalent in *milliliters*.

$$5\ mg = ?\ mL$$

You cancel the *milligrams* and obtain the equivalent quantity in *milliliters*.

$$5\ mg \times \frac{?\ mL}{?\ mg} = ?\ mL$$

The label reads 4 milligrams per *milliliter*, therefore, the unit fraction is $\frac{1\ mL}{4\ mg}$

$$5\ \cancel{mg} \times \frac{1\ mL}{4\ \cancel{mg}} = 1.25\ mL$$

(b)

$4\ mg = 1\ mL$ (strength)

$5\ mg = x\ mL$ (dose)

$$\frac{4\ mg}{1\ mL} = \frac{5\ mg}{x\ mL}$$

$$5 = 4x$$

$$\frac{5}{4} = x$$

$$1.25 = x$$

So, you would administer 1.3 *mL*.

Parenteral Medications Supplied in Powder Form: Reconstitution

Some parenteral medications are unstable when stored in liquid form, so they are packaged in powder form. Before they can be administered, the powder in the vial must be diluted with a liquid (*diluent* or *solvent*). This process is referred to as *reconstitution*.

Sterile water (SW) for injection and 0.9% sodium chloride (NS) are the most commonly used *diluents*. Using the wrong diluent may result in an incompatability resulting in crystallization and/or clumping of the drug in solution form. This can cause problems in the tissue or circulation of the client. Bacteriostatic water for injection is another type of diluent that may NOT be used in place of sterile water for injection. Both the type and the amount of diluent to be used must be determined when reconstituting parenteral medications. This information is found on the medication label or package insert. Because many reconstituted parenteral medications can be administered intramuscularly or intravenously, it is essential to verify the route ordered **before** reconstituting the medication—different routes may require different strengths.

Drugs dissolve completely in the diluent. Some drugs do not add any volume to the amount of diluent added, whereas other drugs increase the amount of total volume. This increase in volume is called the *displacement factor*. For example, directions for a 1 *g* powder medication may state to add 2 *mL* of diluent to provide an approximate volume of 2.5 *mL*. When the 2 *mL* of diluent is added, the 1 *g* of powder drug displaces an additional

0.5 *mL* for a total volume of 2.5 *mL*. The available strength after reconstitution is 1 *g* in 2.5 *mL* or 400 *mg/mL*.

To reconstitute a powder medication:

- Follow the directions on the label or package insert exactly as specified.
- Check the expiration dates of the drug and the diluent.
- Add the diluent to the vial.
- Shake, roll, or invert the vial as directed.
- Make sure that the powder is fully dissolved.

NOTE

If there are no directions for reconstitution on the label or package insert, consult appropriate resources such as the *PDR*, the pharmacist, DailyMed, or the prescribing information on the manufacturer's website before reconstituting.

ALERT

Reconstitution directions on vial labels may be very small and difficult to read. Use great care in identifying both the type and volume of the diluent to be used.

Example 9.7

The prescriber ordered *ceftriaxone* 250 *mg IM stat* to treat a client who has gonorrhea.

Read the label and the directions for reconstitution in Figure 9.9 to determine how to prepare and administer this cephalosporin antibiotic.

Directions for Use

Intramuscular Administration

Reconstitute ceftriaxone for injection powder with sterile water for injection. Inject diluent into vial, and shake vial thoroughly to form solution.

Figure 9.9 Ceftriaxone vial and portion of reconstitution directions.

SOURCE: Pearson Education, Inc.

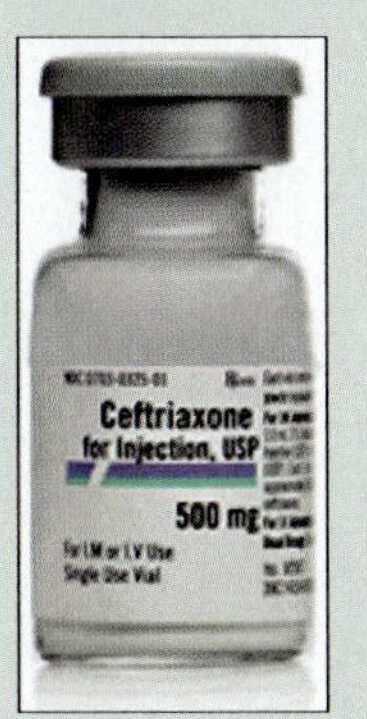

Vial Dosage Size	Amount of Diluent to Be Added	
	250 *mg/mL*	**350 *mg/mL***
250 *mg*	0.9 *mL*	–
500 *mg*	1.8 *mL*	1.0 *mL*
1 *g*	3.6 *mL*	2.1 *mL*
2 *g*	7.2 *mL*	4.2 *mL*

After reconstitution, each 1 *mL* of solution contains approximately 250 *mg* or 350 *mg* equivalent of ceftriaxone, according to the amount of diluent indicated.

As with all intramuscular preparations, ceftriaxone for injection, USP, should be injected well within the body of a relatively large muscle; aspiration helps to avoid unintentional injection into a blood vessel.

To prepare the solution, inject 1.8 *mL* of air into the vial of sterile water for injection and withdraw 1.8 *mL* of sterile water. Then inject the 1.8 *mL* of sterile water into the 500 *mg* ceftriaxone vial and shake well to form a solution. Figure 9.10.

Figure 9.10 Reconstitution of ceftriaxone.

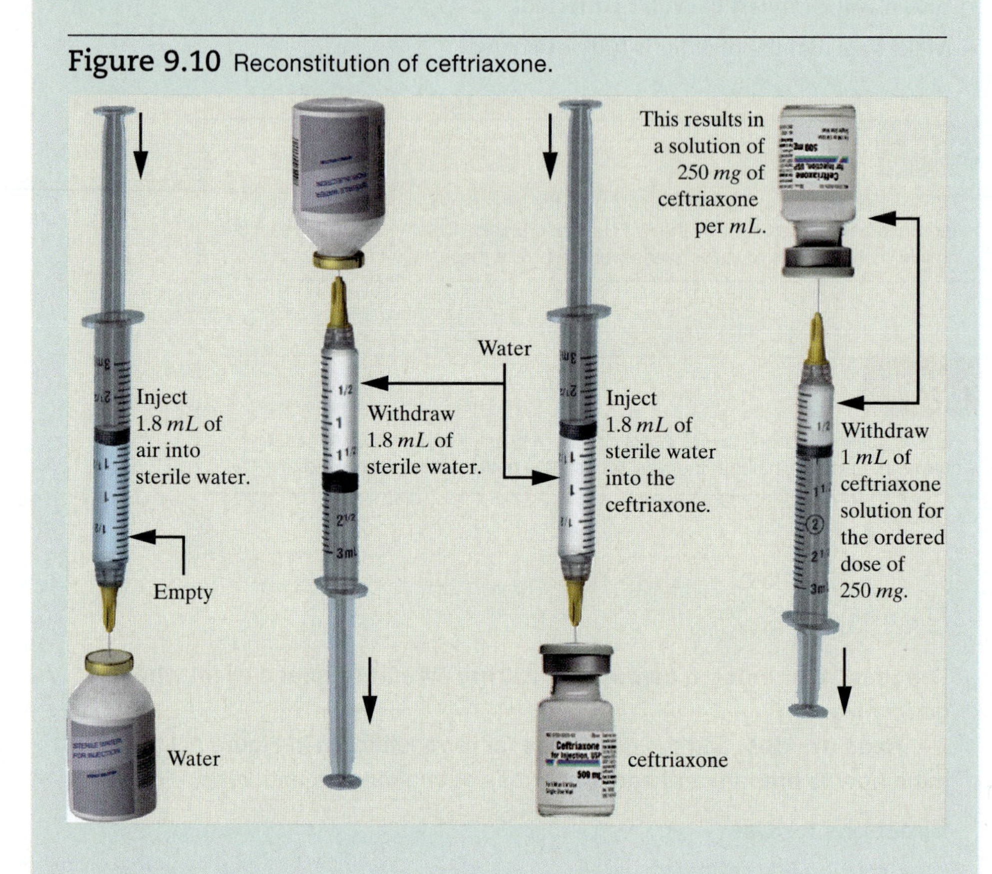

Now the vial contains a reconstituted solution in which 1 *mL* = 250 *mg*.

So, you would withdraw 1 *mL* of ceftriaxone from the vial and administer it to the client.

NOTE

The label in Example 9.7 states that when 1.8 *mL* of diluent is added, the resulting solution has a strength of 250 *mg/mL*. There is an approximate volume of 2 *mL* as a result of the displacement factor of 0.2 *mL*, which adds 0.2 *mL* to the 1.8 *mL* of diluent, to yield a total solution of 2 *mL*.

When you reconstitute a multiple-dose vial of powder medication, it is important that you clearly label the vial with the following:

1. Date and time of preparation
2. Strength of the solution
3. Date and time the reconstituted solution will expire
4. Storage directions
5. Your initials

ALERT

Proper labeling of reconstituted medication is critical for safe administration.

Suppose that at 6:00 P.M. on January 23, 2020, Marie Colon, R.N., reconstitutes a drug to a strength of 50 *mg/mL*, which will retain its potency for one week if kept refrigerated. Nurse Colon would write the following information on the label:

> ***1/23/2020, 1800h, 50 mg/mL,***
> ***Expires 1/30/2020, 1800h,***
> ***Keep refrigerated. MC***

NOTE

If the vial label does not contain reconstitution directions, refer to the drug package insert or contact the pharmacist. If directions are given for both IM and IV reconstitution, be careful to use the directions appropriate for the route prescribed.

Example 9.8

Order: *Unasyn (ampicillin sodium/sulbactam sodium)* 1,700 *mg IM q6h*. Read the drug label and portion of the package insert in Figure 9.11. The package insert indicates that the solution must be used within one hour of preparation.

Figure 9.11 Drug label and portion of package insert for Unasyn.

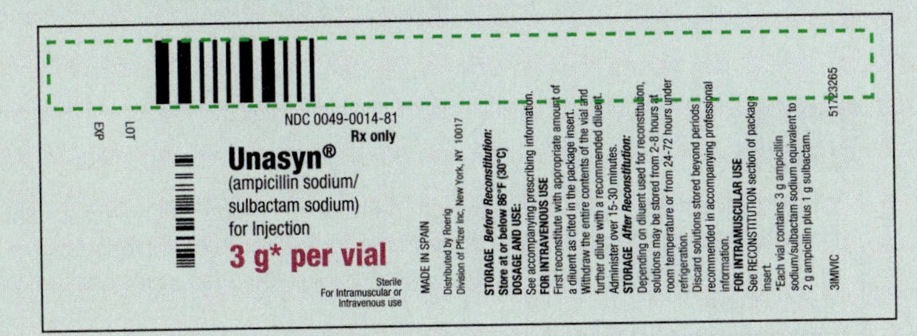

Preparation for Intramuscular Injection

1.5 *g* and 3.0 *g* Standard Vials: Vials for intramuscular use may be reconstituted with Sterile Water for Injection USP, 0.5% Lidocaine Hydrochloride Injection USP or 2% Lidocaine Hydrochloride Injection USP. Consult the following table for recommended volumes to be added to obtain solutions containing 375 *mg* UNASYN per *mL* (250 *mg* ampicillin/125 *mg* sulbactam per *mL*). Note: Use only freshly prepared solutions and administer within one hour after preparation.

UNASYN Vial Size	Volume of Diluent to Be Added	Withdrawal Volume*
	There is sufficient excess present to allow withdrawal and administration of the stated volumes.	
1.5 *g*	3.2 *mL*	4.0 *mL*
3.0 *g*	6.4 *mL*	8.0 *mL*

(a) How much diluent must be added to the vial?

(b) If Nurse Susan Green reconstitutes the Unasyn at 0600h on February 1, 2016, complete the label she will place on the vial.

(c) Determine how many *milliliters* of this antibiotic Nurse Green will give the client.

(Continued)

(a) First, prepare the solution. Because the vial contains 3 *g*, inject 6.4 *mL* of air into a vial of Sterile Water for Injection and withdraw 6.4 *mL* of sterile water. Add the sterile water to the Unasyn 3 *g* vial and be sure the solution is completely mixed.

(b) Nurse Green would write the following on the label:

2/1/2020, 0600h, reconstituted strength 375 mg/mL.
Expires 2/1/2020, 0700h. SG

(c) To calculate the amount of this solution, you need to convert the *milligrams* to *milliliters*.

DIMENSIONAL ANALYSIS

$$1{,}700\ mg \times \frac{?\ mL}{?\ mg} = ?\ mL$$

The vial contains 375 *mg* per 1 *mL*, so the unit fraction is $\frac{1\ mL}{375\ mg}$

$$1{,}700\ \cancel{mg} \times \frac{1\ mL}{375\ \cancel{mg}} = 4.533\ mL$$

FORMULA METHOD

D (desired dose) = 1,700 *mg*
H (dose on hand) = 375 *mg*
Q (dosage unit) = 1 *mL*
X (unknown) = ? *mL*

Fill in the formula $\frac{D}{H} \times Q = X$

$$\frac{1700\ mg}{375\ mg} \times 1\ mL = ?\ mL$$

Cancel $\frac{1700\ \cancel{mg}}{375\ \cancel{mg}} \times 1\ mL = ?\ mL$

Multiply $4.533 \times 1\ mL = 4.533\ mL$

So, Nurse Green would withdraw 4.5 *mL* and administer it to the client in two injections.

NOTE

When reconstituting a multiple-strength parenteral medication, select a solution strength that results in a volume appropriate for the route of administration—for example, a volume of no more than 3 *mL* per IM dose. Also, consider the client's age and size.

NOTE

In Example 9.9, the *stronger* the strength (concentration) of the reconstituted drug, the *smaller* the volume to be administered.

Example 9.9

An order requires 80 *mg* of a drug to be administered IM stat. The vial has the following three choices of strength after reconstitution:

10 *mg/mL*
20 *mg/mL*
40 *mg/mL*

For each of the three strengths:

(a) Determine the required volume of the solution to be administered.

(b) Choose the most appropriate strength.

(a) To calculate the amount of the 10 *mg/mL* solution (weakest strength), you need to convert the *milligrams* prescribed to *milliliters*.

$$80\ mg \times \frac{?\ mL}{?\ mg} = ?\ mL$$

- The vial contains 10 *mg* per 1 *mL*, so the unit fraction is $\frac{1\ mL}{10\ mg}$

$$80\ \cancel{mg} \times \frac{1\ mL}{10\ \cancel{mg}} = 8\ mL$$

- Using the 20 *mg/mL* solution (moderate strength), the unit fraction is $\frac{1\ mL}{20\ mg}$

$$80\ \cancel{mg} \times \frac{1\ mL}{20\ \cancel{mg}} = 4\ mL$$

- Using the 40 *mg/mL* solution (strongest strength), the unit fraction is $\frac{1\ mL}{40\ mg}$

$$80\ \cancel{mg} \times \frac{1\ mL}{40\ \cancel{mg}} = 2\ mL$$

In summary:

(Weakest) **10 *mg/mL* requires 8 *mL***
(Moderate) **20 *mg/mL* requires 4 *mL***
(Strongest) **40 *mg/mL* requires 2 *mL***

(b) **Weakest: 10 *mg/mL*** requires 8 *mL* to be administered. However, IM volumes are generally less that 3 *mL*. Therefore, this strength *should not be selected*.

Moderate: 20 *mg/mL* requires 4 *mL* to be administered. However, IM volumes are generally less that 3 *mL*. Therefore, this strength is a *poor choice*. However, the 4 *mL* could be divided into two syringes and administered at two different sites.

Strongest: 40 *mg/mL* requires 2 *mL* to be administered. This is less than 3 *mL* and is the *best choice*.

Example 9.10

A prescriber ordered *Pfizerpen (penicillin potassium) 200,000 units IM stat and q6h*. Read the label in Figure 9.12 and calculate how many *milliliters* of this penicillin antibiotic you will administer to the client.

Figure 9.12 Drug label for Pfizerpen.

SOURCE: Courtesy of Pfizer, Inc.

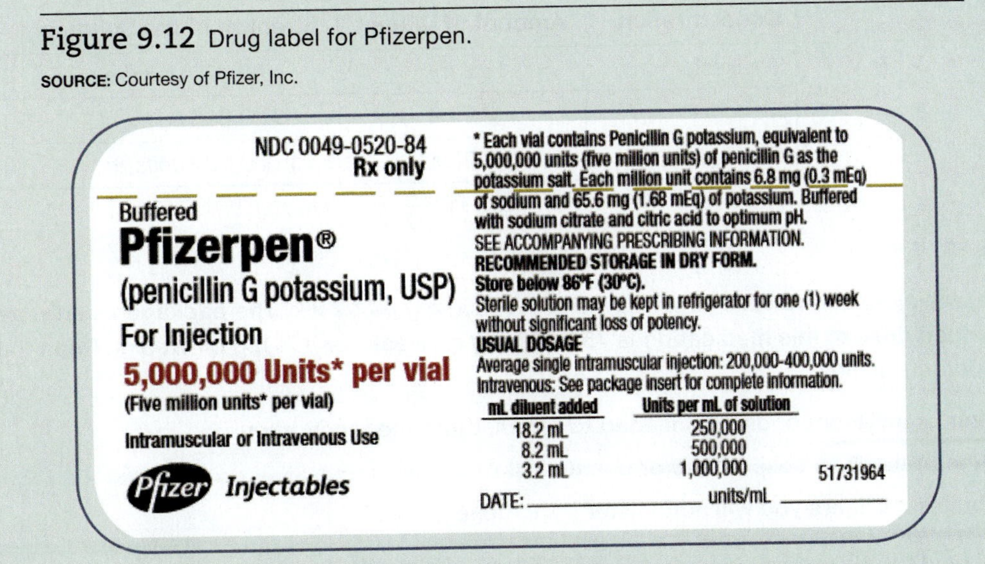

First, reconstitute the solution. The label lists three options: 250,000 *units/mL*; 500,000 *units/mL*; and 1,000,000 *units/mL*. If you choose the first option, 18.2 *mL* of diluent must be added to obtain a dosage strength of 250,000 *units/mL*.

(Continued)

> **NOTE**
>
> After you reconstitute the Pfizerpen, you would write the following information on the label: date, time reconstituted, and strength (1 *mL* = 250,000 *units*).

Now, inject 18.2 *mL* of air into a vial of sterile water for injection and then withdraw 18.2 *mL* of sterile water. Add the sterile water to the Pfizerpen vial and shake well. Now the vial contains a solution in which 1 *mL* = 250,000 *units*.

To calculate the amount of this solution to be administered, you need to convert units to *milliliters*.

FORMULA METHOD

D (desired dose) = 200,000 *units*
H (dose on hand) = 250,000 *units*
Q (dosage unit) = 1 *mL*
X (unknown) = ? *mL*

Fill in the formula $\frac{D}{H} \times Q = X$

$$\frac{200{,}000 \text{ units}}{250{,}000 \text{ units}} \times 1 \text{ mL} = ? \text{ mL}$$

Cancel $\frac{\overset{4}{\cancel{200{,}000}} \cancel{\text{ units}}}{\underset{5}{\cancel{250{,}000}} \cancel{\text{ units}}} \times 1 \text{ ml} = ? \text{ mL}$

Multiply $\frac{4}{5} \times 1 \text{ mL} = 0.8 \text{ mL}$

RATIO & PROPORTION

250,000 *units* = 1 *mL* (strength)
200,000 *units* = *x mL* (dose)

$$\frac{250{,}000 \text{ units}}{1 \text{ mL}} = \frac{200{,}000 \text{ units}}{x \text{ mL}}$$

$$200{,}000 = 250{,}000x$$

$$\frac{200{,}000}{250{,}000} = x$$

$$0.8 = x$$

So, you would withdraw 0.8 *mL* from the vial and administer it to the client.

In Example 9.10, if a *stronger concentration* had been chosen for the reconstitution, then a *smaller volume* of the solution would be administered. The calculations would be similar to those just completed. The bottom two lines of the following table show the volumes for the other two options.

Concentration	Amount of Diluent	Strength of the Solution	Volume to Administer
Weakest	18.2 *mL*	250,000 *units/mL*	0.8 *mL*
Moderate	8.2 *mL*	500,000 *units/mL*	0.4 *mL*
Strongest	3.2 *mL*	1,000,000 *units/mL*	0.2 *mL*

Example 9.11

Order: *olanzapine extended release (Zyprexa Relprevv) 250 mg IM q2 wk*. The package insert notes that the recommended dose of this medication is *150–300 mg q2 weeks or 405 mg q4 weeks*. Read the label in Figure 9.13 and determine:

a. The number of milliliters of diluent needed to reconstitute the medication

b. Whether the prescribed dose is safe or unsafe

c. The number of milliliters you will administer if the dose is safe

a. The label indicates that *1.3 mL* of diluent must be added to the vial.

b. The order prescribes *250 mg*. Because *250 mg* is within the safe dose range of *150–300 mg*, the prescribed dose is safe.

NOTE

Some medications must be reconstituted immediately before administering them because they lose potency rapidly. Zyprexa, for example, must be used within 24 hours of being reconstituted.

Figure 9.13 Drug label and diluent for olanzapine (Zyprexa Relprevv) Extended Release.

SOURCE: © Copyright Eli Lily and Company. All rights reserved. Used with permission.

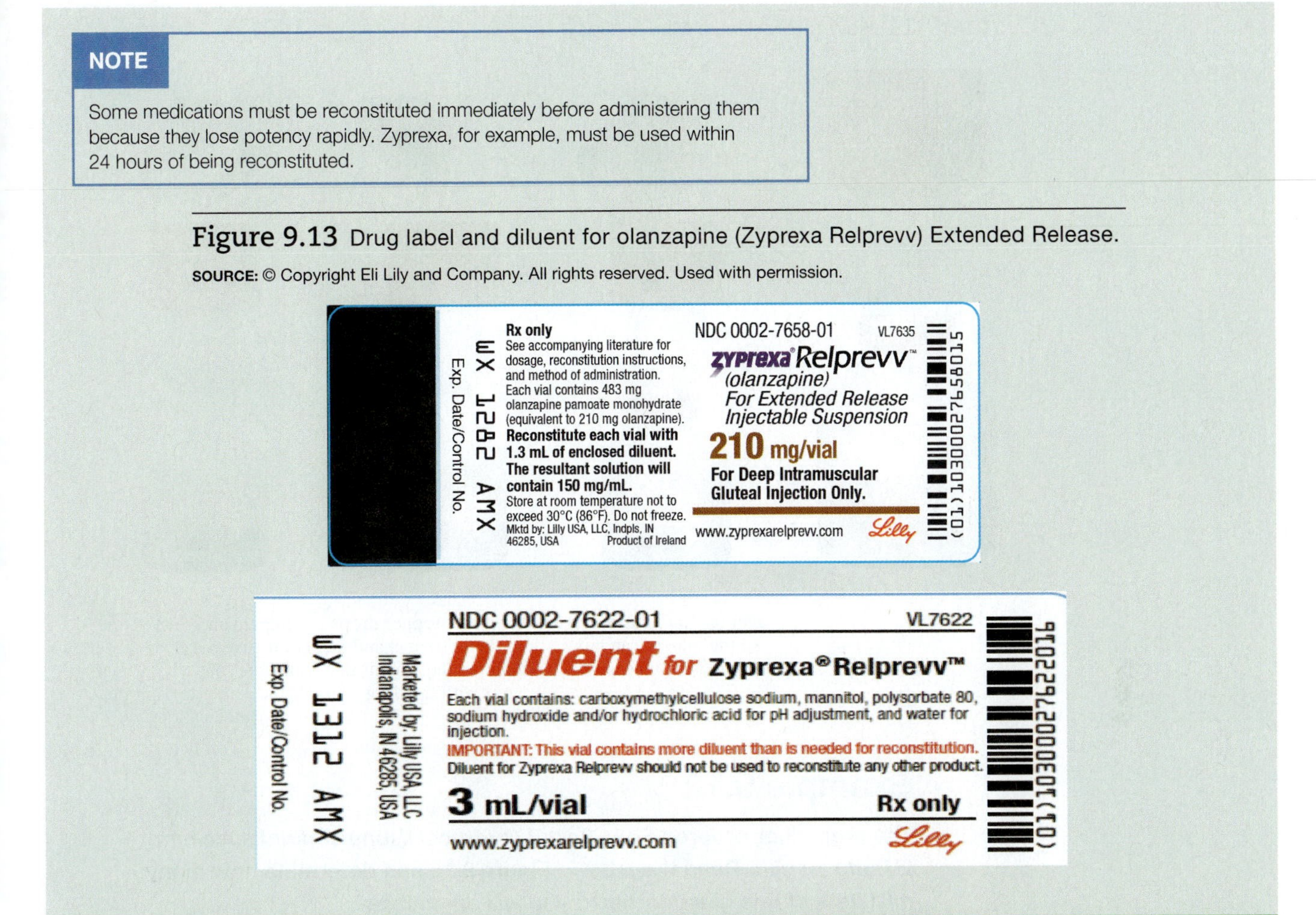

DIMENSIONAL ANALYSIS

To calculate the amount of solution to be administered, you need to convert 250 *mg* to *milliliters*:

$$250\ mg = ?\ mL$$

$$250\ mg \times \frac{?\ mL}{?\ mg} = ?\ mL$$

The vial has a concentration of 150 *mg* per *mL*, so the unit fraction is $\frac{1\ mL}{150\ mg}$.

$$250\ \cancel{mg} \times \frac{1\ mL}{150\ \cancel{mg}} = 1.667\ mL$$

RATIO AND PROPORTION

Think:

$$150\ mg = 1\ mL \text{ (strength)}$$

$$250\ mg = x\ mL \text{ (dose)}$$

$$\frac{150\ mg}{1\ mL} = \frac{250\ mg}{x\ mL}$$

$$250 = 150x$$

$$1.667\ mL = x$$

So, you would administer 1.7 *mL* of the reconstituted Zyprexa to the client.

How to Use a Two-Chambered Vial

Some medications are manufactured in vials (Mix-O-Vial or Act-O-Vial) that have two compartments separated by a rubber stopper. The top compartment contains a sterile liquid (diluent), and the bottom portion contains the medication in powder form. When pressure is applied to the top of the vial, the rubber stopper that separates the medication from the diluent is released. This allows the diluent and powder to mix. Figure 9.14.

Figure 9.14 How to prepare a Mix-O-Vial.

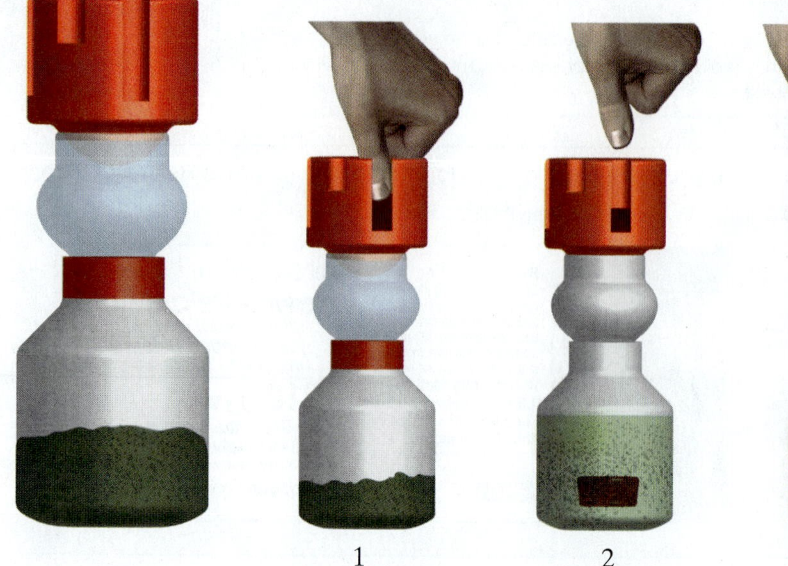

1
Depress the plastic cap so the diluent can mix into the bottom chamber.

2
When the stopper drops into the bottom chamber, it allows the diluent to mix with the drug.

3
Flip up and remove the protective cover, and insert needle squarely through the center to aspirate medication.

Example 9.12

The prescriber ordered *Solu-Cortef (hydrocortisone sodium succinate)* 200 *mg IM q6h*. Read the label in Figure 9.15 and determine how many *milliliters* of this glucocorticoid you will administer.

Figure 9.15 Solu-Cortef Act-O-Vial and drug label.

SOURCE: Courtesy of Pfizer, Inc.

Store at controlled room temperature 20° to 25°C (68° to 77°F) [see USP]. Protect solution from light.
Discard after three days.
Usual adult dose: 250 mg repeated as necessary.
DOSAGE AND USE: See accompanying prescribing information.
Lyophilized in container.
*Each 4 mL (when mixed) contains hydrocortisone sodium succinate equivalent to 500 mg of hydrocortisone.
Reconstituted ______
Distributed by Pharmacia & Upjohn Co
Division of Pfizer Inc, NY, NY 10017

Single-Dose Vial NDC 0009-0016-12
4 mL Act-O-Vial®
Solu-Cortef®
(hydrocortisone sodium succinate for injection, USP)
500 mg*
For intramuscular or intravenous use
Preservative-Free **Rx only**

First, reconstitute the solution:

1. Press down on the plastic activator to force diluent into the lower compartment.
2. Gently agitate to effect solution.

Now the vial contains a solution with the strength of 4 *mL* = 500 *mg*.

To calculate the amount of this solution to be administered, you need to convert the dose of 200 *mg* to *milliliters*.

$$200\ mg \times \frac{?\ mL}{?\ mg} = ?\ mL$$

The vial contains 500 *mg* per 4 *mL*, so the unit fraction is $\frac{4\ mL}{500\ mg}$

$$200\ \cancel{mg} \times \frac{4\ mL}{500\ \cancel{mg}} = 1.6\ mL$$

So, you would administer 1.6 *mL* of Solu-Cortef.

3. Remove the protective cap.
4. Insert needle squarely through center of stopper until tip is just visible. Invert vial and withdraw dose.

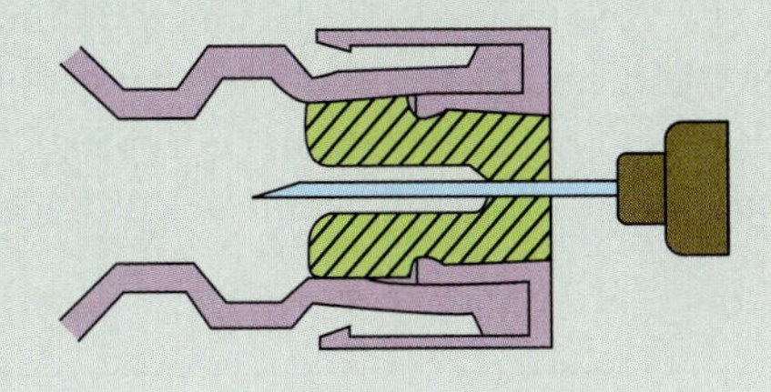

Heparin

Heparin sodium is a potent anticoagulant that inhibits clot formation and blood coagulation. Heparin is a high-alert drug and can be administered subcutaneously or intravenously. It is *never given intramuscularly because of the danger of hematomas*. According to the ISMP, anticoagulant medications are more likely to cause harm resulting from complex dosing, insufficient monitoring, and inconsistent client compliance. The Joint Commission (TJC) now requires a National Patient Safety Goal to reduce the likelihood of client harm associated with use of anticoagulant therapy.

Like insulin, penicillin, and some other medications, heparin is supplied and ordered in units. Heparin is available in single and multi-dose vials, as well as in commercially prepared IV solutions. It is available in a variety of strengths, ranging from 10 *units/mL* to 50,000 *units/mL*. See Figure 9.16. Heparin is also available in prepackaged syringes. Lovenox (enoxaprin) and Fragmin (dalteparin sodium) are examples of low-molecular-weight heparin. They are used to prevent and treat deep vein thrombosis (DVT) following abdominal surgery, hip or knee replacement, unstable angina, and acute coronary syndromes.

When administered as a continuous IV infusion (see Chapter 11), the heparin dosage rate may be ordered as *units* per *hour* (*units/h*) or individualized by weight as *units* per *kilogram* per *hour* (*units/kg/h*). Initially, a bolus dose is administered to achieve a therapeutic blood level. This is followed by a continuous IV infusion. To maintain a constant rate, heparin is always administered by an electronic infusion pump. Dosage rates are adjusted according to lab results. The nurse may have to recalculate the heparin dosage to meet the client's new requirements.

Figure 9.16 Heparin vials.

SOURCE: Pearson Education, Inc.

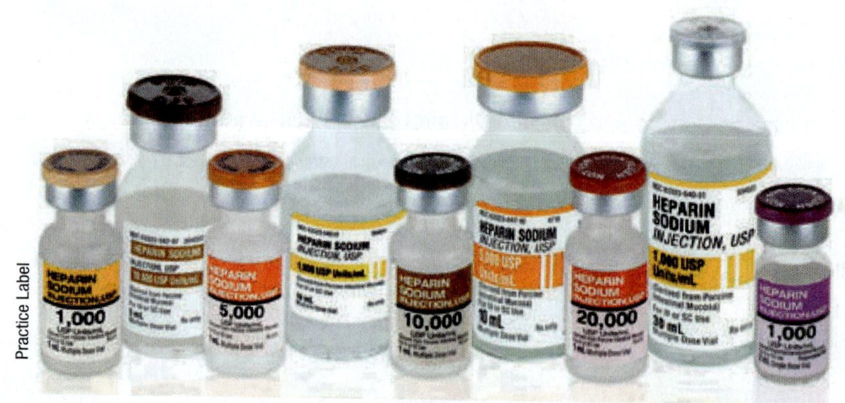

Heparin requires close monitoring of the client's bloodwork because of the bleeding potential associated with anticoagulant drugs. To assure accuracy of dose measurement, a 1 *mL* syringe should be used to administer heparin subcutaneously. Healthcare providers should know and follow agency policies when administering heparin.

Heparin flush solutions (e.g., Hep-Flush or Hep-Lock) are used for maintaining the patency of indwelling IV catheters. These solutions are available in strengths of 10 *units/mL* and 100 *units/mL* (see Figure 9.17). Heparin sodium injections and heparin flush solutions are different and cannot be used interchangeably. Note the large differences in dosage strength between heparin sodium (1,000–50,000 *units/mL*) and heparin flush solutions (10–100 *units/mL*). Thus, the healthcare provider must be careful when preparing heparin.

Figure 9.17 Heparin flush. (For educational purposes only)

SOURCE: Pearson Education, Inc.

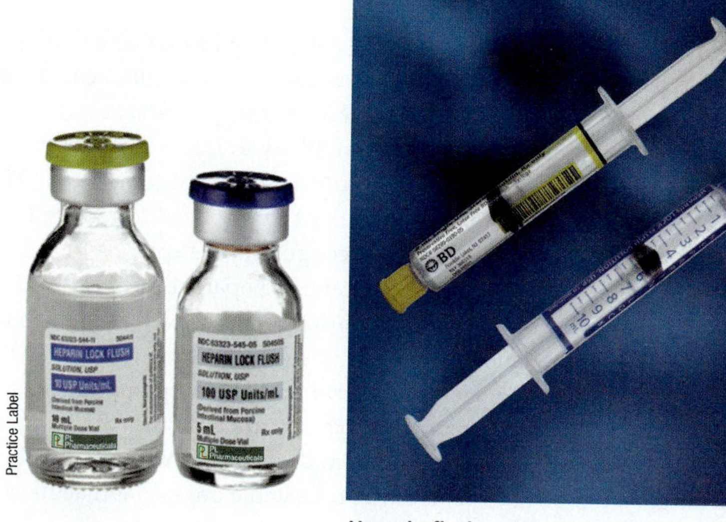

Heparin flush syringes.

ALERT

Fatal hemorrhages have occurred in pediatric clients as a result of medication errors in which 1 *mL* heparin sodium injection vials were confused with 1 *mL* "catheter lock flush" vials. Carefully examine all heparin sodium injection vials to confirm the correct vial choice prior to administration of the drug.

Example 9.13

The prescriber ordered *heparin* 4,000 *units subcut q12h*. Read the drug label in Figure 9.18.

(a) Calculate the number of *milliliters* you will administer to the client.

(b) Indicate the dose on the syringe below.

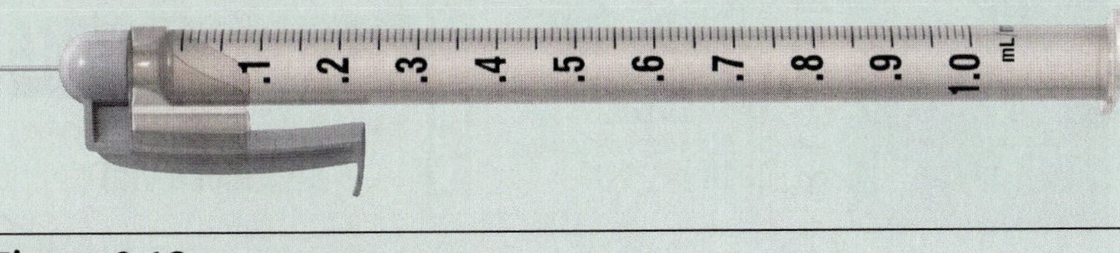

Figure 9.18 Drug label for heparin.

SOURCE: Courtesy of Pfizer, Inc.

NOTE the statement "NOT FOR LOCK FLUSH" on the label

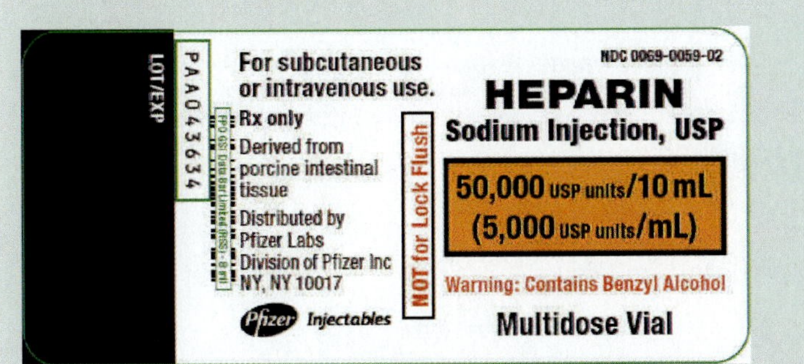

(a) You want to convert units to *milliliters*.

$$4{,}000\ units = ?\ mL$$

You cancel the units and obtain the equivalent amount in *milliliters*.

$$4{,}000\ units \times \frac{?\ mL}{?\ units} = ?\ mL$$

The strength on the vial is 5,000 *units* per *milliliter*, so the unit fraction is

$$\frac{1\ mL}{5{,}000\ units}$$

$$\cancel{4{,}000\ units} \times \frac{1\ mL}{\cancel{5{,}000\ units}} = \frac{4\ mL}{5} = 0.8\ mL$$

So, you would use a 1 *mL* syringe and administer 0.8 *mL* of heparin.

(b)

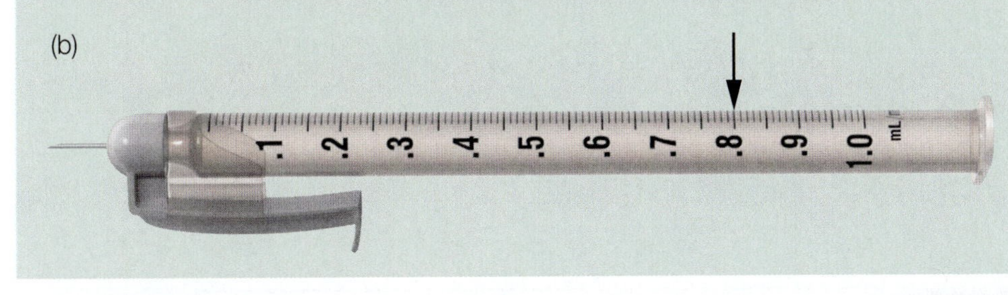

Example 9.14

The prescriber ordered *heparin* 4,000 *units subcut q12h*. Read the drug label in Figure 9.19.

(Continued)

Figure 9.19 Drug label for heparin.

SOURCE: Courtesy of Pfizer, Inc.

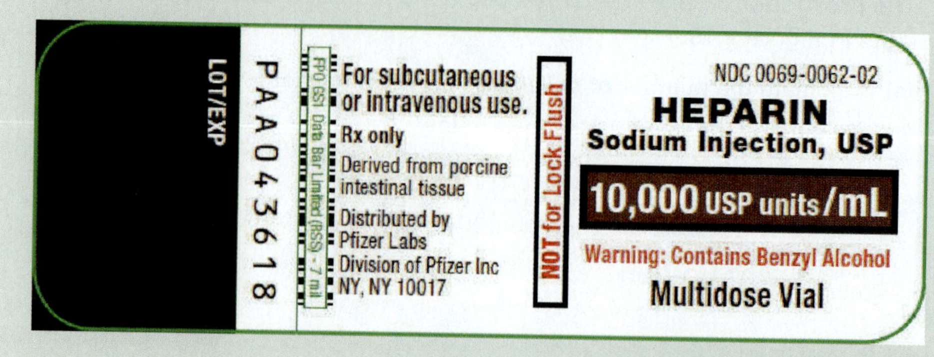

(a) Calculate the number of *milliliters* you will administer to the client.

(b) Indicate the dose on the syringe below.

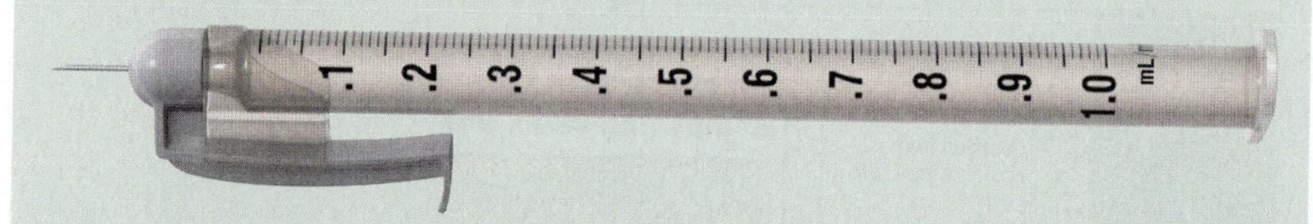

(a) You want to convert units to *milliliters*.

$$4{,}000\ units = ?\ mL$$

You cancel the units and obtain the equivalent amount in *milliliters*.

$$4{,}000\ units \times \frac{?\ mL}{?\ units} = ?\ mL$$

The strength on the vial is 10,000 *units* per *milliliter*, so the unit fraction is

$$\frac{1\ mL}{10{,}000\ units}$$

$$\cancel{4{,}000\ units} \times \frac{1\ mL}{\cancel{10{,}000\ units}} = \frac{4\ mL}{10} = 0.4\ mL$$

So, you would use a 1 *mL* syringe and administer 0.4 *mL* of heparin.

(b)

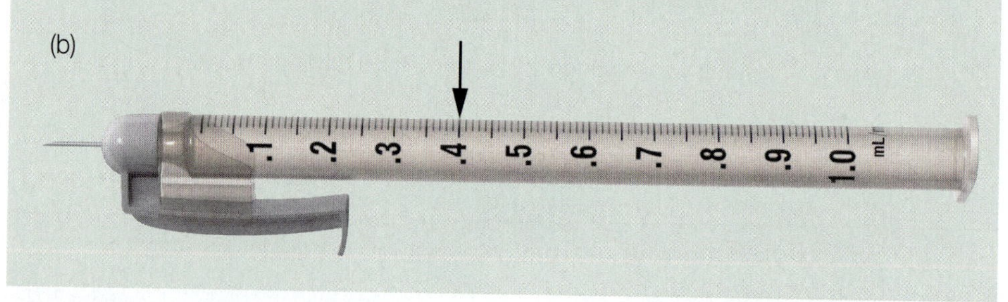

ALERT

Observe that, in Examples 9.13 and 9.14, the order for heparin is exactly the same (4,000 *units* subcutaneously *q12h*). However, the available dosage strengths are different. In Example 9.14 the strength (10,000 *units/mL*) is twice the strength of that in Example 9.13 (5,000 *units/mL*). Therefore, only half the amount of the stronger solution is needed.

Example 9.15

The prescriber ordered *Fragmin (dalteparin sodium) 120 units/kg subcutaneously q12h* for a client who weighs 138 *pounds*. See Figure 9.20 and determine how many *milliliters* of this low-molecular-weight heparin you will need to administer the dose.

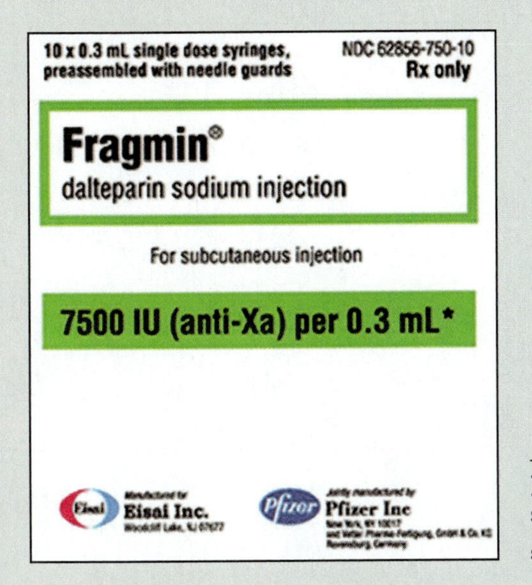

Figure 9.20 Box label for Fragmin single-dose syringes.

SOURCE: Courtesy of Pfizer, Inc.

Because this example contains a lot of information, it is useful to summarize it as follows:

Client:	138 *lb* (single unit of measurement)
Known equivalences:	1 *kg* = 2.2 *lb* (needed to convert *lb* to *kg*)
	120 *units/kg* (order)
	7,500 *units*/0.3 *mL* (strength on the drug label)
Administer:	? *mL*

DIMENSIONAL ANALYSIS

You want to convert a single unit of measurement (138 *lb*) to another single unit of measurement (*mL*).

$$138\ lb = ?\ mL$$

You want to cancel *lb*. To do this you must use a unit fraction containing *lb* in the denominator. Using the equivalence 1 *kg* = 2.2 *lb*, this fraction will be $\frac{1\ kg}{2.2\ lb}$

$$138\ \cancel{lb} \times \frac{1\ kg}{2.2\ \cancel{lb}} = ?\ mL$$

Now, on the left side *kg* is in the numerator. To cancel the *kg* will require a unit fraction with *kg* in the denominator, namely, $\frac{120\ units}{kg}$.

$$138\ \cancel{lb} \times \frac{1\ \cancel{kg}}{2.2\ \cancel{lb}} \times \frac{120\ units}{\cancel{kg}} = ?\ mL$$

FORMULA METHOD

First change the weight of 138 *pounds* to kilograms by dividing by 2.2.

$$\frac{132}{2.2} \approx 62.7$$

So, the client weighs 62.7 *kg*.

Because the order is based on the size of the client, use the formula:

Size of the client × Order = Dose

$$62.7\ kg \times \frac{120\ units}{kg} = 7{,}524\ units$$

Now, you need to convert 7,524 *units* to *milliliters*.

D (desired dose) = 7,524 *units*
H (dose on hand) = 7,500 *units*
Q (dosage unit) = 0.3 *mL*
X (unknown) = ? *mL*

(Continued)

DIMENSIONAL ANALYSIS

Now, on the left side units is in the numerator. To cancel the *units* will require a fraction with *units* in the denominator, namely, $\frac{0.3\ mL}{7{,}500\ units}$.

$$138\ lb \times \frac{1\ kg}{2.2\ lb} \times \frac{120\ units}{kg} \times \frac{0.3\ mL}{7500\ units} = ?\ mL$$

After cancellation, only *mL* remains on the left side. This is what you want. Now multiply the numbers

$$138\ lb \times \frac{kg}{2.2\ lb} \times \frac{120\ units}{kg} \times \frac{0.3\ mL}{7{,}500\ units} = 0.301\ mL$$

FORMULA METHOD

Fill in the formula $\frac{D}{H} \times Q = X$

$$\frac{7{,}524\ units}{7{,}500\ units} \times 0.3\ mL = ?\ mL$$

Cancel $\frac{7{,}524\ units}{7{,}500\ units} \times 0.3\ ml = ?\ mL$

Multiply $1.003 \times 0.3\ mL = 0.3009\ mL$

Therefore, you would need to administer 0.3 *mL*.

Summary

In this chapter, you learned how to calculate doses for administering parenteral medications in liquid form, the procedure for reconstituting medications in powder form, and how to calculate dosages for medications supplied in units.

- Medications supplied in powder form must be reconstituted following the manufacturer's directions.
- You must determine the best dosage strength when there are several options for reconstituting the medication.
- After reconstituting a multiple-dose vial, label the medication vial with the dates and times of both preparation and expiration, storage directions, your initials, and the strength.
- When directions on the label are provided for both IM and IV reconstitution, be sure to read the order and the label carefully to determine the necessary type and amount of diluent to use.
- Heparin is measured in USP units.
- It is especially important that heparin orders be carefully checked with the available dosage strength before calculating the amount to be administered.
- A tuberculin 1 *mL* or a 0.5 *mL* syringe should be used when administering heparin.
- Heparin sodium and heparin flush solutions are different and should never be used interchangeably.

Case Study 9.1

Read the Case Study and answer the questions. Answers can be found in Appendix A.

A 69-year-old male is admitted to the ambulatory surgery unit for a laproscopic repair of a torn meniscus. He reports a past medical history of hypertension, hypercholesterolemia, osteoarthritis, and atrial fibrillation. He has a past surgical history of bilateral repair of rotator cuffs and a right total hip replacement. He is 6 *feet* tall and weighs 175 *pounds*. He denies any allergies to food or drugs. His vital signs are T 98.9° F; B/P 138/90; P 96; R 18.

Pre-op orders:

- NPO
- IV RL @ 25 *mL/h*
- ondansetron hydrochloride 4 *mg* IM stat before anesthesia induction
- fentanyl 75 *mcg* IVP stat
- Transfer to OR

Post-op orders:

- NPO, progress to clear liquids as tolerated
- IV D5NS @ 125 *mL/h* until tolerating liquids
- Nexium (esomeprazole magnesium) 20 *mg* IVP stat
- Morphine sulfate 5 *mg* IM once if needed for pain
- V/S q15 *min* × 4, then q30 *min* × 2*h*, then q1*h* × 2*h*
- Cold compresses to right leg q1*h* × 20 *minutes*
- Discharge when stable

Discharge orders:

- amlodipine 5 *mg*/ valsartan 160 *mg*/ hydrochlorothiazide 25 *mg* po once daily
- lovastatin 20 *mg* PO daily
- escitalopram oxalate 15 *mg* PO daily
- warfarin 3.75 *mg* PO daily
- Nexium (esomeprazole magnesium) 20 *mg* PO 1*h* ac meals
- hydrocodone 5 *mg* PO q6*h* prn pain
- Cold compresses to right leg q1*h* × 20 *minutes*
- Make appointment for follow-up in 1 *week*

Refer to the labels in Figure 9.21 when necessary to answer the following questions.

1. The ondansetron hydrochloride is supplied in vials labeled 32 *mg*/5 *mL*.
   (a) How many *milliliters* are needed for the prescribed dose?
   (b) What type of syringe is needed to administer the dose?
2. The fentanyl is supplied in vials labeled 0.05 *mg/mL*.
   (a) How many *milliliters* are needed for the prescribed dose?
   (b) What type of syringe is needed to administer the dose?
3. The anesthetist will be administering propofol 2 *mg/kg* IV q 10 *seconds* until induction onset.
   (a) How many *milliliters* will the anesthetist prepare?
   (b) What type of syringe will be used to draw up the propofol?
4. The esomeprazole magnesium is supplied in 40 *mg* vials, and the label states to reconstitute the powder with 5 *mL* of normal saline. Calculate how many *milliliters* the client will receive.
5. During your discharge teaching, you are reviewing the client's medication vials and dosages.
   (a) Select the correct label for the amlodipine, valsartan, hydrochlorothiazide order.
   (b) How many tablets should you instruct the client to take?
6. The strength of the lovastatin is 20 *mg* per tablet. How many tablets will you instruct the client to take?
7. The strength of the escitalopram is 5 *mg*/5 *mL*. How many *milliliters* will you instruct the client to take?
8. (a) Select the correct label for the hydrocodone dose.
   (b) How many tablets may the client take in a 24-*hour* period?
9. How many tablets of warfarin should you instruct the client to take each day?
10. How many *milligrams* of esomeprazole magnesium may the client take each day?

Figure 9.21 Drug labels for Case Study.

Cozaar® 100 mg
(Losartan Potassium Tablets)
MERCK & CO., INC., Whitehouse Station, NJ 08889, USA
Losartan Potassium (active ingred.) Made in France
Formulated in USA
Each tablet contains 100 mg of losartan potassium. Store at 25°C (77°F); excursions permitted to 15-30°C (59-86°F) [see USP Controlled Room Temperature]. Keep container tightly closed. Protect from light.
960
90 Tablets
Lot
NDC 0006-0960-54
USUAL ADULT DOSAGE: See accompanying circular.
Rx only
COZAAR is a registered trademark of E.I. du Pont de Nemours and Company, Wilmington, DE
9580001
90 | No.6536
N 3 0006-0960-54 3

SOURCE: Reproduced with permission of Merck Sharp & Dohme Corp., a subsidiary of Merck & Co, Inc., Whitehouse Station, New Jersey, USA. All Rights Reserved.

(a)

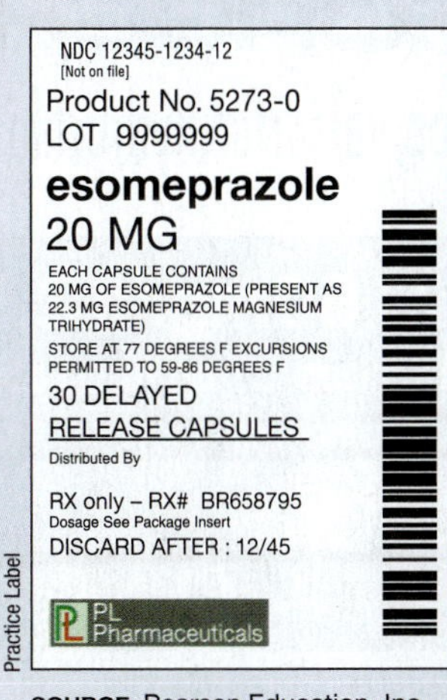

SOURCE: Pearson Education, Inc.

(b) **(For educational purposes only)**

(continued)

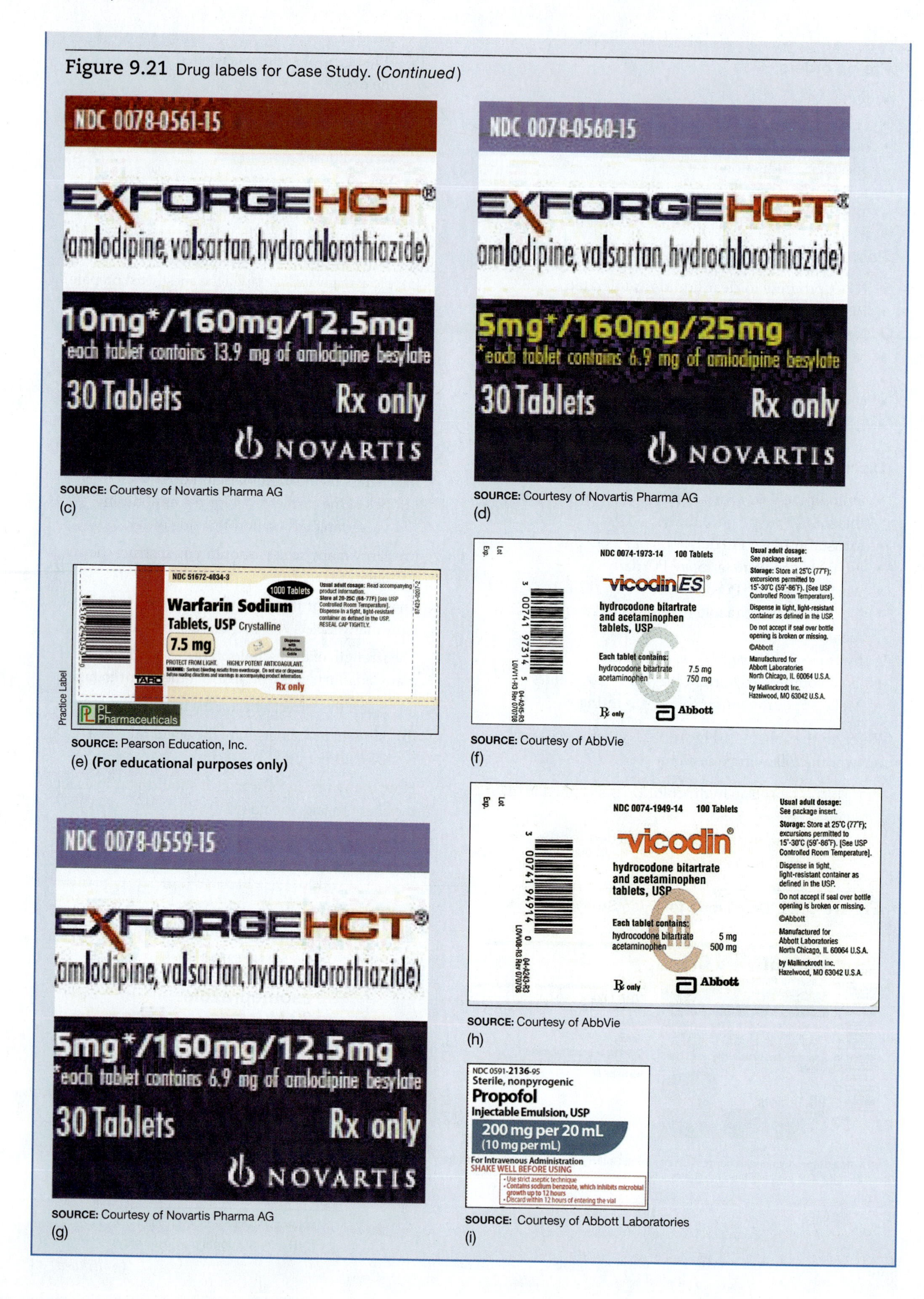

Figure 9.21 Drug labels for Case Study. *(Continued)*

SOURCE: Courtesy of Novartis Pharma AG
(c)

SOURCE: Courtesy of Novartis Pharma AG
(d)

SOURCE: Pearson Education, Inc.
(e) **(For educational purposes only)**

SOURCE: Courtesy of AbbVie
(f)

SOURCE: Courtesy of AbbVie
(h)

SOURCE: Courtesy of Novartis Pharma AG
(g)

SOURCE: Courtesy of Abbott Laboratories
(i)

Practice Sets

The answers to *Try These for Practice, Exercises,* and *Cumulative Review Exercises* are found in Appendix A. Ask your instructor for the answers to the *Additional Exercises.*

Try These for Practice

Test your comprehension after reading the chapter.

1. Order: *ceftriaxone 1 g IM daily in 2 equally divided doses.*

   Read the label in Figure 9.22. How many *mL* will you administer?

Figure 9.22 Drug label for ceftriaxone.

SOURCE: Courtesy of Pfizer, Inc.

Each vial contains: Ceftriaxone sodium USP powder equivalent to 2 g ceftriaxone.
For I.M. Administration: Reconstitute with 4.2 mL 1% Lidocaine Hydrochloride Injection (USP) or Sterile Water for Injection (USP). Each 1 mL of solution contains approximately 350 mg equivalent of ceftriaxone.
For I.V. Administration: Reconstitute with 19.2 mL of an I.V. diluent specified in the accompanying package insert. Each 1 mL solution contains approximately 100 mg equivalent of ceftriaxone. **Withdraw entire** contents and dilute to the desired concentration with the appropriate I.V. diluent.
USUAL DOSAGE: See package insert.
Storage Prior to Reconstitution: Store powder at 20° to 25°C (68° to 77°F) [see USP Controlled Room Temperature].
Protect From Light.
Storage After Reconstitution: See package insert.
Code No.: 78/MD/AP/96/F/B/R Made in India

Single-Use Vial **Rx only**
ceftriaxone for injection, USP
For I.M. or I.V. Use
2 g/vial
Distributed by
Pfizer Labs
Division of Pfizer Inc, NY, NY 10017
10300694483033
P1405091
Lot
EXP

2. Order: *ampicillin 400 mg IM q6h.*

   Read the label in Figure 9.23. How many *milliliters* will you administer?

Figure 9.23 Drug label for ampicillin.

SOURCE: Courtesy of Pfizer, Inc.

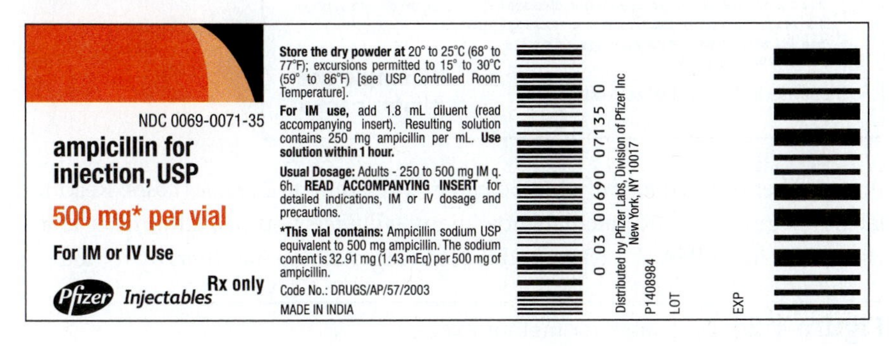

3. Order: *Cleocin Phosphate (clindamycin) 600 mg IM q12h.*

   Read the label in Figure 9.24 and calculate how many *milliliters* of this antibiotic you will administer.

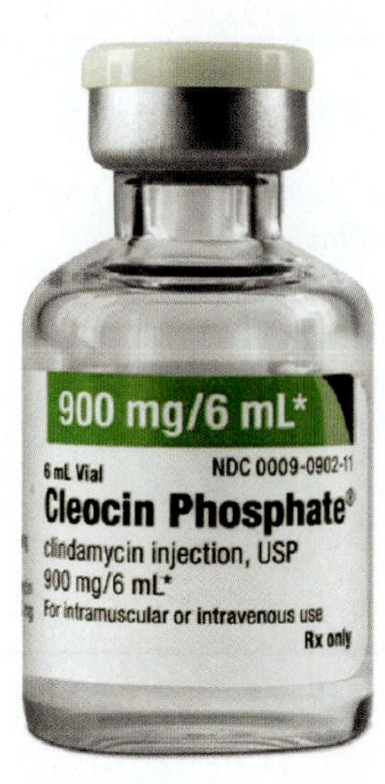

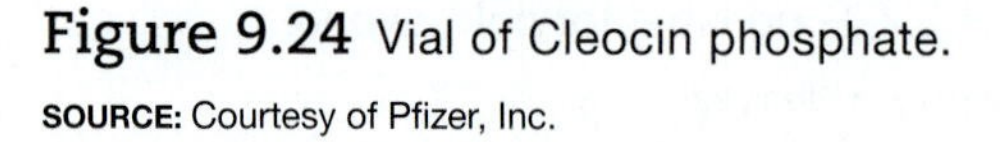

Figure 9.24 Vial of Cleocin phosphate.

SOURCE: Courtesy of Pfizer, Inc.

4. A prescriber ordered *interferon beta-1b (Extavia) 0.25 mg subcut every other day* for a client who has multiple sclerosis. Read the label in Figure 9.25 and calculate how many *milliliters* you will administer.

Figure 9.25 Drug label for interferon beta-1b (Extavia).

SOURCE: Courtesy of Novartis Pharma AG

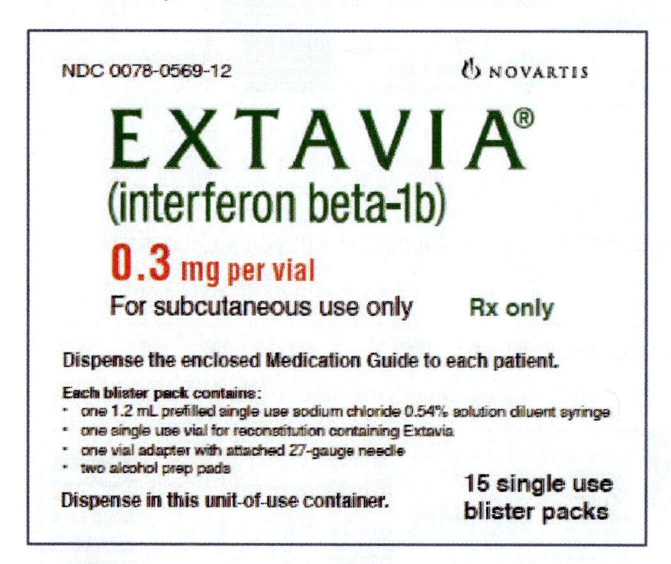

5. A prescriber ordered *methotrexate* 30 *mg*/*m*^{2} *IM weekly in 2 divided doses*. Read the label in Figure 9.26 and calculate how many *milliliters* you will administer to a client who has a BSA of 1.65 *m*^{2} and is receiving maintenance therapy for leukemia.

Figure 9.26 Drug label for methotrexate.

SOURCE: Copyright TEVA, Used with permission

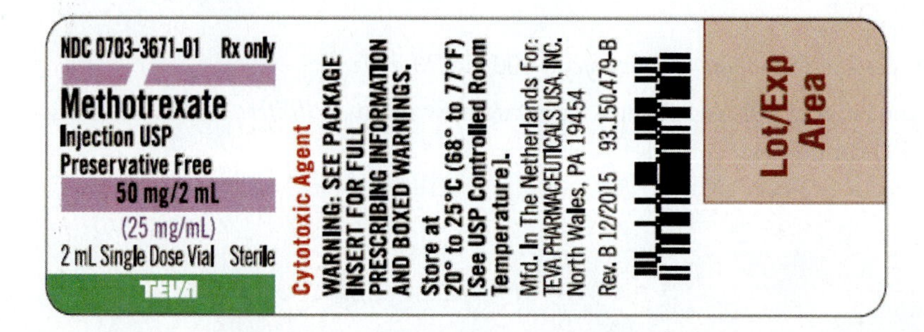

Exercises

Reinforce your understanding in class or at home.

1. Order: *hydralazine hydrochloride* 10 *mg IM q.i.d.*

   The strength in the vial is 20 *mg/mL*. How many *milliliters* of this antihypertensive will you administer?

2. Order: *Robinul (glycopyrrolate)* 4 *mcg/kg IM q3h.*

   The strength in the vial is 0.2 *mg/mL*, and the client weighs 46 *kg*. How many *milliliters* of this preanesthetic will you administer?

3. Order: *Neupogen (filgrastim)* 5 *mcg/kg subcut daily.*

   The strength is 300 *mcg* = 1 *mL* in a single-use vial. The client weighs 39 *kg*. How many *milliliters* of this drug will you administer?

4. Order: *Ticar (ticarcillin disodium)* 1 *g IM q6h.*

   The reconstitution directions on the 3 *g* vial state, "add 6 *mL* sterile water for injection to the vial yielding a concentration of 385 *mg/mL*." How many *milliliters* of this antibiotic drug will you administer?

5. Order: *heparin* 4,000 *units subcut q12h.*

   Read the label in Figure 9.27. How many *milliliters* will you administer?

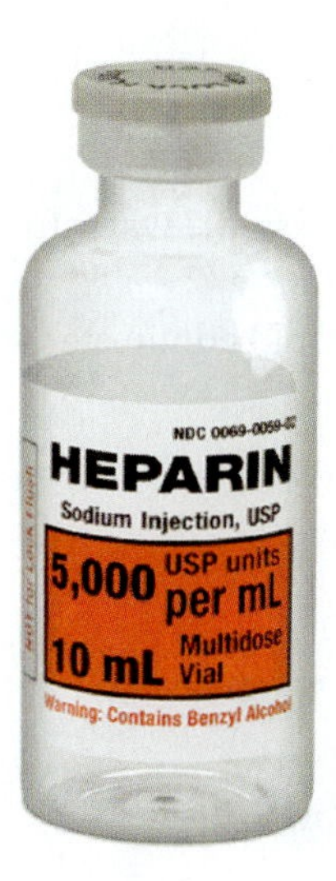

Figure 9.27 Vial of heparin.
(For educational purposes only)

SOURCE: Courtesy of Pfizer, Inc.

6. Order: *penicillin G potassium* 250,000 *units IM q6h.* Read the label in Figure 9.28.
   (a) Calculate the number of *milliliters* of this antibiotic you would administer to the client if you use the 8.2 *mL* of diluent to reconstitute the drug.
   (b) Indicate the dose by placing an arrow on the most appropriate syringe below.

Figure 9.28 Drug label for penicillin G potassium.

SOURCE: Courtesy of Pfizer, Inc.

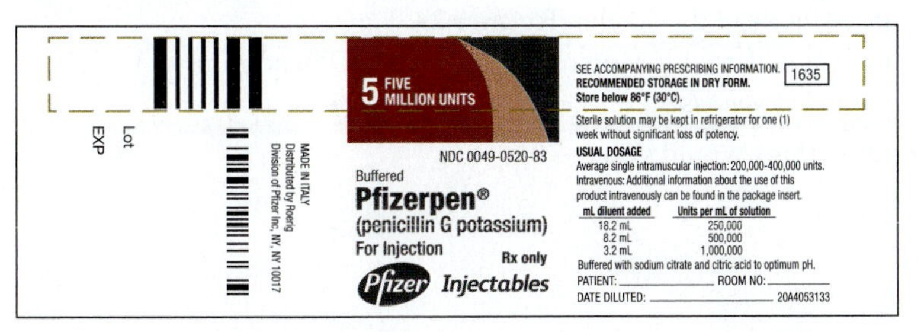

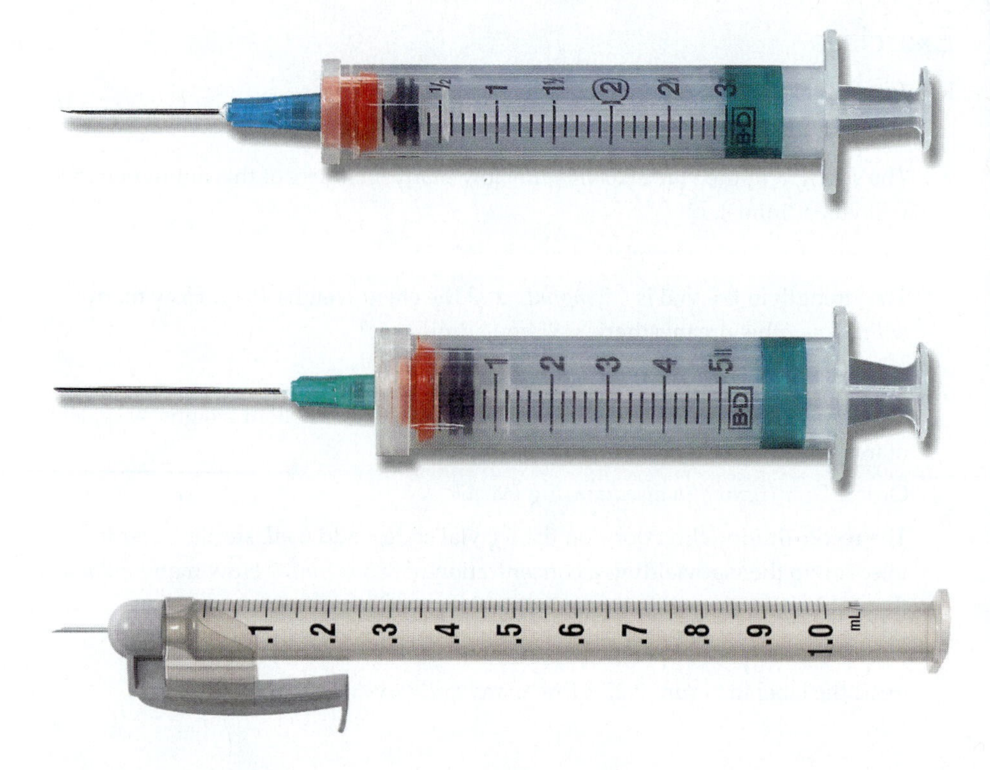

7. Order: *ticarcillin disodium* 1 *g IM q6h*

   The label reads, "reconstitute each 1 *g* of ticarcillin with 2 *mL* of sterile water for injection or NS and use promptly. The resulting concentration is 1 *g*/2.6 *mL*."

   (a) Calculate the number of *milliliters* of this antibiotic you would administer to the client.

   (b) Indicate which size syringe you would use and place arrow at the dosage.

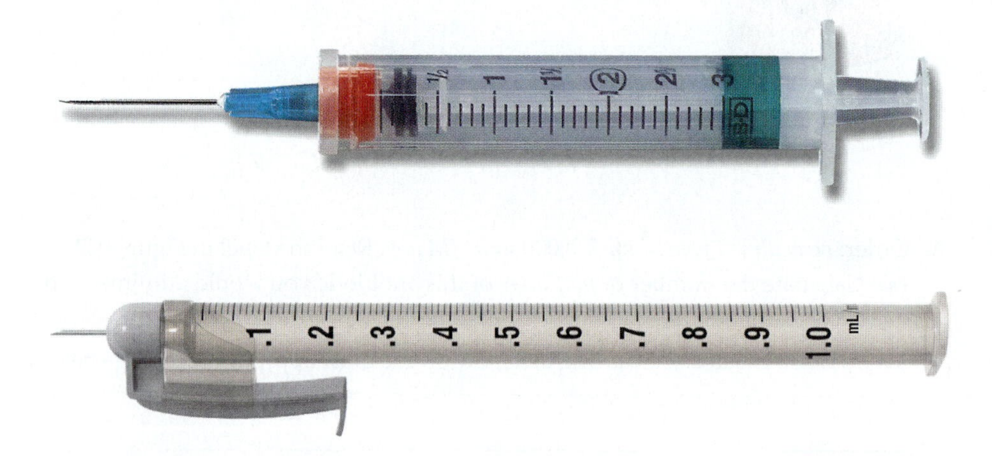

8. The prescriber ordered Dilaudid (HYDROmorphone HCl) 0.01 *mg/kg* subcut q3h prn moderate pain. Read the label in Figure 9.29.

   (a) How many *milliliters* of this opioid analgesic will you administer to a client who weighs 154 *pounds*?

   (b) What size syringe would you use?

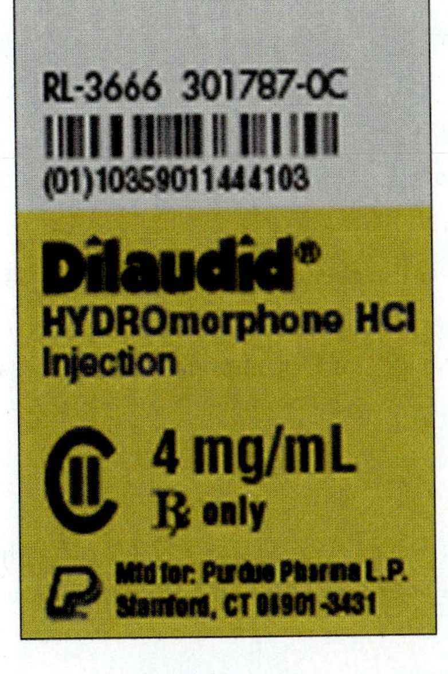

Figure 9.29 Drug label for Dilaudid.

SOURCE: © Purdue, used with permission.

9. The prescriber ordered *Aranesp (darbepoetin alfa)* 0.75 *mcg/kg subcut once every* 2 *weeks*. The client has chronic kidney disease, weighs 110 *pounds*, and is receiving dialysis treatments. The label reads 40 *mcg*/0.4 *mL*.
   (a) Calculate how many *milliliters* you will administer.
   (b) What size syringe will you use?
10. The prescriber ordered *ZYPREXA (olanzapine for injection)* 7.5 *mg IM stat*. The reconstitution directions state that after adding 1.2 *mL* of diluent the resulting strength will be 5 *mg/mL*. Read the information in Figure 9.30.
    (a) How many *milliliters* will you administer?
    (b) What size syringe will you use?

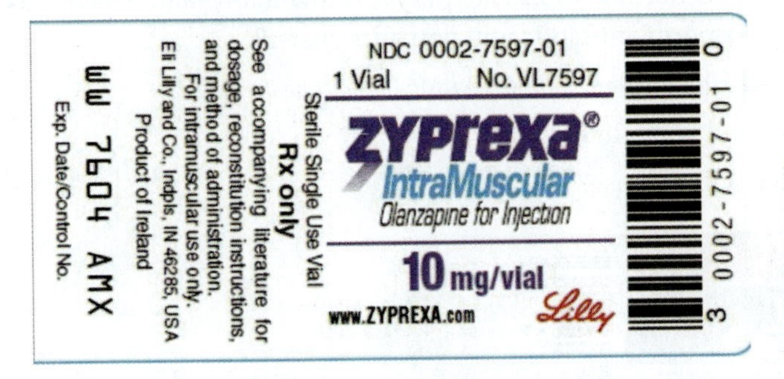

Figure 9.30 Drug information for ZyPREXA.

SOURCE: © Copyright Eli Lily and Company. All rights reserved. Used with permission.

11. The prescriber ordered *Pitocin (oxytocin)* 20 *units IM stat*. Read the label in Figure 9.31.
    (a) Calculate how many *milliliters* you will prepare.
    (b) What size syringe will you use?

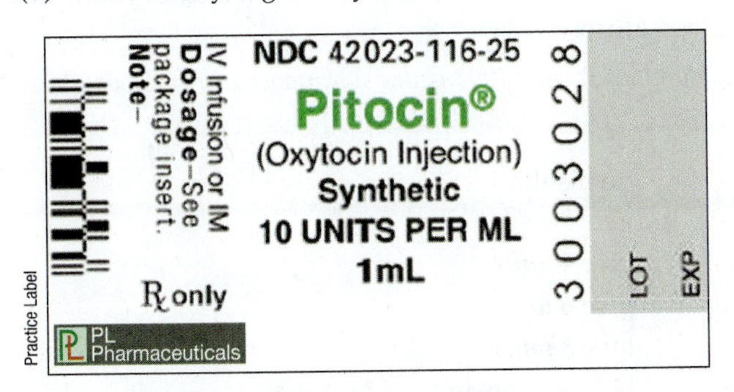

Figure 9.31 Drug label for Pitocin. (For educational purposes only)

SOURCE: Courtesy of JHP Pharmaceuticals and Par Pharmaceutical, Inc.

12. Order: *Epogen (epoetin alfa) 100 units/kg subcut three times a week*. The label reads 10,000 *units* per *mL*, and the client weighs 200 *pounds*.
    (a) How many *milliliters* will you administer?
    (b) What size syringe will you use?
13. Order: *Tigan (trimethobenzamide HCl) 200 mg IM q3h prn nausea and vomiting*. The 20 *mL* multiple-dose vial is labeled 100 *mg* per *mL*.
    (a) How many *milliliters* will you administer?
    (b) What is the maximum number of *milliliters* the client may receive in 24 *hours*?
14. Order: *Neupogen 5 mcg/kg subcut daily*. The client weighs 200 *pounds*. There are two vials; the strength of one vial is 480 *mcg* per 0.8 *mL*, and the strength of the other is 300 *mcg* per *mL*.
    (a) What strength vial will you use?
    (b) How many *milliliters* will you administer?
15. The prescriber ordered: *40 mg of pasireotide (Signifor LAR) IM once q4 weeks*. Use the label in Figure 9.32 to calculate the number of *milliliters* you will administer. Note the prefilled syringe contains 2 *mL* of diluent.

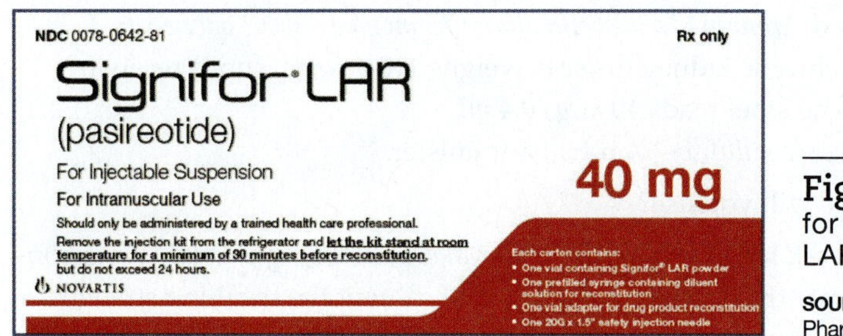

Figure 9.32 Drug label for pasireotide (Signifor LAR).

SOURCE: Courtesy of Novartis Pharma AG

16. Order: *cefazolin sodium 250 mg IM q6h*. The instructions on the 500 *mg* vial are to add 2 *mL* of sterile water for injection or 0.9% Sodium Chloride injection, resulting in a 2.2 *ml* volume with a concentration of 225 *mg* per *mL*. How many *milliliters* of this first-generation cephalosporin antibiotic will you administer?
17. The prescriber ordered *Humalog mix 50/50 12 units subcut ac breakfast*.
    (a) How many units will you administer?
    (b) What size syringe will you use?

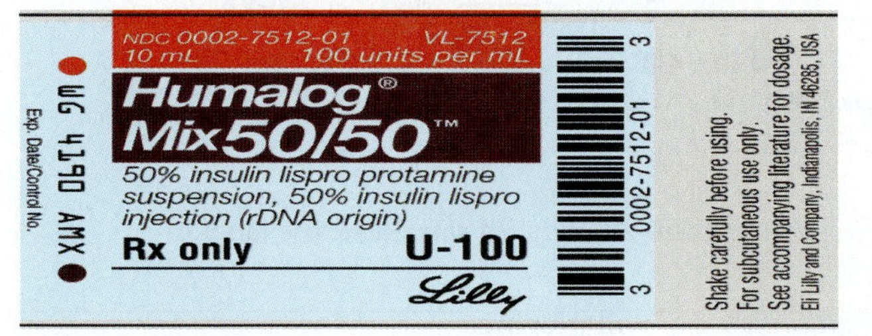

Figure 9.33 Humalog Mix 50/50.

SOURCE: © Copyright Eli Lily and Company. All rights reserved. Used with permission.

18. Use the insulin "sliding scale" below to determine how much insulin you would give to a client whose blood glucose is 265.

    The prescriber ordered *Humulin R Unit 100 insulin subcutaneously for blood-glucose levels as follows:*

Glucose less than 160	no insulin
Glucose 160–220	give 2 *units*
Glucose 221–280	give 4 *units*
Glucose 281–340	give 6 *units*
Glucose 341–400	give 8 *units*
Glucose more than 400	hold insulin and call MD stat

19. A client weighs 210 *pounds*. The daily recommended safe dose for a certain drug is 0.02–0.05 *mg/kg*.
    (a) What is the minimum number of *milligrams* of this drug that this client should receive each day?
    (b) What is the maximum number of *milligrams* of this drug that this client should receive each day?
20. The prescriber ordered *testosterone undecanoate (Aveed) 750 mg IM*. Read the label in Figure 9.34 and determine how many *milliliters* of this androgen you will administer.

Figure 9.34 Drug label for Aveed.

SOURCE: Endo Pharmaceuticals Inc.

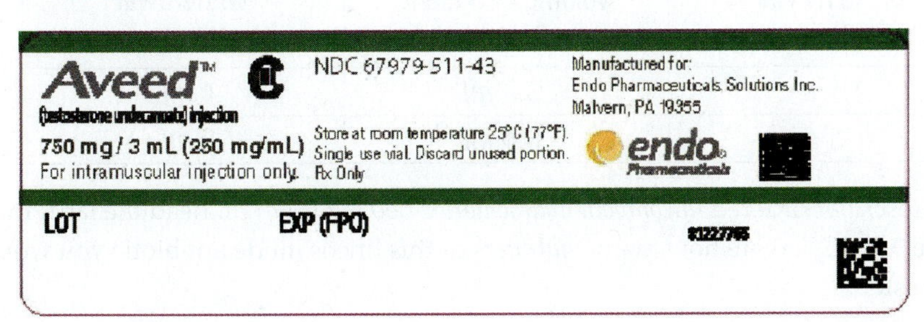

Additional Exercises

Now, test yourself!

1. The prescriber ordered *Navane (thiothixene hydrochloride)* 4 *mg IM B.I.D.* The label on the vial reads 5 *mg/mL*. Calculate how many milliliters of this antipsychotic drug you would administer.
2. The prescriber ordered *Amevive (alefacept)* 15 *mg IM once per week for* 12 *weeks*. The instructions on the 15 *mg* vial states "reconstitute with 0.4 *mL* of the supplied diluent to yield 15 *mg*/0.5 *mL*." How many *milliliters* of this biologic response modifier would you administer?
3. The prescriber ordered *heparin* 8,000 *units subcut q8h*. Read the label in Figure 9.35.
    (a) How many *milliliters* of this anticoagulant will you administer?
    (b) What size syringe will you use?

Figure 9.35 Drug label for heparin.

SOURCE: Courtesy of Pfizer, Inc.

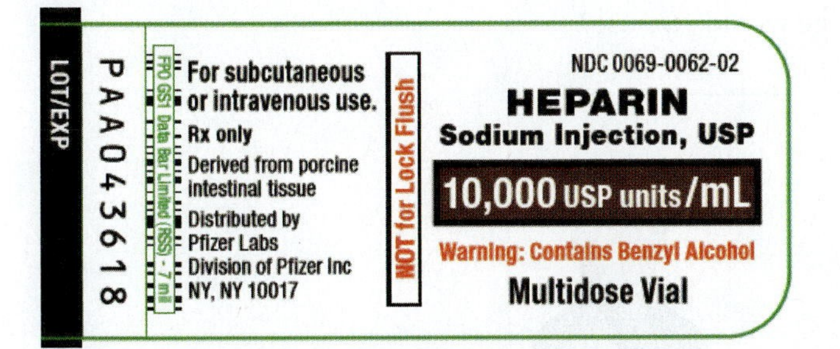

4. The prescriber ordered *Unasyn (ampicillin sodium/sublactam sodium)* 2 *g IM q6h*. Use the information from the package insert in Figure 9.36.
    (a) How much diluent must be added to the vial?
    (b) What is the reconstituted volume in the vial?
    (c) What is the strength of the reconstituted solution?
    (d) How many *milliliters* of this antibiotic will you administer?

Figure 9.36 Drug label and portion of package insert for Unasyn.

SOURCE: Courtesy of Pfizer, Inc.

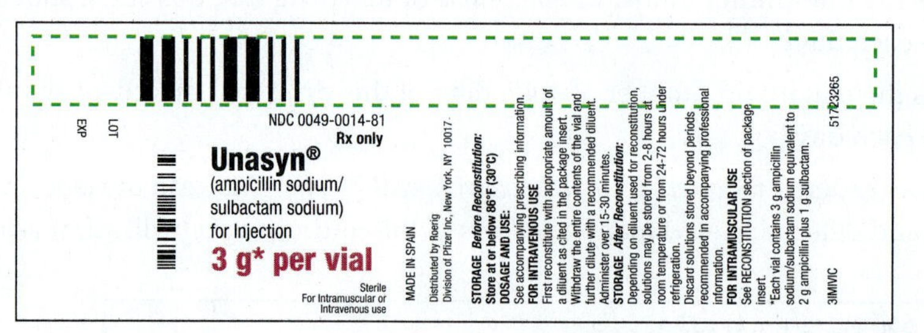

UNASYN Vial Size	Volume of Diluent to Be Added	Withdrawal Volume
1.5 *g*	3.2 *mL*	4 *mL*
3 *g*	6.4 *mL*	8 *mL*

5. The prescriber ordered *lincomycin hydrochloride 600 mg IM q12h*. Read the label in Figure 9.37. Calculate how many *milliliters* of this lincosamide antibiotic you would administer.

Figure 9.37 Drug label for Lincocin.

SOURCE: Courtesy of Pfizer, Inc.

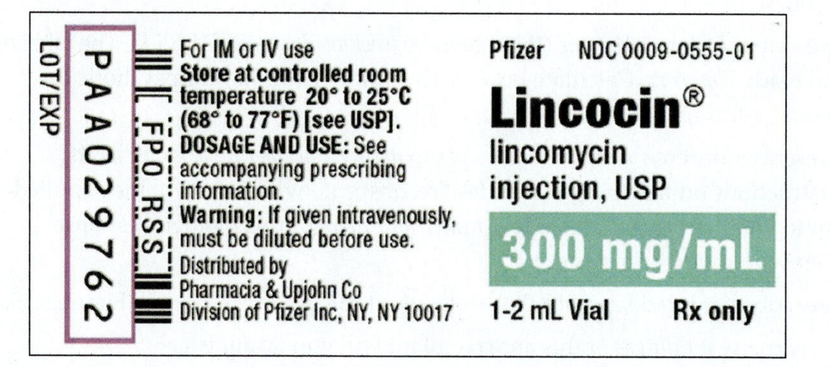

6. The prescriber ordered *Benadryl (diphenhydramine hydrochloride)* 45 *mg IM q4h*. Read the label in Figure 9.38. The manufacturer states not to exceed 400 *mg/day*.
   (a) Is this a safe dose?
   (b) How many *milliliters* of this antihistamine would you administer?
   (c) What size syringe would you use?

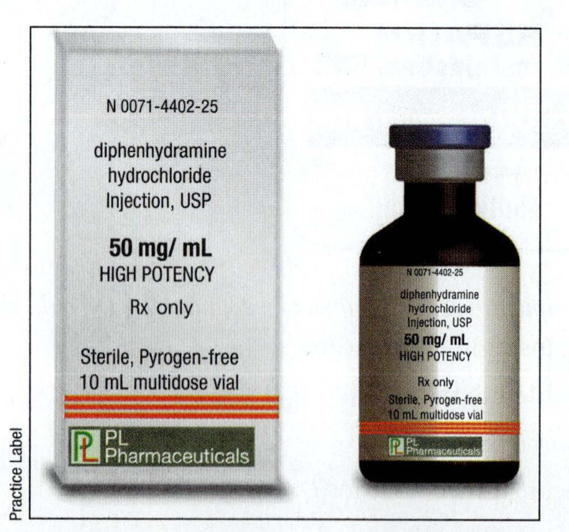

Figure 9.38 Drug box and vial for diphenhydramine hydrochloride. (For educational purposes only)

SOURCE: Pearson Education, Inc.

7. The prescriber ordered *fentanyl citrate* 55 *mcg IM prn pain*. Read the label in Figure 9.39.
   (a) How many *milliliters* of this narcotic analgesic would you administer?
   (b) Which size syringe would you use?

Figure 9.39 Drug label for fentanyl citrate. (For educational purposes only)

SOURCE: Pearson Education, Inc.

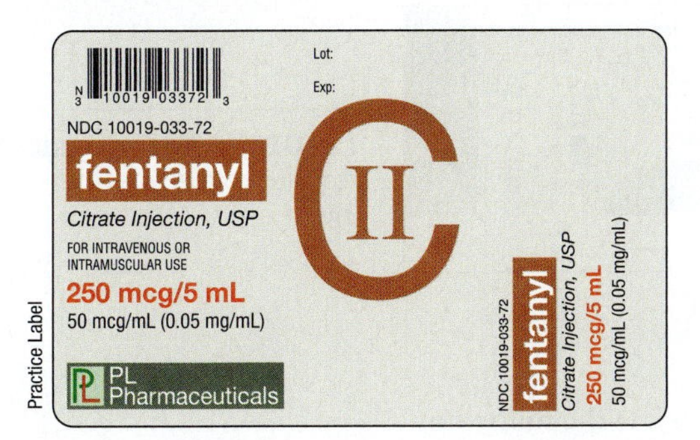

8. The prescriber ordered *ceftriaxone sodium* 1,200 *mg IM q12h for* 4 *days*. The instructions in the package insert state to reconstitute the 1 *g* or 2 *g* vial by adding 2.1 *mL* or 4.2 *mL*, respectively, of sterile water for injection, yields 350 *mg/mL*.
   (a) What vial would you use?
   (b) How many *milliliters* of this cephalosporin antibiotic would you administer?
   (c) What size syringe would you use?
9. The prescriber ordered *morphine sulfate* 0.2 *mg/kg IM q4h prn moderate to severe pain*. Read the label in Figure 9.40.
   (a) How many *milliliters* of this narcotic analgesic would you administer to a client who weighs 154 *pounds*?
   (b) What size syringe would you use?
   (c) The package insert states that the maximum dose is 10 *mg*/24*h*. Is the client receiving a safe dose?

Figure 9.40 Drug label for morphine sulfate. (For educational purposes only)

SOURCE: Pearson Education, Inc.

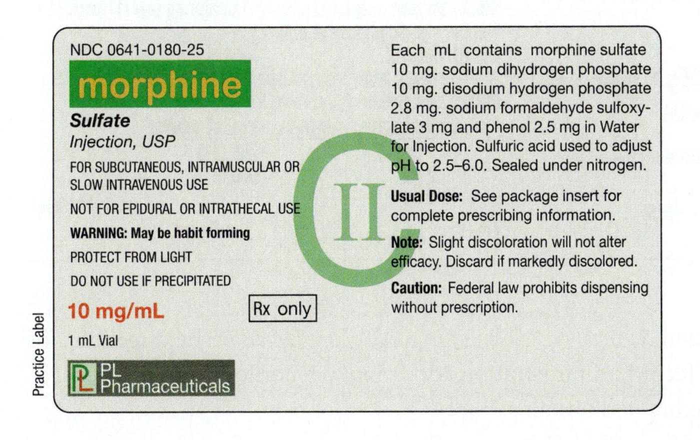

10. The prescriber ordered *Kenalog (triamcinolone)* 15 *mg into the knee joint stat*. The medication is available in a 5 *mL* multi-dose vial with a strength of 10 *mg/mL*.
   (a) How many *milliliters* of this synthetic glucocorticoid will the client receive?
   (b) How many doses of 15 *mg* are contained in the vial?

11. The prescriber ordered *leuprolide acetate injection* 1 *mg subcut now*. Read the information in Figure 9.41.
    (a) How many *milliliters* of this hormone would you prepare?
    (b) What size syringe would you use?
    (c) How many doses are in the vial?

Sterile injection. For subcutaneous injection.
Store below 25°C (77°F). Protect from light. Do Not Freeze.
NDC 0703-4014-11
LEUPROLIDE
Acetate Injection
1 mg/0.2 mL
℞only
2.8 mL Multiple Dose Vial
Usual Dosage: 0.2 mL subcutaneous injection once daily.
See package insert for full prescribing information and patient use information.
Oncology
401413
Practice Label
PL Practice Label Co.

Figure 9.41 Drug label for leuprolide acetate injection.

SOURCE: Pearson Education, Inc.

12. Use the label in Figure 9.42 to answer the following:
    (a) How much diluent must be added to the vial to prepare 500,000 *units/mL* strength?
    (b) What strength would be available if you added 18.2 *mL* of diluent?
    (c) What is the total dose of penicillin G potassium in the vial?
    (d) The prescriber ordered *penicillin G potassium 2 million units IM q4h*. Which dosage strength would you use?
    (e) How many *milliliters* of this antibiotic would you administer?

Figure 9.42 Drug label for Pfizerpen.

SOURCE: Courtesy of Pfizer, Inc.

NDC 0049-0520-84
Rx only
Buffered
Pfizerpen®
(penicillin G potassium, USP)
For Injection
5,000,000 Units* per vial
(Five million units* per vial)
Intramuscular or Intravenous Use
Pfizer Injectables

*Each vial contains Penicillin G potassium, equivalent to 5,000,000 units (five million units) of penicillin G as the potassium salt. Each million unit contains 6.8 mg (0.3 mEq) of sodium and 65.6 mg (1.68 mEq) of potassium. Buffered with sodium citrate and citric acid to optimum pH.
SEE ACCOMPANYING PRESCRIBING INFORMATION.
RECOMMENDED STORAGE IN DRY FORM.
Store below 86°F (30°C).
Sterile solution may be kept in refrigerator for one (1) week without significant loss of potency.
USUAL DOSAGE
Average single intramuscular injection: 200,000-400,000 units.
Intravenous: See package insert for complete information.

mL diluent added	Units per mL of solution
18.2 mL	250,000
8.2 mL	500,000
3.2 mL	1,000,000

51731964
DATE: ______ units/mL ______

13. The prescriber ordered *Ancef (cefazolin sodium)* 250 *mg IM q8h*. The directions for the 1 *g* vial state "for IM administration add 2.5 *mL* of sterile water for injection. Provides an approximate volume of 3 *mL*."
    (a) What is the total amount of Ancef in the vial?
    (b) How many *milliliters* of this cephalosporin antibiotic would you administer?
14. The prescriber ordered *furosemide* 30 *mg IM B.I.D.* Read the label in Figure 9.43.
    (a) How many *milliliters* of this loop diuretic would you administer?
    (b) What size syringe would you use?

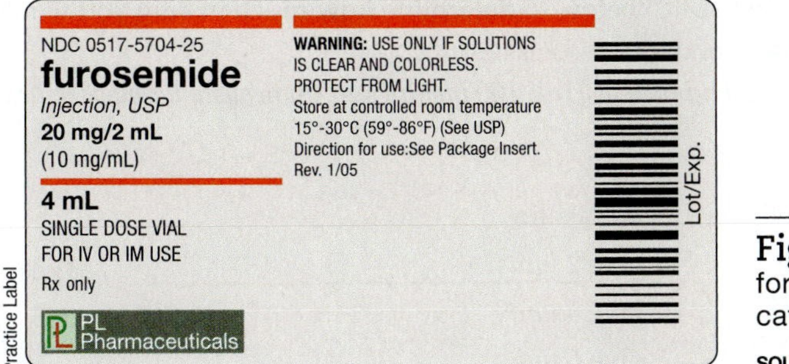

Figure 9.43 Drug label for furosemide. (For educational purposes only)

SOURCE: Pearson Education, Inc.

15. The prescriber ordered *streptomycin 15 mg/kg IM stat*. Use the label in Figure 9.44 to calculate the number of *milliliters* you would administer to a client who weighs 150 *pounds*.

2.5 mL

Streptomycin Sulfate Injection, USP

1 g/2.5 mL

(400 mg/mL)
(of streptomycin)

*For **IM** use only*

Store under refrigeration at 36° to 46°F (2° to 8°C)

CAUTION: Federal law prohibits dispensing without prescription.

LOT 8E31A
EXP

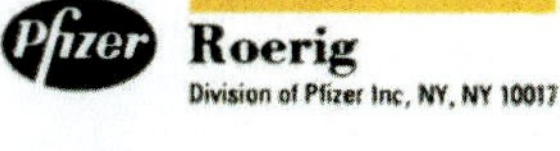

Figure 9.44 Drug label for streptomycin.

SOURCE: Courtesy of Pfizer, Inc.

16. The prescriber ordered *oxacillin 500 mg IM q6h*. The instructions on the 2 *g* vial state to reconstitute the powder with "11.5 *mL* of sterile water for injection, yielding 250 *mg*/1.5 *mL*."
    (a) What is the strength of the reconstituted solution?
    (b) How many *milliliters* would you administer?
17. The prescriber ordered *Humalog Mix 75/25 15 units subcut ac breakfast*. Use the label in Figure 9.45 to determine the following:
    (a) How many units will you administer?
    (b) How many units are contained in the pen?

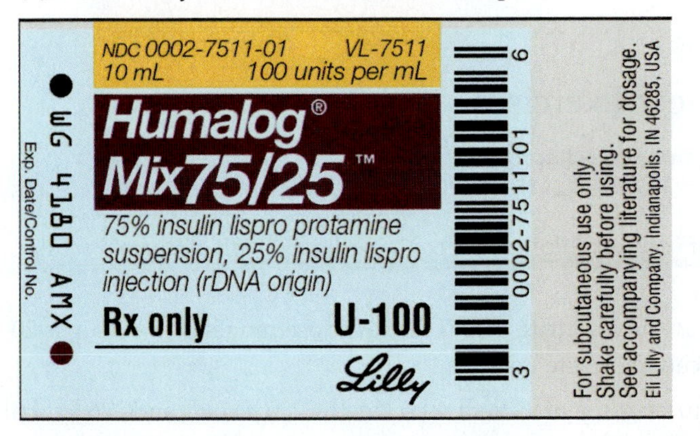

Figure 9.45 Drug label for Humalog Mix 75/25.

18. Use the insulin "sliding scale" below to determine how much insulin you would give to a client whose blood glucose is 244.
    The prescriber ordered *Humulin R Unit 100 insulin subcutaneously for blood-glucose levels as follows:*

Glucose less than 160	no insulin
Glucose 160–220	give 2 *units*
Glucose 221–280	give 4 *units*
Glucose 281–340	give 6 *units*
Glucose 341–400	give 8 *units*
Glucose more than 400	hold insulin and call MD stat

19. A client weighs 110 *pounds*. The daily recommended safe dose range for a certain drug is 0.03–0.04 *mg/kg*.
    (a) What is the minimum number of *milligrams* of this drug that this client should receive each day?
    (b) What is the maximum number of *milligrams* of this drug that this client should receive each day?
20. The prescriber ordered *terbutaline* 0.25 *mg subcut q*15 *to* 30 *minutes, no more than* 0.5 *mg in* 4 *h*. Read the label in Figure 9.46 to answer the following:
    (a) How many *milliliters* would you administer?
    (b) What size syringe would you use?
    (c) What is the maximum number of *milliliters* of this bronchodilator the client may receive in 30 *minutes*?

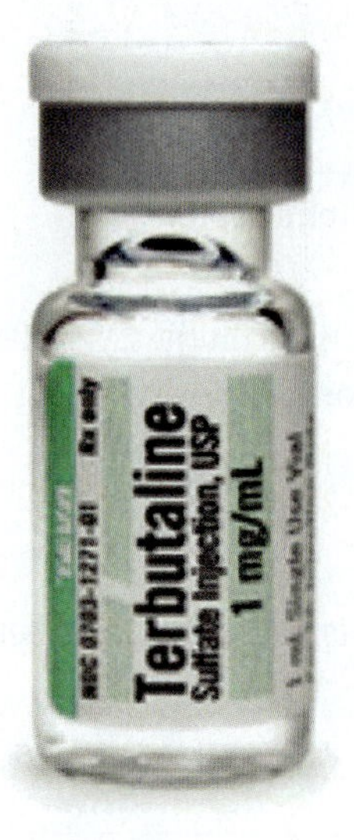

Figure 9.46 Drug label for terbutaline.

SOURCE: © Pearson Education, Inc.

Cumulative Review Exercises

Review your mastery of previous chapters.

1. 330 *lb* = ? *kg*
2. How many grams of sodium chloride are contained in 500 *mL* of normal saline (0.9% NaCl)?
3. A client is receiving 10 *mg* of a drug q4h. If the safe dose range for the drug is 20–40 *mg/d*, is the client receiving a safe dose?
4. Estimate the body surface area of a client who weighs 200 *pounds* and is 6 *feet* tall.

5. Order: *Oxycontin (oxycodone hydrochloride) 10 mg po q6h prn moderate to severe pain.* The strength available is 20 *mg/mL.*
   How many *milliliters* of this analgesic will you administer?

Read the label in Figure 9.47 to answer questions 6 through 10.

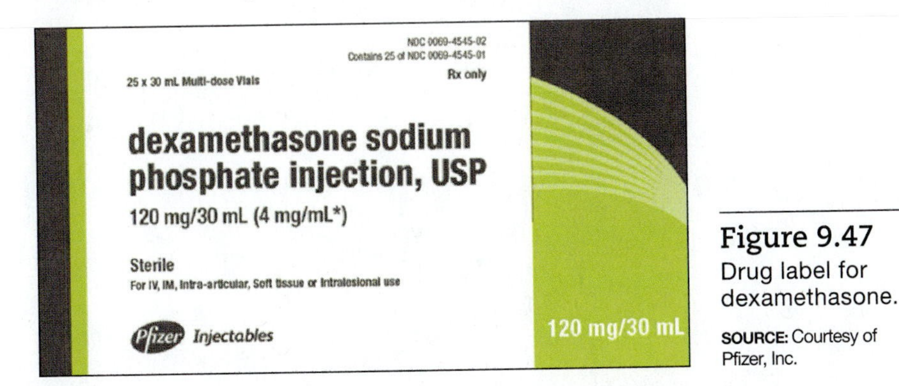

Figure 9.47 Drug label for dexamethasone.

SOURCE: Courtesy of Pfizer, Inc.

6. What is the generic name of this drug?
7. What is the dosage strength?
8. What is the route of administration?
9. A client is to receive 3 *mg* injected into the knee joint. How many *milliliters* will be injected?
10. What is the total volume in the vial?
11. How many *milligrams* of Na Cl are contained in 200 *mL* of a 0.9% NaCl solution?
12. The prescriber ordered *clarithromycin (Biaxin) oral suspension 300 mg PO B.I.D.* Read the label in Figure 9.48 and determine how many *milliliters* of this macrolide antibiotic you will administer.

Figure 9.48 Clarithromycin (Biaxin) label.

SOURCE: Courtesy of AbbVie

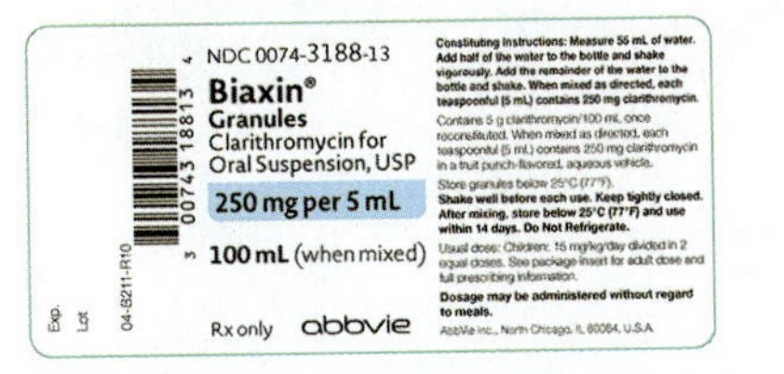

13. The prescriber ordered *duloxetine (Cymbalta) delayed-release capsules 60 mg po once daily* for a client who has fibromyalgia.The strength on the label is 20 *mg* per *cap.* How many capsules will you administer?
14. The prescriber ordered *oxytocin (Pitocin) 20 units IM stat.* The strength on the label is 10 *units* per *mL.*
    (a) How many *milliliters* will you administer?
    (b) What size syringe will you use?
15. The prescriber ordered *epoetin alfa (Epogen) 50 units per kg subcut stat.* The client weighs 150 *pounds* and the strength on the label is 4,000 *units* per *mL.*
    (a) How many *units* will you administer?
    (b) How many *mL* will you administer?
    (c) What size syringe will you use?

Unit 4

Infusions and Pediatric Dosages

Chapter 10

Flow Rates and Durations of Enteral and Intravenous Infusions

Learning Outcomes

After completing this chapter, you will be able to

10.1 Describe the basic concepts and standard equipment used in administering enteral and intravenous (IV) infusions.

10.2 Quickly convert flow rates between *gtt/min* and *mL/h*.

10.3 Calculate the flow rates of enteral and IV infusions.

10.4 Calculate the durations of enteral and IV infusions.

10.5 Determine fluid replacement volumes.

This chapter introduces the basic concepts of enteral and intravenous therapy. For both pumps and gravity systems, you learn how to calculate a flow rate, determine how long an infusion will take, and determine the volume of solution infused. The computations for adjusting flow rates are demonstrated, and fluid balance problems complete the chapter.

Introduction to Enteral and Intravenous Solutions

Fluids can be given to a client slowly over a period of time through a vein (*intravenous*) or through a tube inserted into the alimentary tract (*enteral*). The rate at which these fluids flow into the client is very important and must be controlled precisely.

Enteral Feedings

When a client cannot ingest food or if the upper gastrointestinal tract is not functioning properly, the prescriber may write an order for an *enteral* feeding (*"tube feeding"*). Enteral feedings provide nutrients and other fluids by way of a tube inserted directly into the gastrointestinal system (alimentary tract).

There are various types of tube feedings. A gastric tube may be inserted into the stomach through the nares (**nasogastric,** as shown in Figure 10.1) or through the mouth (**orogastric**). A longer tube may be similarly inserted, but would extend beyond the stomach into the jejunum in the upper small intestine (**nasojejunum** or **orojejunum**).

For long-term feedings, tubes can be inserted surgically or laproscopically through the wall of the abdomen and directly into either the stomach (gastrostomy) or through the stomach and on to the jejunum (jejunostomy). These tubes are sutured in place and are referred to as *percutaneous endoscopic gastrostomy* (*PEG*) tubes and *percutaneous endoscopic jejunostomy* (*PEJ*) *tubes*, respectively (Figure 10.2).

Figure 10.1 A client with a nasogastric tube.

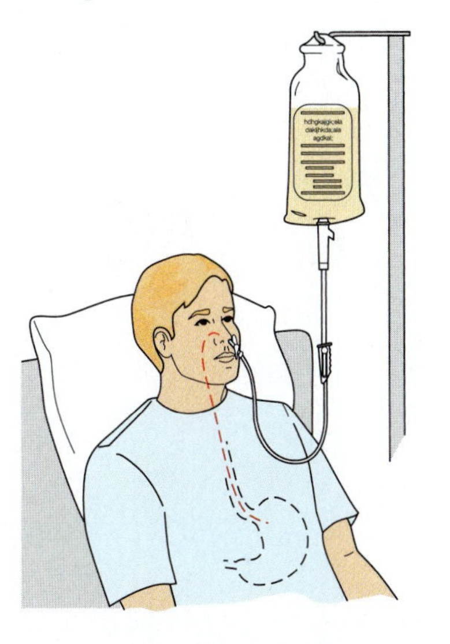

Figure 10.2 A percutaneous endoscopic jejunostomy (PEJ) tube.

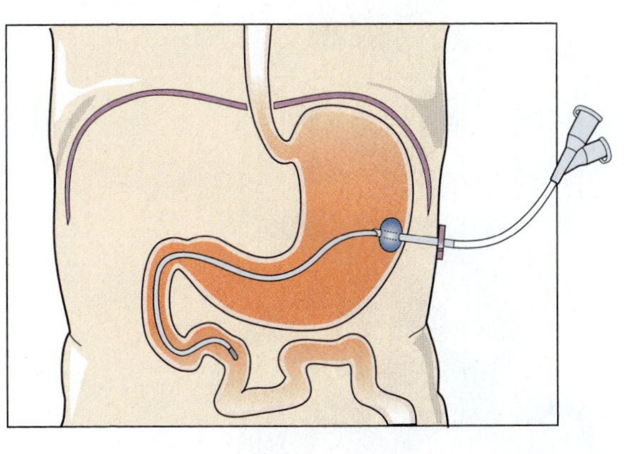

Enteral feedings may be given *continuously* (over a 24-hour period) or *intermittently* (over shorter periods, perhaps several times a day). There are many enteral feeding solutions, including Boost, Compleat, Ensure, Isocal, Resource, and Sustacal. Enteral feedings are generally administered via pump (Figure 10.3).

Orders for enteral solutions always indicate a volume of fluid to be infused over a period of time; that is, a flow rate. For example, a tube feeding order might read ***Isocal 50 mL/h via nasogastric tube for 6 hours beginning 6 A.M.*** This order is for an intermittent feeding in which the name of the solution is Isocal, the rate of flow is 50 *mL/h*, the route of administration is via nasogastric tube, and the duration is 6 *hours*.

Intravenous Infusions

Intravenous (IV) means "through the vein." Fluids are administered intravenously to provide a variety of fluids, including blood, water containing nutrients, electrolytes, minerals, and specific medications to the client. IV fluids can replace lost fluids, maintain fluid and electrolyte balance, or serve as a medium to introduce medications directly into the bloodstream.

Replacement fluids are ordered for a client who has lost fluids through hemorrhage, vomiting, or diarrhea. *Maintenance fluids* help sustain normal levels of fluids and electrolytes. They are ordered for clients who are at risk of becoming depleted; for example, clients who are NPO (nothing by mouth).

Intravenous infusions may be *continuous* or *intermittent*. Continuous IV infusions are used to replace or maintain fluids or electrolytes. Intermittent IV infusions—for example, IV piggyback (IVPB) and IV push (IVP)—are used to administer drugs and supplemental fluids. *Intermittent peripheral infusion devices* (saline locks or heparin locks) are used to maintain venous access without continuous fluid infusion. Intermittent IV infusions are discussed in Chapter 11.

A healthcare professional must be able to perform the calculations to determine the correct rate at which an enteral or intravenous solution will enter the body (*flow rate*).

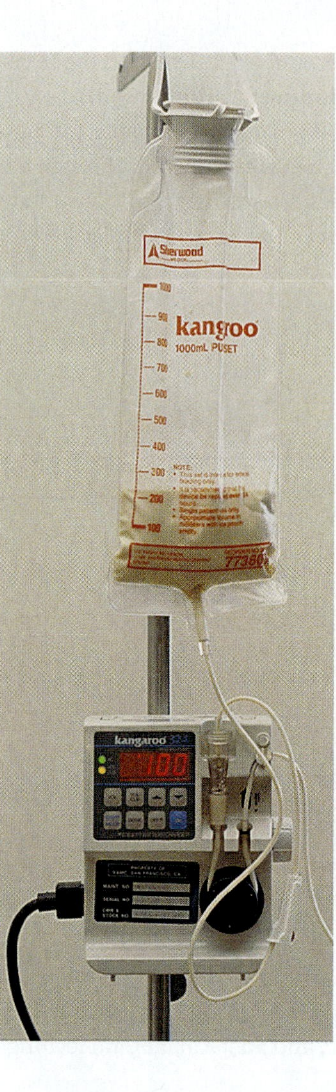

Figure 10.3 Enteral feeding via pump.

SOURCE: Pearson Education, Inc.

Infusion flow rates are usually measured in drops per *minute* (*gtt/min*) or *milliliters* per *hour* (*mL/h*). It is important to be able to convert each of these rates to the other and to determine how long a given amount of solution will take to infuse.

For example, a continuous IV order might read ***IV fluids: D5W 125 mL/h for 8h***. In this case, the order is for an IV infusion in which the name of the solution is 5% dextrose in water, the rate of flow is 125 *mL/h*, the route of administration is intravenous, and the duration is 8 hours.

Intravenous Solutions

A saline solution, which is a solution of *sodium chloride (NaCl)* in sterile water, is commonly used for intravenous infusion. Sodium chloride is ordinary table salt. Saline solutions are available in various concentrations for different purposes. A 0.9% NaCl solution is also referred to as **normal saline (NS)**. Other saline solutions commonly used include **half-normal saline** (0.45% NaCl), written as $\frac{1}{2}$NS; and **quarter-normal saline** (0.225% NaCl), written as $\frac{1}{4}$NS.

Intravenous fluids generally contain dextrose, sodium chloride, or electrolytes:

- D5W, D5/W, or 5% D/W is a 5% dextrose solution, which means that 5 *g* of dextrose are dissolved in water to make each 100 *mL* of this solution (Figures 10.4a and 10.4b).
- NS or 0.9% NaCl is a solution in which each 100 *mL* contain 0.9 *g* of sodium chloride (Figures 10.4c and 10.4d).
- 5% D/0.45% NaCl is a solution containing 5 *g* of dextrose and 0.45 *g* of NaCl in each 100 *mL* of solution (Figure 10.5b).
- Ringer's Lactate (RL), also called Lactated Ringer's solution (LRS), is a solution containing electrolytes, including potassium chloride and calcium chloride (Figure 10.5c).

NOTE

Pay close attention to the abbreviations of the names of the IV solutions. *Letters* indicate the solution compounds, whereas *numbers* indicate the solution strength (e.g., D5W).

Figure 10.4 Examples of IV bags and labels.

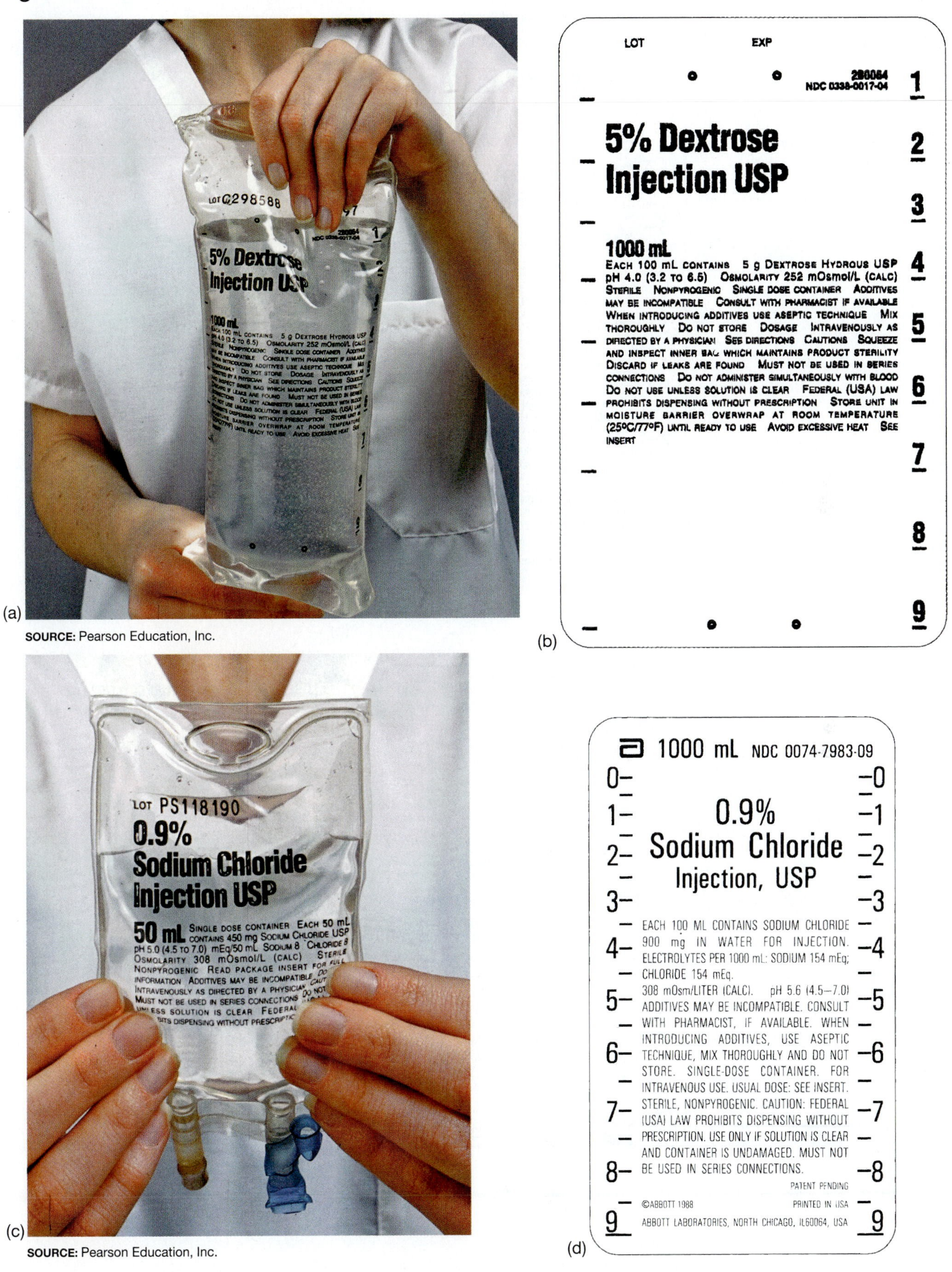

(a) **SOURCE:** Pearson Education, Inc.

(b)

(c) **SOURCE:** Pearson Education, Inc.

(d)

> **ALERT**
>
> In Figures 10.5, solutions (a) and (b) both contain 5% dextrose and $\frac{1}{2}$ NS. However, solution (a) also contains 20 *mEq* of potassium chloride, which is a high-alert medication. Do not confuse these two solutions.

Figure 10.5 Examples of intravenous fluids.

(Reproduced with permission of Abbott Laboratories.)

20 mEq POTASSIUM

1000 mL NDC 0074-7902-09

20 mEq POTASSIUM CHLORIDE

in 5% Dextrose and
0.45% Sodium Chloride Inj., USP

EACH 100 mL CONTAINS POTASSIUM CHLORIDE 149 mg; SODIUM CHLORIDE 450 mg; DEXTROSE, HYDROUS 5 g IN WATER FOR INJECTION. MAY CONTAIN HCl FOR pH ADJUSTMENT. ELECTROLYTES PER 1000 mL (NOT INCLUDING IONS FOR pH ADJUSTMENT): POTASSIUM 20 mEq; SODIUM 77 mEq; CHLORIDE 97 mEq.
447 mOsmol/LITER (CALC). pH 4.2 (3.5 – 6.5)

ADDITIVES MAY BE INCOMPATIBLE. CONSULT WITH PHARMACIST, IF AVAILABLE. WHEN INTRODUCING ADDITIVES, USE ASEPTIC TECHNIQUE, MIX THOROUGHLY AND DO NOT STORE.

SINGLE-DOSE CONTAINER. FOR INTRAVENOUS USE. USUAL DOSE: SEE INSERT. STERILE, NONPYROGENIC. CAUTION: FEDERAL (USA) LAW PROHIBITS DISPENSING WITHOUT PRESCRIPTION. USE ONLY IF SOLUTION IS CLEAR AND CONTAINER IS UNDAMAGED. MUST NOT BE USED IN SERIES CONNECTIONS.
U.S. PAT. NO. 4,368,765
©ABBOTT 1994 PRINTED IN USA
ABBOTT LABORATORIES, NORTH CHICAGO, IL 60064, USA

1 2 3 4 5 6 7 8 9

(a)

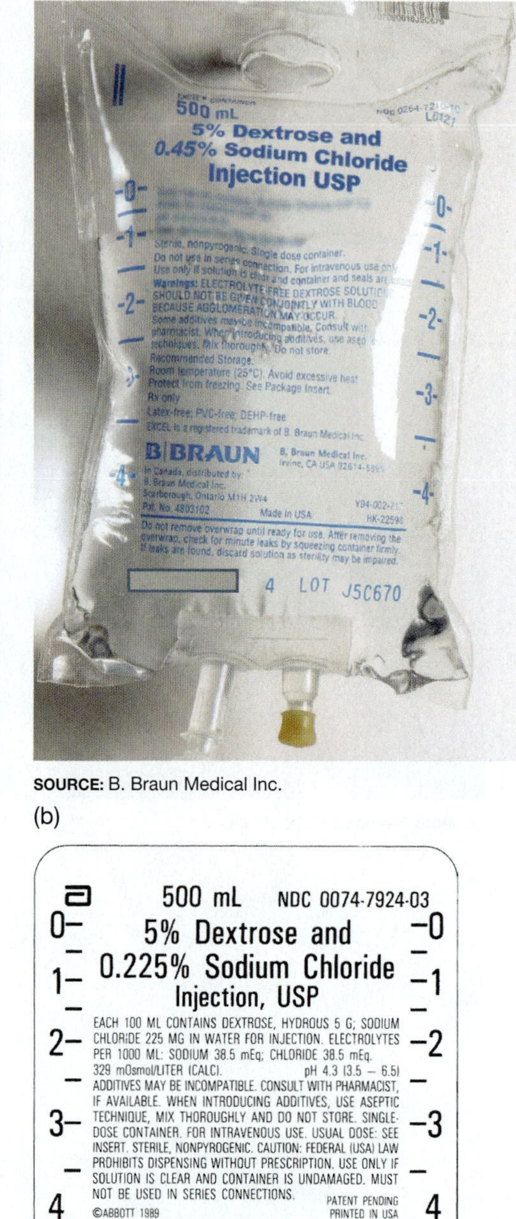

SOURCE: B. Braun Medical Inc.

(b)

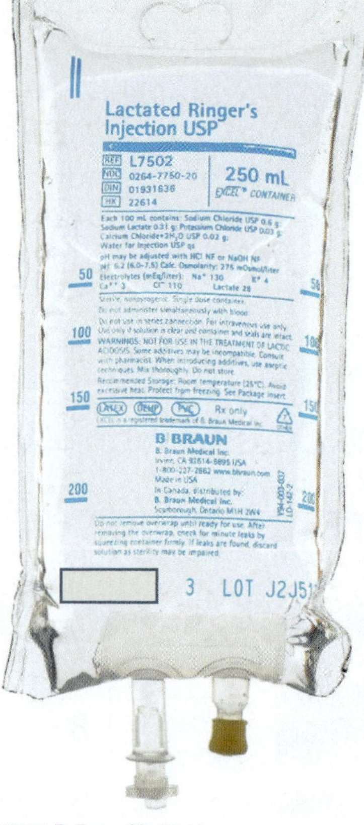

SOURCE: B. Braun Medical Inc.

(c)

500 mL NDC 0074-7924-03

5% Dextrose and
0.225% Sodium Chloride
Injection, USP

EACH 100 ML CONTAINS DEXTROSE, HYDROUS 5 G; SODIUM CHLORIDE 225 MG IN WATER FOR INJECTION. ELECTROLYTES PER 1000 ML: SODIUM 38.5 mEq; CHLORIDE 38.5 mEq.
329 mOsmol/LITER (CALC). pH 4.3 (3.5 – 6.5)
ADDITIVES MAY BE INCOMPATIBLE. CONSULT WITH PHARMACIST, IF AVAILABLE. WHEN INTRODUCING ADDITIVES, USE ASEPTIC TECHNIQUE, MIX THOROUGHLY AND DO NOT STORE. SINGLE-DOSE CONTAINER. FOR INTRAVENOUS USE. USUAL DOSE: SEE INSERT. STERILE, NONPYROGENIC. CAUTION: FEDERAL (USA) LAW PROHIBITS DISPENSING WITHOUT PRESCRIPTION. USE ONLY IF SOLUTION IS CLEAR AND CONTAINER IS UNDAMAGED. MUST NOT BE USED IN SERIES CONNECTIONS.
PATENT PENDING
©ABBOTT 1989 PRINTED IN USA
ABBOTT LABORATORIES, NORTH CHICAGO, IL60064, USA

0 1 2 3 4

(d)

Additional information on the many other IV fluids can be found in nursing and pharmacology textbooks.

Gravity Systems and Pumps

Equipment used for the administration of continuous IV infusions includes the IV solution and IV tubing, a drip chamber, at least one injection port, and a roller clamp. The tubing connects the IV solution to the hub of an IV catheter at the infusion site. The rate of flow of the infusion is regulated by an electronic infusion device (pump or controller) or by gravity (Figures 10.6 and 10.9).

ALERT

No intravenous solution should infuse for more than 24 hours. Be sure to check the institution's policy.

Figure 10.6 Primary intravenous line (gravity flow).

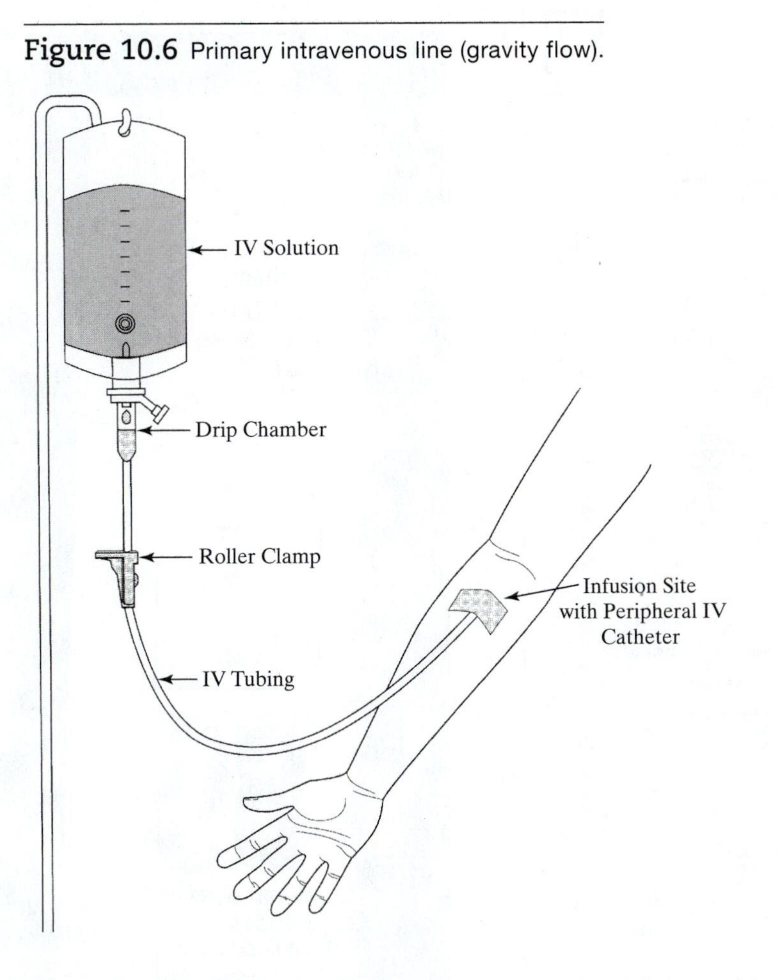

Figure 10.7 Tubing with drip chamber.

SOURCE: Photodisc/Getty Images

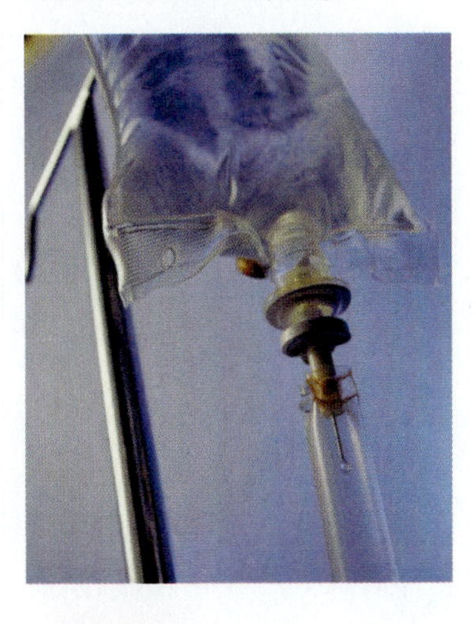

The *drip chamber* (Figure 10.6) is located at the site of the entrance of the tubing into the container of intravenous solution. It allows you to count the number of drops per minute that the client is receiving (flow rate).

A *roll valve clamp or clip* is connected to the tubing and can be manipulated to increase or decrease the flow rate.

ALERT

Be sure to follow the procedures for eliminating all air in the tubing.

The size of the drop that IV tubing delivers is not standard; it depends on the way the tubing is designed (Figure 10.7). Manufacturers specify the number of drops that equal 1 *mL* for their particular tubing. This equivalent is called the tubing's **drop factor** (Figure 10.8 and Table 10.1). You must know the tubing's drop factor when calculating the flow rate of solutions in *drops per minute (gtt/min)* or *microdrops per minute (mcgtt/min)*.

It is difficult to visually make an accurate count of the drops falling per minute when setting the flow rate on a gravity system infusion. In addition, the flow rate of a gravity system infusion depends on the *relative heights* of the IV bag and the infusion site; changes in the relative position of either may cause flow rate changes. Electric IV pumps and controllers now make up the majority of infusion systems in use in healthcare facilities.

> **NOTE**
>
> 60 microdrops = 1 *mL* is a universal equivalent for IV tubing calibrated in microdrops.

Table 10.1 Common Drop Factors

10 *gtt* = 1 *mL* 15 *gtt* = 1 *mL* 20 *gtt* = 1 *mL*	macrodrops
60 *mcgtt* = 1 *mL*	microdrops

Figure 10.8 Samples of IV tubing containers with drop factors of 10 and 60.

SOURCE: Pearson Education, Inc.

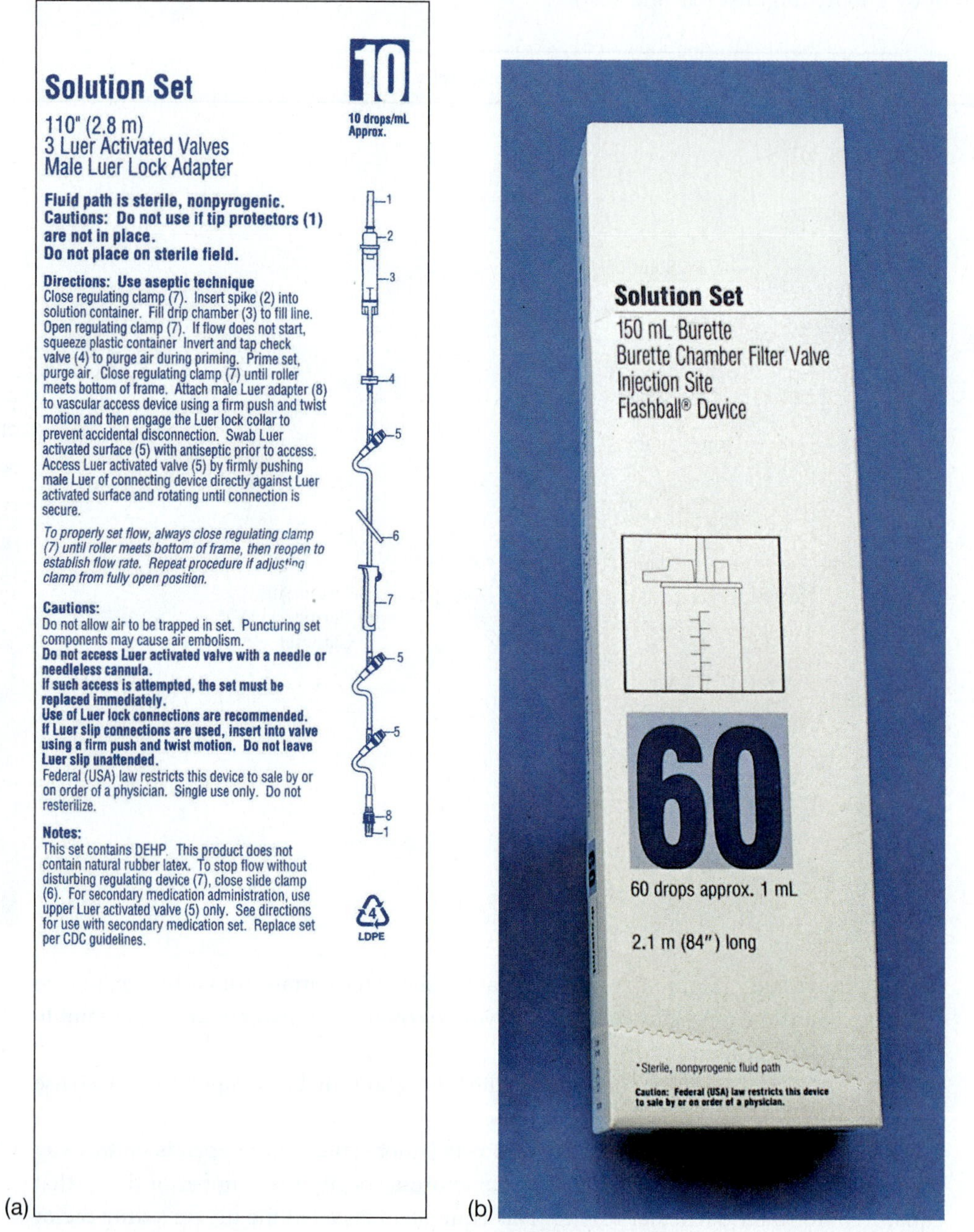

SOURCE: Pearson Education, Inc.

An intravenous infusion can flow solely by the force of gravity or by an electronic infusion pump. There are many different types of electronic infusion pumps (Figure 10.9).

These electrically operated devices allow the rate of flow (usually specified in *mL/h*) to be simply keyed into the device by the user. The pumps can more precisely regulate the flow rate than can the gravity systems. For example, pumps detect an interruption in the flow (constriction) and sound an alarm to alert the nursing staff and the client, sound

Figure 10.9 Volumetric infusion pump.

SOURCE: Pearson Education, Inc.

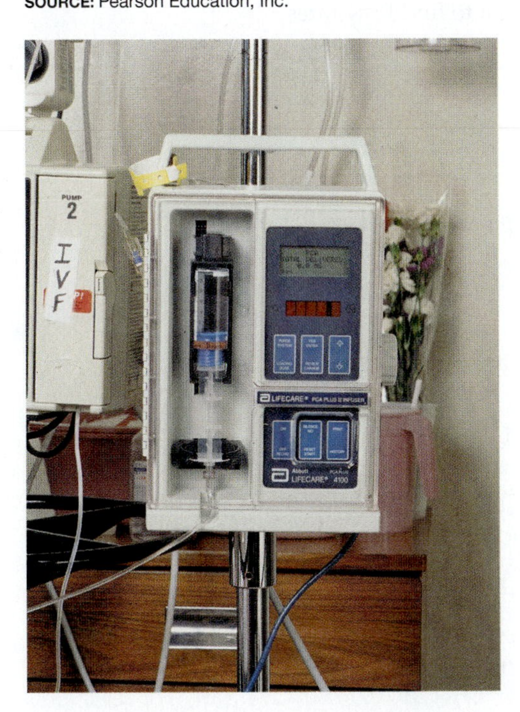

Figure 10.10 Patient-controlled analgesia (PCA) (a) pump and (b) control button.

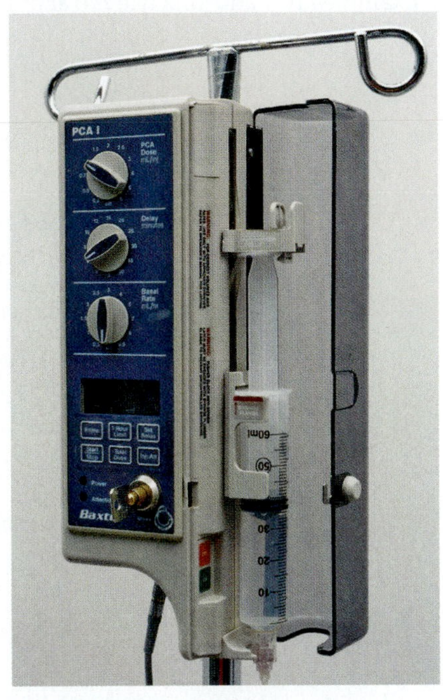

SOURCE: Pearson Education, Inc.
(a)

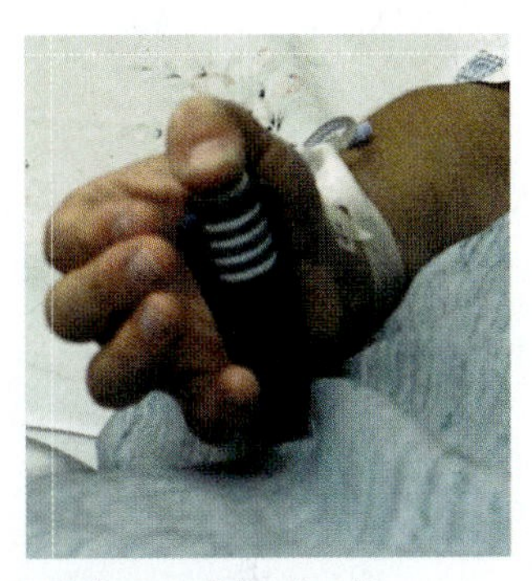

SOURCE: Pearson Education, Inc.
(b)

an alarm when the infusion finishes, indicate the volume of fluid already infused, and indicate the time remaining for the infusion to finish. "Smart" pumps may contain libraries of safe dosage ranges that will help prevent the user from keying in an unsafe dosage.

A ***client-controlled analgesia (PCA) pump*** (see Figure 10.10) allows a client to self-administer pain-relieving drugs. The dose is predetermined by the physician, and the pump is programmed accordingly. To receive the drug when pain relief is needed, the client presses the button on the handset, which is connected to the PCA pump. A lockout device in the pump prevents client overdose.

ALERT

A facility might use many different types of infusion pumps. The healthcare provider must learn how to program all of them. Be sure to use the specific tubing supplied by the manufacturer for each pump.

Calculations for Infusions

Infusions involve three quantitative components: flow rate, volume of fluid infused, and duration of the IV. For most of the calculations involving infusions, two of these three major components are known, and you are asked to find the missing third component. Most intravenous or enteral solutions are administered by using a pump that measures flow rates in *milliliters per hour.* Examples 10.1 through 10.6 illustrate problems where pumps are used.

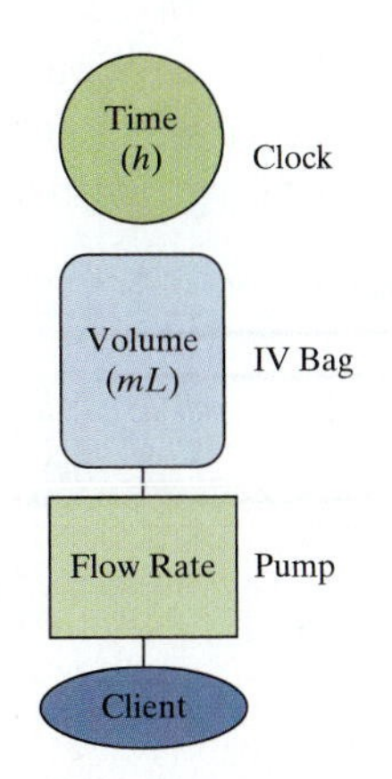

Finding the Flow Rate on a Pump

The **flow rate** of an infusion is the *volume of fluid* that enters the client over a *period of time.* For example, 25 *mL/h* and 15 *gtt/min* are flow rates. The following formula may be used to determine a flow rate.

$$\textit{Flow Rate} = \frac{\textit{Volume}}{\textit{Time}}$$

Examples 10.1 and 10.2 use the above formula to find flow rates.

Example 10.1

Order: *NS 1,000 mL continuous IV for 24 hours.* Find the pump setting in *milliliters per hour*.

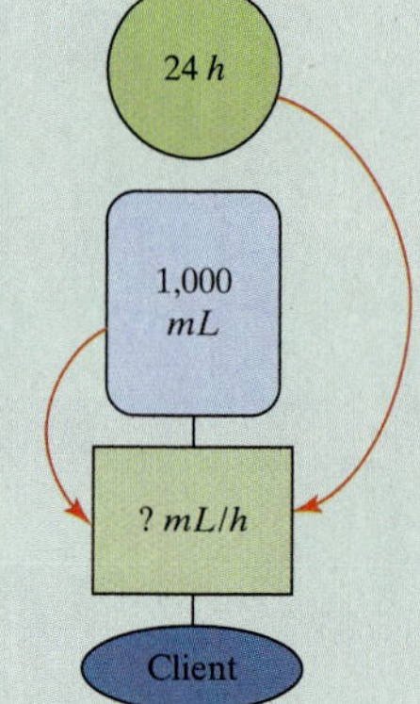

To find the flow rate, use the formula

$$\textit{Flow Rate} = \frac{\textit{Volume}}{\textit{Time}}$$

Substitute 1,000 *mL* for the volume in the bag and 24 *h* for the time.

$$\textit{Flow Rate} = \frac{1{,}000\ mL}{24\ h} = 41.67\ mL/h$$

So, the pump setting is 42 *mL/h*.

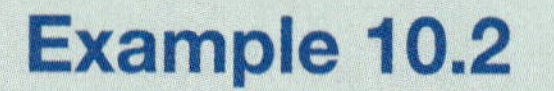

Example 10.2

A client must receive a tube-feeding of *Ensure 120 milliliters in 90 minutes.* Calculate the flow rate in *milliliters per hour.*

Volume to be infused: *120 mL*

Time: *90 min*

Flow rate you want to find: **?** *mL/h*

The flow rate $\frac{\textit{volume}}{\textit{time}}$ can be determined by placing the volume [*120 mL*] over the time [*90 min*].

$$\frac{120\ mL}{90\ min} = ?\ \frac{mL}{h}$$

DIMENSIONAL ANALYSIS

You want to change one flow rate [*mL/min*] to another flow rate [*mL/h*]. Each flow rate has *mL* in the numerator, which is what you want. You want to cancel *min*, which is in the denominator. To do this, you must use a unit fraction containing *min* in the numerator.

Because 1 *h* = 60 *min*, this fraction will be $\frac{60\ min}{1\ h}$

$$\frac{120\ mL}{90\ \cancel{min}} \times \frac{60\ \cancel{min}}{1\ h} = \frac{80\ mL}{1\ h}$$

RATIO & PROPORTION

Because 1 *hour* = 60 *minutes*, the problem becomes

$$\frac{120\ mL}{90\ min} = ?\ \frac{mL}{60\ min}$$

$$\frac{120\ mL}{90\ min} = \frac{x\ mL}{60\ min}$$

$$90\,x = 7{,}200$$

$$x = 80$$

So, the flow rate is *80 milliliters per hour.*

Finding the Volume Infused Using a Pump

In Examples 10.3 and 10.4, you are asked to find the infused volume. This is done by converting the time (*h*) to volume (*mL*) by using the flow rate (*mL/h*) as the unit fraction.

Example 10.3

Order: *Lactated Ringer's at 167 mL/h IV for 6 h.* How many *milliliters* will the client receive in 6 *hours*?

DIMENSIONAL ANALYSIS

Time:	*6 h*	[single unit of measurement]
Flow rate:	*167 mL/h*	[equivalence]
Volume to be infused:	*? mL*	[single unit of measurement]

In this example, you want to change the single unit of measurement [6 *h*] to another single unit of measurement [*mL*].

$$6\ h = ?\ mL$$

The flow rate provides the equivalence [167 *mL* = 1 *h*] for the unit fraction.

$$6\ \cancel{h} \times \frac{167\ mL}{\cancel{h}} = 1{,}002\ mL$$

RATIO & PROPORTION

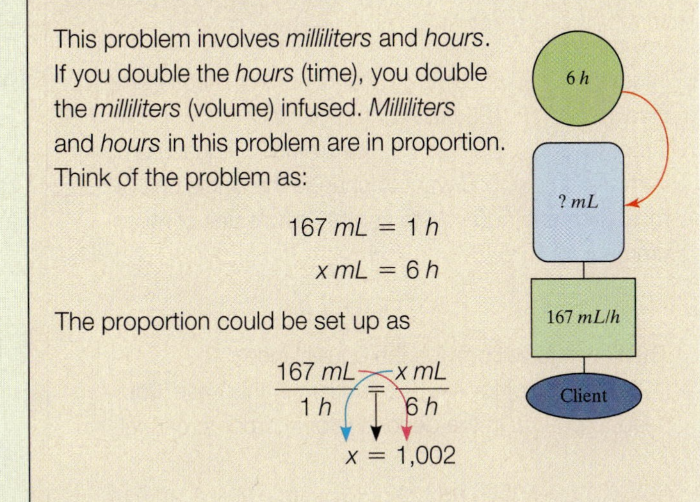

This problem involves *milliliters* and *hours*. If you double the *hours* (time), you double the *milliliters* (volume) infused. *Milliliters* and *hours* in this problem are in proportion. Think of the problem as:

$$167\ mL = 1\ h$$
$$x\ mL = 6\ h$$

The proportion could be set up as

$$\frac{167\ mL}{1\ h} = \frac{x\ mL}{6\ h}$$

$$x = 1{,}002$$

So, the client will receive *1,002 milliliters* of Lactated Ringer's.

Example 10.4

D5/W has been infusing at 30 mL/h IV for 8 hours. How many milliliters have infused?

DIMENSIONAL ANALYSIS

In this example, you change *8 h* to *? mL*, using 30 *mL/h* as the unit fraction.

$$8\ h = ?\ mL$$

$$\frac{8\ \cancel{h}}{1} \times \frac{30\ mL}{\cancel{h}} = 240\ mL$$

RATIO & PROPORTION

Milliliters and *hours* are proportional. Think of the problem as:

$$30\ mL = 1\ h$$
$$?\ mL = 8\ h$$

The proportion could be set up as

$$\frac{30\ mL}{1\ h} = \frac{x\ mL}{8\ h}$$

Cross multiply $x = 240$

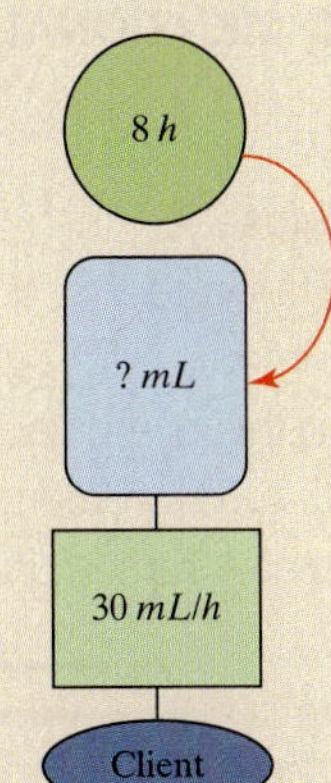

So, *240 mL* of D5/W have infused.

Finding the Duration of an Infusion Using a Pump

In Examples 10.5 and 10.6, you are asked to find the duration of an infusion. This will be done by converting the ***volume (mL)*** to ***time (h)*** by using the flow rate ***(mL/h)*** as the unit fraction.

Example 10.5

Order: ***0.9% NaCl 500 mL IV at 125 mL/h.*** **How long will this infusion take?**

DIMENSIONAL ANALYSIS

Volume to be infused:	*500 mL*	[single unit of measurement]
Flow rate:	*125 mL/h*	[equivalence]
Time:	*? h*	[single unit of measurement]

In this example, you want to change the single unit of measurement [*500 mL*] to another single unit of measurement [*h*].

$$500\ mL = ?\ h$$

The flow rate will provide the equivalence [125 *mL* = 1 *h*] for the unit fraction. In this case, you need to put *mL* in the denominator in order to cancel.

$$500\ \cancel{mL} \times \frac{1\ h}{125\ \cancel{mL}} = 4\ h$$

RATIO & PROPORTION

This problem involves *milliliters* and *hours*. If you double the *hours* (time), you double the *milliliters* (volume) infused. *Milliliters* and *hours* in this problem are in proportion.

Think of the problem as:

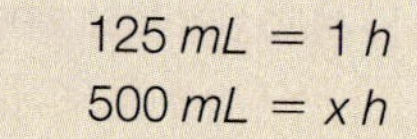

$$125\ mL = 1\ h$$
$$500\ mL = x\ h$$

The proportion could be set up as

$$\frac{125\ mL}{1\ h} = \frac{500\ mL}{x\ h}$$
$$500 = 125x$$
$$4 = x$$

? h

500 mL

125 mL/h

Client

So, the infusion will take *4 hours.*

Example 10.6

Order: $\frac{1}{2}$ ***NS 1,000 mL IV at 50 mL/h.*** **If the IV starts at** ***1200h on Monday,*** **at what time will it finish?**

DIMENSIONAL ANALYSIS

Volume to be infused:	*1,000 mL*	[single unit of measurement]
Flow rate:	*50 mL/h*	[equivalence]
Time:	*? h*	[single unit of measurement]

In this example, you want to change the single unit of measurement [*1,000 mL*] to another single unit of measurement [*h*].

$$1{,}000\ mL = ?\ h$$

The flow rate will provide the equivalence [50 *mL* = 1 *h*] for the unit fraction. In this case, you need to put *mL* in the denominator in order to cancel.

$$1{,}000\ \cancel{mL} \times \frac{1\ h}{50\ \cancel{mL}} = 20\ h$$

RATIO & PROPORTION

Think of the problem as:

$$50\ mL = 1\ h$$
$$1{,}000\ mL = x\ h$$

The proportion could be set up as

$$\frac{50\ mL}{1\ h} = \frac{1{,}000\ mL}{x\ h}$$
$$1{,}000 = 50x$$
$$20 = x$$

? h

1,000 mL

50 mL/h

Client

So, the infusion will take 20 hours.

One way to continue is to add

$$\begin{array}{r} 1200\,h \\ +\ 2000\,h \\ \hline 3200\,h \end{array}$$

Because military time has a 24 clock, you must now subtract 2400 *h*.

$$\begin{array}{r} 3200\,h \\ -\ 2400\,h \\ \hline 0800\,h \end{array}$$

So, the infusion will finish at *0800 h on Tuesday.*

Flow Rate Conversion Number

Flow rates for gravity systems are measured in *drops/minute (gtt/min)*. A quick way to convert flow rates from *mL/h* to *gtt/min*, and vice versa, is to use the flow rate conversion number method.

The **flow rate conversion number,** abbreviated as **FC** (think: flow converter), is equal to the quotient of 60 and the drop factor (DF). That is,

$$FC = \frac{60}{DF}$$

For example, if the DF is 15 *gtt/mL*, then the FC is obtained as follows:

$$FC = \frac{60}{15} = 4$$

Table 10.2 shows the common drop factors and their corresponding flow rate conversion numbers.

Table 10.2 Common Drop Factors and Corresponding Flow Rate Conversion Numbers

Drop Factor	Flow Rate Conversion Number
10	$\frac{60}{10} = 6$
15	$\frac{60}{15} = 4$
20	$\frac{60}{20} = 3$
60	$\frac{60}{60} = 1$

To change flow rates between *mL/h* and *gtt/min* involves simply multiplying or dividing the given flow rate by the flow rate conversion number as follows:

To change from mL/h to gtt/min, divide the given rate by FC.

To change from gtt/min to mL/h, multiply the given rate by FC.

An easy way to remember the FC method is:

When you want *Drops*, *Divide*.

When you want *Milliliters*, *Multiply*.

Both dimensional analysis and FC methods are illustrated in Examples 10.7 through 10.14.

Finding the Flow Rate (Drip Rate) Using a Gravity System

Solutions are also infused using gravity systems that measure flow rates in *drops per minute.* Calculations for gravity systems are similar to those for pumps, except that for *Dimensional Analysis* the drop factor is used as a unit fraction, and for *Ratio & Proportion* the FC method is used to convert flow rates between *gtt/min* and *mL/h.* Examples 10.7 through 10.9 illustrate finding flow rates in drops per minute for gravity systems.

Example 10.7

The prescriber ordered $\frac{1}{4}$ *NS 850 mL IV in 8 hours.* The label on the box containing the intravenous set to be used for this infusion is shown in Figure 10.11. Calculate the flow rate in drops per minute.

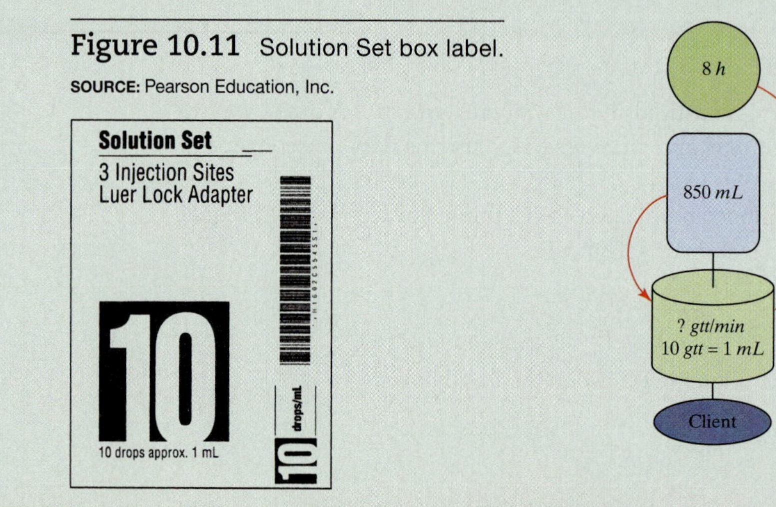

Figure 10.11 Solution Set box label.

SOURCE: Pearson Education, Inc.

DIMENSIONAL ANALYSIS

Given flow rate: 850 *mL*/8 *h*

Known equivalences: 10 *gtt*/*mL* (drop factor)

1 *h* = 60 *min*

Flow rate you want to find: ? *gtt*/*min*

You want to convert the flow rate from *milliliters* per *hour* to *drops per minute*.

$$\frac{850\ mL}{8\ h} = \frac{?\ gtt}{min}$$

You want to cancel *mL*. To do this you must use a unit fraction containing *mL* in the denominator. Using the drop factor, this fraction will be $\frac{10\ gtt}{1\ mL}$

$$\frac{850\ \cancel{mL}}{8\ h} \times \frac{10\ gtt}{1\ \cancel{mL}} = \frac{?\ gtt}{min}$$

Now, on the left side *gtt* is in the numerator, which is what you want. But *h* is in the denominator and it must be cancelled. This will require a unit fraction with *h* in the numerator, namely, $\frac{1\ h}{60\ min}$

Now cancel and multiply the numbers

$$\frac{850\ \cancel{mL}}{8\ \cancel{h}} \times \frac{1\cancel{0}\ gtt}{1\ \cancel{mL}} \times \frac{1\ \cancel{h}}{6\cancel{0}\ min} = 17.7\ \frac{gtt}{min}$$

FC METHOD

The problem is

$$\frac{850\ mL}{8\ h} = ?\ \frac{gtt}{min}$$

Because

$$\frac{850}{8} = 106.25$$

The problem becomes

$$106.25\ \frac{mL}{h} = ?\ \frac{gtt}{min}$$

DF = 10, therefore

$$FC = \frac{60}{10} = 6$$

Because you want *Drops* per minute, Divide the given flow rate by 6

$$\frac{106.25}{6} = 17.7$$

So, the flow rate is 18 *drops per minute*.

Example 10.8

The prescriber orders *D5/0.45% NaCl IV to infuse at 21 drops per minute*. If the drop factor is 20 *drops per milliliter*, how many *milliliters per hour* will the client receive?

Given flow rate: 21 *gtt/min*

Known equivalences: 20 *gtt/mL* (drop factor)

1 *h* = 60 *min*

Flow rate you want to find: ? *mL/h*

You want to convert a flow rate of 21 *drops per minute* to a flow rate in *milliliters per hour*.

$$\frac{21\ gtt}{min} = \frac{?\ mL}{h}$$

21 gtt/min
20 gtt = 1 mL
? mL/h
Client

DIMENSIONAL ANALYSIS

You want to cancel *gtt*. To do this you must use a unit fraction containing *gtt* in the denominator.

Using the drop factor, this fraction is $\frac{1\ mL}{20\ gtt}$

$$\frac{21\ gtt}{min} \times \frac{1\ mL}{20\ gtt} = \frac{?\ mL}{h}$$

Now, on the left side *mL* is in the numerator, which is what you want. But *min* is in the denominator and it must be cancelled. This will require a unit fraction with *min* in the numerator, namely, $\frac{60\ min}{1\ h}$

Now cancel and multiply the numbers

$$\frac{21\ gtt}{min} \times \frac{1\ mL}{20\ gtt} \times \frac{60\ min}{1\ h} = 63\ \frac{mL}{h}$$

FC METHOD

The problem is

$$21\ \frac{gtt}{min} = ?\ \frac{mL}{h}$$

DF = 20, therefore

$$FC = \frac{60}{20} = 3$$

Because you want Milliliters per hour, Multiply the given flow rate by 3

$$21 \times 3 = 63$$

So, the flow rate is 63 *mL* per *hour*.

Example 10.9

The order reads *125 mL D5W IV in 1 hour.* What is the flow rate in *microdrops per minute*?

DIMENSIONAL ANALYSIS

Given flow rate: 125 *mL/h*

Known equivalences: 60 *mcgtt/mL* (drop factor for microdrops)

1 *h* = 60 *min*

Flow rate you want to find: ? *mcgtt/min*

FC METHOD

The problem is

$$\frac{125\ mL}{1\ h} = ?\ \frac{mcgtt}{min}$$

Because this is a conversion from *mL/h* to *gtt/min,* use the FC technique.

(Continued)

You want to change the flow rate from 125 *mL* per *hour* to *microdrops per minute*.

$$\frac{125\ mL}{h} = \frac{?\ mcgtt}{min}$$

You want to cancel *mL*. To do this you must use a unit fraction containing *mL* in the denominator. Using the drop factor, this fraction will be $\frac{60\ mcgtt}{1\ mL}$

$$\frac{125\ \cancel{mL}}{h} \times \frac{60\ mcgtt}{1\ \cancel{mL}} = \frac{?\ mcgtt}{min}$$

Now, on the left side *mcgtt* is in the numerator, which is what you want. But *h* is in the denominator and it must be cancelled. This will require a unit fraction with *h* in the numerator, namely, $\frac{1\ h}{60\ min}$

Now cancel and multiply the numbers

$$\frac{125\ \cancel{mL}}{\cancel{h}} \times \frac{60\ mcgtt}{1\ \cancel{mL}} \times \frac{1\ \cancel{h}}{60\ min} = 125\ \frac{mcgtt}{min}$$

It is standard that 60 *mcgtt* = 1 *mL*, therefore, use DF = 60 to calculate FC.

$$FC = \frac{60}{DF}$$

$$FC = \frac{60}{60} = 1$$

Because you want Drops per minute, Divide the given flow rate by FC

$$\frac{125}{1} = 125$$

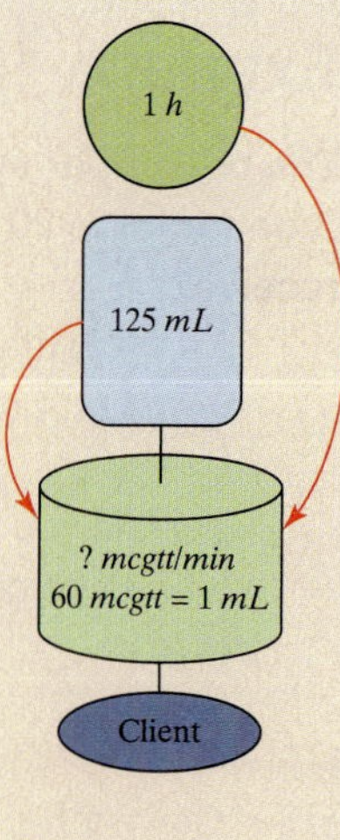

So, 125 *mL* per *hour* is the same rate of flow as 125 *microdrops per minute*.

NOTE

In Example 10.9, it is shown that 125 *mL* per *hour* is the same flow rate as 125 *microdrops per minute* because the 60s always cancel. The flow rates of *milliliters per hour* and *microdrops per minute* are equivalent. Therefore, calculations are not necessary to change *mL/h* to *mcgtt/min*.

Finding the Volume Infused Using a Gravity System

Examples 10.10 and 10.11 illustrate finding infused volumes for gravity systems.

Example 10.10

How many *milliliters* of D5 W will infuse intravenously in 10 *hours* at the rate of 13 *gtt/min*? The drop factor is 15 *gtt/mL*.

DIMENSIONAL ANALYSIS

In this example, you change 10 *h* to ? *mL*, using both the flow rate of 13 *gtt/min* and the drop factor of 15 *gtt/mL* as unit fractions.

$$10\ h = ?\ mL$$

Now, you will have to do the following:

$$10\ h \longrightarrow ?\ min \longrightarrow ?\ gtt \longrightarrow ?\ mL$$

$$\frac{10\ \cancel{h}}{1} \times \frac{60\ \cancel{min}}{\cancel{h}} \times \frac{13\ \cancel{gtt}}{\cancel{min}} \times \frac{mL}{15\ \cancel{gtt}} = 520\ mL$$

RATIO & PROPORTION

The first problem is to convert the flow rate to *mL/h*.

$$13\ \frac{gtt}{min} = ?\ \frac{mL}{h}$$

DF = 15, therefore

$$FC = \frac{60}{15} = 4$$

Because you want Milliliters per hour, Multiply the given flow rate by 4

$$13 \times 4 = 52$$

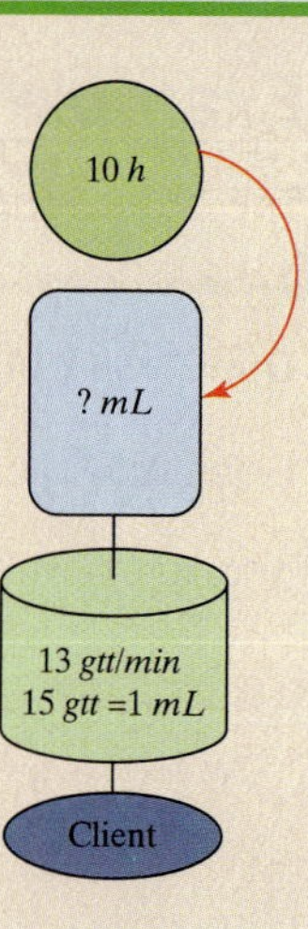

So, the flow rate is 52 *mL/h*.
Mililiters and *hours* are proportional
Think of the problem as:

$$52\ mL = 1\ h$$
$$?\ mL = 10\ h$$

The proportion could be set up as

$$\frac{52\ mL}{1\ h} = \frac{x\ mL}{10\ h}$$

Cross multiply $x = 520$

So, 520 *mL* will infuse in 10 *hours*.

Example 10.11

An IV of 1,000 *mL* D5 and $\frac{1}{2}$ NS has been ordered to infuse at 25 *gtt/min*. The drop factor is 20 *gtt/mL*. If the IV was hung at 10:00 P.M. on Tuesday, how many *milliliters* will have infused by 2:30 A.M. on Wednesday?

DIMENSIONAL ANALYSIS

From 10:00 P.M. Tuesday until 2:30 A.M. Wednesday is $4\frac{1}{2}$ *hours*.
In this example you change $4\frac{1}{2}$ *h* to ? *mL*, using both the flow rate of 25 *gtt/min* and the drop factor of 20 *gtt/mL* as unit fractions.

$$4\tfrac{1}{2}\ h = ?\ mL$$

Now, you will have to do the following:

$$4\tfrac{1}{2}\ h \longrightarrow ?\ min \longrightarrow ?\ gtt \longrightarrow ?\ mL$$

$$\frac{9\ \cancel{h}}{2} \times \frac{60\ \cancel{min}}{\cancel{h}} \times \frac{25\ \cancel{gtt}}{\cancel{min}} \times \frac{mL}{20\ \cancel{gtt}} = 337.5\ mL$$

RATIO & PROPORTION

The first problem is to convert the flow rate to *mL/h*.

$$25\ \frac{gtt}{min} = ?\ \frac{mL}{h}$$

DF = 20, therefore

$$FC = \frac{60}{20} = 3$$

Because you want Milliliters per hour, Multiply the given flow rate by 3

$$25 \times 3 = 75$$

So, the flow rate is 75 *mL/h*.
Milliliters and *hours* are proportional.
Think of the problem as:

$$75\ mL = 1\ h$$
$$?\ mL = 4.5\ h$$

The proportion could be set up as

$$\frac{75\ mL}{1\ h} = \frac{x\ mL}{4.5\ h}$$

Cross multiply $x = 337.5$

So, 338 *mL* will have infused by 2:30 A.M. Wednesday.

Finding the Duration of an IV Using a Gravity System

Examples 10.12 and 10.13 illustrate how to find durations of IV's for gravity systems.

Example 10.12

An infusion of 5% D/W is infusing at a rate of 20 *drops per minute*. If the drop factor is 15 *drops per milliliter*, how many *hours* will it take for the remaining solution in the bag (Figure 10.12) to infuse?

In Figures 10.12 you can see that 500 *mL* of solution were originally in the bag, and that the client has received 200 *mL*. Therefore, 300 *mL* remain to be infused.

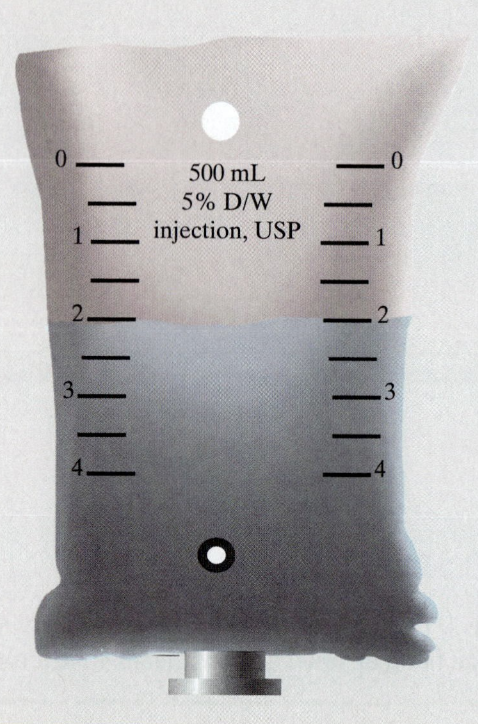

Figure 10.12 5% D/W intravenous solution.

DIMENSIONAL ANALYSIS

Given:	300 *mL* (volume to be infused)
Known equivalences:	15 *gtt/mL* (drop factor)
	20 *gtts/min* (flow rate)
	1 *h* = 60 *min*
Find:	? *h*

You want to convert this single unit of measurement 300 *mL* to the single unit of measurement *hours.*

$$300\ mL = ?\ h$$

You want to cancel *mL*. To do this you must use a unit fraction containing *mL* in the denominator. Using the drop factor, this fraction will be $\frac{15\ gtt}{1\ mL}$

$$300\ \cancel{mL} \times \frac{15\ gtt}{1\ \cancel{mL}} = ?\ h$$

Now, on the left side *gtt* is in the numerator, but you don't want *gtt*. You need a unit fraction with *gtt* in the denominator to cancel.

Using the flow rate, this fraction is $\frac{1\ min}{20\ gtt}$

$$300\ \cancel{mL} \times \frac{15\ \cancel{gtt}}{1\ \cancel{mL}} \times \frac{1\ min}{20\ \cancel{gtt}} = ?\ h$$

Now, on the left side *min* is in the numerator, but you don't want *min*. You need a fraction with *min* in the denominator to cancel, namely, $\frac{1\ h}{60\ min}$

FC METHOD AND PROPORTION

The first problem is to convert the flow rate to *mL/h*.

$$20\ \frac{gtt}{min} = ?\ \frac{mL}{h}$$

DF = 15, therefore

$$FC = \frac{60}{15} = 4$$

Because you want Milliliters per hour, Multiply the given flow rate by 4

$$20 \times 4 = 80$$

So, the flow rate is 80 *mL/h*.

Now use the proportion

$$\frac{80\ mL}{1\ h} = \frac{300\ mL}{x\ h}$$

$$300 = 80x$$

$$3.75 = x$$

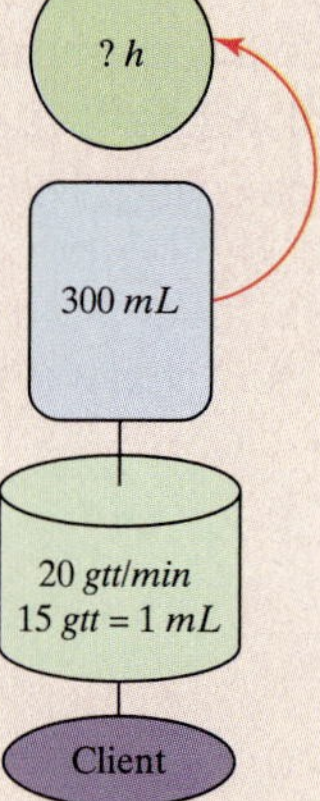

Now cancel and multiply the numbers

$$300\ \cancel{mL} \times \frac{15\ \cancel{gtt}}{\cancel{mL}} \times \frac{\cancel{min}}{20\ \cancel{gtt}} \times \frac{1\ h}{60\ \cancel{min}} = 3.75\ h$$

So, it will take $3\frac{3}{4}$ hours for the remaining solution to infuse.

Example 10.13

An IV of 1,000 *mL* of 5% D/0.9% NaCl is started at 8:00 P.M. The flow rate is 38 *drops per minute*, and the drop factor is 10 *drops per milliliter*. At what time will this infusion finish?

DIMENSIONAL ANALYSIS

Given: 1,000 *mL* (volume to be infused)

Known equivalences: 10 *gtt/mL* (drop factor)
38 *gtt/min* (flow rate)
1 *h* = 60 *min*

Find: ? *h*

You must first find how many *hours* the infusion will take to finish. You want to convert the single unit of measurement 1,000 *mL* to the single unit of measurement *hours*.

$$1{,}000\ mL = ?\ h$$

You want to cancel *mL*. To do this you must use a unit fraction containing *mL* in the denominator. This fraction will be $\frac{10\ gtt}{1\ mL}$

$$1{,}000\ \cancel{mL} \times \frac{10\ gtt}{1\ \cancel{mL}} = ?\ h$$

Now, on the left side *gtt* is in the numerator, but you don't want *gtt*. You need a fraction with *gtt* in the denominator. Using the flow rate, this fraction is $\frac{1\ min}{38\ gtt}$

$$1{,}000\ \cancel{mL} \times \frac{10\ \cancel{gtt}}{1\ \cancel{mL}} \times \frac{1\ min}{38\ \cancel{gtt}} = ?\ h$$

Now, on the left side *min* is in the numerator, but you don't want *min*. You need a fraction with *min* in the denominator, namely, $\frac{1\ h}{60\ min}$ Now, cancel and multiply the numbers.

$$1{,}000\ \cancel{mL} \times \frac{\overset{1}{\cancel{10}}\ \cancel{gtt}}{1\ \cancel{mL}} \times \frac{1\ \cancel{min}}{38\ \cancel{gtt}} \times \frac{1\ h}{\underset{6}{\cancel{60}}\ \cancel{min}} = 4.4\ h$$

You then convert 0.4 *h* to *min*.

$$0.4\ \cancel{h} \times \frac{60\ min}{1\ \cancel{h}} = 24\ min$$

FC METHOD AND PROPORTION

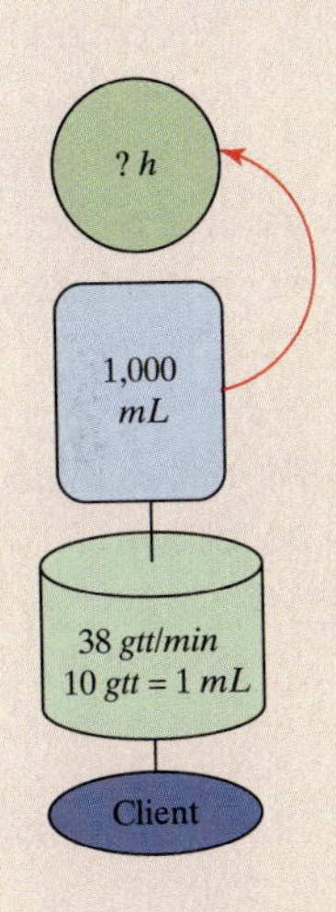

For duration problems, first convert the flow rate to *mL/h*.

$$38\ \frac{gtt}{min} = ?\ \frac{mL}{h}$$

DF = 10, therefore

$$FC = \frac{60}{10} = 6$$

Because you want Milliliters per hour, Multiply the given flow rate by 6

$$38 \times 6 = 228$$

So, the flow rate is 228 *mL/h*.
Now use the proportion

$$\frac{228\ mL}{1\ h} = \frac{1{,}000\ mL}{x\ h}$$

$$1{,}000 = 228\,x$$

$$4.4 \approx x$$

So, it will take 4.4 *hours* for the remaining solution to infuse.
To convert 0.4 *hours* to *minutes*, use the proportion

$$\frac{1\ h}{60\ min} = \frac{0.4\ h}{x\ min}$$

$$24 = x$$

Therefore, 0.4 *hours* equals about 24 *minutes*.

So, the IV will infuse for 4 *hours* and 24 *minutes*. Because the infusion started at 8:00 P.M., it will finish at 12:24 A.M. on the following day.

Adjusting the Flow Rate of an IV

Examples 10.14 and 10.15 illustrate how to adjust the flow rates of IV′-s for gravity systems.

Example 10.14

(a) The order is *500 mL of 5% D/W to infuse IV in 5 hours.* Calculate the flow rate in *drops per minute* if the drop factor is 15 *drops per milliliter.*

(b) When the nurse checks the infusion 2 *hours* after it started, 400 *mL* remain to be absorbed in the remaining 3 *hours*. Recalculate the flow rate in *drops per minute* for the remaining 400 *mL*.

DIMENSIONAL ANALYSIS

(a) Given flow rate: 500 *mL*/5 *h*

Known equivalences: 15 *gtt*/*mL* (drop factor)

1 *h* = 60 *min*

Flow rate you want to find: ? *gtt*/*min*

You want to convert the flow rate from 500 *mL* in 5 *hours* to *drops per minute*.

$$\frac{500\ mL}{5\ h} = \frac{?\ gtt}{min}$$

As in the previous examples, you can do this in one line as follows:

$$\frac{500\ \cancel{mL}}{5\ \cancel{h}} \times \frac{\overset{1}{\cancel{15}}\ gtt}{1\ \cancel{mL}} \times \frac{1\ \cancel{h}}{\underset{4}{\cancel{60}}\ min} = 25\ \frac{gtt}{min}$$

So, the flow rate is 25 *drops per minute*.

(b) When the nurse checks the infusion, 400 *mL* need to be infused in 3 *hours*.

So, you now want to convert 400 *mL* in 3 *hours* to *drops per minute*.

$$\frac{400\ mL}{3\ h} = \frac{?\ gtt}{min}$$

In a similar manner to part (a), you can do this in one line as follows:

$$\frac{400\ \cancel{mL}}{3\ \cancel{h}} \times \frac{\overset{1}{\cancel{15}}\ gtt}{1\ \cancel{mL}} \times \frac{1\ \cancel{h}}{\underset{4}{\cancel{60}}\ min} = 33.3\ \frac{gtt}{min}$$

FC METHOD

(a) The problem is

$$\frac{500\ mL}{5\ h} = ?\ \frac{gtt}{min}$$

Because

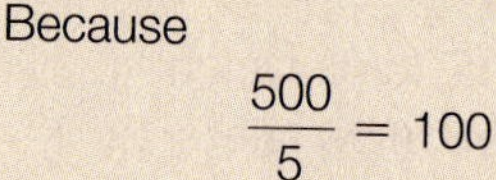

$$\frac{500}{5} = 100$$

The problem becomes

$$100\ \frac{mL}{h} = ?\ \frac{gtt}{min}$$

DF = 15, therefore

$$FC = \frac{60}{15} = 4$$

Because you want Drops per minute, Divide the given flow rate by 4

$$\frac{100}{4} = 25$$

So, the flow rate is 25 *gtt/min*.

(b) When the nurse checks the infusion, 400 *mL* need to be infused in 3 *hours*. So the problem is

$$\frac{400\ mL}{3\ h} = ?\ \frac{gtt}{min}$$

Because

$$\frac{400}{3} \approx 133.3$$

The problem becomes

$$133.3\ \frac{mL}{h} = ?\ \frac{gtt}{min}$$

Because you want Drops per minute, Divide the given flow rate by FC, which is 4.

$$\frac{133.3}{4} = 33.3$$

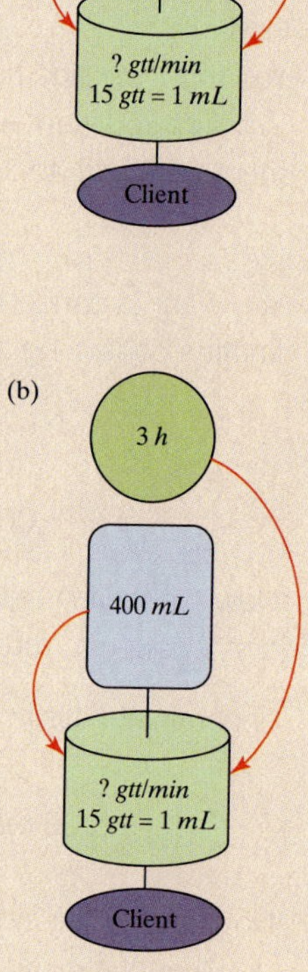

So, in order for the infusion to be completed within the 5-*hour* period as ordered, the flow rate must be increased to 33 *drops per minute*.

NOTE

Sometimes, for a variety of reasons the infusion flow rate can change. A change may affect the prescribed duration of time in which the solution will be administered. For example, with a gravity system, raising or lowering the infusion site or moving the client's body or bed relative to the height of the bag may change the flow rate of the IV infusion. Therefore, the flow rate must be periodically assessed, and adjustments made if necessary. Example 10.14 illustrates the computations involved in this process.

Example 10.15

The order reads: *1,000 mL D5W IV over 8 hours.* The drop factor is 10 *gtt/mL*.

(a) Calculate the initial flow rate in *gtt/min* for this infusion.

(b) After 5 *hours* 700 *mL* remain to be infused. How must the flow rate be adjusted so that the infusion will finish on time?

(c) If the facility has a policy that flow rate adjustments must not exceed 25% of the original rate, was the adjustment required within the guidelines?

DIMENSIONAL ANALYSIS

(a) First, convert the flow rate of 1,000 *mL* in 8 *hours* to *gtt/min*. You can do this in one line as follows:

$$\frac{1{,}000\ \cancel{mL}}{8\ \cancel{h}} \times \frac{1\ \cancel{h}}{60\ min} \times \frac{10\ gtt}{\cancel{mL}} = 20.8\ \frac{gtt}{min}$$

So, the initial flow rate is 21 *gtt/min*.

(b) After 5 *hours*, 700 *mL* remain to be infused in the remaining 3 *hours*. Now, the new flow rate must be calculated. That is, you must convert the flow rate of 700 *mL* in 3 *hours* to *gtt/min*. You can do this in one line as follows:

$$\frac{700\ \cancel{mL}}{3\ \cancel{h}} \times \frac{1\ \cancel{h}}{60\ min} \times \frac{10\ gtt}{\cancel{mL}} = 38.9\ \frac{gtt}{min}$$

So, the adjusted flow rate is 39 *gtt/min*.

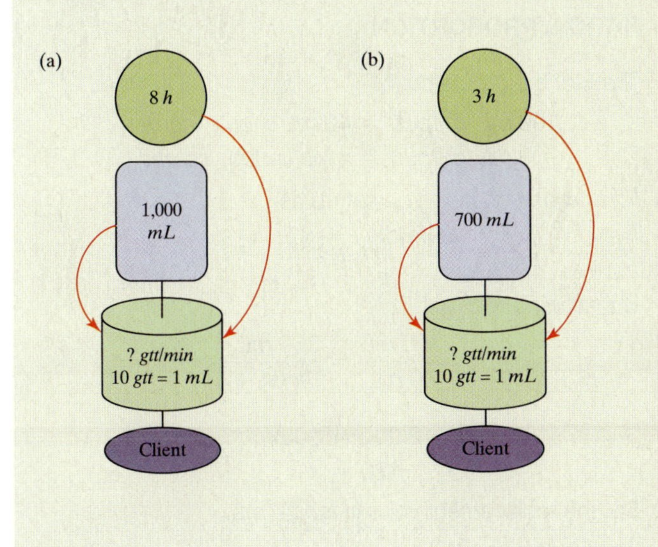

FC METHOD AND PROPORTION

(a) The problem is

$$\frac{1{,}000\ mL}{8\ h} = ?\ \frac{gtt}{min}$$

Because

$$\frac{1{,}000}{8} = 125$$

the problem becomes

$$125\ \frac{mL}{h} = ?\ \frac{gtt}{min}$$

DF = 10, therefore

$$FC = \frac{60}{10} = 6$$

Because you want *Drops per minute*, Divide the given flow rate by 6

$$\frac{125}{6} \approx 20.8$$

So, the new flow rate is 21 *gtt/min*.

(b) After 5 *hours*, 700 *mL* remain to be infused in the remaining 3 *hours*.

The problem is

$$\frac{700\ mL}{3\ h} = ?\ \frac{gtt}{min}$$

Because

$$\frac{700}{3} \approx 233.3$$

then the problem becomes

$$233.3\ \frac{mL}{h} = ?\ \frac{gtt}{min}$$

As in part (a) FC = 6.

(Continued)

(c) Because you want *Drops per minute*, Divide the given flow rate by 6

$$\frac{233.3}{6} \approx 38.9$$

(c) Since the facility has a policy that flow rate adjustments must not exceed 25% of the original rate, you must now calculate 25% of the original rate; that is, 25% of 21 *gtt/min*.

$$25\% \text{ of } 21\ gtt/min = (.25 \times 21)\ gtt/min$$
$$= 5.25\ gtt/min$$

So, the flow rate may not be changed by more than about 5 *gtt/min*. Therefore, the initial flow rate of 21 *gtt/min* can be changed to no less than 16 (21 minus 5) *gtt/min* and no more than 26 (21 plus 5) *gtt/min*.
Since 39 *gtt/min* is outside the acceptable range of roughly 16–26 *gtt/min*, this change is not within the guidelines and the adjustment may not be made. You must contact the prescriber.

Fluid Balance: Intake/Output

To work well, the various body systems need a stable environment in which their tissues and cells can function properly. For example, the body requires somewhat constant levels of temperature, salts, glucose, and, in particular, adequate hydration to maintain homeostasis.

Part of hydration management involves the monitoring of a client's fluid intake and output. This is especially important with pediatric, geriatric, renal, cardiac, and critical care clients.

Fluid intake is the amount of fluid that enters the body (oral and parenteral fluids), whereas **fluid output** is the amount of fluid that leaves the body (urine, sweat, liquid stool, emesis, and drainage).

Fluid replacement is sometimes necessary to avoid dehydration. If (as in Example 10.15) a physician provides an order with a specific ratio comparing the necessary replacement fluid with the client's fluid output and if the client's fluid output is known, then dimensional analysis could be used to determine the volume of replacement fluid to give the client.

Example 10.16

Order: *For every 100 mL of urine output, replace with 40 mL of water via PEG tube q4h.* The client's urine output is 300 *mL*. What is the replacement volume?

DIMENSIONAL ANALYSIS

Think of the problem as:

Output: 300 *mL* (out) [single unit of measurement]
Replacement: 100 *mL* (out)/40 *mL* (in) [equivalence]
Input: ? *mL* (in) [single unit of measurement]

In this example, you want to change the single unit of measurement [*300 mL(out)*] to another single unit of measurement [*mL(in)*].

$$300\ mL(out) = ?\ mL(in)$$

The flow rate provides the equivalence [*100 mL(out)/40 mL(in)*] for the unit fraction.

$$300\ \cancel{mL(out)} \times \frac{40\ mL(in)}{100\ \cancel{mL(out)}} = 120\ mL(in)$$

So, the replacement volume is *120 mL*.

RATIO & PROPORTION

Think of the problem as:

100 *mL (output)* = 40 *mL (input)* [*order*]
300 *mL (output)* = *x mL (input)* [*client*]

The proportion could be set up as

$$\frac{Out}{In} = \frac{Out'}{In'}$$

Substituting, you get

$$\frac{100\ mL}{40\ mL} = \frac{300\ mL}{x\ mL}$$

$$12{,}000 = 100x$$
$$120 = x$$

So, the replacement volume is 120 *mL*.

Summary

In this chapter, the basic concepts and standard equipment used in enteral and intravenous therapy were introduced.

- Fluids can be given to a client slowly over a period of time through a vein (*intravenous*) or through a tube inserted into the alimentary tract (*enteral*).
- Enteral and IV fluids can be administered continuously or intermittently.
- There is a wide variety of commercially prepared enteral and IV solutions.
- In IV solutions, *letters* indicate solution compounds, whereas *numbers* indicate solution concentration.
- Care must be taken to eliminate the air from, and maintain the sterility of, IV tubing.
- An IV infusion can flow solely by the force of gravity or by an electronic infusion pump.
- Use the following formula to determine flow rate:

$$\textit{Flow Rate} = \frac{\textit{Volume}}{\textit{Time}}$$

- Flow rates are usually given as either *mL/h* or *gtt/min*.
- The drop factor of the IV administration set must be known in order to calculate flow rates.
- *Microdrops/minute* are equivalent to *milliliters/hour.*
- For microdrops, the drop factor is 60 *micro-drops* per *milliliter*.
- For macrodrops, the usual drop factors are 10, 15, or 20 *drops per milliliter*.
- The *flow rate conversion number* (*FC*) is the quotient of 60 and the *drop factor* (*DF*); that is, $FC = \frac{60}{DF}$.
- Use the FC technique to convert between the flow rates $\frac{\text{mL}}{\text{h}}$ and $\frac{\text{gtt}}{\text{min}}$:

  To get Drops, Divide by FC.
  To get Milliliters, Multiply by FC.

- To calculate the duration of an IV solution, first determine the flow rate in *ml/h*.
- Know the policy of the facility regarding readjustment of flow rates.

Case Study 10.1

Read the Case Study and answer the questions. Answers can be found in Appendix A.

A 68-yr-old male is brought by ambulance to the hospital from home. He is clammy, has tachypnea, and decreased level of responsiveness. He has no known allergies to food, but is allergic to aspirin and penicillin. He has a history of HTN, DM, COPD, osteoarthritis, and congestive heart failure. He had a right-sided CVA 10 yrs ago, is apha-sic, and has right-sided hemiplegia. He is 6 *feet* 3 *inches* and weighs 140 *pounds,* and has a PEG feeding tube. His vitals are T 102° F, B/P 100/60, P 100, R 26 and shallow. His admitting diagnosis is dehydration, R/O pneumonia, UTI, and sepsis.

His orders include:

- Chest X-ray stat
- Blood cultures stat
- Urine culture stat
- CBC and SMA 12 stat
- Hbg and Hct stat
- NPO
- IV: NS infuse at 90 *mL/h*
- Perative (1,300 cal/L) via PEG 480 *mL* over 6 *h*, flush with 50 *mL* water after feeding and after medication administration
- Check gastric residual every 4 *h*, hold feeding if residual greater than 200 *mL*. Reinfuse residual and recheck in 2 *h*
- O_2 via nasal cannula at 2 *L/min*
- Suprax (cefixime) 400 *mg* via PEG daily
- Cleocin (clindamycin) 360 *mg* via PEG q12h
- enoxaparin 1 *mg*/*kg* subcut q12h
- Humalog 50/50 *mix* 35 *units* subcut before tube feeding
- cimetidine HCl 400 *mg* via PEG at bedtime

1. The label on the Suprax reads 500 *mg*/*mL*. How many *milliliters* will you administer?
2. The IV is infusing via gravity flow. Calculate the rate in *mcgtt/min*.
3. The strength on the enoxaparin label is 300 *mg*/*mL*. How many *milliliters* will you administer?
4. Place an arrow at the correct measurement on the most appropriate syringe to indicate the amount of enoxaparin to be administered.

(*continued*)

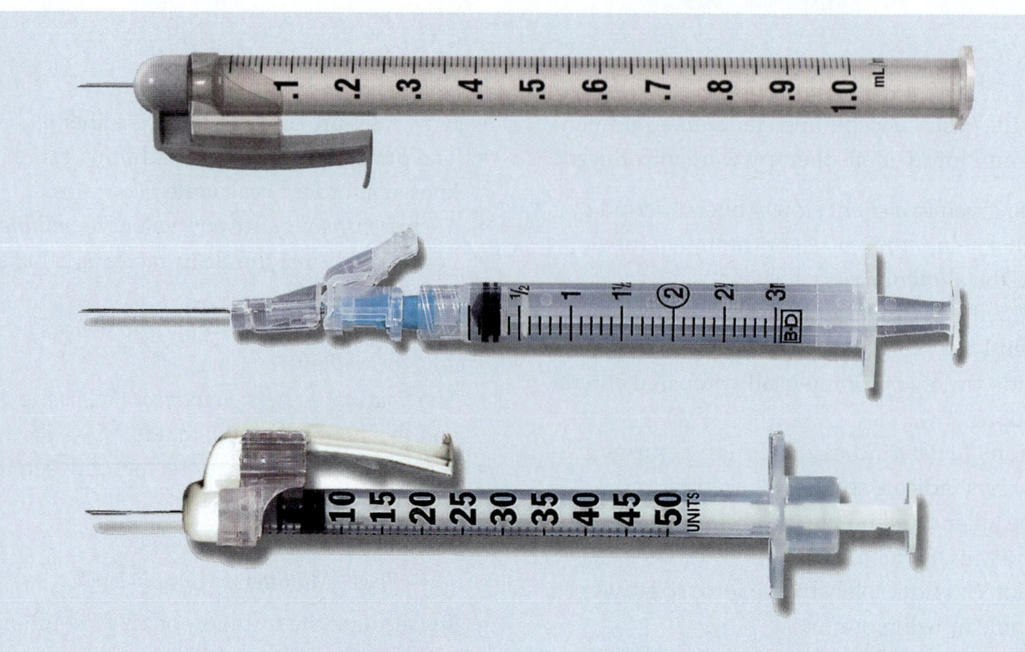

5. How many *milligrams* of enoxaparin is the client receiving each day?
6. Calculate the flow rate of the Perative in *mL/h*.
7. How many *milliliters* of IV fluid is the client receiving in 24 hours?
8. The label on the Cleocin reads 75 *mg*/5 *mL*. How many *milliliters* will you administer?
9. The label on the cimetidine reads 300 *mg*/5 *mL*. How many *milliliters* will you administer?
10. Calculate the total amount of enteral fluid the client will receive in 24 *hours*.

Practice Sets

The answers to *Try These for Practice*, *Exercises*, and *Cumulative Review Exercises*, are found in Appendix A. Ask your instructor for the answers to the *Additional Exercises*.

Try These for Practice

Test your comprehension after reading the chapter.

1. Order: D_5W 500 *mL IV infuse over* 12 *hours*. Find the pump setting in *mL/h*. ____________
2. Order: *NS* 1,000 *mL IV infuse over* 24 *h*. Find the drip rate in *drops per minute* if the drop factor is 15 *gtt/mL*. ____________
3. A continuous IV is infusing at 120 *mL/h*. How many *milliliters* will infuse in *two hours and thirty minutes*? ____________
4. An IV starts at 1800 *h* and runs at 21 *gtt/min* with a drop factor of 10 *gtt/mL*. At what time will the first 200 *mL* have infused into the client?
5. Order: For every 100 *mL* of urine output, replace with 40 *mL* of water via nasogastric tube q6h. If the client's urine output for the past 6 *hours* is 300 *mL*, what is the replacement volume of water needed?

Exercises

Reinforce your understanding in class or at home.

1. Order: *RL* 1,000 *mL IV infuse over* 16 *hours*. What is the pump setting in *mL/h*?

   ____

2. Normal saline is infusing intravenously at 125 *mL/h*. What is the flow rate measured in *mcgtt/min*?

   ____

3. Order: *D5/W* 2,000 *mL IV infuse over* 12 *h*. The drop factor is 10 *gtt/mL*. Calculate the flow rate in *gtt/min*.

   ____

4. Order: *3/4 strength Ensure* 240 *mL via NG tube over* 8 *h*. What is the pump setting in *mL/h*?

   ____

5. How many *mL* of solution will be infused in 4 *hours* if the flow rate is 20 *mL/h*?

   ____

6. Order: *NS* 1,000 *mL IV infuse over* 24 *h*. Find the pump setting in *milliliters per hour.*

   ____

7. Order: D_5W 1,000 *mL IV infuse over* 12 *h*. Find the flow rate in *drops per minute if the drop factor is* 20 *gtt/mL*.

   ____

8. Order: *NS* 800 *mL IV infuse in* 6 *hours*.
   (a) Calculate the initial pump setting in *mL/h*.
   (b) When the nurse checks this infusion 4 *hours* later, 500 *mL* are LIB (left in the bag). Recalculate the pump setting for the remaining 500 *mL*.
   (c) If the facility protocols indicate that flow rate adjustments must not exceed 25% of the original rate, may the adjustment be made?

   ____

9. A 500 *mL* IV starts at 9:00 P.M. and runs at 33 *gtt/min* with a drop factor of 10 *gtt/mL*. At what time will it finish?

   ____

10. How long will it take 1,000 *mL* to infuse if the flow rate is 125 *mL/h*?

    ____

11. How many *milliliters* will infuse in 2 *hours* at the rate of 30 *gtt/min* with a drop factor of 15 *gtt/mL*?

    ____

12. A continuous IV is infusing at 120 *mcgtt/min*. How many *milliliters* will infuse in 4 *hours*?

    ____

13. Order: *NS* 1,000 *mL IV infuse in* 12 *hours*. The drop factor is 20 *gtt/mL*.
    (a) Calculate the initial drip rate in *gtt/min*.
    (b) When the nurse checks this infusion 7 *hours* later, 500 *mL* are LIB (left in the bag). Recalculate the drip rate for the remaining 500 *mL*.
    (c) If the facility protocols indicate that flow rate adjustments must not exceed 20% of the original rate, may the adjustment be made?

14. A continuous IV is infusing at 30 *mL/h*. How many *milliliters* will infuse in 45 *minutes*?

15. Order: *NS 500 mL IV infuse at 50 mL/h stat.* If the IV started at 8:00 P.M. on Monday, at what time and on what day will it finish?
16. Normal saline is infusing with a drip rate of *22 gtt/min*. The tubing set is calibrated to deliver *10 gtt per mL*. What volume of normal saline will infuse in 2 *hours*?
17. Order: *NS 200 mL intravenous over 4 h stat.* At 0700 *h*, *150 mL* has infused. At what time will the infusion finish?
18. At 10:30 A.M. there are 250 *mL* LIB (left in the bag) when a physician reduces the drip rate to *20 gtt/min*. The drop factor is *15 gtt/mL*. At what time and day will the infusion be completed?
19. Order: *800 mL D5NS IV infuse over 8 h stat.* The tubing is rated at *10 gtt/mL*.
    (a) What is the initial flow rate in *gtt/min*?
    (b) After 4 *hours* it is observed that the bag contained 500 *mL* when it should have contained *400 mL*. If the flow rate is reset to have the IV finish on time, what should the new drip rate be in *gtt/min*?
    (c) If the facility allows no more than a 20% change in IV flow rates, is the reset in part (b) allowed?
20. Order: *For every 200 mL of urine output, replace with 40 mL of H_2O via PEG tube q6h.* If urine output for the past 6 *hours* is 500 *mL*, find the replacement fluid volume.

Additional Exercises

Now, test yourself!

1. Order: *5% D 0.45% NaCl* 500 *mL IV over* 3 *hours*. Find the pump setting in *milliliters per hour*.

______

2. Order: *Ringer's Lactate* 500 *mL IV over* 12 *h*. Find the flow rate in *drops per minute* if the drop factor is 15 *gtt/mL*.

______

3. D5/W is infusing at 90 *mL/h* using an electronic controller. How much D5/W will infuse in 90 *minutes*?

______

4. NS is infusing intravenously at 75 *mL/h*. How long will it take for 500 *mL* to infuse?

______

5. Order: 1,000 *mL NS infuse at* 75 *mL/h*. The infusion starts at 7:00 A.M. on Tuesday. When is the infusion scheduled to be completed?

______

6. Order: 500 *mL NS IV run* 75 *mL/h*. How many *milliliters* will infuse in 3 *hours*?

______

7. Order: *NS* 1,500 *mL over* 12 *h*. After 3 *hours* 1,200 *mL* remain in the bag. The facility policy indicates that flow rate adjustments may not exceed 25% of the original rate. Recalculate the flow rate so that the infusion will finish on time, and decide if the adjustment is within the guidelines.

______

8. Find the flow rate in *drops per minute* that is equivalent to a flow rate of 75 *mL/h* when you are using 20 *gtt/mL* macrodrip tubing.

______

9. A pump is set at 200 *mL/h*. Find the flow rate in *gtt/min* if the drop factor is 10 *gtt/mL*.

______

10. Find the flow rate in *microdrops per minute* that is equivalent to a rate of 35 *mL/h*.

11. Order: *For every* 100 *mL of urine output, replace with* 30 *mL of* H_2O *through the percutaneous endoscopic gastrostomy (PEG) tube q4h*. If urine output for the last 4 *hours* is 500 *mL*, find the replacement fluid volume.

12. Determine the completion time of 200 *mL* packed blood cells that ran at 50 *mL/h*. The bag was hung at 3:15 P.M. on Monday.

13. Order: *RL* 375 *mL IV over* 3 *h*. The tubing has a drop factor of 10 *gtt/mL*.
    (a) Calculate the initial flow rate in *gtt/min*.
    (b) After 1 *hour*, 175 *mL* have infused. Determine the adjusted flow rate so that the infusion will finish on time.
    (c) If flow rate adjustments cannot exceed 25% of the original rate, is the adjustment in part (b) within the guidelines?

14. A continuous IV is infusing at 40 *mL/h*. How many *milliliters* will infuse in 30 *minutes*?

15. Order: *NS* 750 *mL IV infuse at* 75 *mL/h*. If the IV started at 11 P.M. on Wednesday, at what time and day will it finish?

16. Order: 1,000 *mL D5* $\frac{1}{2}$ *NS to run at* 90 *mL/h*. Find the drip rate for 15 *gtt/mL* tubing.

17. Order: *NS* 1,000 *mL intravenous over* 10 *h*. At 0700 *h*, 400 *mL* has infused. At what time will the infusion finish?

18. Order: *RL* 1,000 *mL IV* 8 A.M.–8 P.M. What is the pump setting in *mL/h*?

19. Order: 150 *mL NS IV over* 3 *hours*. At how many *mcgtt/min* would you run this infusion?

20. *For every* 200 *mL of urine output, replace with* 40 *mL of* H_2O *through the jejunostomy tube (J-tube) q8h*. If urine output for the past 8 *hours* is 700 *mL*, find the replacement fluid volume.

Cumulative Review Exercises

Review your mastery of previous chapters.

1. Find the height in centimeters of a woman who is 5 *feet* 6 *inches* tall.
2. 120 *mL* = ? *oz*
3. Find the weight in *kilograms* of a man who weighs 187 *pounds*.
4. 5.6 *cm* = ? *mm*
5. Write 4:55 P.M. in military time.
6. How many *milligrams* of sodium chloride are contained in 500 *mL* of a 0.9% NaCl solution?

7. What is the strength expressed as a percent of a 400 *mL* solution that contains 10 *grams* of magnesium sulfate?

____

8. Calculate the BSA of a client who is 150 *cm* tall and weighs 88 *kg*.

____

9. The drug in a vial has a concentration of 40 *mg* per *mL*. If 3 *mL* are withdrawn from this vial into a syringe, what is the concentration of the solution in the syringe?

____

10. A client weighs 100 *lb*. The order calls for 0.6 *mg/kg po daily*. How many *mg* of the drug will the client receive?
11. If the label on a 100 *mL* bottle indicates a stated strength of "*250 mg/5 mL*," which of the following statements must *always* be true?
    (a) There are 5 *mL* of solution in the bottle.
    (b) Each teaspoon of the solution contains 250 *mg* of the drug.
    (c) The strength of the solution is 2%.
    (d) There are 250 *mg* of the drug in the entire bottle.
12. Order: ***phenobarbital 0.09 g po b.i.d***. The strength of phenobarbital is *30 mg per tablet*. The recommended dosage for this client with seizures is *100–300 mg/day in divided doses*. Is the order safe and, if so, how many *tablets* would you administer to the client?
13. *Ondansetron HCl oral solution 6 mg po* has been ordered to prevent chemotherapy-induced nausea and vomiting in a client with cancer. If the drug is supplied as *4 mg/5 mL*, how many *milliliters* will you administer?
14. Ordered for a client with an infection: *oxacillin 500 mg IM stat*. The 1 *gram* vial must be reconstituted by adding *5.7 mL* of sterile water for injection to the vial to yield *250 mg per 1.5 mL*. How many *mL* will you administer?
15. Convert a flow rate of *19 mcgtt/min* to an equivalent flow rate measured in *mL/h*.

Chapter 11

Flow Rates and Dosage Rates for Intravenous Medications

Learning Outcomes

After completing this chapter, you will be able to

11.1 Describe intravenous (IV) medication administration.

11.2 Calculate dosage rates for intravenous piggyback (IVPB) infusions.

11.3 Convert between IVPB dosage rates (drug/time) and flow rates (volume/time).

11.4 Calculate the infused volume and duration of an IVPB infusion.

11.5 Calculate flow rates for IV push medications.

11.6 Calculate the dosage rate when the order involves a compound rate (*mg/kg/min*).

11.7 Perform calculations for infusions when medication must be added to the IVPB bag.

11.8 Construct titration tables.

This chapter extends the discussion of infusions to include the administration of intravenous *medications*.

In the previous chapter the focus was on **flow rates** (*volume of fluid per time*, e.g., *mL/h* or *gtt/min*). However, in this chapter, the infusing solutions will contain medication, so you also calculate **dosage rates** (*amount of drug per time*, e.g., *mg/min* or *units/hr*).

This chapter also introduces orders containing **compound rates** (amount of drug per size of the client per time, e.g., *mg/kg/min* or $mcg/m^2/min$).

The calculations involved in medication administered by **IV push** and **titration** are also introduced.

Intravenous Administration of Medications

Intravenous (IV) administration of medications provides rapid access to a client's circulatory system, thereby presenting potential hazards. Errors in medications, dose, or dosage strength can prove fatal. Therefore, *caution must be taken in the calculation, preparation, and administration of IV medications.*

Typically, a **primary** IV line provides continuous fluid to the client. **Secondary** lines can be attached to the primary line at injection ports, and these lines are often used to deliver *continuous or intermittent* medication intravenously. A secondary line is referred to as a **piggyback** or **intravenous piggyback (IVPB)**. With intermittent IVPB infusions, the bags generally hold 50–250 *mL* of fluid containing dissolved medication and usually require 20–60 *minutes* to infuse. Like a primary line, an IVPB infusion may use a manually controlled gravity system or an electronic infusion device.

A **heplock,** or **saline lock,** is an infusion port attached to an indwelling needle or cannula in a peripheral vein. Intermittent IV infusions can be administered through these ports via IV lines connected to the ports. An **IV push** (IVP), or **bolus,** is a direct injection of medication either into the heplock/saline lock or directly into the vein.

ALERT

Whenever two different medications are infused via the same IV line, consult the proper resource to be sure that the drugs are compatible.

Syringe pumps can also be used for intermittent infusions. A syringe with the medication is inserted into the pump. The medication is delivered at a set rate over a short period of time.

A **volume-control set** is a small container, called a *burette,* that is connected to the IV line. Burettes are often used in pediatric or geriatric care, where accurate volume control is critical. The danger of overdose is limited because of the small volume of solution in the burette. Burettes are discussed in Chapter 12.

Intravenous Piggyback Infusions

Clients can receive a medication through a port in an existing IV line. This is called **intravenous piggyback (IVPB)** (Figure 11.1). The medication is in a secondary bag. Notice in Figure 11.1 that the secondary bag is higher than the primary bag so that the pressure in the secondary line will be greater than the pressure in the primary line. Therefore, the secondary medication infuses first. Once the secondary infusion is completed, the primary line begins to flow. Be sure to keep both lines open because if you close the primary line, the primary line will not flow into the vein when the secondary IVPB is completed.

A typical IVPB order might read: *cimetidine* 300 *mg IVPB q6h in* 50 *mL NS infuse over* 20 *min.* This is an order for an IV piggyback infusion in which 300 *mg* of the drug cimetidine diluted in 50 *mL* of a normal saline solution must infuse in 20 *minutes.* So, the client receives 300 *mg* of cimetidine in 20 *minutes* via a secondary line, and this dose is repeated every 6 *hours.*

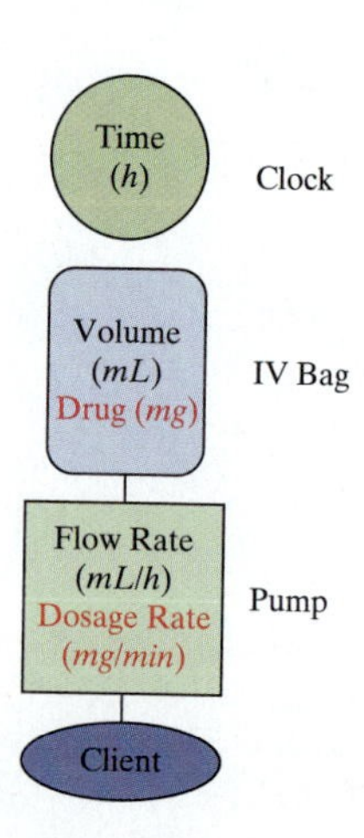

In this chapter, you encounter both flow rates and dosage rates. The following formulas apply:

$$\text{Flow Rate} = \frac{\text{Volume}}{\text{Time}}$$

$$\text{Dosage Rate} = \frac{\text{Drug}}{\text{Time}}$$

The setup shown in Figure 11.1 may look intimidating. However, the mathematics involved in IVPB infusions is simplified by the fact that when the IVPB bag is infusing, the primary bag is not running and may therefore be ignored. In the examples for this chapter, the diagram to the left is used to show the structure of the IVPB infusion.

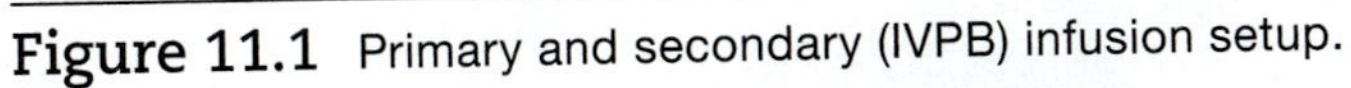

Figure 11.1 Primary and secondary (IVPB) infusion setup.

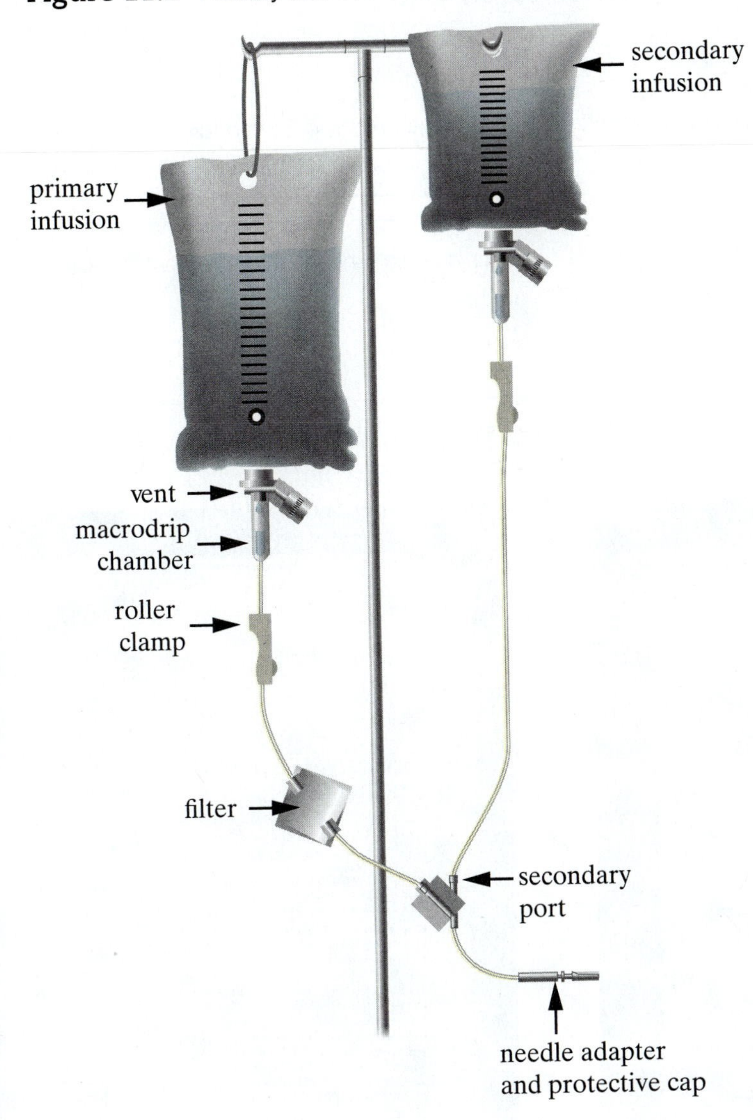

Finding the Dosage Rate

A dosage rate is calculated in Example 11.1.

Example 11.1

Order: *cimetidine 300 mg IVPB q6h in 50 mL NS infuse in 20 min.* Find the

(a) IV flow rate measured in *milliliters/min*.

(b) Dosage rate measured in *milligrams/min*.

(a) To find the flow rate, use the formula from the previous chapter

$$\text{Flow Rate} = \frac{\text{Volume}}{\text{Time}}$$

Substitute 50 *mL* for the volume in the bag, and 20 *min* for the time.

$$\text{Flow Rate} = \frac{50 \text{ mL}}{20 \text{ min}} = 2.5 \text{ mL/min}$$

So, the IV flow rate is 2.5 *mL/min*, which means that the client receives a volume of 2.5 *mL* of solution every minute.

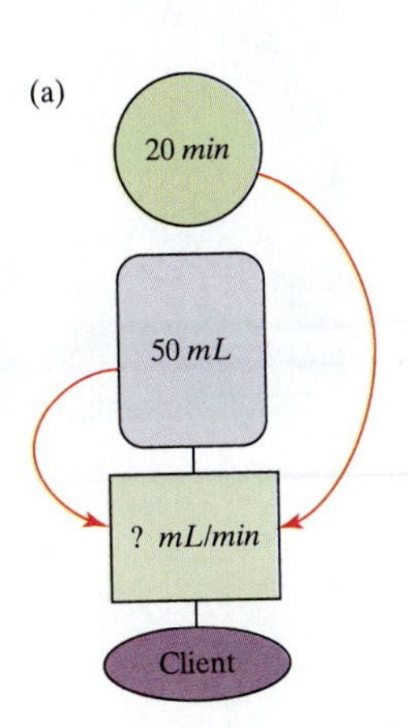

(Continued)

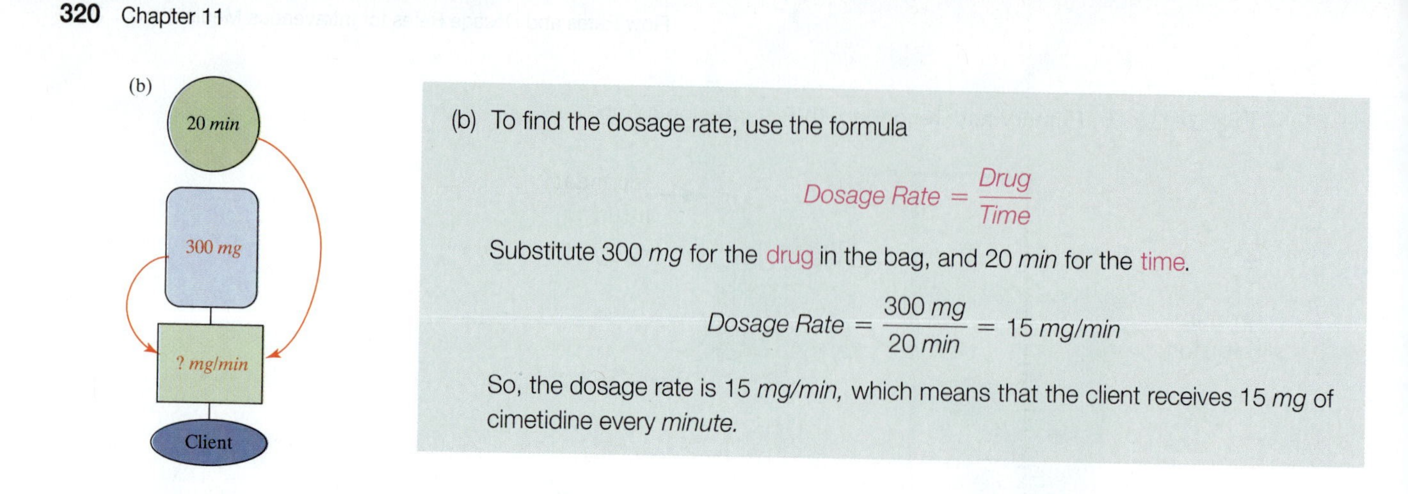

(b) To find the dosage rate, use the formula

$$\text{Dosage Rate} = \frac{\text{Drug}}{\text{Time}}$$

Substitute 300 *mg* for the drug in the bag, and 20 *min* for the time.

$$\text{Dosage Rate} = \frac{300\ mg}{20\ min} = 15\ mg/min$$

So, the dosage rate is 15 *mg/min,* which means that the client receives 15 *mg* of cimetidine every *minute.*

Figure 11.2 Packages of secondary IV tubing: (a) 60 *drops per mL,* (b) 10 *drops per mL.*

SOURCE: Al Dodge/Pearson Education, Inc.

(a)

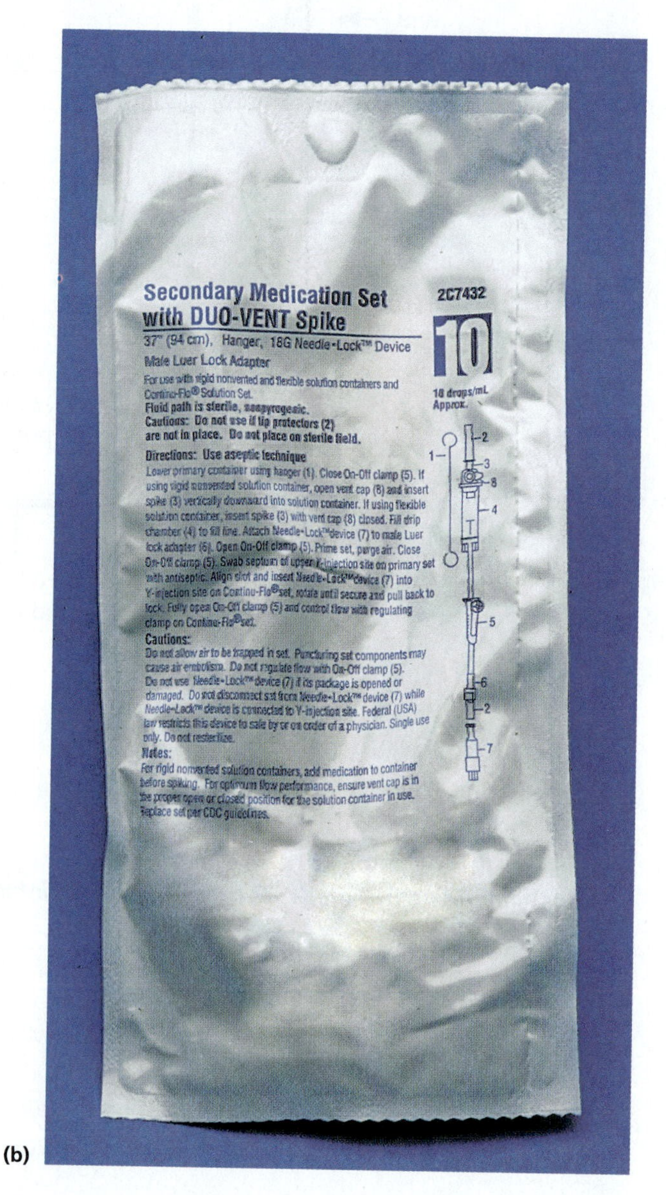

(b)

Converting IV Dosage Rates to Flow Rates

Each of the next three examples (11.2 through 11.4) converts rates from dosage rates (*amount of medication per time*) to IV flow rates (*volume of solution per time*).

Example 11.2

Order: *cefoxitin 1 g IVPB q6h over 30 minutes.* Read the drug label in Figure 11.3.

(a) Find the dosage rate in *grams per hour*.

(b) Change the dosage rate to the flow rate in *milliliters per hour*.

(c) Change the flow rate from *mL/h* to *drops per minute* if the drop factor is 10 *gtt/mL*.

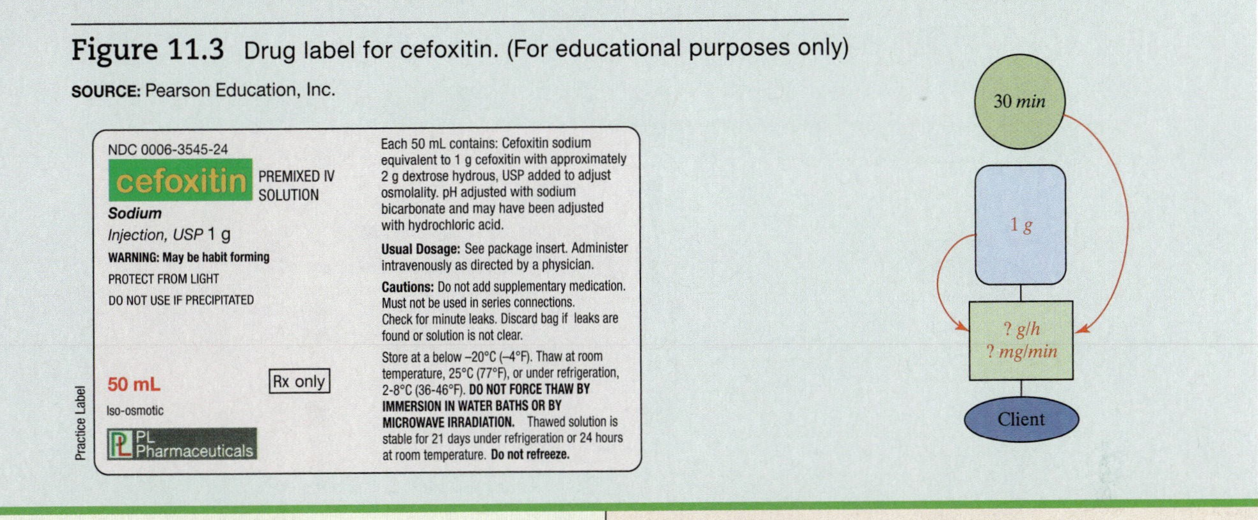

Figure 11.3 Drug label for cefoxitin. (For educational purposes only)

SOURCE: Pearson Education, Inc.

DIMENSIONAL ANALYSIS

(a) Because 1 *gram* must infuse in 30 *minutes*, the dosage rate $\left(\dfrac{\textit{weight of drug}}{\textit{time}}\right)$ is $\dfrac{1\ g}{30\ min}$

$$\frac{1g}{30min} = ?\ \frac{g}{h}$$

To change the *minutes to hours*, use 1 *h* = 60 *min*

$$\frac{1\ g}{30\ \cancel{min}} \times \frac{60\ \cancel{min}}{1\ h} = \frac{2\ g}{h}$$

So, the dosage rate is 2 *grams per hour.*

(b) $\dfrac{2\ g}{h} = ?\ \dfrac{mL}{h}$

Use the strength of the solution 50 *mL* = 1 *g* to form the unit fraction.

$$\frac{2\ \cancel{g}}{h} \times \frac{50\ mL}{1\ \cancel{g}} = \frac{100\ mL}{h}$$

So, the flow rate is 100 *milliliters per hour.*

(c) $\dfrac{100\ mL}{h} = ?\ \dfrac{gtt}{min}$

Use the drop factor of *10 gtt per mL*.

$$\frac{100\ \cancel{mL}}{\cancel{h}} \times \frac{1\ \cancel{h}}{60\ min} \times \frac{10\ gtt}{\cancel{mL}} = \frac{16.7\ gtt}{min}$$

PROPORTION

(a) The dosage rate in the order is $\dfrac{1\ g}{30\ min}$, and this rate must be changed to *g/h*. So the problem is

$$\frac{1\ g}{30\ min} = ?\ \frac{g}{h}$$

One way to do this is to write 30 *minutes* as $^1/_2$ *hour* or 0.5 *h*.

Therefore, $\dfrac{1\ g}{30\ min} = \dfrac{1\ g}{0.5\ h}$

But $\dfrac{1}{0.5} = 2$

So, the dosage rate is 2 *g/h*.

(b) The dosage rate of 2 *g/h* must be changed to *mL/h*. So the problem is

$$2\ g = ?\ mL$$

Because the strength of the solution stated on the IV bag is 1 *g* = 50 *mL*, you can use the proportion

$$\frac{2\ g}{x\ mL} = \frac{1\ g}{50\ mL}$$

$$x = 100$$

So, the IV flow rate is 100 *mL/h*.

(c) Now, change the rate 100 *mL/h* to *gtt/min*, using the FC method.

DF = 10 and *FC* = $\frac{60}{10}$ = 6. You want *Drops per minute*, so Divide.

$$\frac{100}{6} \approx 16.7$$

So, the flow rate is *17 drops per minute.*

Example 11.3

Order: *heparin sodium in dextrose 30,000 units/24 h continuous IV stat*. See Figure 11.4 for a picture of the 500-*mL* heparin bag to be used. Calculate the infusion rate in *milliliters per hour*.

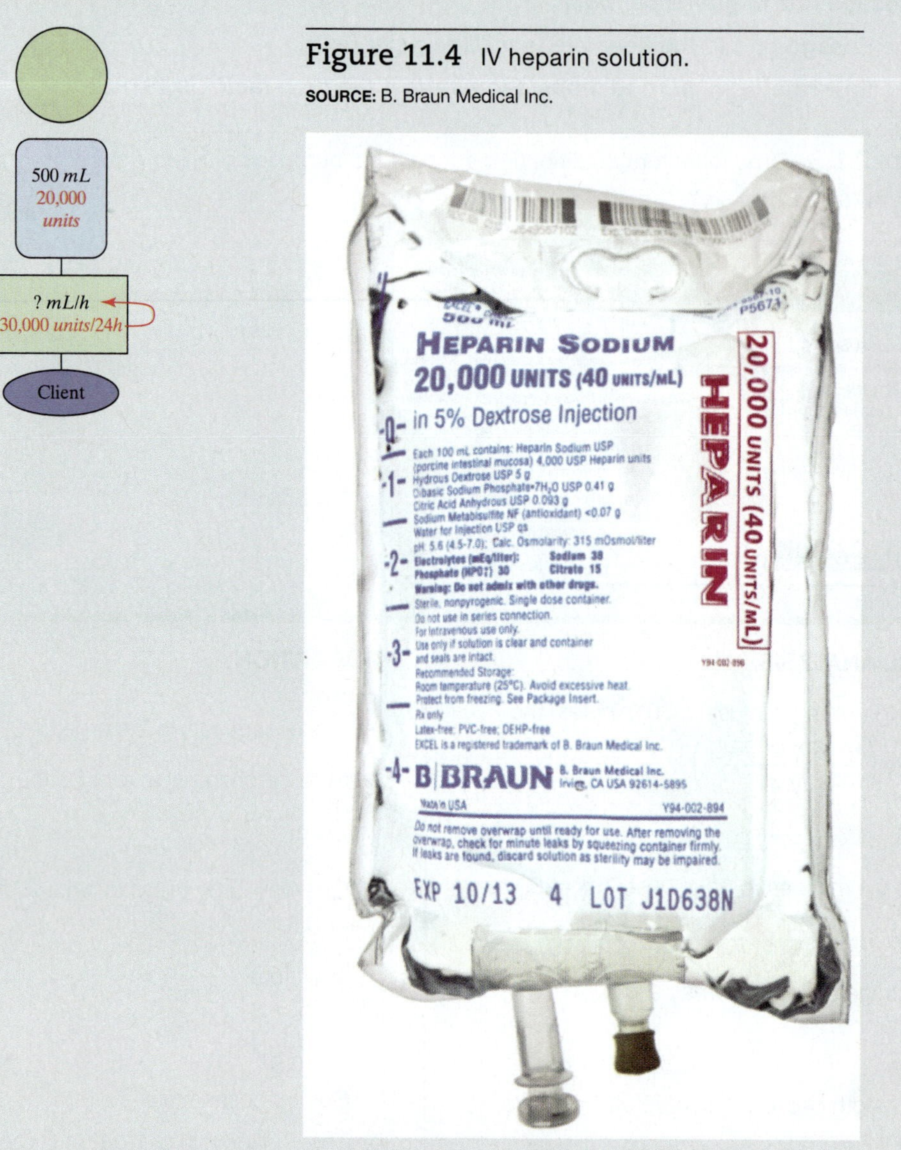

Figure 11.4 IV heparin solution.

SOURCE: B. Braun Medical Inc.

You want to convert the dosage rate of *30,000 units per 24 hours* to a flow rate in *milliliters per hour.* That is,

$$\frac{30{,}000\ units}{24\ h} = ?\ \frac{mL}{h}$$

DIMENSIONAL ANALYSIS

Use the concentration in the bag 20,000 *units*/500 *mL* (or equivalently 40 *units* per *mL*) to construct the unit fraction.

$$\frac{30{,}000\ \cancel{units}}{24\ h} \times \frac{500\ mL}{20{,}000\ \cancel{units}} = 31.25\ \frac{mL}{h}$$

PROPORTION

You need to change the numerator of the fraction from 30,000 *units* of heparin to *milliliters* of solution.

Think:

$$30{,}000\ units = ?\ mL$$

$$40\ units = 1\ mL \quad \text{[strength in the bag]}$$

Use the proportion:

$$\frac{30{,}000\ units}{x\ mL} = ?\ \frac{40\ units}{1\ mL}$$

Cross multiply:

$$40\,x = 30{,}000$$
$$x = 750\ mL$$

But $\frac{750\ mL}{24\ h}$ is equal to 31.25 *mL/h*.

So, the IV infusion rate is 31 *mL/h*.

Example 11.4

The prescriber writes an order for 1,000 *mL* of 5% D/W with 10 *units* of Pitocin (oxytocin). Your client must receive 3 *mU* of this *drug per minute*. Calculate the flow rate in *microdrops per minute*.

DIMENSIONAL ANALYSIS

Given dosage rate: 3 *mU/min*

Known equivalences: 10 *units*/1,000 *mL* (strength)
60 *mcgtt/mL* (standard microdrop drop factor)
1 *unit* = 1,000 *mU*

Flow rate you want to find: ? *mcgtt/min*

You want to change the dosage rate from *milliunits per minute* to a flow rate of *microdrops per minute*.

$$3\,\frac{mU}{min} = ?\,\frac{mcgtt}{min}$$

You want to cancel *mU*. To do this you must use a unit fraction containing *mU* in the denominator. Using the equivalence 1 *mU* = 1,000 units, this fraction will be $\frac{1\ unit}{1{,}000\ mU}$.

$$\frac{3\ mU}{min} \times \frac{1\ unit}{1{,}000\ mU} = ?\,\frac{mcgtt}{min}$$

Now, on the left side, unit is in the numerator, and it must be cancelled. This will require a unit fraction with unit in the denominator. Using the strength, this fraction will be $\frac{1{,}000\ mL}{10\ units}$.

$$\frac{3\ mU}{min} \times \frac{1\ unit}{1{,}000\ mU} \times \frac{1{,}000\ mL}{10\ units} = ?\,\frac{mcgtt}{min}$$

Now, on the left side, *mL* is in the numerator, and it must be cancelled. This will require a unit fraction with *mL* in the denominator. Using the drop factor, this fraction will be $\frac{60\ mcgtt}{mL}$.

Now, cancel and multiply the numbers

$$\frac{3\ mU}{min} \times \frac{1\ unit}{1{,}000\ mU} \times \frac{1{,}000\ mL}{10\ units} \times \frac{60\ mcgtt}{mL}$$
$$= 18\,\frac{mcgtt}{min}$$

So, you will administer 18 *mcgtt/min*.

RATIO & PROPORTION

One way to do the problem is to first change the dosage rate to *mL/h*. The first problem is

$$\frac{3\ mU}{min} = ?\,\frac{mL}{h}$$

Multiply by $\frac{60}{60}$

$$\frac{3\ mU}{min} \times \frac{60}{60} = \frac{180\ mU}{60\ min} = \frac{180\ mU}{1\ h}$$

In the numerator change 180 *mU* to 0.18 *units* by moving the decimal point three places to the left. Now the problem becomes

$$\frac{0.18\ units}{h} = ?\,\frac{mL}{h}$$

To change 0.18 *units* of the drug to *mL* of solution, think:

0.18 *units* = *x mL*
10 *units* = 1,000 *mL* [strength of the solution]

Use the proportion

$$\frac{0.18\ units}{x\ mL} = \frac{10\ units}{1{,}000\ mL}$$
$$10\,x = 180$$
$$x = 18$$

So the flow rate is 18 *mL/h*, which is the same as 18 *mcgtt/min*.

1,000 *mL*
10 *units*
? *mcgtt/min*
3 *mU/min*
60 *mcgtt* = 1 *mL*
Client

NOTE

1 unit = 1,000 *milliunits* (*mU*)

Converting IV Flow Rates to Dosage Rates

Each of the next three examples (11.5 through 11.7) converts infusion rates from IV flow rates (*volume of solution per time*) to dosage rates (*amount of medication per time*).

Example 11.5

Calculate the number of units of regular insulin a client is receiving per hour if the order is *500 mL NS with 300 units of regular insulin and it is infusing at the rate of 12.5 mL per hour via the pump.*

You want to convert the flow rate from *mL* per hour to the dosage rate in *units per hour*.

$$\frac{12.5\ mL}{h} \longrightarrow ?\ \frac{\text{units}}{h}$$

DIMENSIONAL ANALYSIS

Using the strength of the solution (300 units/500 *mL*) you do this in one line as follows:

$$\frac{12.5\ \cancel{mL}}{h} \times \frac{3\cancel{0}\cancel{0}\ \text{units}}{5\cancel{0}\cancel{0}\ \cancel{mL}} = \frac{37.5\ \text{units}}{5\ h}$$

$$\text{or}\quad 7.5\ \frac{\text{units}}{h}$$

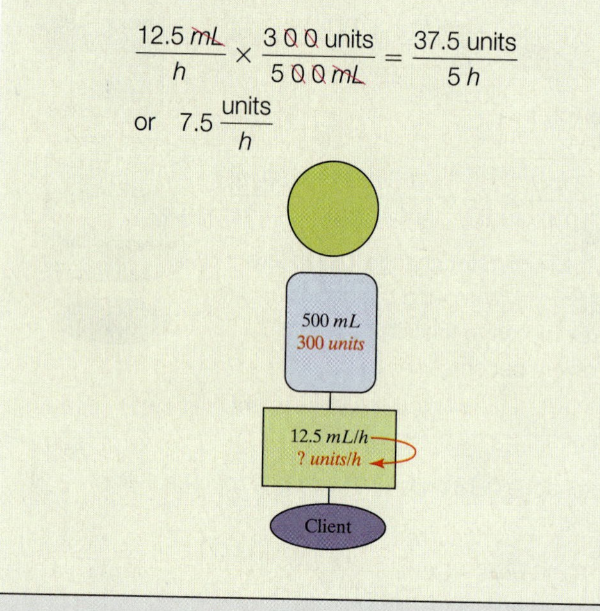

RATIO & PROPORTION

In the numerator, change 12.5 *mL* of solution to units of insulin.

Think:

$$12.5\ mL = x\ units$$
$$300\ mL = 500\ units = \text{[strength of the solution]}$$

Use the proportion

$$\frac{12.5\ mL}{x\ units} = \frac{500\ mL}{300\ units}$$
$$500x = 3{,}750$$
$$x = 7.5$$

This means that 7.5 units of insulin are contained in 12.5 *mL* of the solution.

So, the client is receiving 7.5 *units per hour*.

Safe Dose Range

Examples 11.6 and 11.7 involve determining if an ordered dose is safe.

Example 11.6

An IV bag contains 1,000 *mL* of NS with 500 *mg* of a drug. It is infusing at 12 *gtt/min*. The drop factor is 10 *gtt/mL*.

(a) Find the dosage rate in *mg/min*.

(b) If the recommended dose is *0.5–2.5 mg/min*, is this infusion in the safe dose range?

DIMENSIONAL ANALYSIS

(a) The problem is to change the flow rate of *12 gtt/min* to a dosage rate in *mg/min.*

$$\frac{12\ gtt}{min} = ?\ \frac{mg}{min}$$

(b) The strength of the solution (500 *mg* = 1,000 *mL*) and the drop factor (10 *gtt* = 1 *mL*) will both be used to construct the necessary unit fractions.

$$\frac{12\ \cancel{gtt}}{min} \times \frac{\cancel{mL}}{10\ \cancel{gtt}} \times \frac{500\ mg}{1{,}000\ \cancel{mL}} = \frac{0.6\ mg}{min}$$

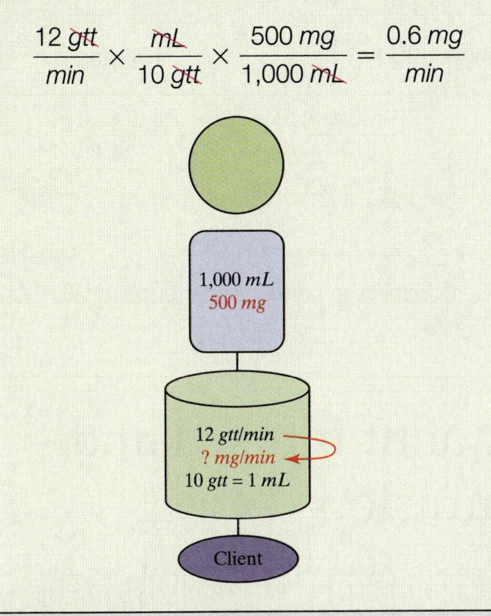

FC & PROPORTION

Change the flow rate of 12 *gtt/min* to *mL/h,* using the FC technique.

DF = 10 and $FC = \frac{60}{10} = 6$. You want *Milliliters per hour*, so Multiply.

$$12 \times 6 = 72$$

Therefore,

$$12\ \frac{gtt}{min} = 72\ \frac{mL}{h}$$

Now, change 72 *mL* to *mg*. Because the strength of the solution is *500 mg/1,000 mL,* you can use the proportion

$$\frac{72\ mL}{x\ mg} = \frac{1{,}000\ mL}{500\ mg}$$

$$1{,}000\,x = 36{,}000$$

$$x = 36$$

So, the dosage rate is $\frac{36\ mg}{1\ h}$. Substituting 60 *minutes* for 1 *hour*, you obtain

$$\frac{36\ mg}{1\ h} = \frac{36\ mg}{60\ min} = 0.6\ \frac{mg}{min}$$

So, the dosage rate is 0.6 *mg/min.*

(b) Because 0.6 is between 0.5 and 2.5, this infusion is in the safe dose range.

Example 11.7

Order: *heparin 40,000 units continuous IV in 1,000 mL of D5W infuse at 30 mL/h*. Find the rate in units/day and determine if it is in the safe dose range—the normal heparinizing range is between 20,000 and 40,000 *units per day*.

You want to convert the flow rate from *milliliters per hour to units per day*.

$$\frac{30\ mL}{1\ h} \longrightarrow ?\ \frac{units}{day}$$

DIMENSIONAL ANALYSIS

Using the strength of the solution (40,000 *units*/1,000 *mL*) and that there are 24 *hours in a day*, you do this on one line as follows:

$$\frac{30\ \cancel{mL}}{\cancel{h}} \times \frac{40{,}\cancel{000}\ units}{1{,}\cancel{000}\ \cancel{mL}} \times \frac{24\ \cancel{h}}{day}$$

$$= 28{,}800\ \frac{units}{day}$$

RATIO & PROPORTION

In the numerator, change 30 mL of solution to units of heparin. Think:

$$30\ mL = x\ units$$

$$1{,}000\ mL = 40{,}000\ units = \text{(strength)}$$

(Continued)

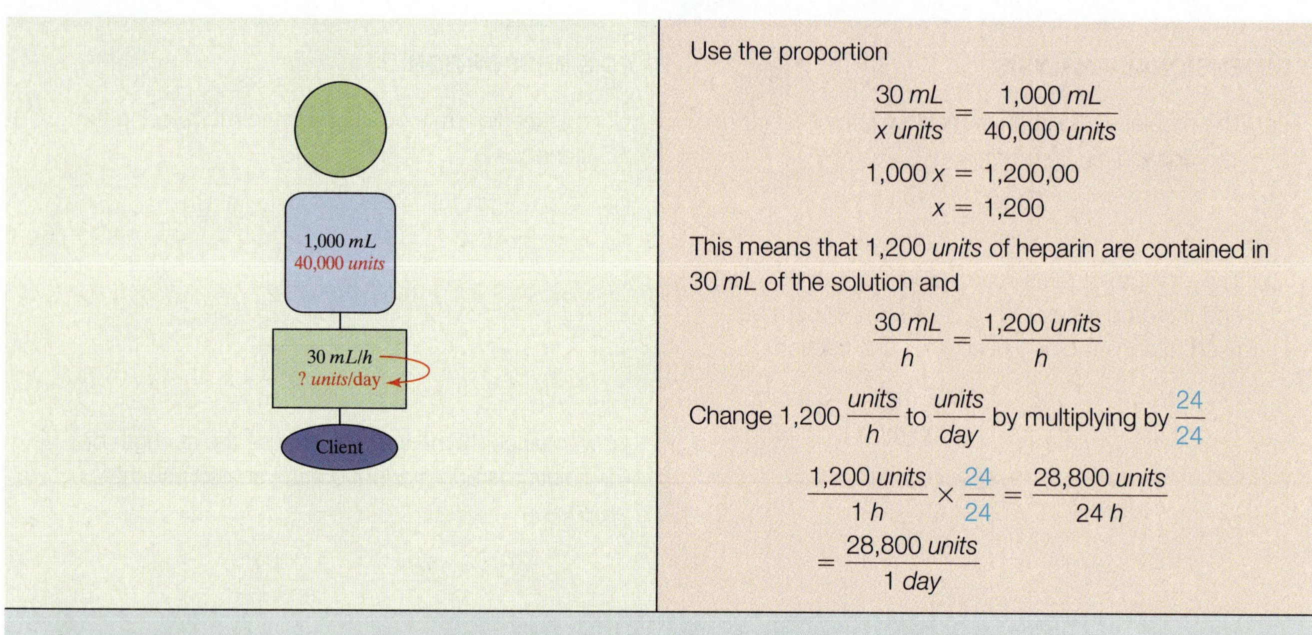

Use the proportion

$$\frac{30\ mL}{x\ units} = \frac{1{,}000\ mL}{40{,}000\ units}$$

$$1{,}000\,x = 1{,}200{,}00$$

$$x = 1{,}200$$

This means that 1,200 *units* of heparin are contained in 30 *mL* of the solution and

$$\frac{30\ mL}{h} = \frac{1{,}200\ units}{h}$$

Change $1{,}200\ \frac{units}{h}$ to $\frac{units}{day}$ by multiplying by $\frac{24}{24}$

$$\frac{1{,}200\ units}{1\ h} \times \frac{24}{24} = \frac{28{,}800\ units}{24\ h}$$

$$= \frac{28{,}800\ units}{1\ day}$$

So, your client is receiving 28,800 *units* of heparin *per day*. This rate is within the safe dosage range of 20,000–40,000 *units per day*.

Determining Amount Infused and Duration of an Infusion

Example 11.8

A client is receiving an infusion at 0.5 *mg/min*. The concentration in the IVPB bag is 100 *mg* in 200 *mL*.

(a) How long will it take for the client to receive 40 *mg*?

(b) How many *milliliters* will the client receive in 30 *minutes?*

DIMENSIONAL ANALYSIS

(a) You are looking for a single unit of measurement (time in *minutes*), so you start with the single unit of measurement that is given, 40 *mg*.

$$40\ mg = ?\ min$$

Use the dosage rate 0.5 *mg/min* to construct the unit fraction.

$$\frac{40\ \cancel{mg}}{1} \times \frac{1\ min}{0.5\ \cancel{mg}} = 80\ min$$

(b) Again, you are looking for a single unit of measurement (volume in *mL*), so you start with the single unit of measurement that is given, the time, 30 *min*.

$$30\ min = ?\ mL$$

You will need both the concentration in the bag, 100 *mg*/200 *mL*, and the dosage rate, 0.5 *mg/min*, to construct the unit fractions.

$$\frac{30\ \cancel{min}}{1} \times \frac{0.5\ \cancel{mg}}{\cancel{min}} \times \frac{200\ mL}{100\ \cancel{mg}} = 30\ mL$$

PROPORTION

(a) Think:

0.5 *mg* infuse in 1 *min* [dosage rate]

40 *mg* infuse in ? *min*

Use the proportion

$$\frac{0.5\ mg}{1\ min} = \frac{40\ mg}{x\ min}$$

Cross multiply

$$0.5\,x = 40$$

$$x = 80\ min$$

So, it takes *80 min* for 40 *mg* to infuse.

(b) Think:

40 *mg* infuse in 80 *min* [from part (a)]

So ? *mg* infuse in 30 *min*

Use the proportion

$$\frac{40\ mg}{80\ min} = \frac{x\ mg}{30\ min}$$

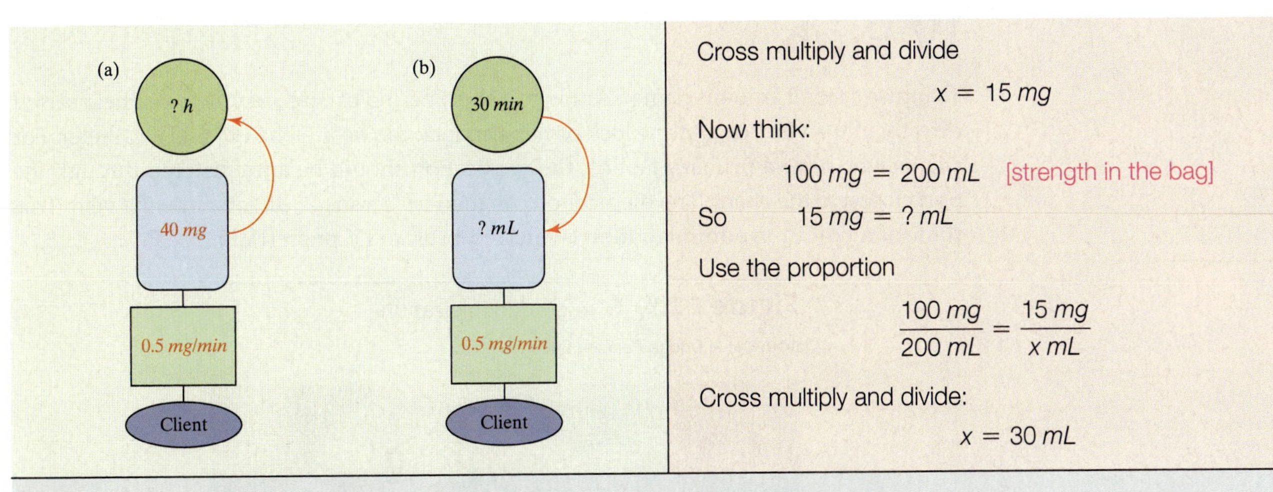

Cross multiply and divide

$$x = 15\ mg$$

Now think:

$100\ mg = 200\ mL$ [strength in the bag]

So $15\ mg = ?\ mL$

Use the proportion

$$\frac{100\ mg}{200\ mL} = \frac{15\ mg}{x\ mL}$$

Cross multiply and divide:

$$x = 30\ mL$$

So, (a) it takes *80 min (or 1 h 20 min)* for 40 *mg* to infuse and (b) *30 mL* will infuse in 30 *min*.

Example 11.9

A client is receiving an infusion of a drug at the rate of 3 *units/min* IVPB. The bag contains 250 *units* of the drug in 100 *mL* of solution.

(a) How many *units* of the drug will the client receive in 20 *minutes?*

(b) How many *minutes* will it take for 50 *mL* of the solution to infuse?

DIMENSIONAL ANALYSIS

(a) You are looking for a single unit of measurement (drug in *units*), so you start with the single unit of measurement that is given, 20 *min*.

$$20\ min = ?\ units$$

Use the dosage rate 3 *units/min* to construct the unit fraction.

$$\frac{20\ \cancel{min}}{1} \times \frac{3\ units}{\cancel{min}} = 60\ units$$

(b) Again you are looking for a single unit of measurement (time in *min*), so you start with the single unit of measurement that is given, 50 *mL*.

$$50\ mL = ?\ min$$

You will need both the concentration in the bag 250 *units*/100 *mL* and the dosage rate 3 units/*min* to construct the unit fractions.

$$\frac{50\ \cancel{mL}}{1} \times \frac{250\ \cancel{units}}{100\ \cancel{mL}} \times \frac{min}{3\ \cancel{units}} = 41.67\ min$$

PROPORTION

You must go from 50 *mL* to ? *units* and then to ? *min*.

(a) Think:

250 *units* are in 100 *mL* [concentration in the bag]

So ? *units* are in 50 *mL*

Use the proportion

$$\frac{250\ units}{100\ mL} = \frac{x\ units}{50\ mL}$$

$$100\ x = 12{,}500\ units$$

$$x = 125\ units$$

(b) Think:

3 *units* infuse in 1 *min* [dosage rate]

So 125 *units* infuse in ? *min*

Use the proportion

$$\frac{3\ units}{1\ min} = \frac{125\ units}{x\ min}$$

$$x = 41.67\ min$$

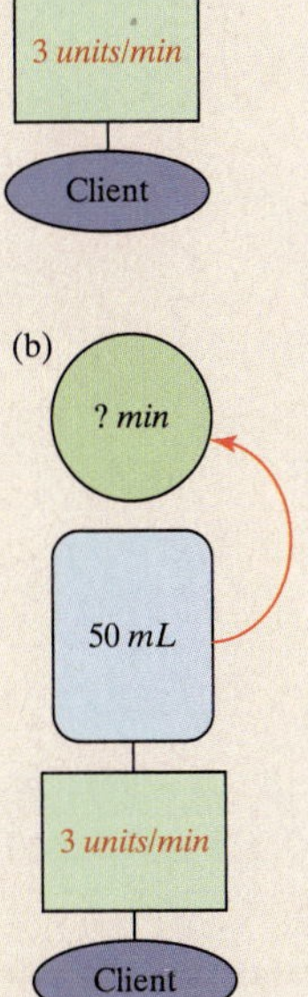

So, (a) in 20 *min* the client will receive *60 units* and (b) it will take *42 minutes* for 50 *mL* to infuse.

IV Push

To infuse a small amount of medication in a short period of time, a syringe can be inserted directly into a vein, or a saline lock or heparin lock can be attached to an IV catheter. For clients who have a primary IV line, the medication should be administered through the port closest to the client. The medication can then be "pushed" directly into the vein. This route of medication administration is referred to as an **IV push (IVP)**. See Figure 11.5.

Figure 11.5 IV push administration.

SOURCE: Al Dodge/Pearson Education, Inc.

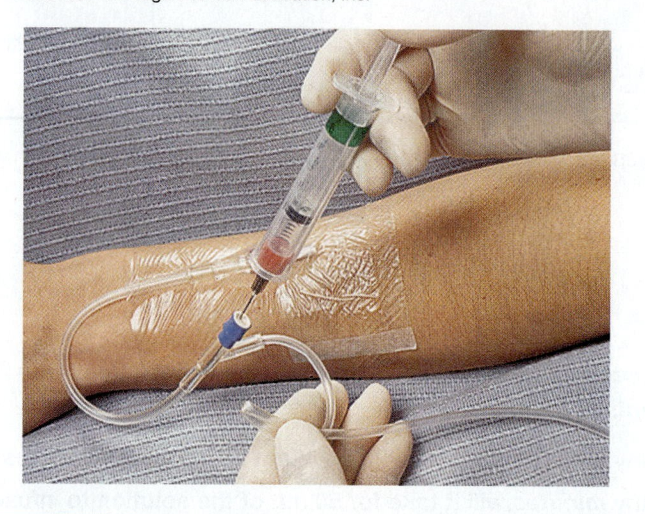

ALERT

An IV push generally involves medications administered over a short period of time. Be sure to verify the following: need for the drug, route, concentration, dose, expiration date, and clarity of the solution. It is also essential to verify the rate of injection with the package insert. Some medications (e.g., adenosine) require rapid administration, whereas others (e.g., verapamil) are administered more slowly.

Because the IVP flow rate is determined by the speed at which the plunger of the syringe is manually pushed, it is important to control that speed. It is difficult to maintain the desired flow rate over the entire infusion. Therefore, the infusion may be mentally divided into smaller segments or pieces to make the flow rate easier to control.

For example, suppose that 4 *mL* of solution must be infused IVP in 1 *minute* (60 *seconds*). Because the total infusion volume (4 *mL*) and duration (60 *sec*) are known, the flow rate is 4 *mL*/60 *sec*. You may choose to divide numerator and denominator of this fraction by any convenient number. By doing so, you will make the numbers in the numerator and denominator smaller and thereby obtain an equivalent infusion rate using the smaller quantities, as shown in the following:

- If you divide both the numerator and denominator of the flow rate of $\frac{4\ mL}{60\ sec}$ by 2, you obtain

$$\frac{4\ mL}{60\ sec} = \frac{4 \div 2\ mL}{60 \div 2\ sec} = \frac{2\ mL}{30\ sec}$$

  and the flow rate of $\frac{4\ mL}{60\ sec}$ is equivalent to $\frac{2\ mL}{30\ sec}$. So, you would push 2 *mL* every 30 *seconds* until the 4 *mL* of medication in the syringe are infused.

- On the other hand, if you divide both the numerator and denominator of the flow rate of $\frac{4\ mL}{60\ sec}$ by 4, you obtain

$$\frac{4\ mL}{60\ sec} = \frac{4 \div 4\ mL}{60 \div 4\ sec} = \frac{1\ mL}{15\ sec}$$

  and the flow rate of $\frac{4\ mL}{60\ sec}$ is equivalent to $\frac{1\ mL}{15\ sec}$. So, you would push 1 *mL* every 15 *seconds* until the 4 *mL* of medication in the syringe are infused.

Example 11.10

750 *mg* of a drug is ordered IVP stat over 5 *minutes*, and the concentration of the drug is 75 *mg/mL*.

(a) Find the total number of *milliliters* you will administer.

(b) Determine the IVP flow rate if you divide the infusion into 5 equal segments.

(c) Determine the IVP flow rate if you divide the infusion into 10 equal segments.

DIMENSIONAL ANALYSIS

(a) The problem is to change the dose of 750 *mg* to the amount of the solution containing this dose measured in *mL*.

$$750\ mg = ?\ mL$$

The strength of 75 *mg* = 1 *mL* will be used to form the unit fraction

$$\frac{750\ \cancel{mg}}{1} \times \frac{1\ mL}{75\ \cancel{mg}} = 10\ mL$$

FORMULA METHOD

(a) D (desired dose) = 750 *mg*
H (dose on hand) = 75 *mg*
Q (dosage unit) = 1 *mL*
X (unknown) = ? *mL*

Fill in the formula $\frac{D}{H} \times Q = X$

$$\frac{750\ mg}{75\ mg} \times 1\ mL = ?\ mL$$

Cancel $\frac{\overset{10}{\cancel{750}}\ \cancel{mg}}{\underset{1}{\cancel{75}}\ \cancel{mg}} \times 1\ mL = 10\ mL$

So, you would administer 10 *mL* over the 5 *minutes*.

(b) In part (a), the rate of infusion is $\frac{10\ mL}{5\ min}$. Because you want to cut the infusion into 5 equal segments, divide both the numerator and denominator of the flow rate by 5.

$$\frac{10\ mL \div 5}{5\ min \div 5} = \frac{2\ mL}{1\ min}$$

So, 2 *mL* will be pushed during *every 1-minute* interval. If a 10 *mL* syringe is used, each tick represents 1 *mL*, and the plunger will move 2 ticks each minute.

(c) In part (a) the flow rate was determined to be 10 *milliliters* in 5 *minutes*. Because you want to cut the infusion into 10 equal segments, divide both the numerator and denominator of the flow rate by 10.

$$\frac{10\ mL \div 10}{5\ min \div 10} = \frac{1\ mL}{0.5\ min}$$

Substitute 30 *seconds* for 0.5 *minutes* to obtain

$$\frac{1\ mL}{0.5\ min} = \frac{1\ mL}{30\ sec}$$

So, each *milliliter* is administered in 30 *seconds*. If a 10 *mL* syringe is used, the plunger will move one tick on the syringe every 30 *seconds*.

Example 11.11

Order: *Cefizox (ceftizoxime sodium) 1,500 mg IVP stat over 4 min.* The 2 *g* Cefizox vial has a strength of 1 *g*/10 *mL*.

(a) Find the total number of *milliliters* you will administer.

(b) Determine the number of *mL* you will push during *each 30-second interval*.

(c) Determine the number of *seconds* needed to deliver each 1 *mL* of the solution.

a. The problem is to change the dose of 1,500 *mg* to a dose measured in *mL*.

$$1{,}500\ mg = ?\ mL$$

(Continued)

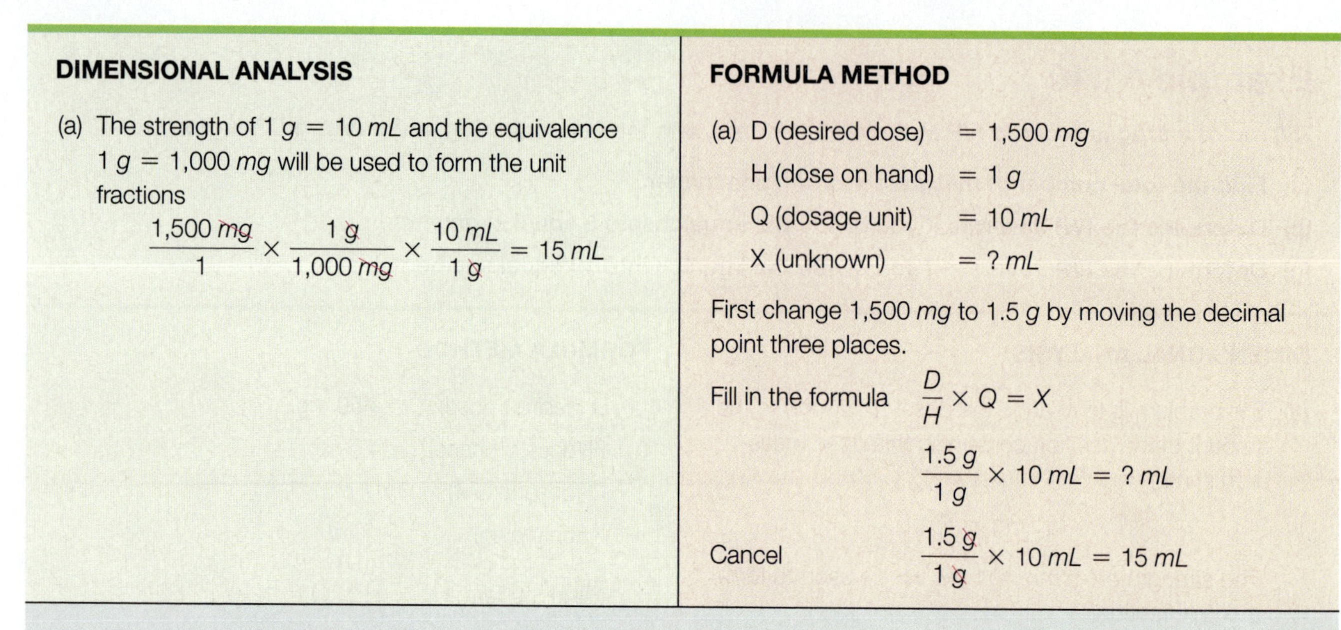

DIMENSIONAL ANALYSIS

(a) The strength of 1 *g* = 10 *mL* and the equivalence 1 *g* = 1,000 *mg* will be used to form the unit fractions

$$\frac{1{,}500\ mg}{1} \times \frac{1\ g}{1{,}000\ mg} \times \frac{10\ mL}{1\ g} = 15\ mL$$

FORMULA METHOD

(a) D (desired dose) = 1,500 *mg*
H (dose on hand) = 1 *g*
Q (dosage unit) = 10 *mL*
X (unknown) = ? *mL*

First change 1,500 *mg* to 1.5 *g* by moving the decimal point three places.

Fill in the formula $\frac{D}{H} \times Q = X$

$$\frac{1.5\ g}{1\ g} \times 10\ mL = ?\ mL$$

Cancel $\frac{1.5\ g}{1\ g} \times 10\ mL = 15\ mL$

So, you would administer a total of 15 *mL* of Cefizox over 4 *minutes*.

(b) In part (a), the rate of infusion is $\frac{15\ mL}{4\ min}$. Because 4 *min* = 240 *sec*, the flow rate is $\frac{15\ mL}{240\ sec.}$ You want to divide the 240-*second* infusion time into 30-*second* segments and

$$\frac{240\ sec}{30\ sec} = 8$$

So, divide both the numerator and the denominator of the flow rate by 8.

$$\frac{15\ mL \div 8}{240\ sec \div 8} = \frac{1.875\ mL}{30\ sec} \approx \frac{1.9\ mL}{30\ sec}$$

So, 1.9 *mL* of Cefizox should be pushed during every 30-*second* interval. This amount cannot be accurately measured on a 20 *mL* syringe; it is only a guideline. Because each tick on a 20 *mL* syringe represents 1 *mL*, the plunger will move about 2 ticks on the syringe each 30 *seconds*.

(c) In part (a) the flow rate was determined to be $\frac{15\ mL}{240\ sec}$

You want to divide the 15 *mL* into 1 *mL* pieces and

$$\frac{15\ mL}{1\ mL} = 15$$

So, both the numerator and denominator of the IVP rate must be divided by 15.

$$\frac{15\ mL \div 15}{240\ sec \div 15} = \frac{1\ mL}{16\ sec}$$

So, 1 *mL* is administered each 16 *seconds*. If a 20 *mL* syringe is used, the plunger will move 1 tick on the syringe every 16 *seconds*.

Compound Rates

In Chapter 6, you calculated dosages based on the *size of the client*, measured in either *kilograms* or *meters squared*. For example, if a client weighing 100 *kg* has an order to receive a drug at the rate of *2 micrograms per kilogram (2 mcg/kg)*, the dose would be obtained by multiplying the size of the client by the rate in the order, as follows:

Size of the client × Order = Dose

$$100\ kg \times \frac{2\ mcg}{kg} = 200\ mcg$$

So, the dose is 200 *mcg*, and the single unit of measurement (*100 kg*) was converted to another single unit of measurement (200 *mcg*).

In this chapter, some IV medications are prescribed not only based on the client's size, but the amount of drug the client receives also depends on *time*. For example, an order might indicate that a drug is to be administered at the rate of 2 *micrograms per kilogram per minute (2 mcg/kg/min)*. This means that, *each minute*, the client is to receive 2 *mcg* of the drug for every kg of body weight. Therefore, the amount of medication the client receives depends on two things: body weight and time.

This new type of rate is called a **compound rate**, and for computational purposes

$$2\ mcg/kg/min \quad \text{is written as} \quad \frac{2\ mcg}{kg \cdot min}$$

where the dot in the denominator stands for multiplication.

Suppose a client weighing 100 *kg* has an order to receive a drug at the compound rate of 2 *mcg/kg/min*. The dosage rate would be obtained by multiplying the size of the client by the compound rate in the order as follows:

Size of the client × Order = Dosage Rate

$$100\ kg \times \frac{2\ mcg}{kg \cdot min} = \frac{200\ mcg}{min}$$

So, the dosage rate is 200 *mcg/min*, and the single unit of measurement (100 *kg*) was converted to a dosage rate (200 *mcg/min*).

Example 11.12

The prescriber ordered: *250 mL 5% D/W with 60 mg of a drug 0.006 mg/kg/min IVPB daily*. The client weighs 75 *kg*, and the drop factor is 20 *gtt/mL*. Calculate the flow rate for this drug in *drops per minute*.

Given: 75 *kg* (weight of the client)

Known equivalences: 0.006 *mg/kg/min* (order)
60 *mg*/250 *mL* (strength)
20 *gtt/mL* (drop factor)

Find: ? *gtt/min* (flow rate)

As shown, multiplying the weight of the client by the order will yield a rate based on *time*. This rate can then be converted to the desired flow rate (*drops per minute*). So you want to start with the weight of the client (*kilograms*) and convert to *drops per minute*.

DIMENSIONAL ANALYSIS

$$75\ kg = gtt/min$$

You want to cancel *kg*. To do this you must use a fraction containing *kg* in the denominator.

Using the order, this fraction will be $\frac{0.006\ mg}{kg \times min}$

$$75\ kg \times \frac{0.006\ mg}{kg \times min} = ?\ \frac{gtt}{min}$$

Now, on the left side *mg* is in the numerator, but you don't want *mg*. You need a fraction with *mg* in the denominator.

Using the strength of the solution, the fraction is $\frac{250\ mL}{60\ mg}$

$$75\ kg \times \frac{0.006\ mg}{kg \times min} \times \frac{250\ mL}{60\ mg} = ?\ \frac{gtt}{min}$$

RATIO & PROPORTION AND FC

Notice that this order involves a compound rate 0.006 *mg/kg/min*. Multiply the size of the client by the order as follows:

$$75\ kg \times \frac{0.006\ mg}{kg \cdot min} = \frac{0.45\ mg}{min}$$

This dosage rate of *0.45 mg/min* must be changed to *mL/h*.

$$\frac{0.45\ mg}{min} = \frac{?\ mL}{h}$$

In the numerator, change *0.45 mg to mL* of solution.

Think:

$$0.45\ mg = x\ mL$$
$$60\ mg = 250\ mL \quad \text{[strength of the solution]}$$

(Continued)

Now, on the left side, *mL* is in the numerator, but you don't want *mL*. To cancel the *mL* you need a fraction with *mL* in the denominator.

Using the drop factor, the fraction is $\frac{20\ gtt}{mL}$.

Now cancel and multiply the numbers.

$$75\ kg \times \frac{0.006\ mg}{kg \times min} \times \frac{250\ mL}{60\ mg} \times \frac{20\ gtt}{mL}$$

$$= 37.5 \frac{gtt}{min}$$

Use the proportion

$$\frac{0.45\ mg}{x\ mL} = \frac{60\ mg}{250\ mL}$$

$$x = 1.875$$

This means that 0.45 *mg* of the drug are contained in 1.875 *mL* of the solution.

The problem becomes

$$\frac{1.875\ mL}{min} = \frac{?\ mL}{h}$$

Change 1.875 $\frac{mL}{min}$ to $\frac{mL}{h}$ by multiplying by $\frac{60}{60}$

$$\frac{1.875\ mL}{min} \times \frac{60}{60} = \frac{112.5\ mL}{60\ min} = \frac{112.5\ mL}{1\ h}$$

Now, change the flow rate of 112.5 *mL/h* to *gtt/min*, using the FC technique.

DF = 20 and $FC = \frac{60}{20} = 3$. You want *Drops per minute*, so Divide.

$$\frac{112.5}{3} = 37.5$$

So, the flow rate is 38 *gtt/min*.

Example 11.13

The prescriber ordered: *Ifex (ifosfamide)* 1.2 *g/m²/day IVPB, infuse over 30 min.* Repeat for 5 consecutive *days*. The IV solution strength is 50 *mg/mL*. The client has BSA of 1.50 *m²*. Find the flow rate in *mL/h*.

Notice that the order contains the compound rate of 1.2 $g/m^2/d$. Multiply the size of the client by this compound rate as follows:

$$1.50\ m^2 \times \frac{1.2\ g}{m^2 \cdot day} = \frac{1.8\ g}{day}$$

This means that the client should receive *1.8 g* of Ifex *per day*. Because the drug must be administered over 30 *minutes*, the dosage rate is $\frac{1.8\ g}{30\ min}$, and it must be changed to $\frac{mL}{h}$.

$$\frac{1.8\ g}{30\ min} = ?\frac{mL}{h}$$

DIMENSIONAL ANALYSIS

Use the concentration *50 mg/mL* to form a unit fraction.

$$\frac{1.8\ g}{30\ min} \times \frac{60\ min}{h} \times \frac{1{,}000\ mg}{1\ g} \times \frac{mL}{50\ mg}$$

$$= 72\frac{mL}{h}$$

RATIO & PROPORTION

$$\frac{1.8\ g}{30\ min} = ?\frac{mL}{h}$$

Replace 1.8 *g* with 1,800 *mg* and 30 *min* with $^1/_2$ *h*.

$$\frac{1.8\ g}{30\ min} = \frac{1{,}800\ mg}{0.5\ h}\ or\ \frac{3{,}600\ mg}{h}$$

The problem becomes

$$\frac{3{,}600\ mg}{h} = \frac{x\ mL}{h}$$

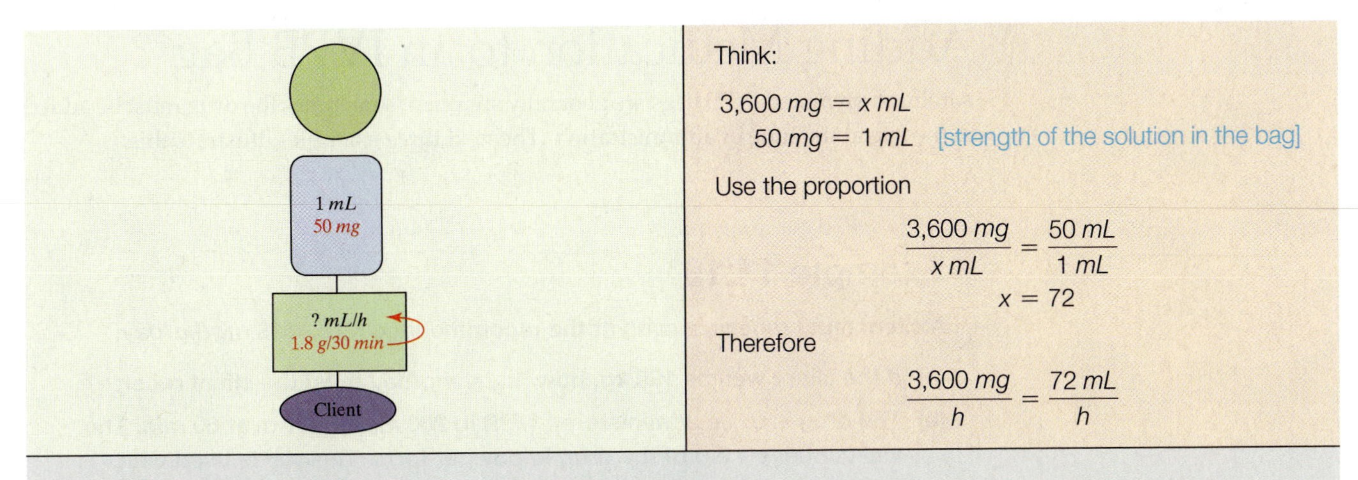

Think:

$$3{,}600\ mg = x\ mL$$
$$50\ mg = 1\ mL$$ [strength of the solution in the bag]

Use the proportion

$$\frac{3{,}600\ mg}{x\ mL} = \frac{50\ mL}{1\ mL}$$
$$x = 72$$

Therefore

$$\frac{3{,}600\ mg}{h} = \frac{72\ mL}{h}$$

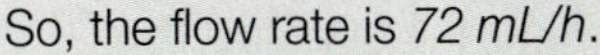

So, the flow rate is *72 mL/h*.

The next example, 11.14 shows how to determine the time it would take a client to receive a given amount of drug when the dosage rate is known.

Example 11.14

The client weighs 80 *kg* and must receive dopamine hydrochloride at the rate of 3 *mcg/kg/min*.

(a) How many *mg/min* should the client receive?

(b) How long will it take for the client to receive 50 *mg* of the drug?

(a) Multiply the size of the client by the order as follows:

$$80\ \cancel{kg} \times \frac{3\ mcg}{\cancel{kg} \cdot min} = \frac{240\ mcg}{min}$$

So, the client should receive the drug at the rate of *240 mcg/min*.

(b) The problem is to find the time (*minutes*) it will take for the client to receive 50 *mg* of the drug.

DIMENSIONAL ANALYSIS

The problem is to change the dose of *50 mg* to time in *minutes*. Use the dosage rate of *240 mcg/min* to form the unit fraction.

$$50\ mg = ?\ min$$

$$\frac{50\ \cancel{mg}}{1} \times \frac{1{,}000\ \cancel{mcg}}{1\ \cancel{mg}} \times \frac{1\ \cancel{min}}{240\ \cancel{mcg}} \times \frac{1\ h}{60\ \cancel{min}} = 3.47\ h$$

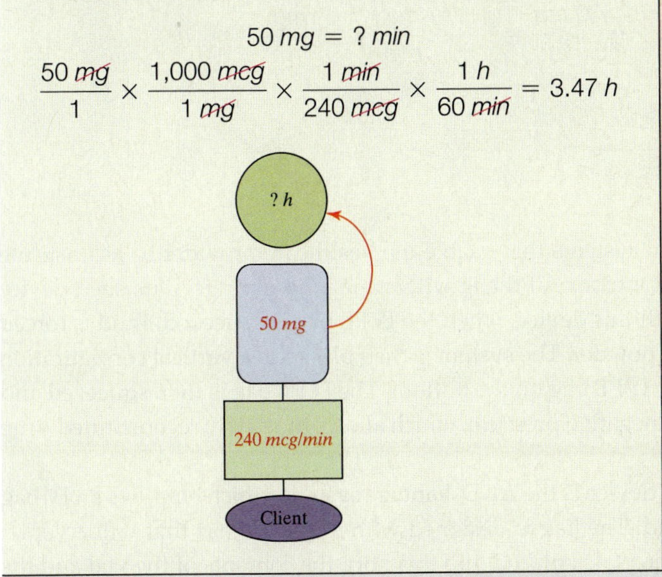

RATIO & PROPORTION

Change 50 *mg* to 50,000 *mcg* by moving the decimal point three places.

Find the time to infuse 50,000 *mcg*.

Think:

$$240\ mcg = 1\ min$$ [dosage rate]
$$50{,}000\ mcg = ?\ min$$

The proportion is $\frac{240\ mcg}{1\ min} = \frac{50{,}000}{x\ min}$

$$240x = 50{,}000$$
$$x = 208.33\ min$$

Now change 208.33 *min* to *hours*.

Think:

$$1\ h = 60\ min$$
$$?\ h = 208.33\ min$$

The proportion is $\frac{1\ h}{60\ min} = \frac{x\ h}{208.33\ min}$

$$60x = 208.33$$
$$x = 3.47\ h$$

So, it will take about $3\frac{1}{2}$ *hours* for the client to receive 50 *mg* of the drug.

Adding Medication to an IVPB Bag

Although premixed IVPB bags are generally supplied, sometimes the drug must be added to the bag at the time of administration. The next three examples illustrate this.

Example 11.15

A client must receive a drug at the recommended rate of 15 *mg/kg/day*.

(a) If the client weighs 100 *kg*, how many *mg/day* must the client receive?

(b) The drug is to be administered IVPB in 200 *mL* D/5/W over 60 *min*. The vial contains 1.5 *g* of the drug in powder form. This vial is used with a reconstitution device similar to that shown in Figure 11.6. Find the IV flow rate in *mL/h*.

(c) How many *mg/min* will the client receive?

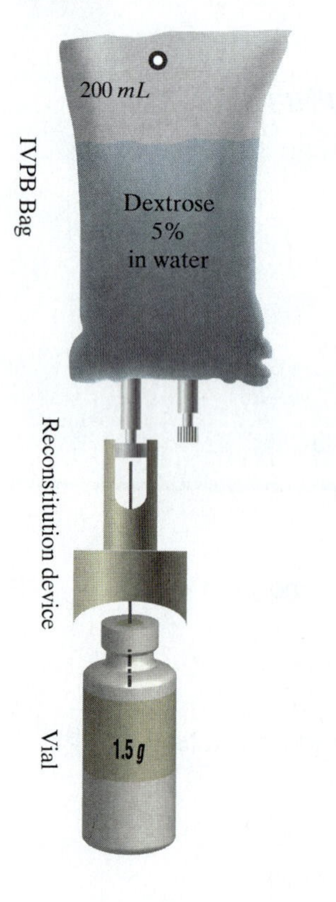

Figure 11.6 Reconstitution system.

(a) Multiply the size of the client by this compound rate as follows:

$$100\ \cancel{kg} \times \frac{15\ mg}{\cancel{kg} \cdot day} = \frac{1{,}500\ mg}{day}$$

This means that the client should receive the dosage rate of 1,500 *milligrams* per day.

(b) Because the drug is dissolved in 200 *mL* and the infusion time is 60 *minutes*, the IV flow rate is

$$\frac{200\ mL}{60\ min}$$

Replace 60 *minutes* by 1 *hour*.

$$\frac{200\ mL}{60\ min} = \frac{200\ mL}{1\ h}$$

So, the IV flow rate is 200 *mL/h*.

(c) The problem is to find the dosage rate in *mg/min*.
Because the client is receiving 1,500 *mg* in 60 *min*, the dosage rate is

$$\frac{1{,}500\ mg}{60\ min} = \frac{1{,}500}{60}\frac{mg}{min} = 25\ \frac{mg}{min}$$

So, the dosage rate is 25 *mg/min*.

There are reconstitution systems that enable the healthcare provider to reconstitute a powder drug and place it into an IVPB bag without using a syringe. One such device is shown in Figure 11.6. With this device, when the IVPB bag is squeezed, fluid is forced into the vial, dissolving the powder. The system is then placed in a vertical configuration with the vial on top and the IVPB bag on the bottom. The IVPB bag is then squeezed and released, thereby creating a negative pressure, which allows the newly reconstituted drug to flow into the IVPB bag.

Another reconstitution device is the ADD-Vantage system, which employs an IV bag containing intravenous fluid. The bag is designed with a special port that will accept a vial of medication. When the vial is placed into this port, the contents of the vial and the fluid mix to form the desired solution. See **Figure 11.7a**.

Figure 11.7a Drug label for an ADD-Vantage® vial.

SOURCE: Courtesy of Pfizer, Inc.

NDC 0409-3378-13

℞ only

Piperacillin and Tazobactam for Injection, USP

3.375 grams*/ADD-Vantage® vial

10 x 3.375 gram Single Dose ADD-Vantage® Vials

ADD-Vantage® Vial

For IV Use

*Each vial provides piperacillin and tazobactam for injection equivalent to 3 g piperacillin, 0.375 g tazobactam and 7.04 mEq (162 mg) of sodium.

Hospira

Contains no preservative.
Usual Dosage: See literature for IV dilution and administration. See instruction sheet for reconstitution, storage and complete directions for use for the ADD-Vantage® system. See literature for stability and storage of ADD-Vantage® solutions after reconstitution. For use only with the ADD-Vantage® diluent container. ADD-Vantage® is a registered trademark of Hospira Inc.
Prior to Reconstitution: Store at 20° to 25°C (68° to 77°F) [See USP Controlled Room Temperature].
Manufactured By:
Sandoz GmbH for Hospira Worldwide, Inc.
Lake Forest, IL 60045 USA.
Made in Kundl, Austria. Product of Spain.
11-2015M RL-5160 46173365

Figure 11.7b shows a DUPLEX® container, which consists of a prefilled, flexible IV bag consisting of two separate compartments: one containing 1 gram of a dry drug and the other containing the diluent. The caregiver simply squeezes the bag to release the seal between the compartments, thereby forming the solution just prior to administration.

Figure 11.7b DUPLEX® IV bag.

SOURCE: B. Braun Medical Inc.

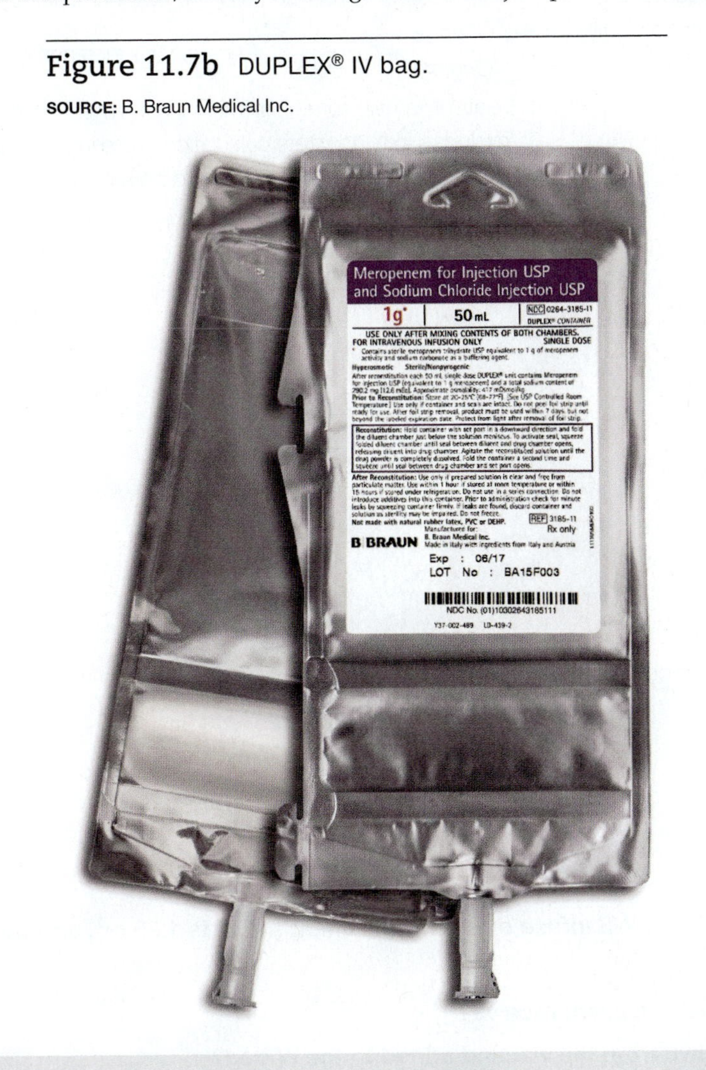

Example 11.16

A client is to receive 150 *mg* of a drug IVPB in 200 *mL* NS over 1 *hour*. The vial of medication indicates a strength of 75 *mg/mL*.

(a) How many *milliliters* must be withdrawn from the vial and added to the IV bag?

(b) At what rate in *mL/h* should the pump be set?

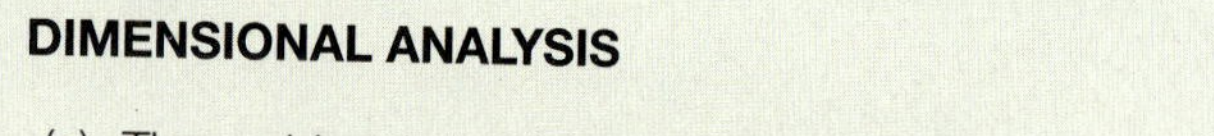

DIMENSIONAL ANALYSIS

(a) The problem is to change the dose of *150 mg* to *mL* of solution to be taken from the vial.

$$150\ mg = ?\ mL$$

In the vial, the strength is *75 mg/mL*; use this to make the unit fraction.

$$\frac{150\ \cancel{mg}}{1} \times \frac{1\ mL}{75\ \cancel{mg}} = \frac{2\ mL}{1}$$

RATIO & PROPORTION

(a) Think:

$$150\ mg = ?\ mL\ [dose]$$
$$75\ mg = 1\ mL\ [strength\ in\ the\ vial]$$

Use the proportion

$$\frac{150\ mg}{x\ mL} = \frac{75\ mg}{1\ mL}$$
$$x = 2$$

So, 2 *mL* of the drug must be withdrawn from the vial and added to the IV bag.

Method 1: *Include the volume of drug added to the IV bag.*

After 2 *mL* of drug are withdrawn from the vial and added to the 200 *mL* of NS, the IVPB bag will then contain (200 + 2) 202 *mL* of solution. Because the infusion will last 1 *hour*, the pump rate would be set at 202 *mL/h*.

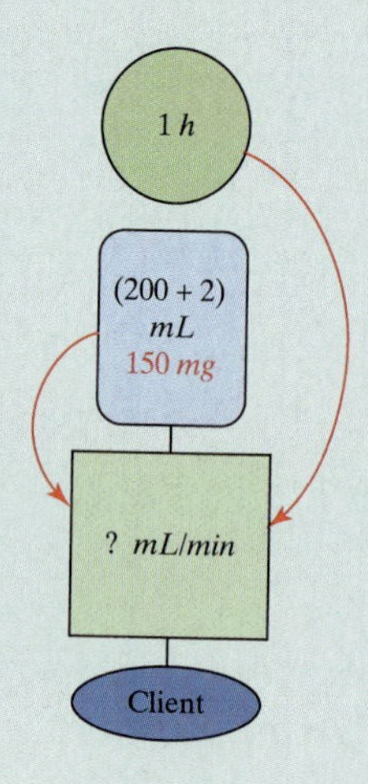

Method 2: *Do not include the volume of drug added to the IV bag.*

When the 2 *mL* of drug from the vial are added to the 200 *mL* of NS, the volume of the bag increases by $\left(\frac{Change}{Original} = \frac{2}{200}\right)1\%$. Because this increase in volume is relatively small, some institutional guidelines permit it to be excluded in IV flow rate calculation. If the increase in volume is excluded, the pump rate would be set at 200 *mL/h*.

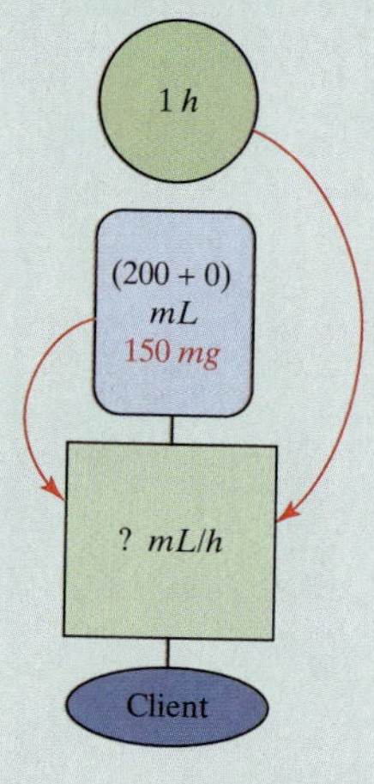

Consult facility protocols to determine which calculation method to use. In the worked-out solutions to the Practice Sets, Method 1 will be used.

Example 11.17

The order is *a drug* 100 *mg/m*^{2} *IVPB in 250 mL NS infuse over 3 h*. The client's BSA is 1.65 *m*^{2}, and the drug is available in a vial labeled 60 *mg/mL*.

(a) How many *milligrams* of the drug must the client receive?

(b) How many *milliliters* must be withdrawn from the vial and added to the IV bag?

(c) The order indicates that the drug should be added to 250 *mL* of NS. At what rate in *mL/h* should the pump be set?

(a) Multiply the size of the client by the order.

$$1.65\ \cancel{m^2} \times \frac{100\ mg}{\cancel{m^2}} = 165\ mg$$

So, the client should receive 165 *mg* of the drug.

(b) The problem is to change the dose of *165 mg* to *mL* of solution to be taken from the vial.

$$165\ mg = ?\ mL$$

DIMENSIONAL ANALYSIS

Use the strength in the vial, *60 mg/mL*, to make the unit fraction

$$\frac{165\ \cancel{mg}}{1} \times \frac{1\ mL}{60\ \cancel{mg}} = 2.75\ mL$$

FORMULA

D (desired dose) = 165 *mg*
H (dose on hand) = 60 *mg*
Q (dosage unit) = 1 *mL*
X (unknown) = ? *mL*

Fill in the formula $\frac{D}{H} \times Q = X$

$$\frac{165\ mg}{60\ mg} \times 1\ mL = ?\ mL$$

Cancel $\frac{165\ \cancel{mg}}{60\ \cancel{mg}} \times 1\ mL = 2.75\ mL$

So, 2.8 *mL* of the drug must be withdrawn from the vial and added to the IV bag.

(c) If the additional volume of the drug is added to the volume of the IVPB bag, the bag will contain (250 + 2.8) 252.8 *mL*, and the pump rate would be set at $\frac{252.8\ mL}{3\ h} = 84.3\ \frac{mL}{h}$. So, the pump would be set at the rate of 84 *mL/h*.
If only the volume of the IV solution (250 *mL*) is considered, the pump rate would be set at $\frac{250\ mL}{3\ h} \approx 83.3\ \frac{mL}{h}$. So, the pump would be set at the rate of 83 *mL/h*.

Example 11.18

A client who weighs 55 *kg* is receiving a medication at the rate of 30 *mL/h*. The concentration of the medication is 400 *mg* in 500 *mL* of D5W. The recommended dose range for the drug is 2–5 *mcg/kg/min*. Is the client receiving a safe dose?

First, use the *minimum* recommended dose of *2 mcg/kg/h* to determine the minimum IV rate in *mL/h* that the client may receive. Multiply the size of the client by the order.

$$55\ \cancel{kg} \times \frac{2\ mcg}{\cancel{kg} \cdot min} = \frac{110\ mcg}{min}$$

Change the dosage rate of 110 *mcg/min* to an IV rate in *mL/h*.

$$\frac{110\ mcg}{1\ min} = ?\ \frac{mL}{h}$$

DIMENSIONAL ANALYSIS

Use the strength of the solution (400 *mg* = 500 *mL*) to form a unit fraction.

$$\frac{110\ \cancel{mcg}}{1\ \cancel{min}} \times \frac{1\ \cancel{mg}}{1{,}000\ \cancel{mcg}} \times \frac{500\ mL}{400\ \cancel{mg}} \times \frac{60\ \cancel{min}}{1\ h}$$

$$= \frac{8.25\ mL}{1\ h}$$

RATIO & PROPORTION

Multiply $\frac{110\ mcg}{1\ min}$ by $\frac{60}{60}$ to change to *mcg/h* as follows:

$$\frac{110\ mcg}{1\ min} \times \frac{60}{60} = \frac{6{,}600\ mcg}{60\ min} = \frac{6{,}600\ mcg}{1\ h}$$

Convert 6,600 *mcg to 6.6 mg* by moving the decimal point 3 places to the left, and the problem becomes:

$$\frac{6.6\ mg}{h} = ?\ \frac{mL}{h}$$

(Continued)

So, the *minimum* IV flow rate is 8.25 *mL/h*.

Now use the *maximum* recommended dose of 5 *mcg/kg/h* to determine the *maximum* IV flow rate in *mL/h* that the client should receive. It can be done in one line as follows:

$$\frac{55\ \cancel{kg}}{1} \times \frac{5\ \cancel{mcg}}{\cancel{kg}\cdot\cancel{min}} \times \frac{1\ \cancel{mg}}{1{,}000\ \cancel{mcg}} \times \frac{500\ mL}{400\ \cancel{mg}} \times \frac{60\ \cancel{min}}{1\ h} = \frac{20.625\ mL}{1\ h}$$

Think:

$$6.6\ mg = x\ mL$$
$$400\ mg = 500\ mL \text{ [strength of the solution]}$$

Use the proportion

$$\frac{6.6\ mg}{x\ mL} = \frac{400\ mg}{500\ mL}$$
$$x = 8.25$$

So, the *minimum IV flow rate* is 8 *mL/h*.

Now, use the *maximum* recommended dose of 5 *mcg/kg/h* to determine the maximum IV rate in *mL/h* the client should receive. You could follow a procedure similar to what was done for the minimum, but it is easier to use a single proportion, as follows:

Think:

2 *mcg/kg/h* results in 8.3 *mL/h*
5 *mcg/kg/h* results in *x mL/h*

Use the proportion

$$\frac{2\ mcg/kg/min}{8.3\ mL/h} = \frac{5\ mcg/kg/min}{x\ mL/h}$$
$$20.75 = x$$

So, the *maximum flow rate* is 21 *mL/h*.

The safe dose range of 2–5 *mcg/kg/min* is equivalent to the flow rate range of *8–21 mL/h* for this client. The client is receiving an IV rate of 30 *mL/h*. Because 30 *mL/h* is larger than the maximum allowable flow rate of 21 *mL/h*, the client is not receiving a safe dose. The client is receiving an overdose. Turn off the IV and contact the prescriber.

ALERT

Whenever your calculations indicate that the prescribed dose is not within the safe range, you must verify the order with the prescriber.

Titrated Medications

The process of adjusting the dosage of a medication based on client response is called **titration**. Orders for titrated medications are often prescribed for critical-care clients. Such orders require that therapeutic effects, such as pain reduction, be monitored. The dose of the medication must be adjusted accordingly until the desired effect is achieved.

An order for a titrated medication generally includes a purpose for titrating and a maximum dose. If either the initial dose or directions for subsequent adjustments of the initial dose are not included in the order, the medication cannot be given, and you must contact the prescriber.

Dosage errors with titrated medications can quickly result in catastrophic consequences. Therefore, a thorough knowledge of the particular medication and its proper dosage adjustments is crucial. Dosage increment choices are medication-specific and depend on many factors that go beyond the scope of this book.

ALERT

Drugs that are titrated are administered according to protocol. Therefore, it is imperative to know the institution's protocols.

Suppose an order indicates that a certain drug must be administered with an initial dosage rate of 10 *mcg/min*, and that the rate should be increased by 5 *mcg/min* every 3–5 *min* for chest pain until response, up to a maximum rate of 30 *mcg/min*. The IV bag has a strength of 50 *mg*/250 *mL*.

To administer the drug, first determine the IV rate in *mL/h* for the initial dose rate of 10 *mcg/min*.

The problem is

$$\frac{10\ mcg}{min} = ?\ \frac{mL}{h}$$

DIMENSIONAL ANALYSIS

Use the strength of the solution (50 *mg* = 250 *mL*) to form a unit fraction

$$\frac{10\ mcg}{1\ min} \times \frac{1\ mg}{1{,}000\ mcg} \times \frac{250\ mL}{50\ mg} \times \frac{60\ min}{1\ h}$$

$$= \frac{3\ mL}{1\ h}$$

RATIO & PROPORTION

Change 10 *mcg* to 0.01 *mg* by moving the decimal 3 places to the left, and the problem becomes

$$\frac{0.01\ mg}{min} = ?\ \frac{mL}{h}$$

Multiplying $\frac{0.01\ mg}{min}$ by $\frac{60}{60}$ will convert the minutes to hours.

$$\frac{0.01\ mg}{min} \times \frac{60}{60} = \frac{0.6\ mg}{60\ min} = \frac{0.6\ mg}{1\ h}$$

The problem becomes

$$\frac{0.6\ mg}{h} = \frac{?\ mL}{h}$$

Now convert 0.6 *mg* in the numerator to *mL*. Think:

$$0.6\ mg = x\ mL$$
$$50\ mg = 250\ mL \quad \text{[strength of the solution]}$$

Use the porportion

$$\frac{0.6\ mg}{x\ mL} = \frac{50\ mg}{250\ mL}$$
$$x = 3$$

So, the initial IV rate is 3 *mL/h*.

After the initial dose is administered, the client is monitored. If the desired response is not achieved, the order indicates to increase the dose rate by 5 *mcg/min*. This requires that you find the corresponding IV rate in *mL/h* for the new dosage rate. This titration may also require other dosage changes. Every time the dose rate is changed, recalculation of the corresponding IV rate is necessary. Rather than performing such calculations each time a dose is modified, it is useful to compile a *titration table* that will quickly provide the IV rate for any possible drug dosage rate choice.

Construction of the titration table for each incremental dose change of 5 *mcg/min*, up to the maximum rate of 30 *mcg/min*, could be accomplished by repeating a procedure similar to that which was used to determine the initial flow rate. Instead, however, the table can be quickly compiled by first finding the incremental IV flow rate for a dosage rate change of 5 *mcg/min*.

DIMENSIONAL ANALYSIS

$$5\ \frac{mcg}{min} = ?\ \frac{mL}{h}$$

Use the strength of the solution (50 *mg* = 250 *mL*) to form a unit fraction

$$\frac{5\ mcg}{1\ min} \times \frac{1\ mg}{1{,}000\ mcg} \times \frac{250\ mL}{50\ mg} \times \frac{60\ min}{1\ h}$$

$$= \frac{1.5\ mL}{1\ h}$$

RATIO & PROPORTION

Think:

$$10\ \frac{mcg}{min} = 3\ \frac{mL}{h} \quad \textit{[initial rate]}$$

$$5\ \frac{mcg}{min} = x\ \frac{mL}{h} \quad \textit{[incremental rate]}$$

The proportion is

$$\frac{10\ mcg/min}{3\ mL/h} = \frac{5\ mcg/min}{x\ mL/h}$$
$$x = 1.5$$

(Continued)

So, for each change of *5 mcg/min*, the incremental IV flow rate is *1.5 mL/h*.

Table 11.1 shows the titration table for the order. It contains the various dosage rates in *mcg/min* and their corresponding flow rates. As you move down the columns, the dosage rate increases in 5 *mcg/min* increments, whereas the corresponding flow rate increases in 1.5 *mL/h* increments.

Table 11.1 Titration Table

Dosage Rate (*mcg/min*)	Flow Rate (*mL/h*)
10 *mcg/min* (initial)	3 *mL/h*
15 *mcg/min*	4.5 *mL/h*
20 *mcg/min*	6 *mL/h*
25 *mcg/min*	7.5 *mL/h*
30 *mcg/min* (maximum)	9 *mL/h*

Example 11.19

The order is: *Pitocin (oxytocin) start at 1 mU/min IV, may increase by 1 mU/min q 15 min to a max of 10 mU/min*. The IV strength is 10 *mU/mL*.

(a) Calculate the initial pump setting in *mL/h*.

(b) Construct a titration table for this order.

(a) Determine the flow rate in *mL/h* for the initial dosage rate of 1 *mU/min*. The problem is

$$\frac{1\ mU}{min} = ?\ \frac{mL}{h}$$

DIMENSIONAL ANALYSIS

Use the strength of the solution (10 *mU* = 1 *mL*) to form a unit fraction

$$\frac{1\ \cancel{mU}}{1\ \cancel{min}} \times \frac{1\ mL}{10\ \cancel{mU}} \times \frac{60\ \cancel{min}}{1\ h} = \frac{6\ mL}{1\ h}$$

Therefore,

$$1\ \frac{mU}{min} = 6\ \frac{mL}{h}$$

and the initial flow rate is 6 *mL/h*.

RATIO & PROPORTION

Multiplying $\frac{1\ mU}{min}$ by $\frac{60}{60}$ will convert the minutes to hours.

$$\frac{1\ mU}{min} \times \frac{60}{60} = \frac{60\ mU}{60\ min} = \frac{60\ mU}{1\ h}$$

The problem becomes

$$\frac{60\ mU}{h} = \frac{?\ mL}{h}$$

Convert 60 *mU* in the numerator to *mL* using a proportion. Think:

$$60\ mU = x\ mL$$
$$10\ mU = 1\ mL \quad \text{[strength]}$$

The proportion is

$$\frac{60\ mU}{x\ mL} = \frac{10\ mU}{1\ mL}$$
$$x = 6\ mL$$

Therefore,

$$1\ \frac{mU}{min} = 6\ \frac{mL}{h}$$

and the initial flow rate is 6 *mL/h*.

(b) The order indicates that the dosage rate may be changed in $1\ \frac{mU}{min}$ increments. Because in part (a) it was shown that $1\ \frac{mU}{min} = 6\ \frac{mL}{h}$, the flow rate increments are also 6 *mL/h*.

Table 11.2 shows the entire titration table. Notice that the dose rates increase in 1 *mU/min* increments, while the flow rates increase in 6 *mL/h* increments.

Table 11.2 Titration Table for example, 11.18

Dosage Rate (*mU/min*)	Flow Rate (*mL/h*)
1 *mU/min* (initial)	6 *mL/h*
2 *mU/min*	12 *mL/h*
3 *mU/min*	18 *mL/h*
4 *mU/min*	24 *mL/h*
5 *mU/min*	30 *mL/h*
6 *mU/min*	36 *mL/h*
7 *mU/min*	42 *mL/h*
8 *mU/min*	48 *mL/h*
9 *mU/min*	54 *mL/h*
10 *mU/min* (maximum)	60 *mL/h*

Summary

In this chapter, the IV medication administration process was discussed. IVPB and IVP infusions were described, and orders based on body weight and body surface area were illustrated.

- A secondary line is referred to as an IV piggyback.
- IV push, or bolus, medications can be injected into a heplock/saline lock or directly into the vein.
- In a gravity system, the IV bag that is hung highest will infuse first.
- An order containing a compound rate of the form *mg/kg/min* directs that each minute the client must receive the stated number of *milligrams* of medication for each *kilogram* of the client's body weight.
- For calculation purposes, write *mg/kg/min* as $\frac{mg}{kg \cdot min}$.
- When the size of the client is multiplied by a compound rate, the dosage rate is obtained.
- When titrating medications, the dose is adjusted until the desired therapeutic effect is achieved.

Case Study 11.1

Read the Case Study and answer the questions. Answers can be found in Appendix A.

A woman is admitted to the labor room with a diagnosis of preterm labor. She states that she has not seen a physician because this is her third baby and she "knows what to do while she is pregnant." Her initial workup indicates a gestational age of 32 weeks, and she tests positive for chlamydia and Strep-B. Her vital signs are T 100°F; P 98; R 18; B/P 140/88. The fetal heart rate is 140–150. The orders include the following:

- NPO
- IV fluids: D5/RL 1,000 *mL* q8h
- Continuous electronic fetal monitoring
- Vital signs q4h
- Dexamethasone 6 *mg* IM q12h for 2 doses
- Brethine (terbutaline sulfate) 0.25 *mg* subcutaneous q30 *minutes* for 2h
- Rocephin (ceftriaxone sodium) 250 *mg* IM stat
- Penicillin G 5 million units IVPB stat; then 2.5 *million units* q4h
- Zithromax (azithromycin) 500 *mg* IVPB stat and daily for 2 *days*

1. Calculate the rate of flow for the D5/RL in *mL/h*.
2. The label on the dexamethasone reads 8 *mg/mL*. How many *milliliters* will you administer?
3. The label on the terbutaline reads 1 *mg/mL*. How many *milliliters* will you administer?
4. The label on the ceftriaxone states to reconstitute the 1 *g* vial with 2.1 *mL* of sterile water for injection, which results in a strength of 350 *mg/mL*. How many *milliliters* will you administer?
5. The instructions state to reconstitute the penicillin G (use the minimum amount of diluent), add to 100 *mL* D5W, and infuse in 1 *hour*. The drop factor is 15. What is the rate of flow of the stat dose in *gtts/min?* See the label in Figure 11.8.

(*continued*)

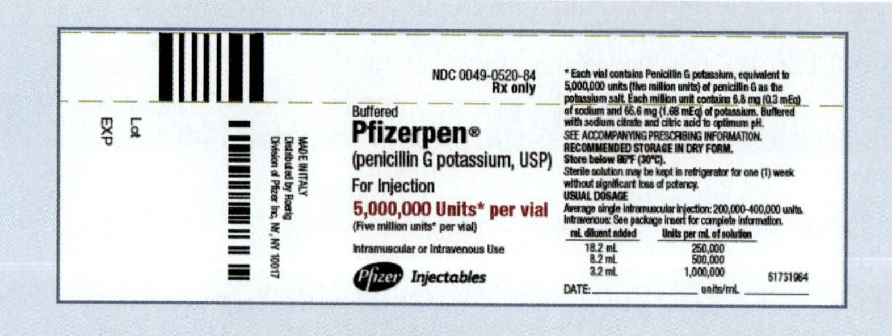

Figure 11.8 Drug label for penicillin G.

SOURCE: Courtesy of Pfizer, Inc.

6. The instructions for the azithromycin state to reconstitute the 500 *mg* vial with 4.8 *mL* until dissolved, to yield a strength of 100 *mg/mL*, and then to add it to 250 *mL* of D5W and administer over at least 60 *minutes*. At what rate will you set the infusion pump if you choose to administer the medication over 90 *minutes?*
7. The client continues to have uterine contractions, and a new order has been written: *magnesium sulfate 4 g IV bolus over* 20 *minutes, then* 1 *g/h.*

   The label on the IV bag states "magnesium sulfate 40 *g* in 1,000 *mL*."
   - What is the rate of flow in *mL/h* for the bolus dose?
   - What is the rate of flow in *mL/h* for the maintenance dose?

The client continues to have contractions and her membranes rupture. The following orders are written:

- Discontinue the magnesium sulfate.
- Pitocin (oxytocin) 10 *units*/1,000 *mL* RL, start at 0.5 *mU/min* increase by 1 *mU/min* q20 *minutes.*
- Stadol (butorphanol tartrate) 1 *mg* IVP stat.

8. What is the rate of flow in *mL/h* for the initial dose of Pitocin?
9. The Pitocin is infusing at 9 *mL/h*. How many *mU/h* is the client receiving?
10. The vial of butorphanol tartrate is labeled 2 *mg/mL*. How many *milliliters* will you administer?

Practice Sets

The answers to *Try These for Practice, Exercises,* and *Cumulative Review Exercises* are found in Appendix A. Ask your instructor for the answers to the *Additional Exercises.*

Try These for Practice

Test your comprehension after reading the chapter.

1. An IV bag contains 600 *mg* of a drug in 200 *mL* of NS, and it must infuse over 2 *hours*. Find the flow rate in *mL/h* and the dosage rate in *mg/min*.
2. Order: *Alimta* 500 *mg*/m^2 *IV on day* 1 *of a 21-day cycle infuse in* 10 *min*. Read the label in Figure 11.9. The directions on the package insert of this antineoplastic drug state: "reconstitute the vial with 20 *mL* NS and further dilute with NS for a total volume of 100 *mL*." The client has BSA of 1 m^2. Find the
   (a) Pump setting in *mL/h*
   (b) Dosage rate in *mg/min*

Figure 11.9 Drug label for Alimta.

SOURCE:

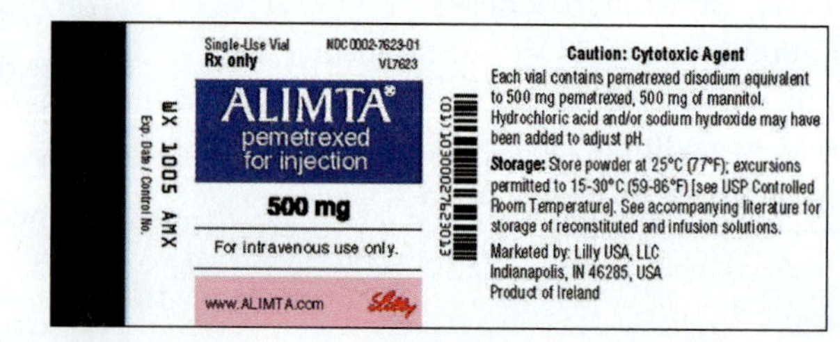

3. An IVPB bag containing 50 *mg* of drug in 100 *mL* of solution must infuse at the rate of 2 *mg/min*. If the infusion begins at 0800 *h*, when will it finish?
4. The order indicates that the client must receive a drug at 1.5 *mcg*/m^2/*min IVPB stat*. The client has BSA of 1.85 m^2, and the strength of the drug in the IV bag is 500 *mcg in* 100 *mL NS*. Find the pump rate in *mL/h*.
5. An intravenous drug must be administered with an initial dosage rate of 0.2 *mg/min*. The order indicates that the dosage rate may be increased by 0.04 *mg/min* every 15 minutes for pain until response up to a maximum of 0.4 *mg/min*. The IV bag contains 200 *mg in* 500 *mL*. Construct a titration table.

Exercises

Reinforce your understanding in class or at home.

1. An IV is infusing at 300 *milliunits per minute*. The solution available is 20 *units* in 250 *mL* D5W. The drop factor is 15 *gtt/mL*. What is the drip rate in *gtt/min?*
2. An IVPB is infusing at 20 *gtt/min*. The concentration of the solution is 40 *mg* of drug in 250 *mL* of D5W. The drop factor is 10 *gtt/mL*. What is the dosage rate in *mcg/min?*
3. An IVPB is infusing at 0.5 *mcg/min*. The solution concentration is 50 *mcg* in 100 *mL* NS. What is the pump setting in *mL/h?*
4. An IVPB is infusing at 120 *mL/h*. The concentration is 50 *mg* in 100 *mL* of NS. What is the dosage rate in *mg/min?*
5. Order: *Gemzar (gemcitabline HCl)* 1,000 *mg*/m^2 *IVPB add to* 200 *mL NS infuse in* 30 *min*. The BSA is 0.91 m^2. Read the label of this antineoplastic drug in Figure 11.10 and determine the
   (a) Number of *mL* of diluent you would add to the Gemzar vial
   (b) Number of *mL* you would take from the Gemzar vial
   (c) Pump setting in *mL/h*
   (d) Dosage rate in *mg/min*

Figure 11.10 Drug label for Gemzar.

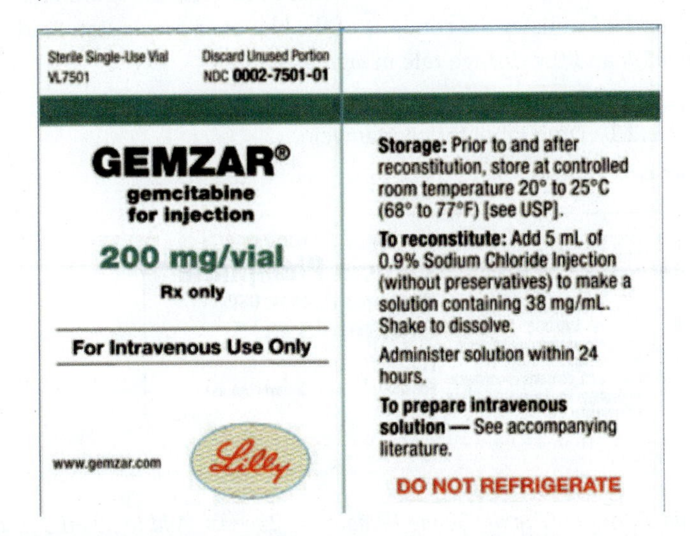

6. Order: *ampicillin sodium* 500 *mg IVPB q6h infuse in* 15 *min*. Find the dosage rate of this antibiotic in *mg/min*.
7. A client with a systemic infection must receive 500 *mg* of ampicillin sodium IV over 60 *minutes*. The concentration of the IV solution is 30 *mg/mL*. What is the flow rate of this antibiotic drug in *mcgtt/min?*

8. Order: *morphine sulfate 4 mg IVP over 5 minutes.* Directions: Further dilute with NS to 5 *mL*. The concentration in the morphine sulfate vial is 10 *mg/mL*.
   (a) How many milliliters will be withdrawn from the vial?
   (b) Find the flow rate in *mL/min*.
   (c) How many *mL* will be administered every 30 *seconds?*
   (d) Using a 12 *mL* syringe, find the number of *seconds* for each calibration on the syringe. [Hint: Each *milliliter* on the 12 *mL* syringe is divided into 5 segments.]
9. Order: *Paraplatin (carboplatin) 360 mg/m^2 IVPB over 15 minutes once q4wk.* The BSA of the client is $1.39\ m^2$. The Paraplatin vial has a concentration of 10 *mg/mL*. Directions: Further dilute medication to 0.5 *mg/mL*.
   (a) How many *mg* must be administered?
   (b) How many *milliliters* must be withdrawn from the vial.
10. A drug is ordered at 0.3 *mg/kg/min*. If the client weighs 148 *pounds,* find the dosage rate in *mg/min*.
11. A drug is ordered at 0.3 *mg/kg/min*. If the client weighs 148 *kilograms,* find the dosage rate in *mg/min*.
12. An IVPB bag contains 200 *mg* of drug in 100 *mL* of solution. If the medication will infuse at the rate of 10 *mg/min,* how long will the infusion take?
13. An IVPB bag contains 400 *mg* of drug in 50 *mL* of solution. If the medication will infuse at the rate of 50 *mg/min,* how many *mL* will infuse in 2 *minutes?*
14. A drug is ordered to start at a rate of 3 *mcg/min IV.* This rate may, depending on the response of the client, be increased by 2 *mcg/min q15 min* to a maximum of 11 *mcg/min*. The IV has a concentration of 5 *mcg/mL*.
   (a) Calculate the initial pump setting in *mL/h*.
   (b) Construct the titration table.
15. Order: *nitroprusside sodium (Nitropress) 5 mcg/kg/minute via continuous infusionstat.* The client weighs 80 *kg*. Find the dosage rate for this client in *mcg/min*.
16. A lidocaine drip is infusing at 30 *mL/hr* via infusion pump. The strength in the IV bag is 800 *mg* lidocaine in 100 *mL* D5W. How many *mg/minute* is the client receiving?
17. An administrator must add the total contents of the vial in Figure 11.11 to a 100 *mL* bag of NS and administer the contents of the bag over 1 *hour* stat. Find the pump setting in *mL/h* and the dosage rate in *mg/min*.

Figure 11.11 Drug label for clindamycin.

SOURCE: Courtesy of Pfizer, Inc.

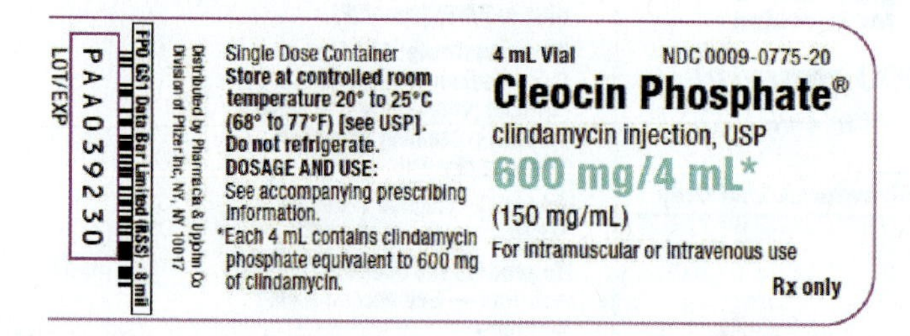

18. Order: *anidulafungin (Eraxis) 50 mg IV daily for 2 weeks. Add to 50 mL NS and infuse over 60 minutes*. Read the label in Figure 11.12.
   (a) How many *mL* of diluent must be added to the vial?
   (b) How many *mL* will be taken from the vial and added to the 50 *mL* bag of NS?
   (c) What is the dosage rate in *mg/min?*

Figure 11.12 Drug label for anidulafungin.

SOURCE: Courtesy of Pfizer, Inc.

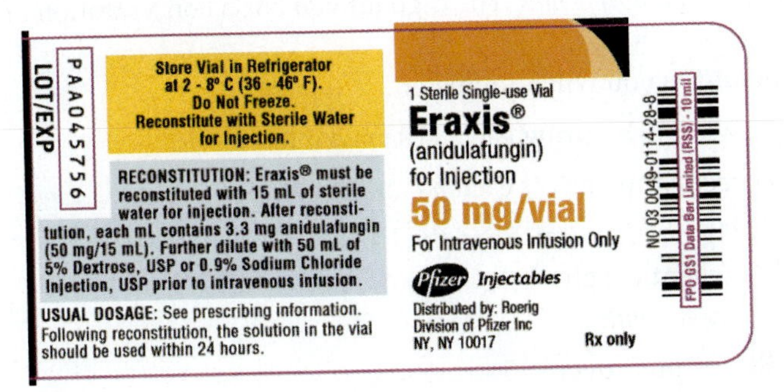

19. Reconstitute the piperacillin and tazobactam by adding 22.5 *mL* NS to the vial. See Figure 11.13. The total contents of the reconstituted vial is then added to an IV bag of 100 *mL* NS. What will be the strength in the bag in *mg/mL*?

Figure 11.13 Drug label for piperacillin and tazobactam.

SOURCE: B. Braun Medical Inc.

NDC 0409-3390-04
℞ only
Piperacillin and Tazobactam for Injection, USP
4.5 grams*/vial
10 x 4.5 gram Single Dose Vials
For IV Use Only
*Each vial provides piperacillin and tazobactam cryodesiccated powders for injection equivalent to 4 g piperacillin, 0.5 g tazobactam and 9.39 mEq (216 mg) of sodium.
Hospira
Contains no preservative. See package insert for reconstitution instructions and complete directions for use.
Prior to Reconstitution: Store at 20° to 25°C (68° to 77°F) [See USP Controlled Room Temperature].
After Reconstitution: Discard any unused portion after 24 hours if stored at room temperature or after 48 hours if refrigerated. See package insert.
Manufactured By: Sandoz GmbH, for Hospira Worldwide, Inc., Lake Forest, IL 60045 USA.
Made in Kundl, Austria. Product of Spain.
11-2015M RL-5156 46173361

20. Ten *milliliters* of a solution must be administered IVP over 2 *minutes*. How many *milliliters* will be pushed every 30 *seconds*?

Additional Exercises

Now, test yourself!

1. An IV is infusing at 80 *mL/h*. The concentration in the IV bag is 40 *mg* in 200 *mL* NS. What is the dosage rate in *mg/min?*
2. An IV is infusing at 0.5 *mg/min*. The concentration in the IV bag is 25 *mg* in 200 *mL* 0.9% NaCl. What is the pump setting in *mL/h?*
3. An IV is infusing at 15 *gtt/min*. The concentration in the IV bag is 40 *mg* in 250 *mL* NS. The drop factor is 10 *gtt/mL*. What is the dosage rate in *mg/min?*
4. An IV is infusing at 40 *milliunits/min*. The concentration in the IV bag is 10 units in 250 *mL* D5W. The drop factor is 10 *gtt/mL*. What is the drip rate in *gtt/min?*
5. The concentration in the IV bag is 150 *mg* in 200 *mL*. If the IV begins on Monday at 0800 *hours* and it must infuse with a dosage rate of 1.5 *mg/min*, then
   (a) what should be the pump setting in *mL/h?*
   (b) when will the IV finish?
6. Order: *lidocaine drip* 0.75 *mg/kg IV in* 500 *mL D5W stat*. The client weighs 169 *pounds*.
   (a) How many *milliliters* of lidocaine 2% will be added to prepare the IV solution?
   (b) Calculate the flow rate in *mL/h* in order for the client to receive the dosage rate of 5 *mg/h*.

7. An IVPB infusion begins at 8:00 P.M. The bag contains 150 *mg* of drug in 200 *mL* of NS. The client is receiving 3 *mg/min*. In military time, when will the infusion finish?

8. Order: *digoxin* 0.75 *mg IVP stat over* 5 *min*. The digoxin vial has a concentration of 0.1 *mg/mL*. Find the
   (a) Total number of *milliliters* you will administer
   (b) Number of *mL* you will push during each 30-*second* interval
   (c) Number of *seconds* needed to deliver each *mL* of the solution

9. Order: *adenosine* 140 *mcg/kg/min IVP stat*. Read the label for this antiarrhythmic drug in Figure 11.14. The client weighs 43 *kg*.
   (a) Find the dosage rate in *mg/min*.
   (b) How many *mL* will you push every 15 *seconds?*

Figure 11.14 Adenosine prefilled syringe.

SOURCE: Pearson Education. Inc.

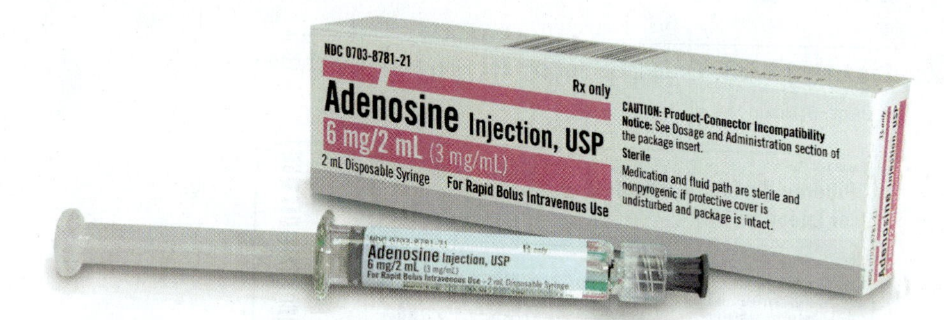

10. The prescriber orders the cardiac stimulant dopamine hydrochloride at a rate of 3 *mcg/kg/min*. The client weighs 155 *lb*. The pharmacist sends a solution of dopamine hydrochloride 200 *mg* in 250 *mL* of D5W.
    (a) How many *mcg/min* will the client receive?
    (b) How many *mL/h* will the client receive?

11. Order: *heparin 1,500 units/h via infusion pump stat*. The premixed IV bag is labeled heparin 25,000 *units* in 500 *mL* 0.45% Sodium Chloride. At what rate will you set the infusion pump in *mL/h*?

12. The prescriber ordered an insulin drip to run at 10 *units per hour*. The IV bag is labeled 100 *units* regular insulin in 250 *mL* NS.
    (a) At what rate will you set the infusion pump in *mL/h*?
    (b) How many *hours* will the IV run?

13. The prescriber ordered Covert *(ibutilide fumarate)* 0.01 *mg/kg IVPB in* 50 *mL of* 0.9% *NaCl to infuse in* 10 *min stat*. The vial label reads 1 *mg*/10 *mL*. The client weighs 125 *pounds*.
    (a) How many *milliliters* of this antiarrhythmic drug will you need?
    (b) Calculate the flow rate in *milliliters per minute*.

14. Order: *desmopressin acetate* 0.3 *mcg/kg IVPB infuse over* 30 *minutes stat*. The vial label reads 4 *mcg/mL* and the client weighs 80 *kg*.
    (a) Calculate the dose of this antidiuretic in *mcg*.
    (b) Add the dose to 50 *mL* 0.9% NaCl; calculate the flow rate in *milliliters/hour*.

15. The physician orders *morphine sulfate* 200 *mg IVPB in NS* 1,000 *mL to be infused at a rate of* 20 *mcg/kg/h stat*. The client weighs 134 *kg*.
    (a) How many *mg*/h of this narcotic analgesic will the client receive?
    (b) How many *mL/h* of the solution will the client receive?

16. Order: *Elspar (asparaginase)* 200 *units/kg/day IV over* 60 *min for* 28 *days*. Add 10,000 *units* to 100 *mL* of D5W. The client weighs 196 *lb*. Calculate the dosage rate for this antineoplastic enzyme in *units/day*.

17. Order: *Humulin R* 100 *units IVPB in* 500 *mL NS infuse at* 0.1 *unit/kg/h stat*. The client weighs 46 *kg*. How long will it take for the infusion of this U-100 insulin to complete?

18. Order: *amikacin sulfate* 7.5 *mg/kg IVPB q8h in* 200 *mL D5W to infuse in* 30 *min*. The vial reads 500 *mg*/2 *mL*. Calculate the flow rate of this aminoglycoxide antibiotic drug in *mL/h* for a client whose weight is 144 *lb*.

19. A drug must be administered IVPB at the initial rate of 2 *mg/min*, and the rate may be increased as needed every *hour* thereafter by 3 *mg/min*, up to a maximum of 20 *mg/min*. The strength of the IV solution is 300 *mg* in 100 *mL D5W*. Make a titration table showing the dosage rate *(mg/min)* and flow rate *(mL/h)*.

20. The physician ordered *Platinol (cisplatin)* 100 mg/m^2 *IV to infuse over* 6 *hours once every* 4 *weeks* for a client who has a BSA of 1.66 m^2.
    (a) How many *mg* of this antineoplastic drug should the client receive?
    (b) If the dose of cisplatin were administered in 1,000 *mL D5 1/2 NS*, at how many *mL/h* would the IV run?

Cumulative Review Exercises

Review your mastery of previous chapters.

1. What is the reading at the arrow on this scale in *mL*? ________

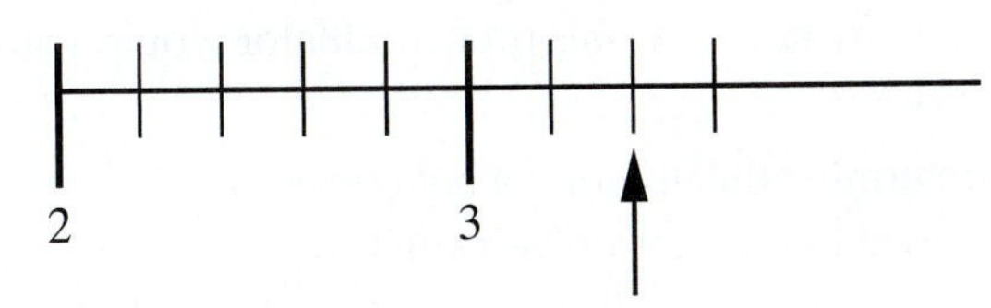

2. What is the weight in pounds and ounces of a neonate who weighs 4,773 *g*? ________

3. Order: *methotrexate* 3.3 $mg/m^2/day$ *IM* × 4 *wk*. The client has BSA of 1.66 m^2. See the label in Figure 11.15 and determine the number of *mL* to take from the vial.

Figure 11.15 Drug label for methotrexate.

SOURCE: Copyright TEVA, Used with permission

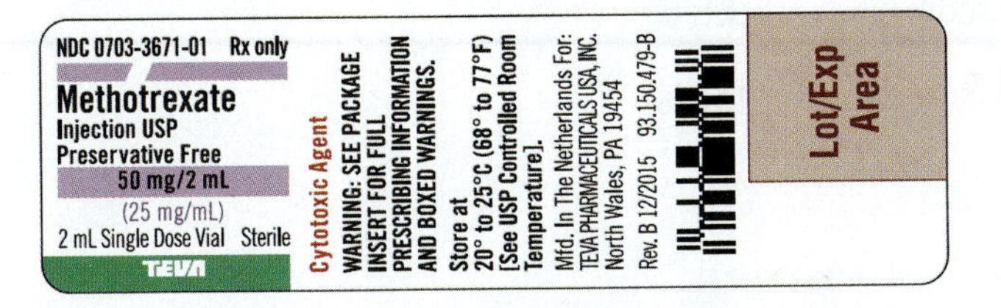

4. Estimate the BSA of a person who is 161 *cm* tall and who weighs 89 *kg*.

5. A client who has hypertension and weighs 154 *pounds* is to receive an infusion of Nitropress (nitroprusside sodium) at a rate of 1 *mL/h*, to be followed by upward titration. The solution contains 50 *mg* of Nitropress in 500 *mL* of D5W. The safe dose range for this drug is 0.3–10 *mcg/kg/min*. Is this initial dose safe?

Figure 11.16 Drug label for levothyroxine.

SOURCE: Courtesy of AbbVie

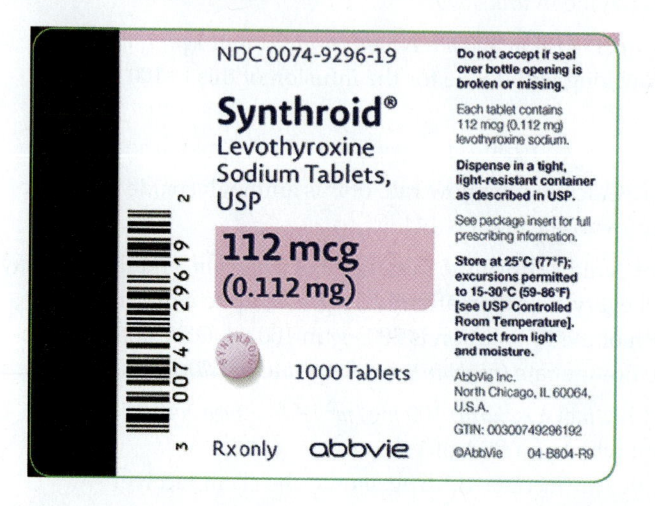

6. Order: *levothyroxine sodium (Synthroid) 224 mcg PO daily*. How many tablets will you administer?
7. A wound has a diameter of 42 *mm*. What is the diameter in *centimeters*? __________
8. Three teaspoons equal how many *milliliters*? __________
9. Your calculations lead to a result of 3.88 *mL*.
   - Round off this calculation to one decimal place. __________
   - Round down this calculation to one decimal place. __________
10. Order: *Uniphyl (theophylline) 5 mg/kg po loading dose stat*. The strength of the Uniphyl is 400 *mg* per tablet. How many tablets of this bronchodilator would you administer to a client who weighs 76 *kg*? __________
11. Read the label in Figure 11.17 to determine the number of *milligrams* of hydrochlorothiazide that are contained in 4 tablets of DiovanHCT.

Figure 11.17 Drug label for valsartan and hydrochlorothiazide.

SOURCE: Courtesy of Novartis Pharma AG

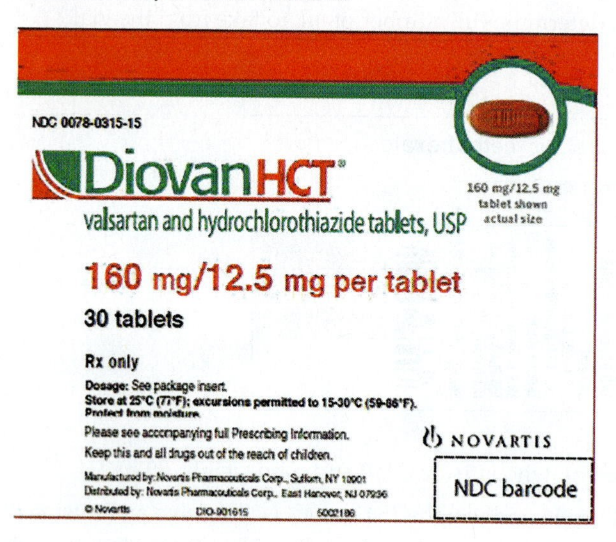

12. Order: ***phenobarbital 0.9 g po b.i.d.*** The recommended dosage for this client with seizures is 100–300 *mg/day in divided doses*. Is the order safe and, if so, how tablets would you administer to the client?

13. The label in Figure 11.18 indicates that the vial contains 0.5 *milligrams* and, equivalently, 500,000 *nanograms* (*ng*). How many *micrograms* (*mcg*) are contained in the vial?

Figure 11.18 Drug label for epoprostenol sodium.

SOURCE: Copyright TEVA, Used with permission

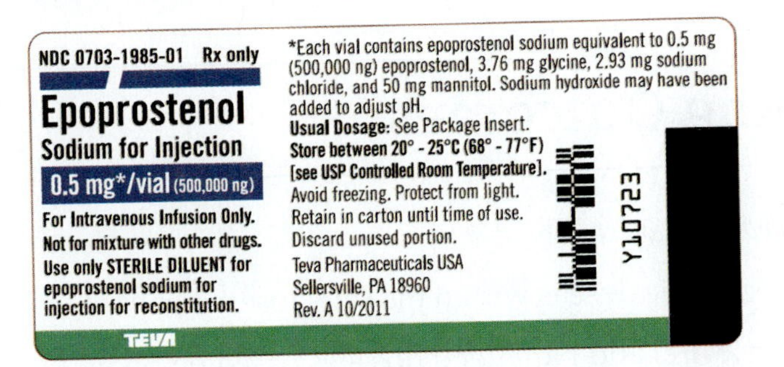

14. A 200 *mg* vial must be reconstituted by adding 9.7 *mL* of sterile water to the vial to yield 20 *mg per mL*. If you need to administer 97 *mg*, how many *mL* will you withdraw from the vial?

15. The flow rate on a pump is 30 *mL/h*. What would be the equivalent flow rate on a gravity system if the drop factor were 20 *gtt/mL*?

Chapter 12
Pediatric Dosages

Learning Outcomes

After completing this chapter, you will be able to

12.1 Determine if a pediatric dose is within the safe dose range.

12.2 Calculate pediatric oral and parenteral dosages based on body weight.

12.3 Calculate pediatric oral and parenteral dosages based on body surface area (BSA).

12.4 Perform calculations necessary for administering medications using a volume-control chamber.

12.5 Calculate daily fluid maintenance.

Because the metabolism and body mass of children are different from those of adults, children are at greater risk of experiencing adverse effects of medications. Refer to your pharmacology and pediatric texts for a complete discussion of the physiological and developmental considerations of administering medications to children. Therefore, with pediatric and high-risk medications, it is essential to *carefully calculate* the dose, determine if the dose is in the *safe dose range* for the client, and *validate your calculations* with another healthcare professional. As always, before administering any medication it is imperative to know its *indications, uses, side effects,* and possible *adverse reactions.*

In this chapter, you are applying many of the techniques you have already learned in the previous chapters to the calculation of pediatric dosages.

Pediatric dosages are generally based on the weight of the child. It is important to *verify* that the dose ordered is safe for the particular child. Pediatric dosages are sometimes rounded down, instead of rounded off, because of the danger that overdose poses to infants and children. Consult your facility's policy on rounding pediatric dosages. In this chapter, dosages are rounded down (rather than rounded off) to provide practice in rounding down.

Pediatric Drug Dosages

Most pediatric doses are based on body weight. Body surface area (BSA) is also used, especially in pediatric oncology and critical care. You must be able to determine whether the amount of a prescribed pediatric dosage is within the recommended range. To do this, you must compare the child's ordered dosage to the recommended safe dosage as found in a reputable drug resource. The recommended dose or dosage range can be found in the package insert, hospital formulary, *Physician's Desk Reference (PDR), United States Pharmacopeia,* manufacturer's website prescribing information, or drug guide books. In order to reduce the chance of errors, the trend is for the pharmacy to supply medication in unit doses. However, the nurse is still responsible for verifying the accuracy of the prepared drug dose, form, and route of administration.

Oral Medications

When prescribing medications for the pediatric population, the oral route is preferred. However, if a child cannot swallow or the medication is ineffective when given orally, the parenteral route is used.

The developmental age of the child must be taken into consideration when determining the device needed to administer oral medication. For example, an older child may be able to swallow a pill or drink a liquid medication from a cup. Children younger than five years of age, however, generally are not able to swallow tablets and capsules. Therefore, most medications for these children are in the form of elixirs, syrups, or suspensions. An *oral syringe, calibrated dropper,* or *measuring spoon* can be selected when giving medication to an infant or younger child. Do NOT mix medications in essential foods or fluids (milk, juice, or formula). If the child does not like the taste, he or she may refuse to accept the food or fluid again. Medications should be placed in the smallest amount of nonessential food or fluid to ensure that the child will take the entire amount. An oral syringe is different from a parenteral syringe in two ways. Generally, an oral syringe does not have a Luer-Lok™ hub and has a cap on the tip that must be removed before administering a medication. Because a needle does not fit on an oral syringe, the chance of administering a medication via a wrong route is decreased. See **Figures 12.1** and **12.2**.

NOTE

Many oral pediatric medications are suspensions. Remember to shake them well immediately before administering.

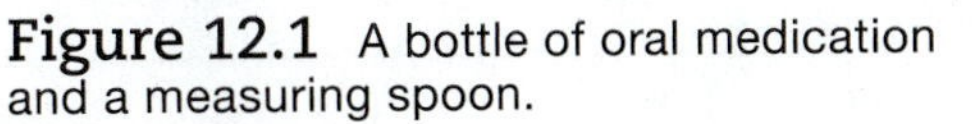

Figure 12.1 A bottle of oral medication and a measuring spoon.

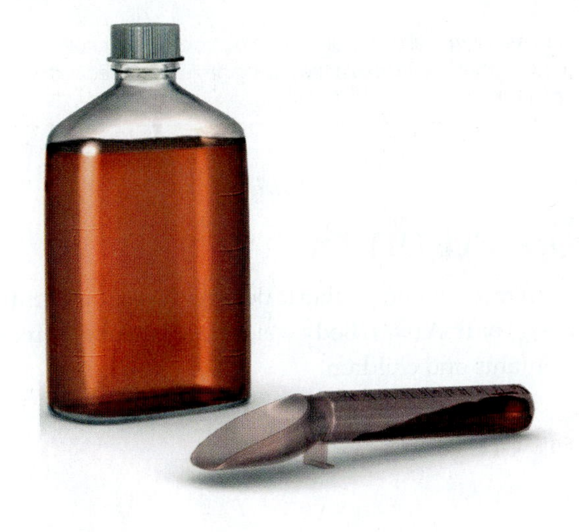

Parenteral Medications

Subcutaneous or intramuscular routes may be necessary, depending on the type of medication to be administered. For example, many childhood immunizations are administered subcutaneously or intramuscularly. Intramuscular injections are rarely ordered on a routine basis for children because of limited sites, developmental considerations, and the possibility of trauma. Because of the small muscle mass of children, the amount injected is usually not more than 2 *mL*. You should consult a current pediatric text for the equipment, injection sites, and procedure.

Figure 12.2 Liquid medication administration devices: Two droppers, an oral syringe, and a measuring spoon.

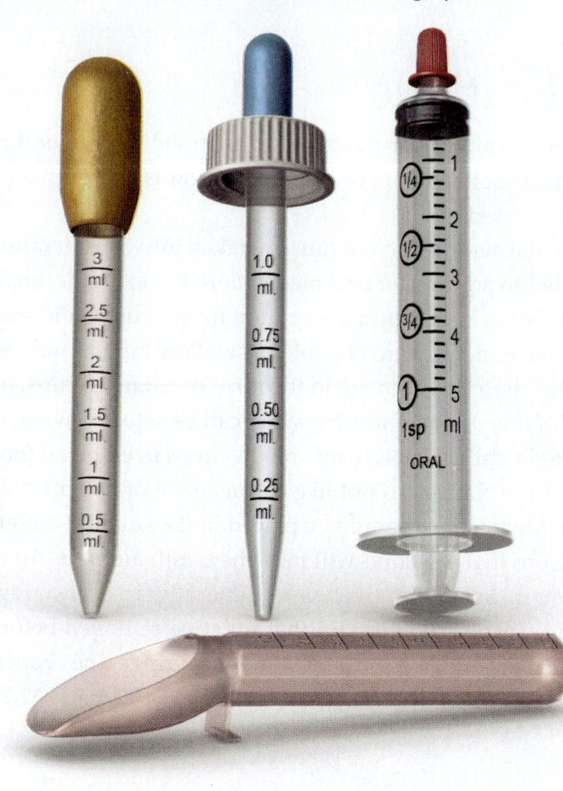

ALERT

Currently, devices used to measure oral doses are not standardized. Therefore, to prevent overdosing or underdosing, never use a measuring device supplied with one medication for a different medication.

Dosages Based on Body Size

Drug manufacturers can recommend pediatric dosages based on client size, as measured by either body weight (*kg*) or BSA (m^2). Body weight in particular is frequently used when prescribing drugs for infants and children.

Dosages Based on Body Weight

Example 12.1

The prescriber ordered *Biaxin (clarithromycin) oral suspension* 15 *mg/kg/day po divided in two equal doses.* Read the label in Figure 12.3 and calculate how many *milliliters* of this macrolide antibiotic a child who weighs 30 *kg* will receive.

The child's weight is 30 *kg*, and the order is for 15 *mg/kg/d* in two equally divided doses. Multiply the *size of the client by the order* to determine the dose of Biaxin.

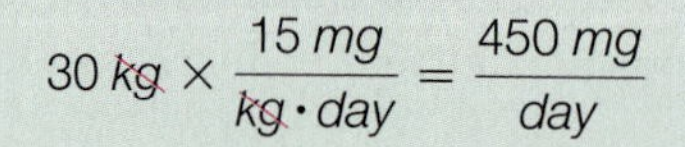

$$30\ \cancel{kg} \times \frac{15\ mg}{\cancel{kg} \cdot day} = \frac{450\ mg}{day}$$

Figure 12.3 Drug label for Biaxin.

SOURCE: Courtesy of AbbVie

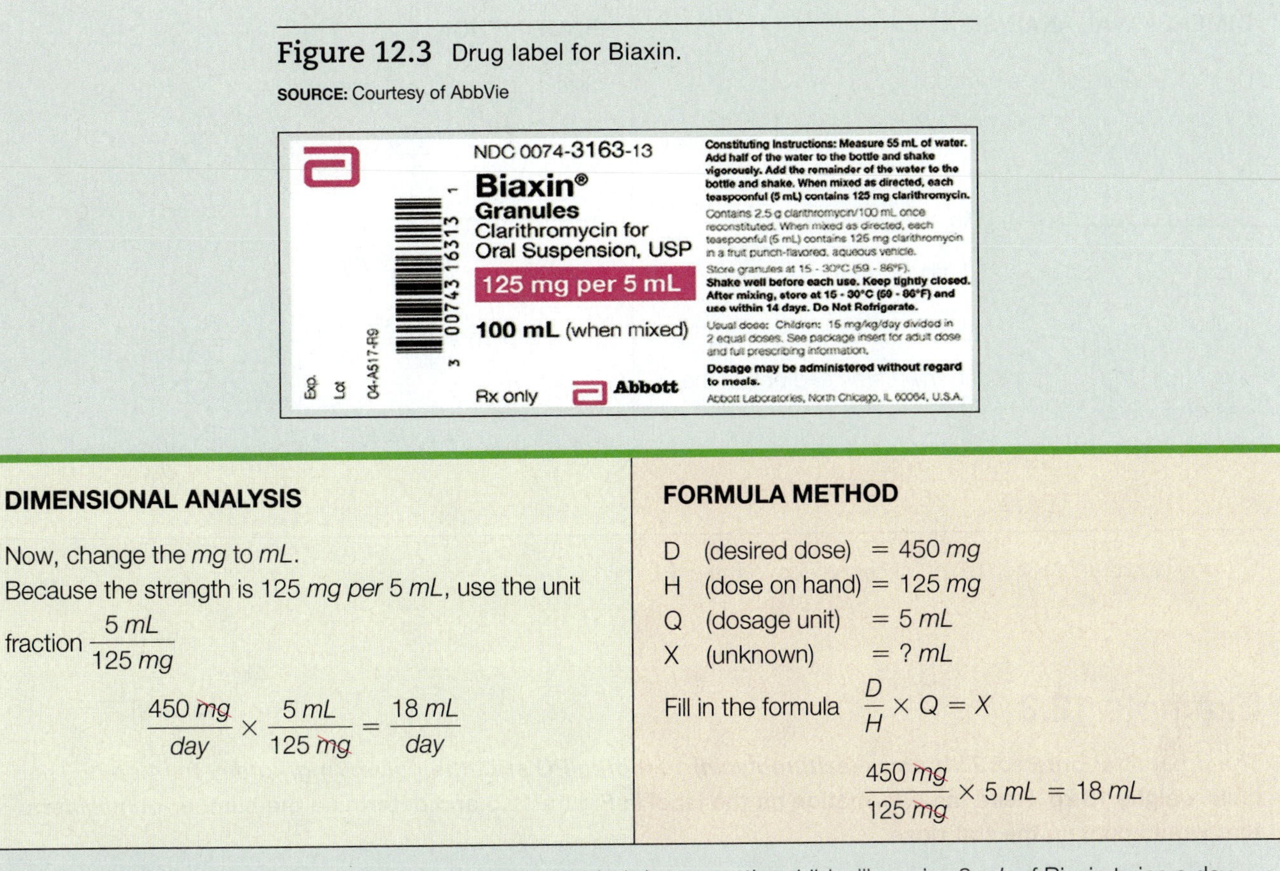

DIMENSIONAL ANALYSIS

Now, change the *mg* to *mL*.

Because the strength is 125 *mg per* 5 *mL*, use the unit fraction $\frac{5\ mL}{125\ mg}$

$$\frac{450\ \cancel{mg}}{day} \times \frac{5\ mL}{125\ \cancel{mg}} = \frac{18\ mL}{day}$$

FORMULA METHOD

D (desired dose) = 450 *mg*

H (dose on hand) = 125 *mg*

Q (dosage unit) = 5 *mL*

X (unknown) = ? *mL*

Fill in the formula $\frac{D}{H} \times Q = X$

$$\frac{450\ \cancel{mg}}{125\ \cancel{mg}} \times 5\ mL = 18\ mL$$

The medication is to be administered in two equally divided doses, so the child will receive 9 *mL* of Biaxin twice a day.

Example 12.2

The prescriber ordered *cephalexin 19 mg/kg PO oral suspension q8h* for a child who weighs 50 *kg* and has otitis media. Read the label in Figure 12.4 and calculate the number of *milliliters* of this cephalosporin antibiotic the child will receive.

Figure 12.4 Drug label for cephalexin.

SOURCE: Copyright TEVA, Used with permission

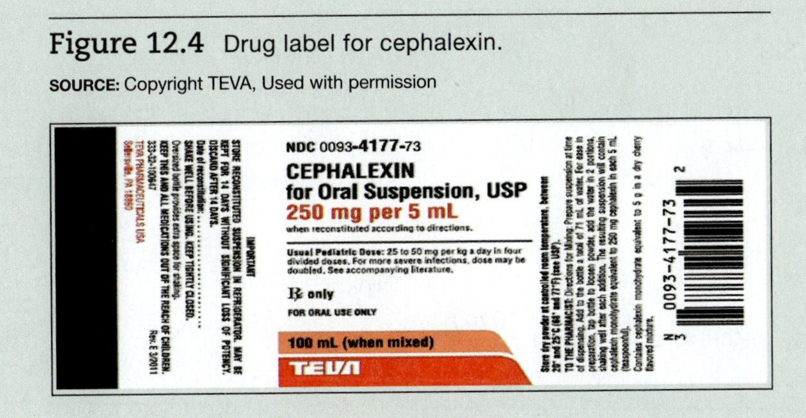

You want to convert the body weight to the dose in *milliliters*.

$$50\ kg \longrightarrow ?\ mL$$

(Continued)

DIMENSIONAL ANALYSIS

Do this problem on one line as follows:

$$50\ kg \times \frac{?\ mg}{?\ kg} \times \frac{?\ mL}{?\ mg} = ?\ mL$$

Because the order is 19 *mg/kg*, the first unit fraction is $\frac{19\ mg}{1\ kg}$

Because the strength is 250 *mg*/5 *mL*, the second unit fraction is $\frac{5\ mL}{200\ mg}$

You cancel the *kilograms* and *milligrams* and obtain the dose in *milliliters*.

$$50\ \cancel{kg} \times \frac{19\ \cancel{mg}}{1\ \cancel{kg}} \times \frac{5\ mL}{250\ \cancel{mg}} = 19\ mL$$

PROPORTION

Size of the client × Order = Dose

$$\frac{50\ \cancel{kg}}{1} \times \frac{19\ mg}{\cancel{kg}} = 950\ mg$$

Think: 950 *mg* = ? *mL*
250 *mg* = 5 *mL*

Make a proportion $\frac{950\ mg}{x\ mL} = \frac{250\ mg}{5\ mL}$

Cross multiply $250x = 4{,}750$

$x = 19\ mL$

So, you would administer 19 *mL* of cephalexin to the child.

Example 12.3

The prescriber ordered: *Zithromax (azithromycin) 10 mg/kg PO stat, then give 5 mg/kg/day for 4 days*. The child weighs 18 *kg*. Read the information on the label in Figure 12.5 and determine the number of *milliliters* that would contain the stat dose.

Figure 12.5 Drug label for Zithromax.

SOURCE: Courtesy of Pfizer, Inc.

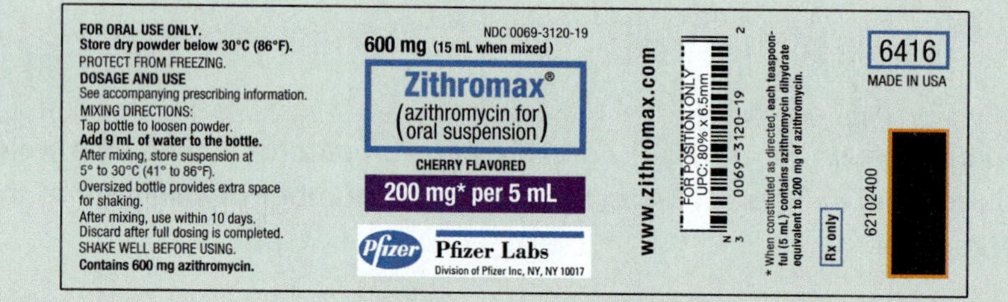

DIMENSIONAL ANALYSIS

You want to convert the body weight to a dose in *milliliters*.

$$18\ kg \longrightarrow ?\ mL$$

Do this on one line as follows:

$$18\ kg \times \frac{?\ mg}{?\ kg} \times \frac{?\ mL}{?\ mg} = ?\ mL$$

Because the order is 10 *mg/kg*, the first unit fraction is $\frac{10\ mg}{kg}$

Because the strength is 200 *mg per* 5 *mL*, the second unit fraction is $\frac{5\ mL}{200\ mg}$

$$18\ \cancel{kg} \times \frac{10\ \cancel{mg}}{\cancel{kg}} \times \frac{5\ mL}{200\ \cancel{mg}} = 4.5\ mL$$

RATIO & PROPORTION

The clients weight is 18 *kg*, and the stat dose is 10 *mg/kg*. Multiply the *size of the client by the order* to determine how many *milligrams* of Zithromax to give the child.

$$18\ \cancel{kg} \times \frac{10\ mg}{\cancel{kg}} = 180\ mg$$

Think:

180 *mg* = ? *mL* (dose)
200 *mg* = 5 *mL* (strength)

One way to set up the proportion is

$$\frac{180\ mg}{x\ mL} = \frac{200\ mg}{5\ mL}$$

$$200x = 900$$

$$x = 4.5$$

So, 4.5 *mL* would contain the stat dose.

Example 12.4

The recommended dose of amikacin sulfate for neonates is 7.5 *mg/kg* IM q12h. If an infant weighs 2,600 *grams*, how many *milligrams* of amikacin would the neonate receive in 1 *day*?

DIMENSIONAL ANALYSIS

You want to convert the body weight to the dose in *milligrams*.

$$2{,}600\ g\ \text{(body weight)} \longrightarrow ?\ mg\ \text{(drug)}$$

Do this problem on one line as follows:

$$2{,}600\ g \times \frac{?\ kg}{?\ g} \times \frac{?\ mg}{?\ kg} = ?\ mg$$

Because 1 kg = 1,000 g, the first unit fraction is $\frac{1\ kg}{1{,}000\ g}$

Because the recommended dose is 7.5 mg/kg, the second unit fraction is $\frac{7.5\ mg}{1\ kg}$

$$2{,}600\ \cancel{g} \times \frac{1\ \cancel{kg}}{1{,}000\ \cancel{g}} \times \frac{7.5\ mg}{\cancel{kg}} = 19.5\ mg\ \text{per dose}$$

FORMULA METHOD AND MOVING THE DECIMAL POINT

The client's weight is 2,600 g. Convert this weight to *kilograms* by moving the decimal point three places to the left. Therefore, the neonate weighs 2.6 kg, and the order is for 7.5 mg/kg. Multiply the size of the neonate by the order to determine how many *milligrams* of amikacin sulfate are needed.

$$2.6\ \cancel{kg} \times \frac{7.5\ mg}{\cancel{kg}} = 19.5\ mg\ \text{per dose}$$

Because the neonate receives two doses per day, the total daily dose is 39 mg.

Dosages Based on BSA

Pediatric dosages may also be based on body surface area (BSA). For example, antineoplastic agents used in the treatment of cancer are often ordered using the BSA. To calculate the BSA accurately, it is important that the *actual* height and weight be assessed, not just estimated. In most instances, the prescriber will calculate the BSA. However, it is the responsibility of the person who administers the drug to verify that the BSA is correct and that the dose is within the safe dosage range.

ALERT

When calculating BSA, be sure to check your calculations with another professional.

Example 12.5

The prescriber ordered *Cytarabine* 200 mg/m^2 *IV over 24h*. Read the label in Figure 12.6 and determine how many *milliliters* of this bone marrow suppressant you will need for a child who has a BSA of 0.49 m^2.

Figure 12.6 Drug label for Cytarabine injection.

SOURCE: Courtesy of Pfizer, Inc.

NDC 0069-0152-01
5 mL Single-Dose Vial
Cytarabine Injection
100 mg/5 mL
(20 mg/mL)
Cytotoxic Agent
Sterile
Isotonic
For Intravenous, Intrathecal, or Subcutaneous Use Only
Rx only

Store at 20 °C to 25 °C (68 °F to 77 °F) [USP Controlled Room Temperature].
Protect from light. Retain in carton until time of use.
Discard unused solution.
Each ml contains: Active: Cytarabine, USP 20 mg;
Inactives: Sodium chloride 0.68% and Water for Injection q.s. When necessary, the pH is adjusted with Hydrochloric acid and/or Sodium hydroxide q.s. to a target pH of 7.4.
Contains approximately 0.12 mEq sodium per mL;
Preservative: None. 1017905
Lot:
Exp.:
MADE IN INDIA
(01)00300690152011
Distributed by Pfizer Labs
Division of Pfizer Inc, New York, NY 10017
Code No.: KR/DRUGS/KTK/28/381/2008

(Continued)

The child's BSA is 0.49 m^2. *Multiply the BSA of the child by the order* to determine how many *milligrams* of Cytarabine are needed.

$$0.49\, \cancel{m^2} \times \frac{200\, mg}{\cancel{m^2}} = 98\, mg$$

DIMENSIONAL ANALYSIS

Now, convert 98 *milligrams* to *mL*. Because the strength on the label is 100 *mg per* 5 *mL*, use the unit fraction $\frac{5\, mL}{100\, mg}$

$$98\, \cancel{mg} \times \frac{5\, mL}{100\, \cancel{mg}} = 4.9\, mL$$

FORMULA METHOD

D (desired dose) = 98 *mg*
H (dose on hand) = 100 *mg*
Q (dosage unit) = 5 *mL*
X (unknown) = ? *mL*

Fill in the formula $\frac{98\, mg}{100\, mg} \times 5\, mL = ?\, mL$

Cancel $\frac{98\, \cancel{mg}}{100\, \cancel{mg}} \times 5\, mL = 4.9\, mL$

So, 4.9 *mL* of Cytarabine are required.

Example 12.6

Order: linezolid 600 mg IV q12h over 120 min. **Read the label in Figure 12.7 and calculate the flow rate in *mL/h* and dosage rate in *mg/min*.**

Figure 12.7

SOURCE: Copyright TEVA, Used with permission

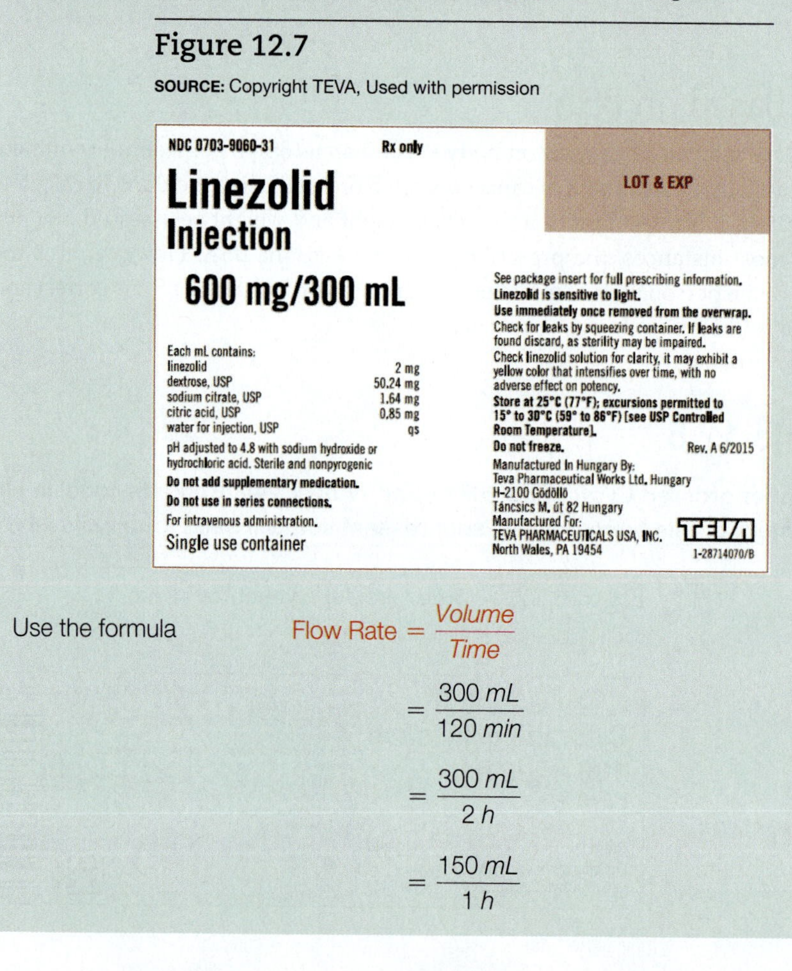

Use the formula

$$\text{Flow Rate} = \frac{Volume}{Time}$$

$$= \frac{300\, mL}{120\, min}$$

$$= \frac{300\, mL}{2\, h}$$

$$= \frac{150\, mL}{1\, h}$$

Use the formula $\text{Dosage Rate} = \frac{\textit{Drug}}{\textit{Time}}$

$$= \frac{600\ mg}{120\ min}$$

$$= 5\ \frac{mg}{min}$$

So, the flow rate is 150 *mL/h* and the dosage rate is 5 *mg/min*.

ALERT

Both overdoses and underdoses are dangerous. Too much medication results in the risk of possible life-threatening effects, whereas too little medication risks suboptimal therapeutic effects.

Determining Safe Dosage Range

The following example illustrates that pediatric dosage orders should always be compared with recommended dosages, as found in reputable drug references such as the *PDR* and drug package inserts.

Example 12.7

The prescriber ordered *Dilantin (phenytoin)* 100 *mg oral suspension PO daily*. The recommended daily maintenance dosage is 4–8 *mg/kg/d*. Is the ordered dose safe for a child who weighs 30 *kg*?

Use the *minimum* recommended dosage of 4 *mg/kg* to determine the minimum number of *milligrams* the child should receive daily.

Multiply the size of the client by the minimum daily recommendation.

$$30\ \cancel{kg} \times \frac{4\ mg}{\cancel{kg}} = 120\ mg$$

So, the *minimum daily safe dose* is 120 *mg*.

Now use the *maximum* recommended dosage of 8 *mg/kg* to determine the maximum number of *milligrams* the child should receive daily.

Multiply the size of the client by the maximum daily recommendation.

$$30\ \cancel{kg} \times \frac{8\ mg}{\cancel{kg}} = 240\ mg$$

So, the *maximum daily safe dose* is 240 *mg*.

The recommended dosage of 4–8 *mg/kg/d* is equivalent to a dose range of 120–240 *mg* daily for this child. The ordered dose of 100 *mg* is smaller than the minimum recommended dose of 120 *mg*. Therefore, the ordered dose is not in the safe dose range, and it should not be administered. The healthcare provider must contact the prescriber.

Example 12.8

The prescriber ordered *gentamicin* 60 *mg IM q8h* for a child who weighs 60 *lb*. The recommended dosage is 6–7.5 *mg/kg/day* in 3 divided doses.

(a) What is the recommended dosage in *mg/day*, and is the order safe?

(b) The strength on the vial is 80 *mg*/2 *mL*. Determine the number of *milliliters* you would administer.

DIMENSIONAL ANALYSIS

(a) You want to convert the body weight in *pounds* to *kilograms*, and then convert the body weight in *kilograms* to the recommended dose in *milligrams* of gentamicin *per day*.

60 *lb* (body weight) ⟶ *kg* (body weight) ⟶ *mg* (drug)

Do this on one line as follows:

$$\frac{60\ lb}{1} \times \frac{?\ kg}{?\ lb} \times \frac{?\ mg}{?\ kg \times day} = \frac{?\ mg}{day}$$

Because 1 *kg* = 2.2 *lb*, the first unit fraction is $\frac{1\ kg}{2.2\ lb}$

Because the *minimum recommended* dose is 6 *mg/kg per day*, the second unit fraction is $\frac{6\ mg}{kg \times day}$

$$\frac{60\ lb}{1} \times \frac{1\ kg}{2.2\ lb} \times \frac{6\ mg}{kg \cdot day} = \frac{163.6\ mg}{day}$$

So, the minimum safe dose is 163.6 *mg/d*. Now, use the *maximum recommended* dose of 7.5 *mg/kg* to determine the maximum number of *milligrams* the child may receive. Because the *maximum recommended* dose is 7.5 *mg/kg per day*, the second unit fraction is $\frac{7.5\ mg}{kg \times day}$

$$\frac{60\ lb}{1} \times \frac{1\ kg}{2.2\ lb} \times \frac{7.5\ mg}{kg \cdot day} = \frac{204.5\ mg}{day}$$

So, the maximum safe dose is 204.5 *mg/d*. The safe dose range of *6–7.5 mg/kg/d* is equivalent to a dose range of *163.6–204.5 mg/d* for this child.

The ordered dose of 60 *mg q8h* is a total of 180 *mg/d* and is within the recommended safe dose range.

RATIO & PROPORTION

(a) The child's weight is 60 *lb*. Divide by 2.2 to convert this weight to *kg*.

$$\frac{60\ lb}{2.2} \approx 27.3\ kg$$

Multiply the weight of the child by the minimum and maximum recommended doses to determine the *safe dose range for this child in milligrams*.

$$27.3\ kg \times \frac{6\ mg}{kg \cdot day} \approx 164\ mg/day \quad \text{[min]}$$

$$27.3\ kg \times \frac{7.5\ mg}{kg \cdot day} \approx 205\ mg/day \quad \text{[max]}$$

The safe dose range for this child is 164–205 *mg/d*. Because the ordered dose of 60 *mg* three times a day (180 *mg/d*), the ordered dose is safe.

(b) Convert the ordered dose of 60 *mg* to *milliliters*. Think:

60 *mg* = ? *mL*

80 *mg* = 2 *mL* [strength on the label]

One way to set up the proportion is

$$\frac{60\ mg}{x\ mL} = \frac{80\ mg}{2\ mL}$$

$$80x = 120$$

$$x = 1.5$$

(b) You want to convert the ordered dose in *milligrams* to *milliliters*.

$$mg \text{ (drug)} \longrightarrow mL \text{ (drug)}$$

Do this on one line as follows:

$$60\ mg \times \frac{?\ mL}{?\ mg} = ?\ mL$$

Because the strength of the gentamicin is 80 *mg*/2 *mL*, the unit fraction is $\frac{2\ mL}{80\ mg}$

$$\frac{60\ \cancel{mg}}{1} \times \frac{2\ mL}{80\ \cancel{mg}} = 1.5\ mL$$

So, you would administer 1.5 *mL* of gentamicin IM q8h.

Example 12.9

Valium (diazepam) 3.75 *mg* *IVP* stat was ordered for a child with status epilepticus. The package insert says that the recommended dose is 0.2–0.5 *mg/kg/d* IVP slowly. The child weighs 33 *lb*, and the label on the vial reads 5 *mg/mL*.

(a) Is the ordered dose within the safe range?

(b) How many *milliliters* would you administer?

DIMENSIONAL ANALYSIS

(a) You want to convert the body weight in *pounds* to *kilograms*; then convert the body weight in *kilograms* to a recommended dose in *milligrams*.

$$33\ lb \text{ (body weight)} \longrightarrow ?\ kg \text{ (body weight)} \longrightarrow ?\ mg \text{ (drug)}$$

Do this on one line as follows:

$$33\ lb \times \frac{?\ kg}{?\ lb} \times \frac{?\ mg}{?\ kg} = ?\ mg$$

Because 1 *kg* = 2.2 *lb*, the first unit fraction is $\frac{1\ kg}{2.2\ lb}$

Because the recommended dosage is 0.2 *mg* to 0.5 *mg/kg* per day, you need to find the minimum and the maximum recommended doses in *milligrams* for this client. Use the unit fractions $\frac{0.2\ mg}{kg}$ and $\frac{0.5\ mg}{kg}$

$$\frac{33\ \cancel{lb}}{1} \times \frac{1\ \cancel{kg}}{2.2\ \cancel{lb}} \times \frac{0.2\ mg}{\cancel{kg}} = 3\ mg \text{ the minimum dose}$$

$$\frac{33\ \cancel{lb}}{1} \times \frac{1\ \cancel{kg}}{2.2\ \cancel{lb}} \times \frac{0.5\ mg}{\cancel{kg}} = 7.5\ mg \text{ the maximum dose}$$

The safe dose range for this client is 3–7.5 *mg*. Because the ordered dose of 3.75 *mg* is between 3 *mg* and 7.5 *mg*, it is a safe dose.

RATIO & PROPORTION

(a) The child's weight is 33 *lb*. Divide by 2.2 to convert this weight to *kg*.

$$\frac{33\ lb}{2.2} = 15\ kg$$

Multiply the *weight of the child* by the *minimum and maximum recommended doses* to determine the *safe dose range for this child in milligrams.*

$$15\ \cancel{kg} \times \frac{0.2\ mg}{\cancel{kg}} = 3\ mg \quad \text{[min]}$$

$$15\ \cancel{kg} \times \frac{0.5\ mg}{\cancel{kg}} = 7.5\ mg \quad \text{[max]}$$

But 7.5 *mg* is above the recommended maximum of 5 *mg* as stated in the example, therefore the *safe dose range for this child is 3–5 mg*. Because the ordered dose of 3.75 *mg* is between 3 *mg* and 5 *mg*, the ordered dose is safe.

(b) Convert the ordered dose of 3.75 *mg* to *milliliters*. Think:

$$3.75\ mg = ?\ mL \quad \text{(dose)}$$
$$5\ mg = 1\ mL \quad \text{[strength on the label]}$$

One way to set up the proportion is

$$\frac{3.75\ mg}{x\ mL} = \frac{5\ mg}{1\ mL}$$
$$5x = 3.75$$
$$x = 0.75$$

(Continued)

(b) You want to convert the ordered dosage in *milligrams* to the liquid *daily dose in milliliters*.

$$3.75\ mg \text{ (drug)} \longrightarrow ?\ mL \text{ (drug)}$$

Do this on one line as follows:

$$3.75\ mg \times \frac{?\ mL}{?\ mg} = ?\ mL$$

Because the vial label says that 5 *mg/mL*., the unit fraction is $\frac{1\ mL}{5\ mg}$

$$\frac{3.75\ \cancel{mg}}{1} \times \frac{1\ mL}{5\ \cancel{mg}} = 0.75\ mL$$

So, you would administer 0.75 *mL* of the Valium IVP slowly.

Intravenous Medications

When a child is to have nothing by mouth (NPO), needs pain relief, or needs a high concentration of a medication, the intravenous (IV) route is the most effective route to use. In addition, when the duration of the therapy is long term, or when gastrointestinal absorption is poor, the IV route is indicated.

Methods of intravenous infusions include peripheral intravenous catheters, peripherally inserted central catheters (PICCs), central lines, and long-term central venous access devices (VADs) or ports. The method chosen is based on the age and size of the child and the duration of therapy.

Most IV medications must be further diluted once the correct dose is calculated. Follow the directions precisely for the reconstitution process. An electronic infusion device and a volume-control chamber should always be used to administer IV fluids and intravenous piggyback (IVPB) medications, especially high-alert drugs, to infants and children.

ALERT

An excessively high concentration of an IV drug can cause irritation to the vein and have potentially life-threatening toxic effects. Read the manufacturer's directions carefully.

NOTE

Know the facility's policy concerning the amount of fluid used to flush the VCC tubing.

Using a Volume-Control Chamber

To avoid fluid overload, pediatric IV medications are frequently administered using a volume-control chamber (VCC) (burette, Volutrol, Buretrol, Soluset).

A VCC is calibrated in 1 *mL* increments and has a capacity of 100–150 *mL*. It can be used as a primary or secondary line. When administering IVPB medications, the medication is added to the top injection port of the VCC. Fluid is then added from the IV bag to further dilute the medication. After the infusion is complete, additional IV fluid is added to the VCC to flush any remaining medication left in the tubing. See **Figure 12.8**.

Figure 12.8 Volume-control chamber.

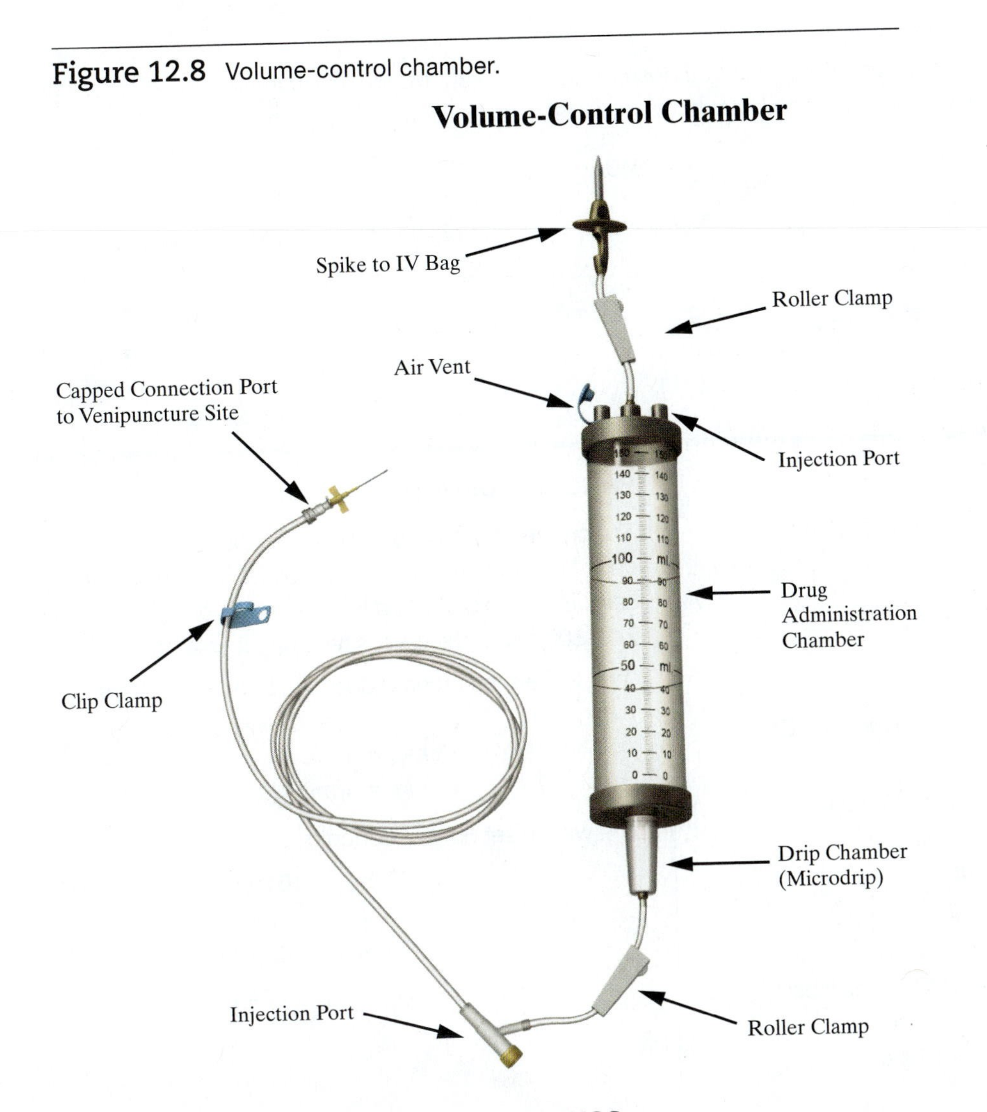

The following example illustrates the use of a VCC.

Example 12.10

Order: ***sulfamethoxazole and trimethoprim (SMZ-TMP) 75 mg in 100 mL*** D_5 ***W IVPB q6h*****. The recommended dose is 6–10** ***mg/kg/day every 6 hours*****. The child weighs 40** ***kg*****.**

(a) Is the prescribed dose in the safe range?

(b) Read the label in Figure 12.9. The manufacturer directions state that "weight-based doses are calculated on the TMP component." How many ***milliliters*** **will you withdraw from the vial?**

(c) Using a volume-control chamber, how many ***milliliters*** **of IV solution will you add?**

> **NOTE**
>
> In Example 12.10, following the infusing of the 100 *mL*, the tubing must be flushed; be sure to follow the institution's policy.

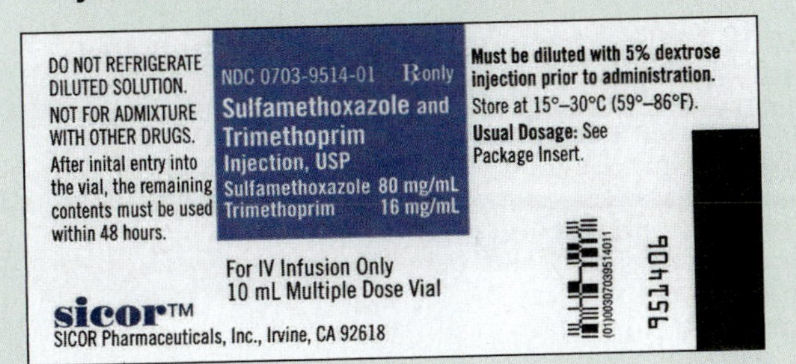

Figure 12.9 Drug label for Sulfamethoxazole and Trimethoprim.

SOURCE: Copyright TEVA, Used with permission

(Continued)

(a) Convert both the *safe dose range* and the *prescribed dose* to *mg/day*. First, use the *minimum safe dose (6 mg/kg/day)* to determine how many *mg/day* the child should minimally receive, as follows:

$$40 \cancel{kg} \times \frac{6\ mg}{\cancel{kg} \cdot day} = 240\ \frac{mg}{day} \quad \text{Minimum}$$

Now, use the *maximum safe dose (10 mg/kg/day)* to determine how many *mg/day* the child should maximally receive, as follows:

$$40 \cancel{kg} \times \frac{10\ mg}{\cancel{kg} \cdot day} = 400\ \frac{mg}{day} \quad \text{Maximum}$$

So, the safe dose range for this child is 240–400 *mg/day*.

DIMENSIONAL ANALYSIS

The ordered dose is 75 *mg* every 6 *hours*. Convert this to *mg/day* as follows:

$$\frac{75\ mg}{6\ \cancel{h}} \times \frac{24\ \cancel{h}}{day} = 300\ \frac{mg}{day}$$

The ordered dose is equivalent to 300 *mg/day*. This is within the safe dose range of 240–300 *mg/day*. So, the child is receiving a safe dose.

(b) You want to convert the order of 75 *mg* to *mL*.

$$75\ mg \longrightarrow ?\ mL$$

$$75\ mg \times \frac{?\ mL}{?\ mg} = ?\ mL$$

The directions state to use the trimethoprim (TMP) component. The strength of the TMP on the label is 16 *mg/mL*. So, the unit fraction is $\frac{1\ mL}{16\ mg}$

$$\frac{75\ \cancel{mg}}{1} \times \frac{1\ mL}{16\ \cancel{mg}} = 4.6875\ mL$$

RATIO & PROPORTION

The ordered dose is 75 *mg* every 6 *hours* (4 *times per day*). Therefore, the ordered dose is (75 × 4) 300 *mg daily*. Because 300 *mg/d* is in the range of 240–300 *mg/d*, the child is receiving a safe dose.

(b) Convert the ordered dose of 75 *mg* to *milliliters*. Think:

$$75\ mg = ?\ mL$$

$$16\ mg = 1\ mL \quad \text{[strength]}$$

One way to set up the proportion is

$$\frac{75\ mg}{x\ mL} = \frac{16\ mg}{1\ mL}$$

$$16x = 75$$

$$x = 4.6875$$

So, you would withdraw 4.6 *mL* of sulfamethoxazole and trimethoprim from the vial. Note that rounding *down* was used here.

(c) You would add *4.6 mL* of sulfamethoxazole and trimethoprim to the VCC, then add D5W to the *100 mL* mark.

Example 12.11

The prescriber ordered *doxycycline hyclate* 100 mg *IVPB daily. Infuse in* 100 *mL D5W over one hour*. The recommended dose is 2.2–4.4 *mg/kg/day*. The child weighs 45 *kg*.

(a) Is the prescribed dose in the safe range?

(b) Read the label in Figure 12.10. The manufacturer directions state that the medication "must be reconstituted with 10 *mL* of sterile water for injection." How many *milliliters* must be withdrawn from the doxycycline vial and added to the VCC?

(c) How many *milliliters* of IV solution will you add to the volume-control chamber?

(d) At what rate will you set the IV pump?

Figure 12.10 Drug label for doxycycline.

SOURCE: Courtesy of Pfizer, Inc.

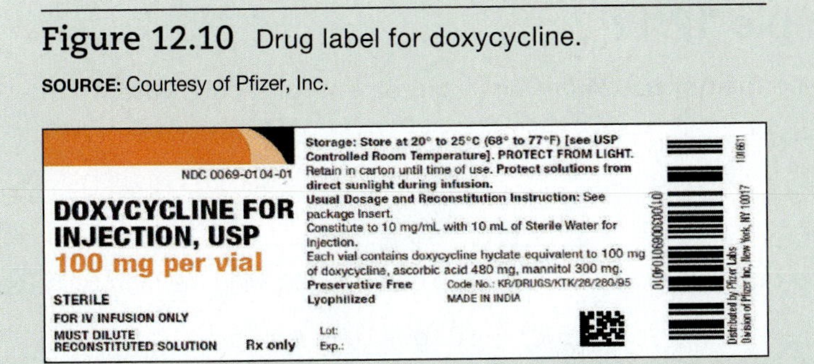

(a) Convert both the *recommended dose range* and the *prescribed dose to mg/day*. First, use the *minimum recommended dose* (2.2 *mg/kg/day*) to determine how many *mg/day* the child should minimally receive as follows:

$$45\ \cancel{kg} \times \frac{2.2\ mg}{\cancel{kg} \cdot day} = 99\ \frac{mg}{day} \quad \text{Minimum}$$

Now, use the *maximum recommended dose* (4.4 *mg/kg/d*) to determine how many *mg/day* the child should maximally receive as follows:

$$45\ \cancel{kg} \times \frac{4.4\ mg}{\cancel{kg} \cdot day} = 198\ \frac{mg}{day} \quad \text{Maximum}$$

So, the safe dose range for this child is 99–198 *mg/day*. The ordered dose of 100 *mg/day* is within the safe dose range. So, the child is receiving a safe dose.

(b) The directions state to reconstitute the 100 *mg* vial of doxycycline with 10 *mL* of sterile water for injection. The strength of the reconstituted solution will then be 100 *mg* per 10 *mL*. Because the ordered dose is 100 *mg*, the entire 10 *mL* of solution must be withdrawn from the vial and added to the VCC.

(c) Because the directions say to infuse in 100 *mL* of D5W, add 100 *mL* of D5W to the VCC.

(d) The VCC contains 10 *mL* of doxycycline and 100 *mL* of D5W, for a total of 110 *mL*. The infusion must last 1 *hour*. So, you would set the pump rate to 110 *mL/h*.

Calculating Daily Fluid Maintenance

The administration of pediatric IV medication requires careful and exact calculations and procedures. Infants and severely ill children are not able to tolerate extreme levels of hydration and are quite susceptible to dehydration and fluid overload. Therefore, you must closely monitor the amount of fluid a child receives. The fluid a child requires over a 24-*hour* period is referred to as *daily fluid maintenance needs*. Daily fluid maintenance includes both oral and parenteral fluids. The amount of maintenance fluid required depends on the weight of the client (see the formula in Table 12.1). The daily maintenance fluid does not include body fluid losses through vomiting, diarrhea, or fever. Additional fluids referred to as *replacement fluids* (usually Lactated Ringer's or 0.9% NaCl) are used to replace fluid losses and are based on each child's condition (e.g., if 20 *mL* are lost, then 20 *mL* of replacement fluids are usually added to the daily maintenance).

Table 12.1 Daily Fluid Maintenance Formula

Pediatric Daily Fluid Maintenance Formula		
For the *first*	10 *kg* of body weight:	100 *mL/kg*
For the *next*	10 *kg* of body weight:	50 *mL/kg*
For *each kg above*	20 *kg* of body weight:	20 *mL/kg*

Example 12.12

Determine the normal 24 *hr* fluid requirement for a child who weighs 33 *lb*.

First, convert the child's weight to *kilograms*.

$$\frac{33\ lb}{1} \times \frac{1\ kg}{2.2\ lb} = 15\ kg$$

Divide the weight (in *kilograms*) into three portions, following the formula in Table 12.1.

$$15\ kg = 10\ kg + 5\ kg + 0\ kg$$

For each of these portions, the number of *milliliters* must be calculated. A table is useful for organizing the calculations (see Table 12.2).

Table 12.2 Daily Fluid Maintenance Computations for Example 12.12

1st Portion	10 *kg*	×	$\frac{100\ mL}{kg}$	=	1,000 *mL*
2nd Portion	5 *kg*	×	$\frac{50\ mL}{kg}$	=	250 *mL*
3rd Portion	0 *kg*	×	$\frac{20\ mL}{kg}$	=	0 *mL*
Total	15 *kg*				1,250 *mL*

So, the child who weighs 33 *lb* has a daily fluid requirement of 1,250 *mL*.

Example 12.13

If the order is *half-maintenance* for a child who weighs 35 *kg*, at what rate should the pump be set in *mL/h*?

Because the child weighs 35 *kg*, this weight would be divided into three portions following the formula in Table 12.1, as follows:

$$35\ kg = 10\ kg + 10\ kg + 15\ kg$$

For each of these three portions, the number of *milliliters* must be calculated. A table will be useful for organizing the calculations (Table 12.3). The daily "maintenance" was determined to be 1,800 *mL*. "Half-maintenance" ($\frac{1}{2}$ of maintenance) is, therefore, $\frac{1}{2}$ of 1,800 *mL*, or 900 *mL*.

Table 12.3 Daily Fluid Maintenance Computations for Example 12.13

1st Portion	10 *kg*	×	$\frac{100\ mL}{kg}$	=	1,000 *mL*
2nd Portion	10 *kg*	×	$\frac{50\ mL}{kg}$	=	500 *mL*
3rd Portion	15 *kg*	×	$\frac{20\ mL}{kg}$	=	300 *mL*
Total	35 *kg*				1,800 *mL*

Now, you must change $\frac{900\ mL}{1\ day}$ to $\frac{mL}{h}$.

Replace 1 day with 24 *hours* to obtain

$$\frac{900\ mL}{1\ day} = \frac{900\ mL}{24\ h} = 37.5\ \frac{mL}{h}$$

So, the pump would be set at the rate of 37 *mL/h*.

Summary

In this chapter, you learned to calculate oral and parenteral dosages for pediatric clients. Some dosages were based on the size of the client: body weight (*kg*) or BSA (m^2). The calculations needed for the use of the volume-control chamber, as well as the method for determining daily fluid maintenance, were explained.

- Taking shortcuts in pediatric medication administration can be fatal to a child.
- Always verify that the order is in the safe dose range.
- Consult a reliable source when in doubt about a pediatric medication order.
- Question the order or check your calculations if the ordered dose differs from the recommended dose.
- Pediatric dosages are sometimes rounded down (truncated) to avoid the danger of an overdose.
- Know your institution's policy on rounding.
- IV bags of no more than 500 *mL* should be hung for pediatric clients.
- No more than 2 *mL* should be given intramuscularly to a pediatric client.
- Because accuracy is crucial in pediatric infusions, electronic control devices or volume-control chambers should always be used.
- Minimal and maximal dilution volumes for some IV drugs are recommended to prevent fluid overload, minimize irritation to veins, and reduce toxic effects.
- When preparing IV drug solutions, the smallest added volume (minimal dilution) results in the strongest concentration; the largest added volume (maximal dilution) results in the weakest concentration.
- For a volume-control chamber, a flush is always used to clear the tubing after the medication is infused.
- Know the facility policy regarding the inclusion of medication volume as part of the total infusion volume.
- Daily fluid maintenance depends on the weight of the child and includes both oral and parenteral fluids.

Case Study 12.1

Read the Case Study and answer the questions. Answers can be found in Appendix A.

An 8-year-old boy is admitted to the hospital with a diagnosis of sickle cell crisis and pneumonia. He complains of pain in his legs and abdomen, wheezing, and pain in his chest. He has a history of asthma and epilepsy and is allergic to peanuts, tomatoes, and aspirin. He is 40 *inches* tall and weighs 55 *pounds*. Vital signs are T 102° F; B/P 90/66; P 112; R 30. Chest X-ray confirms right upper-lobe pneumonia, and the throat culture is positive for Group A streptococcus. His orders include the following:

- Bed Rest
- Diet as tolerated, encourage PO fluids
- IV D5 $\frac{1}{3}$ NS @ 110 *mL/h*
- morphine sulfate 0.025 *mg/kg/h* IV
- penicillin G 100,000 *units/kg/day* divided q6h, infuse via pump in 100 *mL* D5W, over 1 *hour*
- methylprednisolone 1 *mg/kg* IM now, then 1 *mg/kg* PO daily in the A.M.
- Flovent HFA (fluticasone propionate) inhalation aerosol 2 puffs B.I.D.
- Folic acid 1 *mg* PO daily
- Depakene (valproic acid) 30 *mg/kg* PO b.i.d.
- Tylenol (acetaminophen) 12 *mg/kg* PO q4h prn temp over 101° F
- montelukast 5 *mg* PO qhs
- albuterol 2 *mg* PO T.I.D.

Use the labels in Figure 12.11 to answer the following questions:

1. Calculate the child's 24-*hour* fluid requirement.
2. How many *milliliters* of diluent will you add to the Pfizerpen vial to obtain a strength of 250,000 *units/mL*,

(continued)

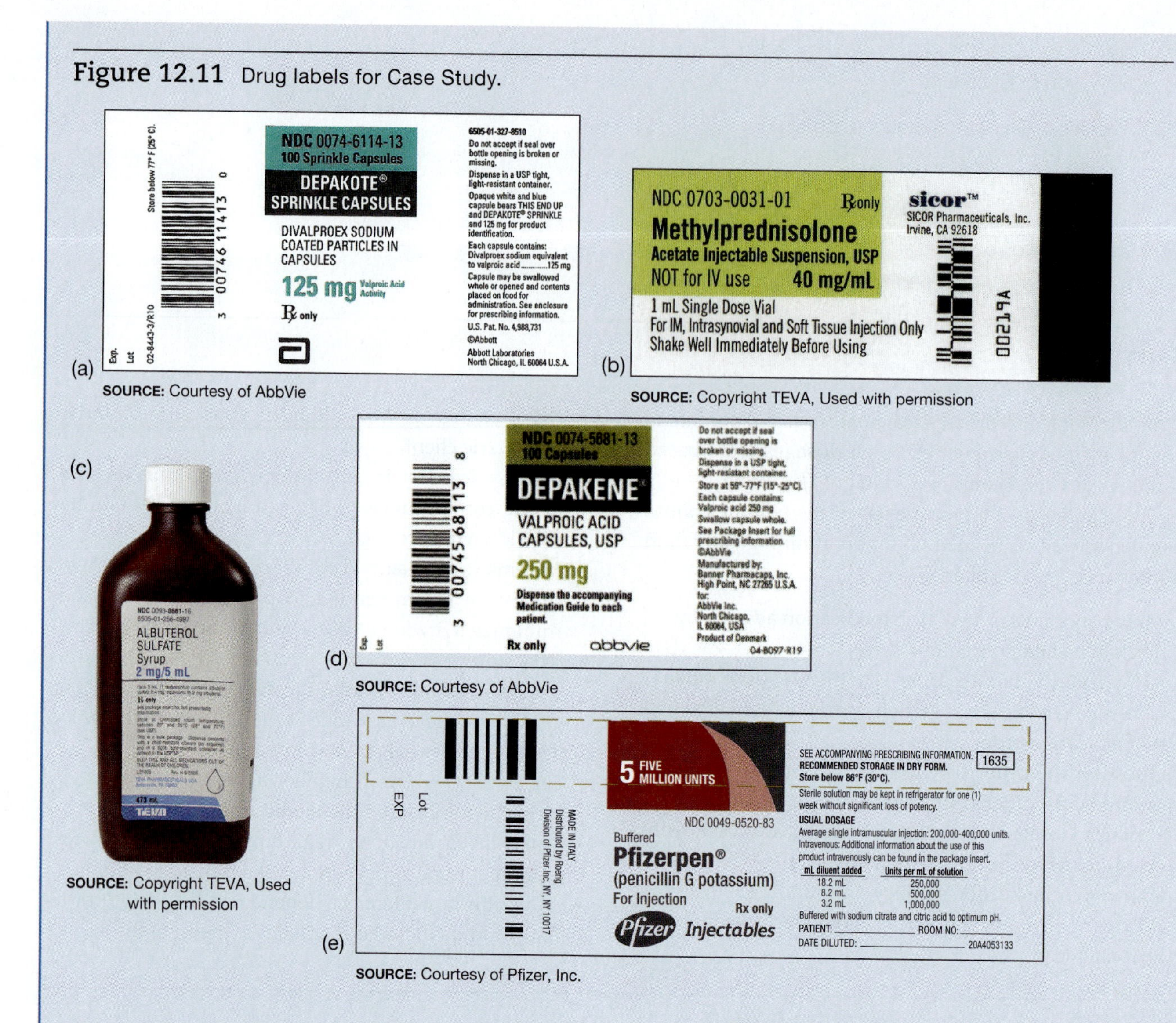

Figure 12.11 Drug labels for Case Study.

(a) **SOURCE:** Courtesy of AbbVie

(b) **SOURCE:** Copyright TEVA, Used with permission

(c) **SOURCE:** Copyright TEVA, Used with permission

(d) **SOURCE:** Courtesy of AbbVie

(e) **SOURCE:** Courtesy of Pfizer, Inc.

and how many *milliliters* will you withdraw to obtain the prescribed dose?

3. At what rate will you set the pump to infuse the Penicillin G?
4. The recommended dose for morphine is 0.05–0.1 *mg/kg IV q4h*. Is the prescribed dose safe?
5. How many *milliliters* of methylprednisolone will you administer for the IM dose?
6. Select the correct label for valproic acid, and determine how many capsules you will administer.
7. The folic acid is available in 1 *mg* tablets. How many *micrograms* is the child receiving per day?
8. If the strength of the montelukast is 5 *mg* per tablet, determine how many tablets you will administer.
9. The Tylenol available is labeled 160 *mg/5 mL*. How many *milliliters* will the child receive for a temperature of 102°F?
10. Select the correct label for albuterol, and determine how many *milliliters* you will administer.
11. The strength of the Flovent is 44 *mcg/inhalation*. How many *mcg* is the client receiving/day?

Practice Sets

The answers to *Try These for Practice*, *Exercises*, and *Cumulative Review Exercises* are found in Appendix A. Ask your instructor for the answers to the *Additional Exercises*.

Try These for Practice

Test your comprehension after reading the chapter.

1. Order: *Dycill (dicloxacillin sodium)* 50 *mg po q6h*. The recommended dosage for a 35-*pound* child is 12.5–25 *mg/kg/day in* 4 *equally divided doses*. Is the prescribed order safe for this child and, if so, how many *milligrams* will you administer?
2. Order: *penicillin G potassium* 125,000 *units IV q6h*. The infant weighs 2,500 *grams*. The recommended dose for infants is 150,000–300,000 *units/kg/day* divided in equal doses q4–6h. Is the ordered dose safe?
3. Order: *Proventil (albuterol)* 2 *mg PO T.I.D*. The recommended dosage range is 0.1–0.2 *mg/kg* t.i.d. max 4 *mg/dose*. The child weighs 32 *pounds*. The label reads 2 *mg* / 5 *mL*. If the dose is safe, how many teaspoons of this bronchodilator will the child receive?
4. The prescriber ordered *cefdinir (Omnicef)* 7 *mg/kg PO q12h for 10 days* for a child who has tonsillitis. The child weighs 80 pounds and the strength on the label is 250 *mg* / 5 *mL*. How many *milliliters* of this cephalosporin antibiotic will you administer?
5. The prescriber ordered furosemide 2 *mg/kg* PO stat. The strength on the label is 10 *mg/mL*. If the child weighs 100 pounds, how many *milliliters* will the child receive?

Exercises

Reinforce your understanding in class or at home.

1. Order: *D_5NS with* 40 *mg gentamicin IV infuse at* 30 *mL/h over* 30 *min q8h*. A volume-control chamber is used with an electronic infusion pump. How many *milliliters* will be infused 1 one day?
2. Order: *cefaclor oral suspension* 200 *mg po q8h* for a child who has otitis media and weighs 33 *pounds*. The recommended dose is 40 *mg/kg/day* in 3 divided doses. Is the ordered dose safe?
3. Order: *Rocephin (ceftriaxone)* 1 *g IV q12h*. The client is a child who has an infection and weighs 30 *pounds*. The recommended dose is 50–75 *mg/kg/day* given once a day, or daily in 2 equally divided doses, not to exceed 2 *g/day*. Is the prescribed order safe?
4. Order: *Narcan (naloxone hydrochloride)* 0.01 *mg/kg subcut stat* for a neonate who weighs 3,300 *g*. The strength available is 0.4 *mg/mL*. How many *milliliters* will you administer?
5. A seven-year-old client weighs 66 *pounds*. The recommended dose of Kantrex (kanamycin) is 15 *mg/kg/day* IM in equally divided doses q8–12h. How many *milligrams* will the prescriber order per day?
6. Order: *Omnicef (cefdinir) oral suspension* 7 *mg/kg q12h for* 10 *days*. Read the information on the label in Figure 12.12. Calculate the number of *milliliters* of this cephalosporin antibiotic you would administer to a child who weighs 77 *pounds*.
7. Calculate the daily fluid maintenance and the hourly flow rate for a child who weighs 17 *kg*.
8. Order: *aminophylline* 27 *mg/kg/day po divided in* 6 *doses*. The strength on the label is 105 *mg* / 5 *mL*. Calculate how many *milliliters* of this bronchodilator you will administer to a child who weighs 45 *pounds*.
9. Order: *Pediapred (prednisolone sodium phosphate)* 60 *mg* / *m^2* / *day PO in three divided doses for* 4 *weeks*. Calculate how many *milliliters* of this anti-inflammatory agent you will administer to a child who has nephrotic syndrome and weighs 30 *pounds* and is 36 *inches* tall. The strength on the vial is 5 *mg per* 5 *mL*.

Figure 12.12 Drug label for Omnicef.

SOURCE: Courtesy of AbbVie

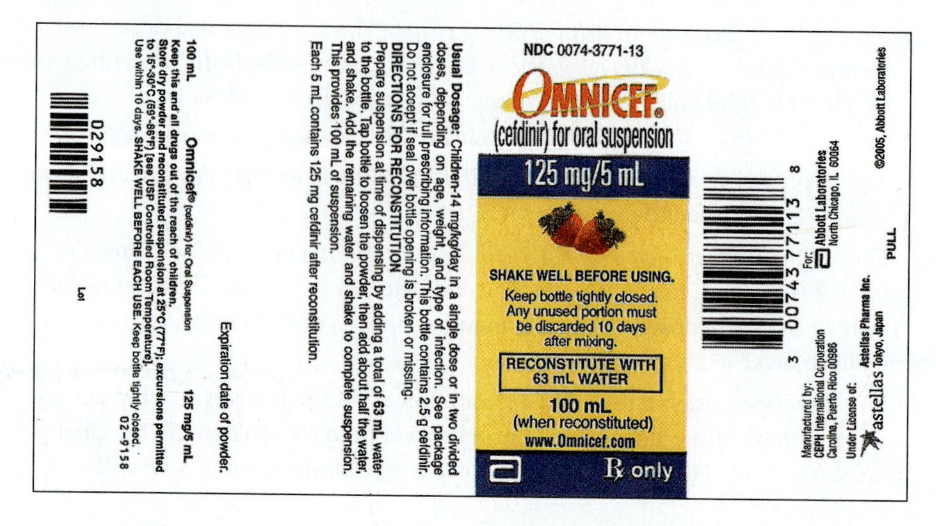

10. Order: *aminophylline* 5 *mg/kg IV loading dose to infuse in* 250 *mL D5W over* 30 *min*.
    (a) Calculate how many *mg* of aminophylline a child who weighs 30 *pounds* will receive.
    (b) At what rate will you set the pump in *mL/h*?
11. Order: *ampicillin* 50 *mg/kg/day in* 4 *equally divided doses IVPB in* 50 *mL NS infuse over* 30 *minutes*. The directions state to "reconstitute the 1 *g* vial with 10 *mL* of NS." The child weighs 40 *kilograms*. How many *milliliters* of this antibiotic will you withdraw from the vial?
12. Order: *ProQuad* 1 *dose subcut now*. The label reads Single-Dose 0.5 *mL* vial. Draw a line on the most appropriate syringe indicating the number of *milliliters* you will administer to a 12-month-old infant in Figure 12.13.

Figure 12.13 Box label for Syringes for question 12.

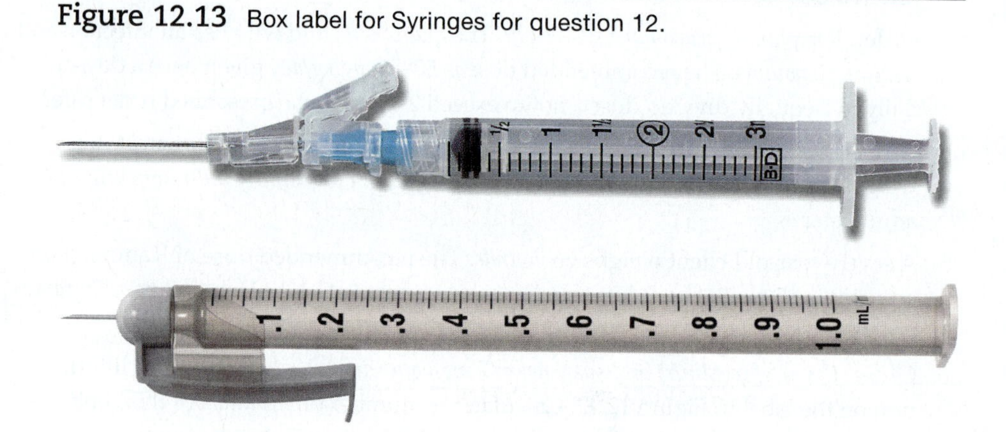

13. The prescriber ordered half-maintenance for a child who weighs 15 *kg*. Calculate the rate at which the pump should be set in *mL/h*.
14. Order: *Morphine sulfate* 3 *mg IVP q3h prn severe pain*. Dilute in 5 *mL* sterile water for injection and administer slowly over 5 minutes. Find the number of *milliliters* you will push every minute.
15. The prescriber ordered half daily fluid maintenance for a child who weighs 30 *kg*. Calculate the rate at which the infusion pump should be set in *mL/h*.
16. Order: *ampicillin sodium and sulbactam sodium (Unasyn)* 300 *mg/kg/day IV in equally divided doses q6h*. The directions on the 1.5 *g* vial state to reconstitute with 3 *mL* of

sterile water for injection, which yields a concentration of 375 *mg/mL*.The child weighs 15 *kg*; how many *milliliters* of this antibiotic will you withdraw?

17. The prescriber ordered *cephalexin for oral suspension 150 mg PO q6h* for a child who weighs 35 *pounds*. The manufacturer states that the usual daily dose for children is 20–50 *mg/kg/day* in 4 divided doses. The strength on the label of this cephalosporin antibiotic is 250 *mg/5 mL*.
    (a) What is the safe dosage range for this child?
    (b) Is the dose ordered safe?
    (c) If the order is safe, how many *milliliters* will you administer?
18. The prescriber ordered *gentamicin 5.2 mg IM q12h* for a child. The strength on the label of gentamicin pediatric is 20 *mg/2 mL*. How many *milliliters* of this aminoglycoside antibiotic will you administer; and what size syringe will you use?
19. The prescriber ordered: *insulin 0.1 units/kg/h IV* for a child who weighs 33 *kg* and is in diabetic ketoacidosis (DKA). The pharmacy sent an IV bag of NS 500 *mL* with 50 units regular insulin. What rate in *mL/h* will you set the infusion pump?
20. Order: *famotidine oral suspension 0.5 mg/kg/dose PO daily*. This is prescribed for an infant who has GERD. The infant weighs 15 *pounds* and the strength on the label is 40 *mg/5 mL*. Calculate the number of *milliliters* you will administer.

Additional Exercises

Now, test yourself!

1. The prescriber ordered *dicloxacillin* 75 *mg oral suspension PO q6h* for a child who weighs 38 *kg*. The recommended dose for a child is 12.5–25 *mg/kg/day* in divided doses q6h. Is the prescribed dose of this penicillin antibiotic safe?
2. Order: *Biaxin (clarithromycin) oral suspension* 7.5 *mg/kg PO q12h*. Read the label in Figure 12.14, and calculate the number of *milliliters* of this macrolide antibiotic you would administer to a child who weighs 18 *pounds*.

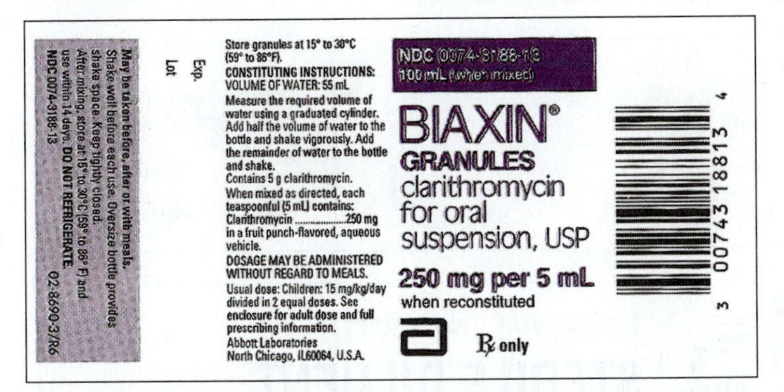

Figure 12.14 Drug label for Biaxin.

SOURCE: Courtesy of AbbVie

3. Order: *theophylline* 300 *mg PO q6h*. The strength available is 150 *mg/15 mL*. How many *milliliters* of this bronchodilator will you administer to the child?
4. The prescriber ordered *cephradine* 275 *mg IVPB q6h* for a child who weighs 31 *pounds*. The recommended dose is 50–100 *mg/kg/day* divided in four doses (maximum 8 *g/day*). Is the prescribed dose of this cephalosporin antibiotic safe?
5. Order: *acyclovir* 250 mg/m^2 *IV q8h*. The child has a BSA of 0.8 m^2, and the vial is labeled "50 *mg/mL*." How many *milliliters* of this antiviral will you prepare?

6. What is the daily fluid maintenance for a child who weighs 82 *pounds*?
7. Order: *Humatrope (somatropin) 0.18 mg/kg/week subcut divided into equal doses give on Mon/Wed/Fri*. Read the label in Figure 12.15 and calculate how many *milliliters* of this growth hormone you will administer to a child who weighs 40 *pounds*. The package insert states to "reconstitute the 5 *mg* vial with 5 *mL* of diluent."

Figure 12.15 Drug label for Humatrope.

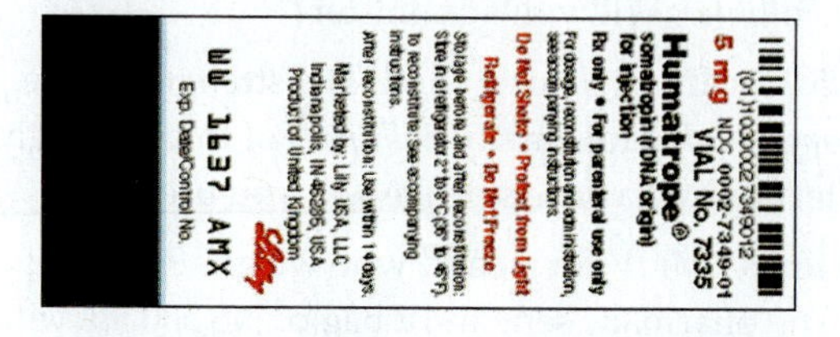

8. Order: *Tavist (clemastine fumarate) 0.05 mg/kg/day PO divided into 2 doses*. The label states "0.67 *mg*/5 *mL*." Calculate how many *milliliters* of this antihistamine you will administer to a child who weighs 35 *pounds*.
9. Order: *Dilantin (phenytoin) 150 mg IVP stat*. The package insert states give 1 *mg/kg/min*, and the label reads 250 *mg*/5 *mL*. Over how many *minutes* should you administer this anticonvulsant to a child who weighs 10 *kg*?
10. Order: *Cefadyl (cephapirin sodium) 40 mg/kg/day IVPB divided into 4 doses. Infuse in 50 mL D5W over 30 min*. The child weighs 20 *kg*, and the directions state to reconstitute the 500 *mg* vial with 1 *mL* of diluent, yielding 500 *mg*/1.2 *mL*. How many *mL/h* of this cephalosporin antibiotic will you infuse?
11. Order: *Zostavax (zoster vaccine live) 1 dose subcut now* has been prescribed for a child. Read the information on the labels in Figure 12.16, and use the diluent supplied to reconstitute the vaccine. Draw a line on the appropriate syringe in Figure 12.17 indicating the number of *milliliters* of this reconstituted vaccine you will administer.

Figure 12.16 Drug labels for Zostavax and Diluent.

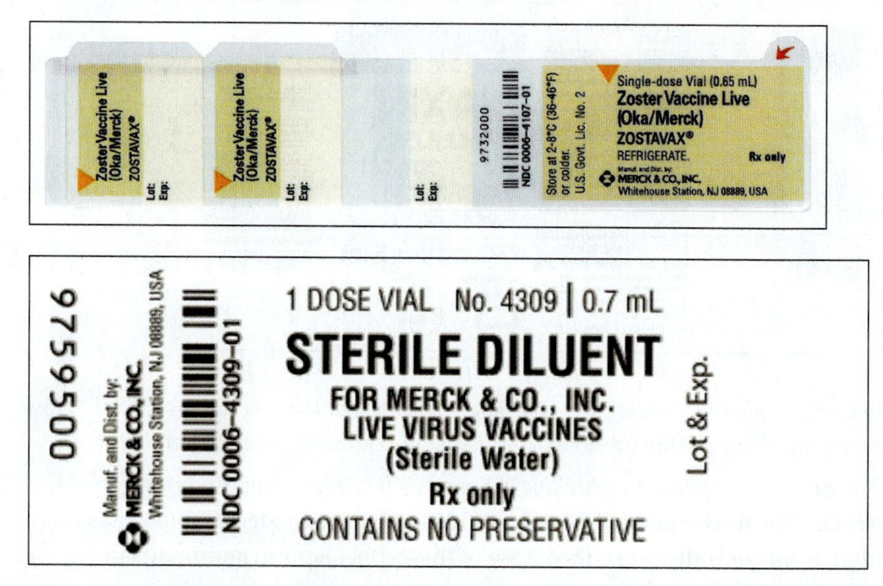

Figure 12.17 Syringes for Question 11.

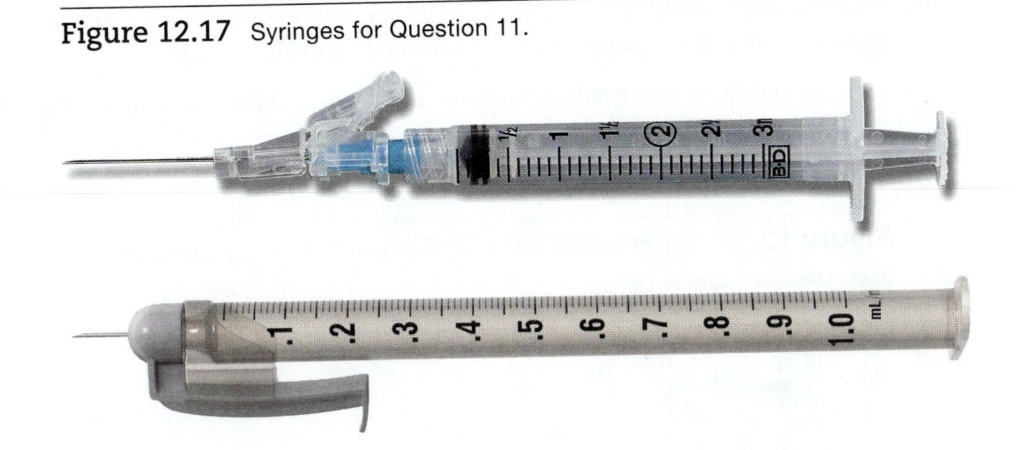

12. Order: *IV D5 $\frac{1}{3}$ NS, infuse at* 40 *mL/h*. What is the rate in *microdrops per minute*?
13. The prescriber ordered 1/3 maintenance for a child who weighs 10 *kg*. Calculate the rate at which the pump should be set in *mL/h*.
14. A child who weighs 33 *pounds* has diarrhea. To prevent dehydration, his fluid requirements are 100 *mL/kg/day*. The pediatrician tells the mom to give the child Pedialyte solution or "freezer pops." The label on the box states "62.5 *mL* per pop." What is the maximum number of Pedialyte freezer pops that the child may have in 1 *hour*?
15. Order: *albuterol sulfate syrup* 3 *mg PO T.I.D*. The recommended dose is 0.1–0.2 *mg/kg* T.I.D (max 4 *mg/dose*).
    (a) Is this a safe dose for a child who weighs 60 *pounds*?
    (b) If the dose is safe, read the label in Figure 12.18 and calculate the number of *milliliters* of this bronchodilator you would administer.

Figure 12.18 Bottle of albuterol sulfate.

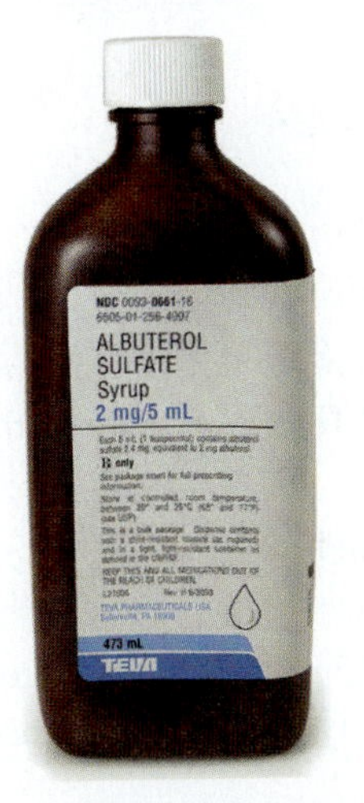

16. Order: *Children's Motrin (ibuprofen)* 400 *mg PO q4h prn temp over* 101°*F*. The recommended dose range is 5–10 *mg/kg* q4–6h up to 40 *mg/kg/day*. Is the ordered dose of this NSAID safe for a child who weighs 45 *kg*?
17. Order: *Cleocin (clindamycin phosphate)* 600 *mg IVPB q8h, infuse in* 50 *mL of D5W over* 20 *minutes*. At what rate in *mL/h* will you set the pump to infuse this cephalosporin antibiotic?

18. Order: *granisetron HCl* 10 *mcg/kg IVPB, 30 minutes before chemotherapy. Infuse in* 20 *mL of D5W over* 15 *minutes*. Read the information in Figure 12.19.

    (a) Calculate how many *milliliters* of this antiemetic a child who weighs 10 *kg* will need.

    (b) At what rate will you set the infusion to run in *mL/h*?

Figure 12.19 Vial of granisetron HCl. (For educational purposes only)

SOURCE: Pearson Education, Inc.

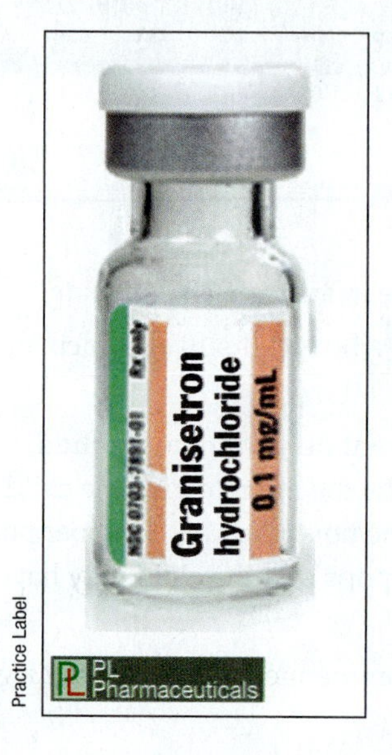

19. The prescriber ordered 2,000 $units/m^2/h$ IVPB of a drug. The solution is labeled 10,000 *units* in 100 *mL* D5W. Calculate the flow rate in *mL/h* for a child who has a BSA of 1.2 m^2.

20. Order: 150 *units of regular insulin in* 250 *mL NS, infuse at* 6 *mL/h*. Calculate the number of units of insulin the child is receiving per hour.

Cumulative Review Exercises

Review your mastery of previous chapters.

1. 42 mm = ? cm
2. How many *grams* of sodium chloride are contained in 1 *liter* of 0.9% NaCl?
3. An IV is infusing at 120 *mL/h* via a pump. If this infusion were switched to a gravity system, what would be the flow rate in *drops per minute*? The drop factor of the tubing is 15 *gtt/mL*.
4. An IVPB bag with a concentration of 300 *milligrams* of a drug in 200 *mL* of D_5W is infusing at the rate of 90 *mL/h*. What is the dosage rate in *mg/min*?
5. Order: *Cefizox (ceftizoxime)* 1,500 *mg IV push q8h infuse over* 7.5 *minutes*. The concentration available is 1 *gram* in 10 *mL* of sterile water. How many *mL* will you infuse every 15 *seconds*?
6. Order: *Nipride (nitroprusside sodium)* 2 *mcg/kg/min IV stat for hypertensive crisis*. The pharmacy has sent an IV labeled Nipride 50 *mg*/250 *mL* NS. The client weighs 250 *pounds*. Calculate the rate at which you will set the IV pump in *milliliters per hour*.
7. Order: *D5W*/0.45% *NaCl* 1,000 *mL infuse at* 25 *gtt/min*. Calculate the number of *hours* it will take for this solution to infuse. The drop factor is 15 *gtt/mL*.

8. The physician ordered *Mirapex (pramipexole dihydrochloride)* 0.125 *mg PO T.I.D.* for a client who has Parkinson's disease. How many *milligrams per day* is the client receiving?
9. The prescriber ordered *Hemabate (carboprost tromethamine)* 250 *mcg deep IM stat. Repeat q15 min not to exceed* 8 *doses*. What is the maximum number of *milligrams* that may be administered in total?
10. What is the BSA of a person who is 75 *inches* tall and weighs 210 *pounds*?
11. A client is receiving an infusion of heparin 25,000 *units* in D5W 500 *mL* at 18 *mL/hr*. How many *units per hour* is the client receiving?
12. Order: *infuse D5W 1,500 mL IV in 12 h*. What rate will you set the infusion pump in *mL/h*?
13. Order: $^3/_4$ *strength Isomil* 4 *oz PO q4h for* 24 *h*. How would you prepare the $^3/_4$ strength solution for the 24 *h*?
14. Order: *amoxicillin/clavulanate potassium oral solution* 500 *mg PO q12h*. The strength on the label is 400 *mg*/57 *mg per* 5 *mL*. How many *milliliters* of this Beta-Lactam antibiotic will you administer?
15. The prescriber ordered *misoprostol (Cytotec)* 200 *mcg PO with food Q.I.D.* to reduce the risk of NSAID-induced gastric ulcers in a client. The strength on the label is 200 *mcg* per tab. How many *milligrams* will the client receive in 1 day?

Comprehensive Self-Tests

Comprehensive Self-Test 1

Answers to *Comprehensive Self-Tests* 1–4 can be found in Appendix A at the back of the book.

1. Order: *Omnicef (cefdinir) for oral suspension* 300 *mg PO q12h for* 10 *days.* Read the label in Figure S.1 and calculate how many *grams* of this antibiotic the client will receive.

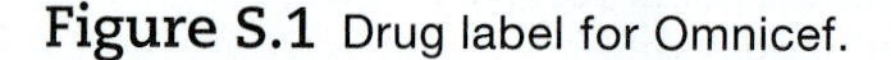

Figure S.1 Drug label for Omnicef.

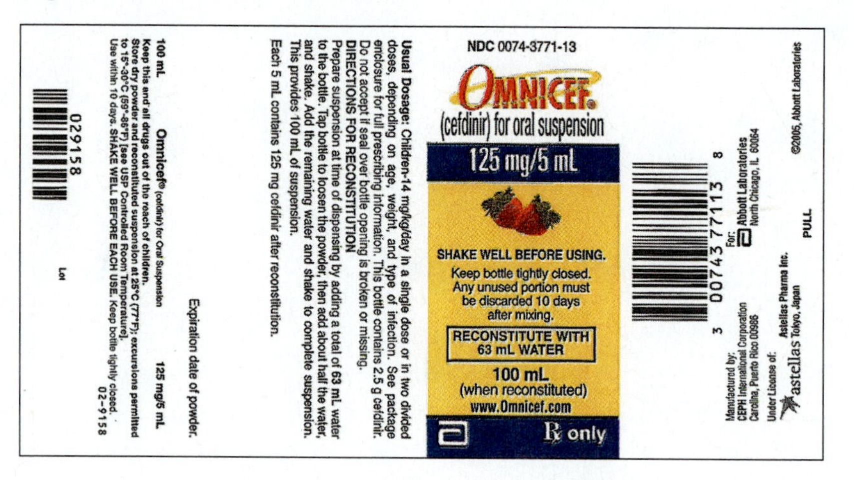

2. Order: *Kaletra (lopinavir/ritonavir)* 400 *mg lopinavir*/100 *mg ritonavir PO b.i.d.* Read the label in Figure S.2 and calculate how many *milliliters* of this antiviral drug you will administer.
3. Order: *Ativan (lorazepam) 2 mg IVP stat inject slowly over 1 minute.* The label on the 10 *mL* multiple-dose vial reads 2 *mg/mL*.
   (a) How many *milliliters* of this anxiolytic will you prepare?
   (b) How many *milliliters* will you administer every 15 *seconds?*
4. Order: *morphine sulfate 10 mg IM stat.* The label reads 15 *mg per mL*.
   (a) How many *milliliters* of this analgesic will you administer?
   (b) What size syringe will you use?
5. *Dopamine hydrochloride* 5 *mcg/kg/min via continuous IV infusion* is ordered for a client who weighs 176 *pounds*. The premixed IV solution reads dopamine 200 *mg* in D_5W 250 *mL* and is infusing via pump at 30 *mL/h*. How many *milligrams per hour* of this sympathomimetic agent is the client receiving?

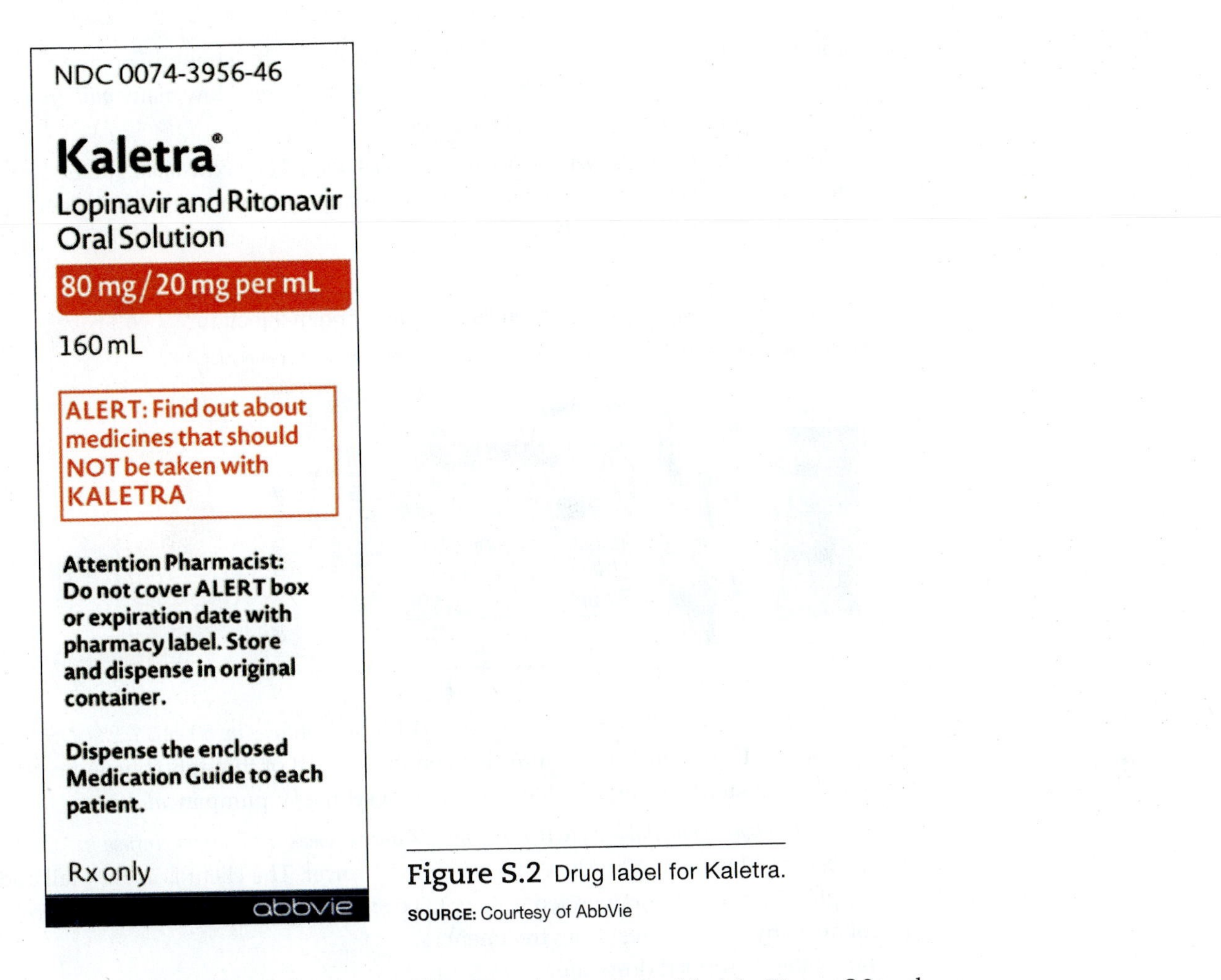

Figure S.2 Drug label for Kaletra.

SOURCE: Courtesy of AbbVie

6. Order: *Depakene (valproic acid)* 15 *mg/kg/day PO*. Read the label in Figure S.3 and calculate how many capsules of this antiseizure medication you will administer to a client who weighs 34 *pounds*.

Figure S.3 Drug label for Depakene.

SOURCE: Courtesy of AbbVie

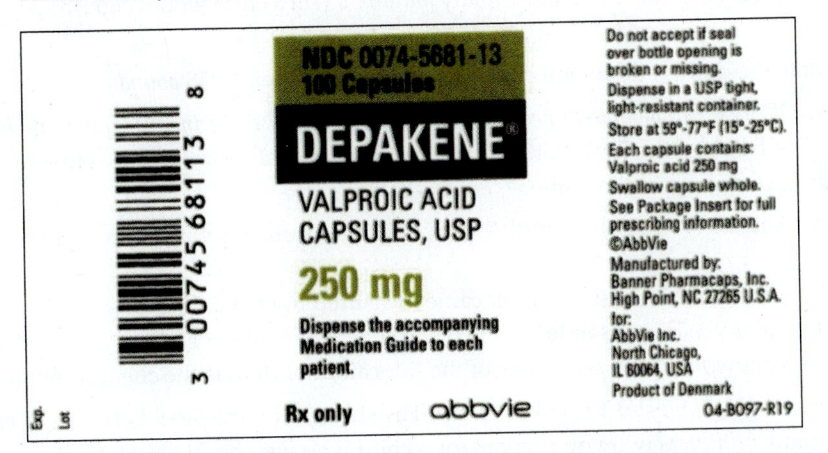

7. Order: *vasopressin* 5 *units IM stat, then* 10 *units IM q4h*. The client has abdominal distention. The label on the vial reads 20 *units/mL*.
   (a) How many *milliliters* of this antidiuretic will you administer for the stat dose?
   (b) What size syringe will you use?

8. Order: *vinblastine sulfate* 5.5 *mg/m*^{2} *IV for one dose.* The strength on the 10 *mL* multiple-dose vial is 1 *mg/mL*. The client has BSA of 1.66 *m*^{2}. How many *milligrams* of this antineoplastic drug will the client receive?
9. Order: *insulin lispro (rDNA origin) injection* 0.4 *units/kg subcut daily.* Refer to the information in Figure S.4 and calculate how many *units* you will administer to a client who weighs 150 *pounds.*

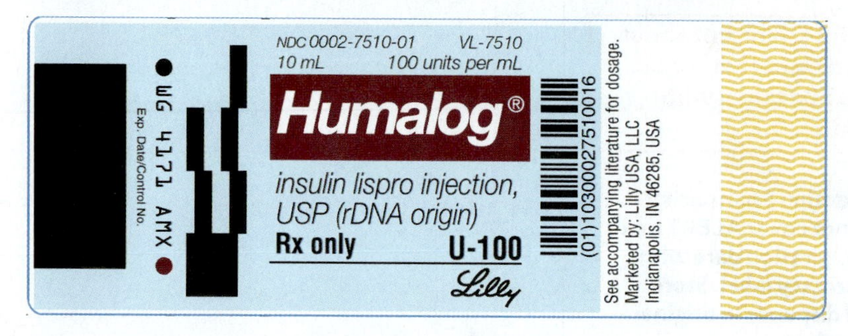

Figure S.4 Drug label for insulin lispro (rDNA origin) injection.

SOURCE: © Copyright Eli Lily and Company. All rights reserved. Used with permission.

10. Order: *Pipracil (piperacillin sodium) 1.5 g IVPB q6h, infuse in* 50 *mL 0.9% NS over* 20 *minutes.* The reconstitution directions on the 3 *g* vial of this antibiotic indicate to add 5 *mL* of sterile water. At what rate will you set the IV pump in *mL/h?*
11. Order: *Gemzar (gemcitabine HCl)* 1,390 *mg IV once a week for* 7 *weeks, infuse in* 100 *mL of NS over* 30 *minutes.* The client has pancreatic cancer. The client is 155 *cm* tall and weighs 45 *kg*. The recommended dose is 1,000 *mg/m*^{2} once weekly for up to 7 *weeks,* followed by 1 *week* of rest from treatment.
    (a) Is the prescribed dose safe?
    (b) At what rate will you set the infusion pump in *mL/h?*
12. Order: *gentamycin sulfate* 3 *mg/kg IV daily in three equally divided doses. Infuse in* 50 *mL NS over* 60 *min.* The client weighs 154 *pounds.* How many *mcgtt/min* of this aminoglycoside will the client receive?
13. Order: *Flumadine (rimantadine hydrochloride) syrup* 5 *mg/kg PO twice a day.* The strength on the label is 50 *mg per* 5 *mL*. How many *milliliters* will a child who weighs 54 *pounds* receive?
14. Calculate the daily fluid maintenance for a child who weighs 58 *pounds.*
15. Order: *DDAVP (desmopressin acetate)* 0.2 *mL nasal spray daily in two equally divided doses.* The label on the 5 *mL* bottle states the strength is 10 *mcg*/0.1 *mL*. How many doses are contained in the bottle?
16. A client has an IV of 250 *mL* with 1 *g* of lidocaine infusing via pump at a rate of 10 *mL/h.*
    (a) What is the concentration of lidocaine measured in *mg/mL?*
    (b) How many *milligrams* of lidocaine is the client receiving per hour?
    (c) How many *milliliters per minute* of the lidocaine solution is the client receiving?
17. Order: *Motrin (ibuprofen) 10 mg/kg PO q8h.* The strength on the label is 100 *mg*/5 *mL*. How many *milliliters* will you prepare for a child who weighs 70 *pounds?*
18. Order: *hyoscyamine sulfate oral solution* 0.025 *mg PO* 1 *h before meals and at bedtime.* The recommended dose for this anticholinergic drug is 0.0625–0.125 *mg* q4h prn (max: 0.75 *mg/d*).
    (a) Is the prescribed dose safe?
    (b) If the dose is safe, how many *milliliters* will you administer? The label reads 0.125 *mg/mL* (0.2 *mL*).

19. The prescriber ordered *Vitamin B_{12} alpha (hydroxocobalamin) 34 mcg IM/month* for a child who weighs 20 *kg*. The label reads 1,000 *mcg/mL*.
    (a) How many *milliliters* will the child receive?
    (b) What size syringe will you use?
20. The prescriber ordered *Zanosar (streptozocin)* 500 $mg/m^2/d$ *IV for* 5 *days*. Read the label in Figure S.5.
    (a) How many *grams* will a client who has a BSA of 1.8 m^2 receive in 5 *days?* The medication is to be infused in 250 *mL* of D5W over 50 *minutes* via pump.
    (b) At what rate will you set the pump in *mL/h?*

Figure S.5 Drug label for Zanosar.

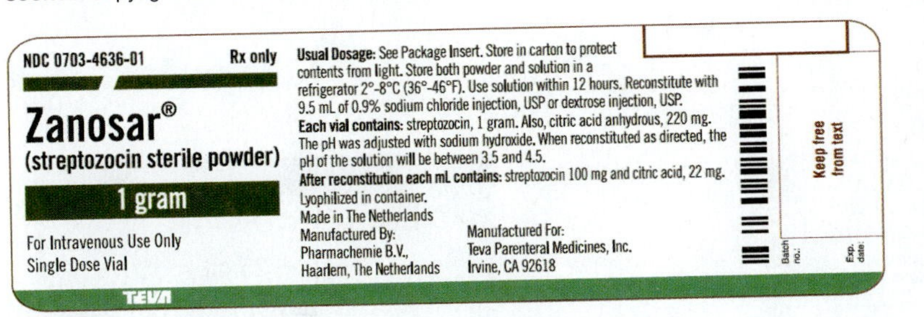

21. Order: *Tegopen (cloxacillin) oral suspension* 400 *mg PO q6h*. The label reads 125 *mg/5 mL*, and the recommended dose is 12.5 *mg*–25 *mg/kg/q6h* (max: 4 *g/d*).
    (a) Is the prescribed dose safe for a child who weighs 66 *pounds?*
    (b) If the dose is safe, how many *milliliters* will the child receive?
22. The recommended dose of Alimta is 500 mg/m^2 administered IVPB over 10 *minutes*. The vial shown in Figure S.6 must be reconstituted with 20 *mL* NS, an appropriate volume of the reconstituted solution must then be withdrawn from the vial and added to 100 *mL* NS. The client has BSA of 1.4 m^2. How many vials will be needed to prepare this infusion?

Figure S.6 Drug label for premetrexed (Alimta).

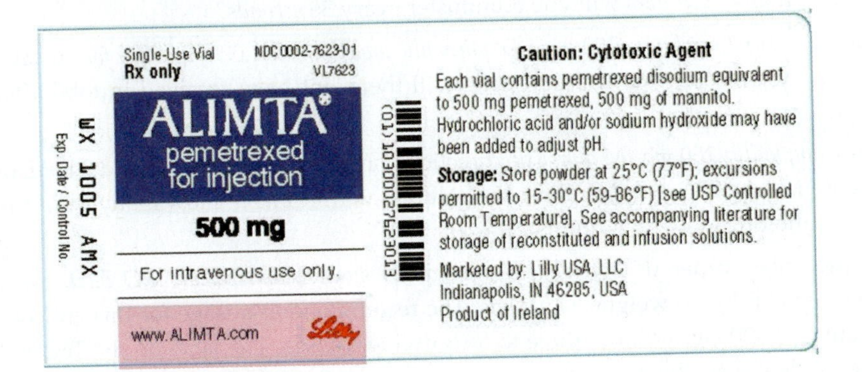

23. Order: *Prinvil (lisinopril)* 0.07 *mg/kg PO daily*. The label reads 1 *mg/mL*. Calculate the number of *milliliters* of this angiotensin-converting enzyme (ACE) inhibitor you will administer to a child who weighs 70 *pounds*.
24. Order: *Ativan (lorazepam)* 3 *mg IV push stat*. The strength on the vial is 4 *mg/mL*. The package insert recommends diluting the medication with an equal volume of compatible solution and to infuse slowly at a maximum rate of 2 *mg/min*.
    (a) How many *milliliters* of Ativan (lorazepam) will you prepare?
    (b) Over how many *minutes* will you administer the Ativan (lorazepam)?

25. Order: *heparin* 1,000 *units in* 500 *mL 0.9% NaCl, infuse at* 100 *mL/h.* How many *units per hour* is the client receiving?

Comprehensive Self-Test 2

Answers to *Comprehensive Self-Tests* 1–4 can be found in Appendix A at the back of the book.

1. Order: *Biaxin (clarithromycin)* 500 *mg PO q12h.* Read the label in Figure S.7 and determine how many *milliliters* of this antibiotic you will administer. Draw a line at the appropriate measurement on the medication cup in Figure S.8.

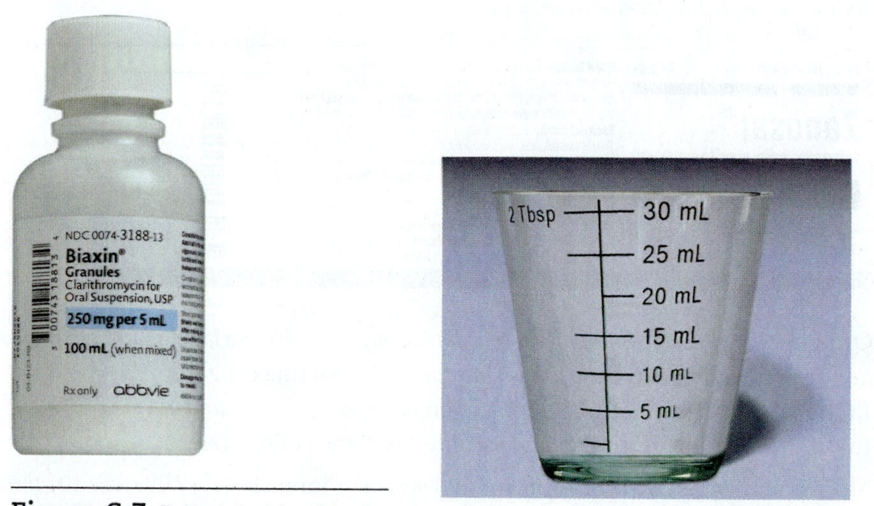

Figure S.7 Drug label for Biaxin.

SOURCE: Courtesy of AbbVie

Figure S.8 Medication cup.

2. The prescriber ordered *acetazolamide* 500 *mg IVP over* 1 *minute* preoperatively for a client who has secondary glaucoma. The directions on the 500 *mg* vial state to reconstitute with 5 *mL* of sterile water for injection.
   (a) How many *milliliters* of this diuretic will you prepare?
   (b) How many *milliliters* will you administer every 30 *seconds?*
3. Order: *Zovirax (acyclovir)* 200 *mg PO q4h while awake (max* 1,000 *mg/day) for* 10 *days.* How many *grams* of this antiviral drug will the client have received in total after 7 *days?*
4. Order: *ampicillin* 250 *mg IM q6h.* The directions on the 1 *g* vial state to add 3.5 *mL* of diluent yielding 250 *mg/mL* and use the solution within 1 *hour.* How many *milliliters* of this antibiotic will you administer?
5. The prescriber ordered *Tegretol (carbamazepine) suspension* 150 *mg PO b.i.d.* for a 5-year-old child who weighs 50 *pounds.* The recommended dosage for this anticonvulsant is 10–20 *mg/kg/day* in three to four divided doses. The label on the Tegretol bottle reads 100 *mg*/5 *mL.*
   (a) Is the ordered dose safe?
   (b) If it is safe, how many *milliliters* will you administer?
6. The prescriber ordered *Myleran (busulfan)* 2.1 mg/m^2 *PO daily* for a child who is 42 *inches* tall and weighs 70 *pounds.* How many *milligrams* of this antineoplastic drug will you administer?
7. The prescriber ordered *Enbrel (etanercept)* 0.4 *mg/kg subcut two times a week* for a child who has rheumatoid arthritis and weighs 40 *pounds.* The label on the vial reads 25 *mg/mL.* How many *milliliters* will you administer?

8. Order: *amoxicillin oral suspension* 120 *mg PO q8h*. The recommended dosage is 20–40 *mg/kg/day*.
   (a) Is this a safe dose for a child who weighs 37 *pounds?*
   (b) If the dose is safe, refer to the information on the label in Figure S.9 and calculate how many *milliliters* of this antibiotic the child would receive.

Figure S.9 Drug label for amoxicillin.

SOURCE: Copyright TEVA, Used with permission

NDC 0093-4155-73
AMOXICILLIN
for Oral Suspension, USP
equivalent to
250 mg per 5 mL
amoxicillin when reconstituted according to directions.
See accompanying literature.
WARNING: NOT FOR INJECTION
℞ only
100 mL (when mixed)
TEVA

Amoxicillin trihydrate equivalent to 5 g amoxicillin.
Usual Dosage: Adults – 250 mg - 500 mg every eight hours, depending on type and severity of infection.
Children – 20 mg - 40 mg/kg/day in divided doses every eight hours, depending on type and severity of infection.
Store dry powder at 20° to 25°C (68° to 77°F) [See USP Controlled Room Temperature].
TO THE PHARMACIST: Prepare suspension at time of dispensing. Add to the bottle a total of 60 mL of water. For ease in preparation, tap bottle to loosen powder, add the water in two portions, shaking well after each addition. The resulting suspension will contain amoxicillin trihydrate equivalent to 250 mg amoxicillin in each 5 mL (teaspoonful).
IMPORTANT
When stored at room temperature or in refrigerator discard unused portion of reconstituted suspension after 14 days.
Date of reconstitution:..................
Shake well before using. Keep tightly closed.
KEEP THIS AND ALL MEDICATIONS OUT OF THE REACH OF CHILDREN.
Manufactured In Canada By:
TEVA CANADA LIMITED
Toronto, Canada M1B 2K9
Manufactured For:
TEVA PHARMACEUTICALS USA
Sellersville, PA 18960
N 3 0093-4155-73 0
361-32-669656240A Rev. 00 Rev. F 7/2010

9. Order: *Doxycin (doxycycline hyclate)* 100 *mg IVPB q12h. Infuse in* 100 *mL D5W over* 1 *hour.* At what rate in *drops per minute* will you set the infusion for this antibiotic if the drop factor is 10 *gtt/mL?*
10. Order: *amlodipine besylate* 10 *mg PO daily*. Read the information in Figure S.10 and calculate how many *tablets* of this calcium channel blocking agent the client will receive in 1 *week*.

Figure S.10 Drug label for amlodipine besylate.

SOURCE: Copyright TEVA, Used with permission

NDC 0093-0083-98
Amlodipine Besylate Tablets USP
2.5 mg*
PHARMACIST: PLEASE DISPENSE WITH ATTACHED PATIENT INFORMATION LEAFLET
℞ only
90 TABLETS
TEVA

*Each tablet contains amlodipine besylate, USP equivalent to 2.5 mg amlodipine.
Usual Dosage: See package insert for full prescribing information.
Store at 20° to 25°C (68° to 77°F) [See USP Controlled Room Temperature].
PROTECT FROM LIGHT.
Dispense in a tight, light-resistant container as defined in the USP, with a child-resistant closure (as required).
KEEP THIS AND ALL MEDICATIONS OUT OF THE REACH OF CHILDREN.
Manufactured In Israel By:
TEVA PHARMACEUTICAL IND. LTD.
Jerusalem, 9777402, Israel
Manufactured For:
TEVA PHARMACEUTICALS USA, INC.
North Wales, PA 19454
N 3 0093-0083-98 3
323K303240515 Rev. E 4/2015

11. Order: *heparin* 30,000 *units IV in* 500 *mL of D5W, infuse at* 1,500 *units/h*. Calculate the flow rate in *mL/h*.
12. Order: *heparin* 50,000 *units in* 500 *mL of NS, infuse at* 25 *mL/h*. Calculate the number of *units per hour* of this anticoagulant the client is receiving.
13. The prescriber ordered an *insulin drip of Humulin R Regular insulin* 50 *units IV in* 100 *mL 0.9% NaCl, infuse at* 6 *mL/h*. How many *units* of insulin *per hour* is the client receiving?
14. The prescriber ordered *morphine sulfate* 4 *mg IVP stat, give slowly over* 5 *minutes*. The strength on the label is 10 *mg/mL*, and the directions state to dilute to 5 *mL* of sterile water.
    (a) How many *milliliters* of this narcotic analgesic will be withdrawn from the vial?
    (b) How many *milliliters* will be administered every 30 *seconds?*

15. Order: *Primaxin (imipenem-cilastatin sodium) 500 mg IVPB q6h.* The recommended dosage is 15–25 *mg/kg* q6h. Is the prescribed dose of this antibiotic safe for a child who weighs 55 *pounds?*
16. Calculate the daily fluid maintenance requirements for a child who weighs 33 *kg*.
17. The prescriber ordered *Azactam (aztreonam) 1 g IV q6h* for a child who has cystic fibrosis. The recommended dosage range is 50–200 *mg/kg* q6h (maximum 8 *g/day*). Is the prescribed dose safe for a child who weighs 70 *pounds?*
18. The prescriber ordered *dopamine* 2 *mcg/kg/min IV* for a client who weighs 110 *pounds.* The label on the IV bag reads dopamine 200 *mg*/250 *mL* D5W. At what rate will you set the infusion pump in *mL/h?*
19. Order: *Solu-Cortef (hydrocortisone sodium succinate)* 150 *mg IM stat.* The strength on the label is 250 *mg*/2 *mL*. How many *milliliters* will the client receive?
20. Order: *Dynapen (dicloxacillin sodium) mg 500 mg PO q6h.* The recommended dosage range for a child with a severe infection is 50–100 *mg/kg/day* divided into doses given q6h. Is the prescribed dose of this antibiotic safe for a child who weighs 77 *pounds?*
21. The prescriber ordered *Mannitol* 12.5 *g IVP stat.* The label on the 50 *mL* vial reads 25%. How many *milliliters* of this osmotic diuretic will you prepare?
22. Order: *Norvir (ritonavir)* 250 mg/m^2 *PO B.I.D.* How many *milligrams* are required for a child who weighs 15 *kg* and is 77 *cm* tall?
23. Order: *D5W* 500 *mL IV, infuse over* 5 *hours.* Calculate the flow rate in *drops per minute.* The drop factor is 15 *gtt/mL.*
24. The prescriber ordered *Synthroid (levothyroxine sodium)* 0.05 *mg PO daily.* The strength on the label is 25 *mcg* (0.025 *mg)/tab.* Calculate how many tablets you will administer.
25. Order: *heparin 8,000 units subcut q12h.* The strength on the vial is 10,000 *units/mL.* How many *milliliters* will you administer?

Comprehensive Self-Test 3

Answers to *Comprehensive Self-Tests* 1–4 can be found in Appendix A at the back of the book.

1. The prescriber ordered *dobutamine* 10 *mcg/kg/min via continuous IV infusion* for a client who weighs 143 *pounds.* The IV is labeled D5/W 500 *mL* with dobutamine 250 *mg.* How many *micrograms* of this beta-adrenergic agent is the client receiving *per minute*?
2. Order: *Vistaril (hydroxyzine pamoate) 75 mg PO Q.I.D.* Read the label in Figure S.11 and calculate how many *milliliters* of this anxiolytic medication you will administer.

Figure S.11 Drug label for Vistaril.

SOURCE: Courtesy of Pfizer, Inc.

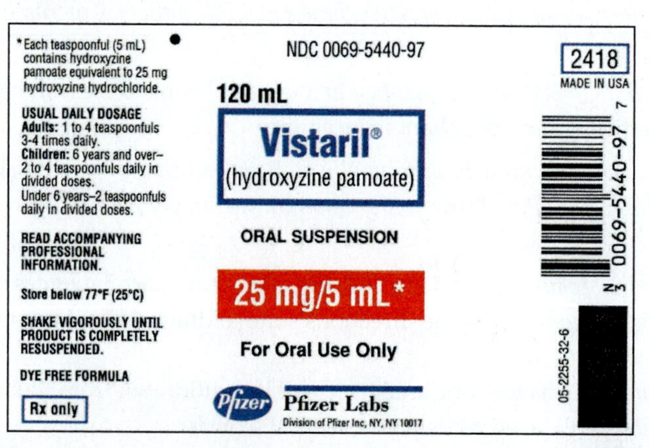

3. You need to prepare 15 *mg* of lidocaine HCl injection. The label reads lidocaine 2%. How many *milliliters* of this antiarrhythmic will you prepare?
4. Order: *heparin 4,000 units subcut q12h.* The label on the 10 *mL* multi-dose vial reads 10,000 *units per mL.* How many *milliliters* of this anticoagulant will you administer?
5. Order: *D_5NS 150 mL IV infuse in 1 hour.* The drop factor is 15 *gtt/mL.* Calculate the flow rate in *drops per minute.*
6. Calculate the number of grams of dextrose in 500 *mL* of D10W.
7. Order: *Humulin Regular insulin U-100* 8 *units and Humulin NPH insulin* 12 *units subcutaneous ac breakfast.* Read the labels in Figure S.12 and place an arrow on the syringe, indicating the total amount of insulin you will give.

Figure S.12 Drug labels for Humulin R and Humulin N and syringe.

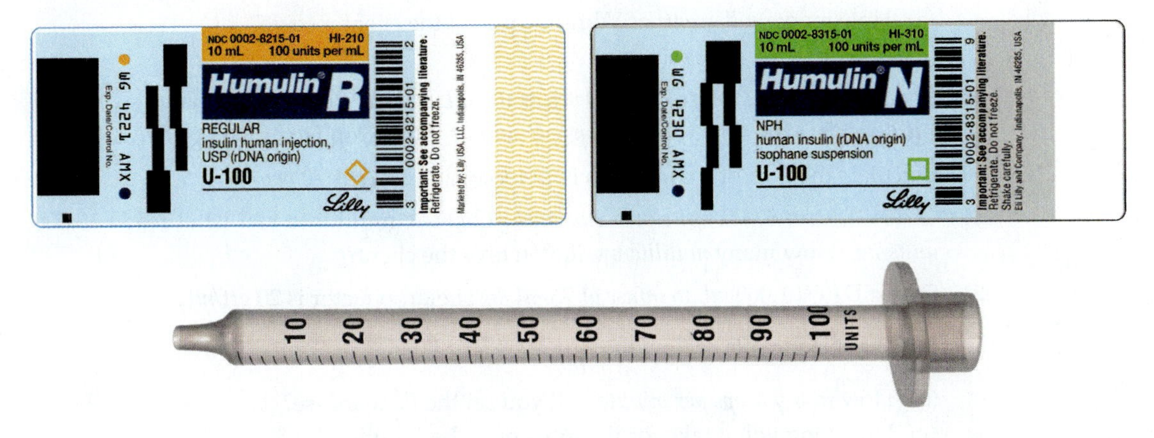

8. The prescriber ordered *Dilaudid (hydromorphone HCl) oral solution 4 mg PO q6h.* The label on the bottle states that each teaspoon contains 5 *mg* of the drug. How many milliliters of this narcotic analgesic will you administer?
9. The prescriber ordered *ampicillin sodium 500 mg IVPB q6h to infuse in* 100 *mL of D5W over* 30 *minutes.*
   (a) Calculate the flow rate in milliliters per hour.
   (b) How many grams of this antibiotic will the client receive per day?
10. Order: *Dilaudid HP (HYDROmorphone HCl)* 1 *mg subcut q2h prn moderate pain.* The strength on the vial is 4 *mg* per *mL.* Calculate the dose in milliliters of this narcotic analgesic and place an arrow on the syringe below, indicating the dose.

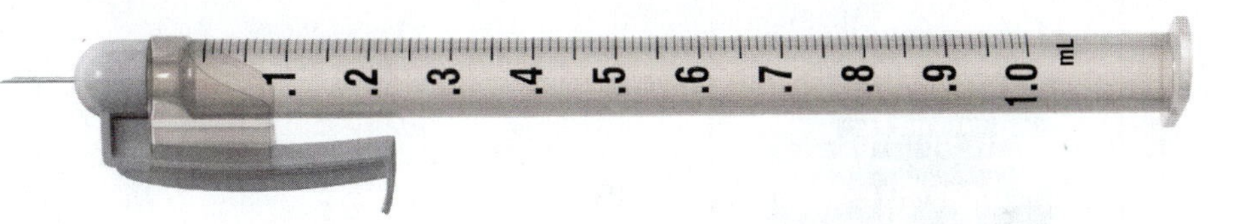

11. Order: *Adrenalin (epinephrine)* 0.3 *mg subcut stat.* The strength on the label is 1:1000. How many *milliliters* of this sympathomimetic catecholamine will you administer?
12. Order: *dopamine hydrochloride* 200 *mg in* 500 *mL NS, infuse at* 2 *mcg/ kg/min for systolic B/P less than* 90. *Increase rate up to*10 *mcg/kg/min as needed.* The client weighs 165 *pounds.* At what flow rate in *milliliters* per hour will you begin the infusion of this cardiac stimulant?
13. Order: *Humulin R insulin* 100 *units in* 100 *mL NS, infuse at* 0.2 *unit/kg/h.* The client weighs 200 *pounds.* How many *units per hour* is the client receiving?

14. Order: *ZyPREXA (olanzapine) 10 mg IM stat.* Reconstitution instructions on the 10 *mg* vial state to "add 2.1 *mL* of sterile water for injection and dissolve contents completely. Each *milliliter* will contain 5 *mg*. Solution must be used within 1 *hour.*" How many *milliliters* of this antipsychotic drug will you administer to the client?
15. Order: *Sandostatin (octreotide acetate) 0.25 mg subcut daily.* The label states that the strength is 500 *mcg* per *mL*. How many milliliters will the client receive?
16. Order: *EryPED200 (erythromycin ethylsuccinate) oral suspension 120 mg PO q4h.* The child weighs 32 *pounds* and the recommended dose is 30–50 *mg/kg/day.*
    (a) What is the minimum daily dose in *mg/day?*
    (b) What is the maximum daily dose in *mg/day?*
    (c) Is the ordered dose of this antibiotic safe?
17. *Vibramycin (doxycycline hyclate) 4.4 mg/kg IVPB daily* is ordered for a child who weighs 80 *pounds.* The premixed IV solution bag is labeled Vibramycin 200 *mg*/250 *mL* D5W to infuse in 4 *hours.*
    (a) How many *milligrams* of Vibramycin will the client receive?
    (b) Calculate the flow rate in *mL/h.*
18. Order: *Levaquin (levofloxacin) 500 mg in 100 mL D5W IVPB daily for 14 days to infuse in 1 h.* Calculate the flow rate in *drops per minute* if the drop factor is 15 *gtt/mL.*
19. Calculate the BSA of a child who is 44 *inches* and weighs 72 *pounds.*
20. Order: *heparin 5,000 units subcutaneous q12h.* The multidose vial label reads 10,000 *units/mL.* How many *milliliters* will you give the client?
21. Order: *D10W 1,000 mL to infuse at 75 mL/h.* The drop factor is 20 *gtt/mL.*
    (a) What is the rate of flow in $\frac{mL}{min}$?
    (b) How many *drops per minute* will you set the IV to infuse?
    (c) How long will it take for the infusion to be complete?
22. Calculate the total daily fluid maintenance for a child who weighs 45 *kg.*
23. Order: *Keflex (cephalexin) oral suspension 50 mg/kg PO q6h.* The label reads 125 *mg*/5 *mL.* The client weighs 33 *pounds.* How many *milliliters* will you give?
24. Read the label in Figure S.13.
    (a) How many *milligrams* of furosemide are in 1 *mL?*
    (b) How many *milliliters* of furosemide are in the *bottle?*

Figure S.13 Drug label for furosemide.

SOURCE: Pearson Education, Inc.

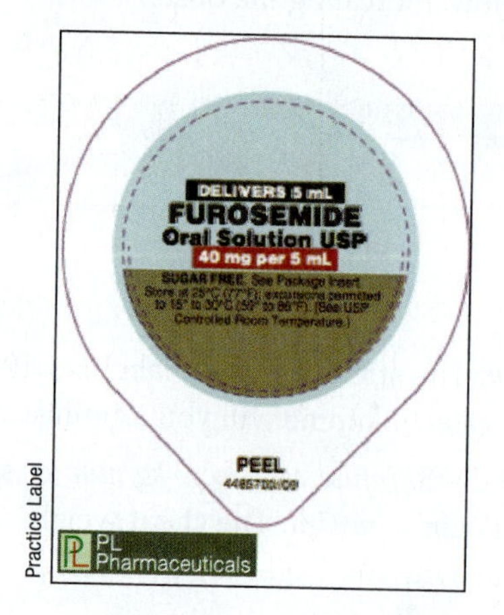

25. The prescriber ordered *ReoPro (abciximab) 0.125 mcg/kg/min IV* for a client who weighs 75 *kg.* Calculate the dosage rate in *micrograms per minute.*

Comprehensive Self-Test 4

Answers to *Comprehensive Self-Tests* 1–4 can be found in Appendix A at the back of the book.

1. A client has an IV of 250 *mL* 0.9% NaCl with 25,000 *units* of heparin infusing at 15 *mL/h*. How many *units* of heparin is the client receiving *per hour*?
2. The prescriber ordered *Phenergan (promethazine HCl) 20 mg IM q6h prn nausea* for a child who weighs 45 *kg*. The recommended dosage of this antiemetic drug is 0.25–0.5 *mg/kg* q4–6h prn (max: 25 *mg/dose*). The label reads 25 *mg/mL*.
   (a) Is the dose safe?
   (b) If the dose is safe, how many *milliliters* will you administer?
3. Order: *vinblastine sulfate 3.7 mg/m² IVP infuse over 1 minute once a week.* The client's BSA is 1.66 *m²*. The package insert states to reconstitute the 10 *mg* vial with 10 *mL* NS, yielding a concentration of 1 *mg/mL*.
   (a) How many *milligrams* of this antineoplastic drug will the client receive?
   (b) How many *milliliters* contain the dose?
   (c) How many *milliliters* will you push every 15 *seconds?*
4. Order: *midazolam HCl 20 mcg/kg IM 1 hour before surgery.* The label on the vial reads 1 *mg/mL*. How many *milliliters* of this central nervous system agent will you prepare for a client who weighs 150 *pounds?*
5. Order: *verapamil ER 120 mg PO daily each morning.* Calculate the *dose* of this calcium channel blocker in *grams*.
6. An IV of D_5RL (1,000 *mL*) is infusing at 50 *mL/h*. The infusion started at 1500 *h*. What time will it finish?
7. A client is to receive *Zofran (ondansteron HCl) 8 mg PO 30 minutes before chemotherapy, then 8 mg 8 hr later, followed by 8 mg q12h for 24 hours.* The label reads 4 *mg per tab.* How many tablets of this antiemetic drug will the client receive in total?
8. The physician ordered *methotrexate 15 mg PO daily* for a child who has leukemia. The child has a BSA of 1.10 *m²*. The recommended daily dosage is 7.5–30 *mg/m²*. Is the prescribed dose safe?
9. Order: *Haldol LA (haloperidol decanoate) 60 mg IM stat.* The strength on the label is 50 *mg/mL*.
   (a) How many *milliliters* will you administer?
   (b) Place an arrow on the syringe, indicating the dose.

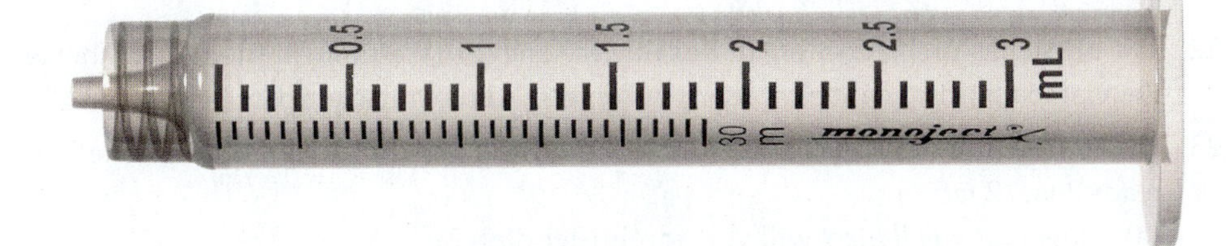

10. The prescriber ordered *Tagamet (cimetidine) 165 mg PO q6h* for a child who weighs 48 *pounds.* The recommended dose is 20–40 *mg/kg/day* divided into 4 *doses.* The strength on the label is 300 *mg* per 5 *mL*.
    (a) Calculate the minimum safe daily dose in *mg/day*.
    (b) Calculate the maximum safe daily dose in *mg/day*.
    (c) Calculate how many *milliliters* of this histamine H2-antagonist you will administer.
11. Calculate how many *grams* of lidocaine are contained in 100 *mL* of 2% lidocaine solution.

12. A client has an IV infusing at 25 *gtt/min*. How many *mL/h* is the client receiving? The drop factor is 20 *gtt/mL*.
13. Calculate the total volume and hourly IV flow rate for a child who weighs 70 *kg* and is receiving maintenance fluids.
14. Order: *nicardipine 25 mg in 250 ml NS infuse at 80 mL/h. The recommended dosage range* is 3–15 *mg/min*. Is the prescribed dose of this calcium channel blocker safe?
15. Order: *dobutamine 250 mg in 50 mL NS, infuse at 5 mcg/kg/min*. Calculate the flow rate in *milliliters per hour* of this beta-adrenergic agonist. The client weighs 165 *pounds*.
16. Order: *Humulin R insulin 100 units in 100 mL NS, infuse at 6 units per hour*. Calculate the *milliliters per hour* at which you will set the IV pump.
17. Order: *Ticar (ticarcillin disodium) 1 g IM q6h*. The package insert states to reconstitute each 1 *g* vial with 2 *mL* of sterile water for injection. Each 2.5 *mL* = 1 *g*. How many *milliliters* will you administer?
18. Order: *Indocin SR (indomethacin) 150 mg PO t.i.d. for 7 days*. The label reads Indocin SR 75-*mg* capsules.
    (a) How many capsules will you give the client for each dose?
    (b) Calculate the entire 7-*day* dosage in *grams*.
19. Order: *Colace (docusate sodium) syrup 100 mg via PEG t.i.d.* The label reads 50 *mg*/15 *mL*. How many *mL* will you give?
20. Order: *theophylline 0.8 mg/kg/h IV via pump*. The premixed IV bag is labeled theophylline 800 *mg* in 250 *mL* D5W. The client weighs 185 *pounds*. At how many *mL/h* will you set the pump?
21. Order: *cefazolin 1 g IVPB q6h, add to 50 mL D5W and infuse over 20 minutes*. Read the reconstitution information from the cefazolin label in Figure S.14.
    (a) How many milliliters of diluent will you add to the vial, so that 1 *gram* of cefazolin is contained in 5 *mL* of the solution?
    (b) Based on the answer in part (a), calculate the flow rate in *milliliters per minute*.

Figure S.14 Reconstitution information from the cefazolin label.

Total Amount of Diluent	Approximate Concentration
45 *mL*	1 *g*/5 *mL*
96 *mL*	1 *g*/10 *mL*

22. The nurse has prepared 7 *mg* of dexamethasone for IV administration. The label on the vial reads 10 *mg/mL*. How many *milliliters* did the nurse prepare?
23. Order: *Cogentin (benztropine mesylate) 2 mg IM stat and then 1 mg IM daily*. The label reads 2 *mg*/2 *mL*.
    (a) How many *milliliters* will you administer daily?
    (b) What size syringe will you use?
24. Order: $\frac{2}{3}$ *strength Sustacal 900 mL via PEG give over 8 h*. How will you prepare this solution?
25. An IV of 250 *mL* NS is infusing at 25 *mL/h*. The infusion began at 1800 *h*. What time will it be completed?

Appendices

Appendix A

Diagnostic Test of Arithmetic

1. $\frac{3}{8}$
2. 0.285
3. 6.5
4. 0.83
5. 3.2
6. 3.8
7. 0.0639
8. 500
9. 2
10. $\frac{1}{4}$ and 0.25
11. $2\frac{1}{3}$
12. $\frac{1}{25}$
13. $\frac{9}{20}$
14. 0.025
15. $\frac{18}{7}$
16. 12
17. 7.6
18. 6
19. 0.4
20. $\frac{3}{4}$

Chapter 1

Try These for Practice

1. 0.44
2. 13.5
3. $\frac{3}{5}$ 0.6 60%
$\frac{9}{20}$ 0.45 45%
$\frac{3}{100}$ 0.03 3%
4. 1
5. $\frac{1}{8}$

Exercises

1. $\frac{11}{20}$
2. 8
3. $1\frac{1}{3}$
4. $\frac{11}{28}$
5. 40
6. $1\frac{3}{5}$
7. $\frac{1}{6}$
8. 0.37
9. 0.64
10. 6.7
11. 0.015
12. 0.21
13. 0.457
14. 0.0131
15. 0.84
16. 0.6
17. 0.9
18. 0.17
19. 0.009
20. 0.27
21. 65.7
22. 0.047
23. 52.94
24. 0.02
25. $7\frac{1}{3}$, 7.3
26. $1\frac{3}{4}$, 1.8
27. $\frac{7}{9}$, 0.8
28. $\frac{1}{8}$, 0.1
29. $\frac{3}{40}$, 0.1
30. $\frac{5}{4}$, 1.3
31. $\frac{7}{8}$
32. 3
33. 9
34. 160
35. 24.74
36. 1.998
37. 0.9
38. 6
39. 100%
40. 50%

Chapter 2

Try These for Practice

1. Xanax
2. intravenous
3. indinavir sulfate
4. 100 *mg*
5. 5 *mcg/cap*

Exercises

1. Xanax
2. 4 *mL*
3. 200 *mg/cap*
4. 25 *mg*
5. indinavir sulfate

6. (a) Levemir and Tylenol with codeine #3
   (b) 1000 *h*, 1400 *h*, 1800 *h*
   (c) Four
   (d) Subcutaneous
   (e) Neurontin, digoxin, Norvasc

7. (a) metoclopramide HCl
   (b) digoxin, Mevacor, Cozaar,
   (c) two times a day
   (d) IVP (intravenous push)
   (e) Up to a maximum of 8 *times per day*

8. (a) olanzapine tablet
   (b) acute agitation associated with schizophrenia and bipolar I mania
   (c) orthostatic hypotension
   (d) 5-10 *mg* once daily
   (e) no

9.

Standard time	Military time
7:30 A.M.	0730 *h*
4:20 P.M.	1620 *h*
5:25 A.M.	0525 *h*
8:10 P.M.	2010 *h*
12:59 P.M.	1259 *h*
12 noon	1200 *h*
10:30 A.M.	1030 *h*
5:41 P.M.	1741 *h*
7:15 P.M.	1915 *h*
5:00 A.M.	0500 *h*

10. Interpret the following medication orders:
    (a) *Administer 81 milligrams of aspirin by mouth every day.*
    (b) *Administer 40 milligrams of atorvastatin (Lipitor) by mouth at bedtime.*
    (c) *Administer 500 milligrams of ampicillin by mouth immediately, then give 250 milligrams of ampicillin by mouth four times a day.*
    (d) *Administer four 300 mg cap of gabapentin (Neurontin) by mouth every 8 hours.*
    (e) *Administer 40,000 units of epoetin alfa (Epogen) subcutaneously weekly.*

11. Determine the missing component(s) for each of the following medication orders:
    (a) Dosage and frequency
    (b) Route and frequency
    (c) Dosage and route
    (d) Route
    (e) Route

12. (a) 20 *milligrams* daily
    (b) 20 *milligrams* two times a day
    (c) 20 *milligrams* every 12 *hours*
    (d) 10 *milligrams* twice a day

Chapter 3

Try These for Practice

1. 390 *sec*
2. 170 *oz*
3. $1\frac{1}{2}$ *hours*
4. 48 *drops/min*
5. 3.5 *lb/wk*

Exercises

1. 12 *min*
2. 18 *mon*
3. 66 *h*
4. 84 *oz*
5. 900 *sec*
6. 12 *in/min*
7. 60 *ft/hr*
8. 12 *hours*

9. 30 pt/h 10. 70 oz 11. $\frac{1}{4}h$ 12. 6 *cups*
13. 604,800 *sec* 14. 42 *in* 15. 4 pt/min 16. 120 qt/h
17. 240 pt/h 18. 3 in/min 19. 5.25 lb/wk 20. 4 T/day

Chapter 4

Try These for Practice

1. (a) 1,000 *mL*
   (b) 1 *cc*
   (c) 1,000 cm^3
   (d) 1,000 *g*
   (e) 1,000 *mg*
   (f) 1,000 *mcg*
   (g) 10 *mm*
   (h) 2 *pt*
   (i) 2 *cups*
   (j) 8 *oz*
   (k) 2 *T*
   (l) 3 *t*
   (m) 12 *in*
   (n) 16 *oz*

2. 15,000 *mcg* 3. 0.03 *mg* 4. 9 *g* 5. 96 *oz*

Exercises

1. 56,000 *mcg* 2. 0.6 *g* 3. 4 *qt* 4. 56 *mm*
5. 72 *oz* 6. 10,000 *mcg* 7. 0.84 *g/wk* 8. 0.65 *g*
9. 1.4 *L* 10. 42 *mg* 11. 2.65 *kg* 12. 9 *pt*
13. 80,000 *mcg* 14. 1.5 *g* 15. 125 *mcg* 16. 250 *mg*
17. 0.08 *g* 18. 0.05 *g* 19. 3.2 *kg* 20. order is safe

Cumulative Review Exercises

1. 8.8 *cm* 2. 2.5 *lb* 3. 3,700 *mL*
4. 15 *t* 5. 60 *in* 6. 140 oz/wk
7. 0.9 *g* 8. 2 *cups* 9. 10 *mg*
10. Route of administration 11. 50 *mg* 12. 50 *mg*
13. 25 *mg* 14. 1044 *h* 15. 1:40 a.m. Tuesday

Chapter 5

Try These for Practice

1. (a) 1,000 *mL*
   (b) 1,000 *g*
   (c) 1,000 *mg*
   (d) 1,000 *mcg*
   (e) 10 *mm*
   (f) 2 *pt*
   (g) 2 *cups*
   (h) 8 *oz*
   (i) 2 *T*
   (j) 3 *t*
   (k) 16 *oz*
   (l) 12 *in*
   (m) 2.5 *cm*
   (n) 2.2 *lb*
   (o) 5 *mL*
   (p) 15 *mL*
   (q) 30 *mL*
   (r) 240 *mL*
   (s) 500 *mL*
   (t) 1,000 *mL*
   (u) 2, 6, 30
   (v) 2, 4, 32, 1,000

2. 158 *cm* 3. 1 *t* 4. 240 *mL* 5. $2\frac{1}{2}$ *quarts*

Exercises

1. 20 *mL*
2. 240 *mL*
3. 3 *T*
4. $\frac{1}{2}$ *cup*
5. 68.2 *kg*
6. 1 *t*
7. 2 *in*
8. 8 *T*
9. 4 *oz*
10. 23 *full t*
11. 6 *ft* 2 *in*
12. 0.2 *g*
13. 6 *lb* 13 *oz*
14. 1 *t*
15. 2 *tab*
16. 40 *oz*
17. 0.325 *g*
18. Thomas
19. 31 *doses*
20. 191 *kg*

Cumulative Review Exercises

1. 80 *kg*
2. 0.08 *g*
3. 2,000 *mL*
4. 0.12 *L*
5. 2,273 *g*
6. 1$\frac{1}{2}$ *pt/day*
7. 105 *mL/wk*
8. 0.84 *g*
9. 1330 *h*
10. No
11. 2035 *hours*
12. 20 *mL/h*
13. 8 *mg*
14. No
15. 3 *cm*

Chapter 6

Case Study

1. E, 1 *tab*
2. K, 4 *cap*
3. H, 1 *tab*
4. 2 *tab*
5. 6 *cap*
6. J, 2,600 *mg*
7. A, 1 *tab*

Practice Reading Labels

1. 250 *mg per* 5 *ml*; 15 *mL*
2. 125 *mg per* 5 *mL*; 20 *mL*
3. 350 *mg per tab*; 1 *tab*
4. 500 *mg*/125 *mg per tab*; 2 *tab*
5. 20 *mg/mL*; 6 *mL*
6. 100 *mg*/5 *mL*; 10 *mL*
7. 15 *mg per* ER *tab*; 1 *tab*
8. 100 *mg per* 5 *mL*; 10 *mL*
9. 30 *mg per tab*; 2 *tab*
10. 100 *mg*/5 *mL*; 4*t*
11. 200 *mg per* 5 *mL*; 10 *mL*
12. 1 *mg per cap*; 2 *cap*
13. 250 *mg*/5 *mL*; 10 *mL*
14. 2.5 *mg*/325 *mg per tab*; 2 *tab*
15. 5 *mg per tab*; 2 *tab*
16. 10 *mg/mL*; 12 *mL*
17. 80 *mg per mL*; 7.5 *mL*
18. 250 *mg per tab*; 1 *tab*
19. 125 *mg per* 5 *mL*; 4 *mL*
20. 4 *mg per tab*; 3 *tab*
21. 250 *mg per cap*; 2 *cap*
22. 250 *mg per* 5 *mL*; 10 *mL*
23. 600 *mg*/42.9 *mg per* 5 *mL*; 10 *ml*
24. 600 *mg per tab* 2 *tab*
25. 10 *mg/mL*; 10 *mL*
26. 5 *mg*/12.5 *mg per tab*; 2 *tab*
27. 0.5 *mg per tab*; 2 *tab*
28. 20 *mg per cap*; 3 *cap*
29. 50 *mg*/1,000 *mg per tab*; 2 *tab*
30. 600 *mg per tab*; 2 *tab*
31. 1,000 *mg*/20 *mg per tab*; 2 *tab*
32. 400 *mg*/80 *mg per tab*; 2 *tab*
33. 125 *mg*/5 *mL*; 20 *mL*
34. 125 *mg per* DR *tab*; 2 *tab*
35. 2 *mg*/5 *mL*; 15 *mL*
36. 500 *mg per* ER *tab*; 2 *tab*

37. 25 *mg per cap*; 2 *cap*
38. 100 *mg/mL*; 28 *mL*
39. (600 *mg*) 8 *mEq per cap*; 2 *cap*
40. 50 *mg/5 mL*; 5 *mL*
41. 80 *mg/20 mg per mL*; 2 *mL*
42. 200 *mg per tab*; 3 *tab*
43. 20 *mg per tab*; 3 *tab*
44. 2.5 *mg/tab* ; 2 *tab*
45. 150 *mcg per* buccal film; 1 buccal film
46. 75 *mg per tab*; 4 *tab*
47. 5 *mg per tab*; 2 *tab*
48. 5 *mg per tab*; 3 *tab*
49. 2.5 *mg per tab*; 2 *tab*
50. 125 *mg/5 mL*; 20 *mL*

Try These for Practice

1. 1.75 m^2
2. 2 *t*
3. 20 *mL*
4. 2.1 *g*
5. 15 *mL*

Exercises

1. 3 *tab*
2. 4 *t*
3. 2.2–2.6 *mg/day*
4. No, it is an overdose.
5. 2 *t*
6. 1.92 m^2
7. Yes, the order of 200 *mg/day* is in the recommended range.
8. 2.4 *g*
9. 3 *cap/day*
10. 9 *mL*
11. 2 *tab*
12. 0.25 *mL*
13. 1 *tab*
14. Prescribed dose is not safe, contact the prescriber
15. 28.8 *g*
16. 2.20 m^2
17. 26.6 *mL*
18. 2 *cap*
19. 1 *cap*
20. 2 *tab*

Cumulative Review Exercises

1. 60 *mL*
2. 20 *kg*
3. 30 *pt*
4. 4.7 *cm*
5. 4 *mL*
6. 2 *tab*
7. 20 *mL*

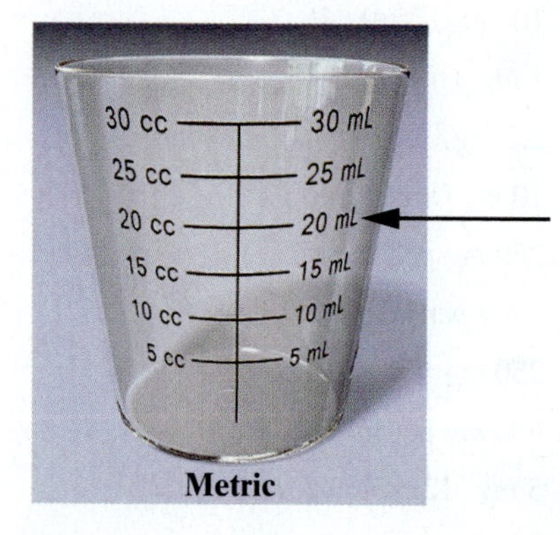

8. 3.3 *mL*
9. 2.19 m^2
10. Tristan
11. 20 *mL*
12. 22.5 *mL*
13. 0207 *h*
14. 6 *kg*
15. 4 *tab*

Chapter 7

Case Study 7.1

1. (a) 0.4 *mL*
   (b) the 1-*mL* syringe

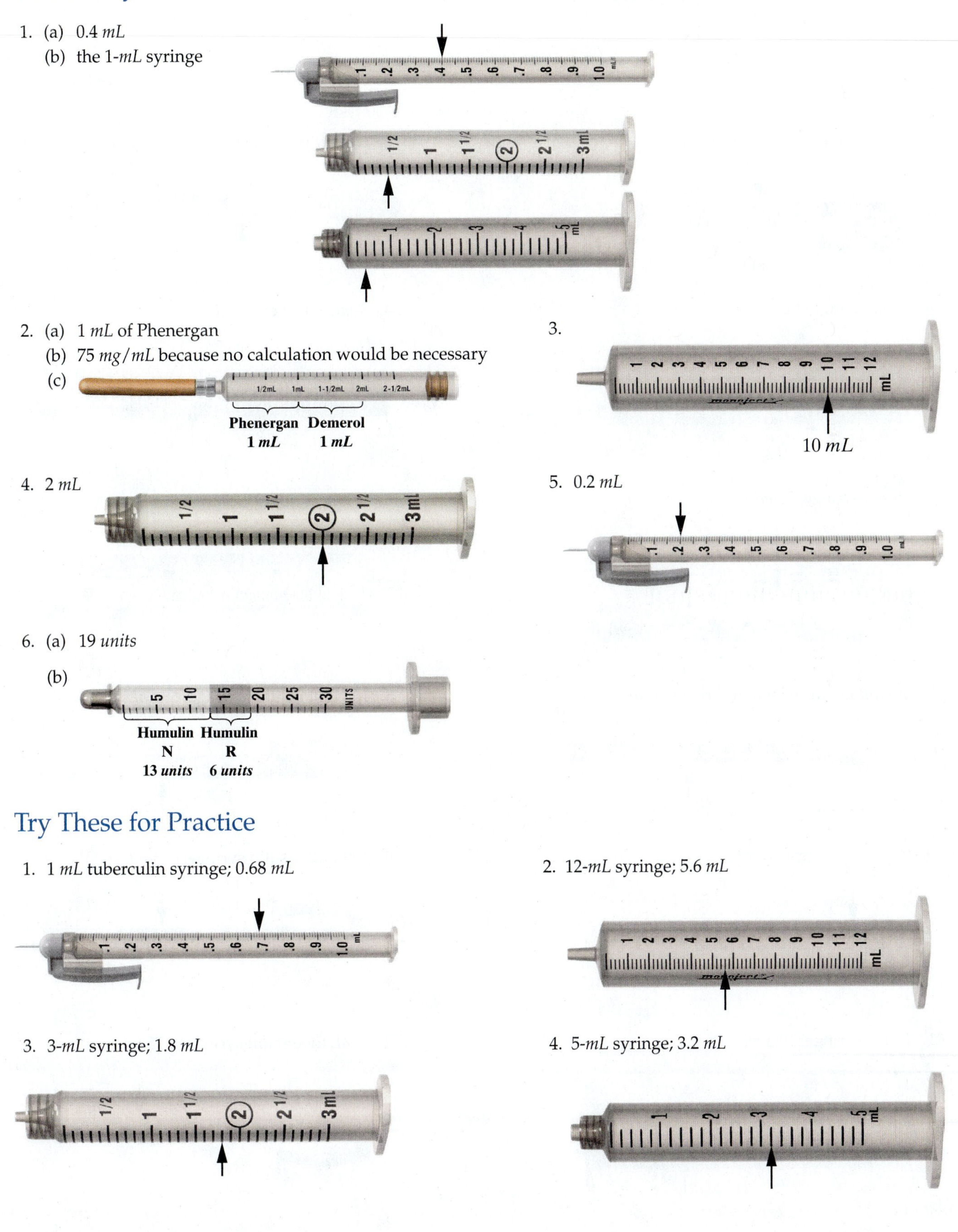

2. (a) 1 *mL* of Phenergan
   (b) 75 *mg/mL* because no calculation would be necessary
   (c)

3.

4. 2 *mL*

5. 0.2 *mL*

6. (a) 19 *units*
   (b)

Try These for Practice

1. 1 *mL* tuberculin syringe; 0.68 *mL*

2. 12-*mL* syringe; 5.6 *mL*

3. 3-*mL* syringe; 1.8 *mL*

4. 5-*mL* syringe; 3.2 *mL*

5. 2 *mL*

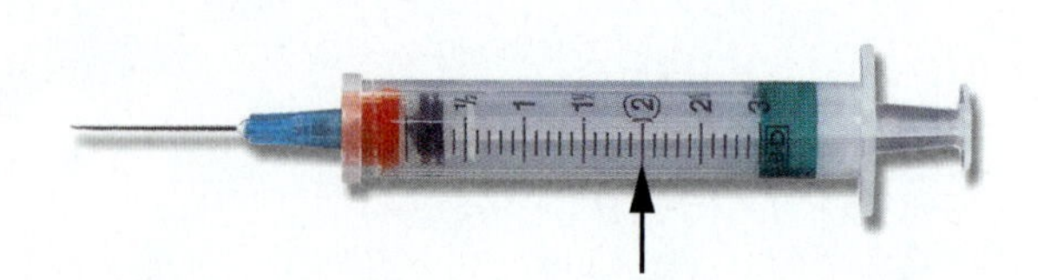

Exercises

1. 1-*mL* tuberculin syringe; 0.45 *mL*

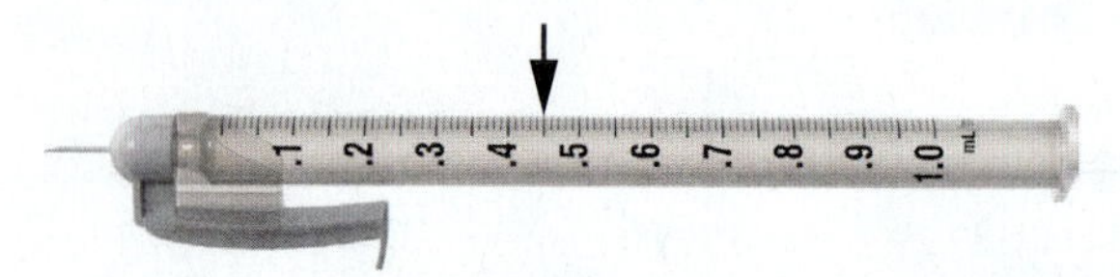

2. 30-*unit* Lo-Dose insulin syringe; 17 *units*

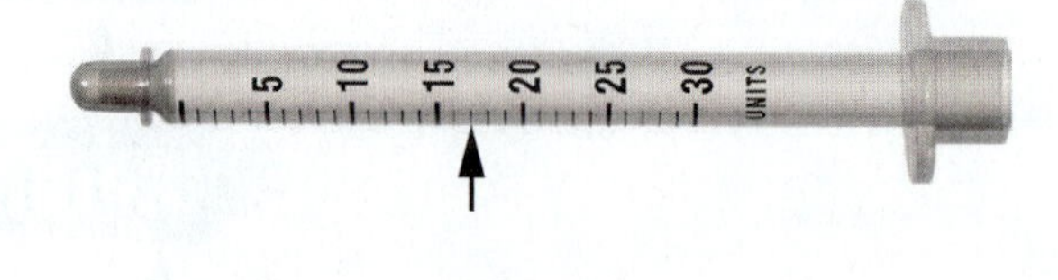

3. 5-*mL* syringe; 1.8 *mL*

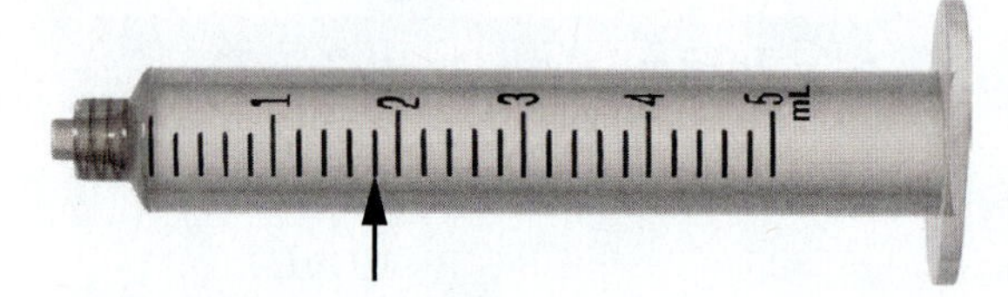

4. 3-*mL* syringe; 1.8 *mL*

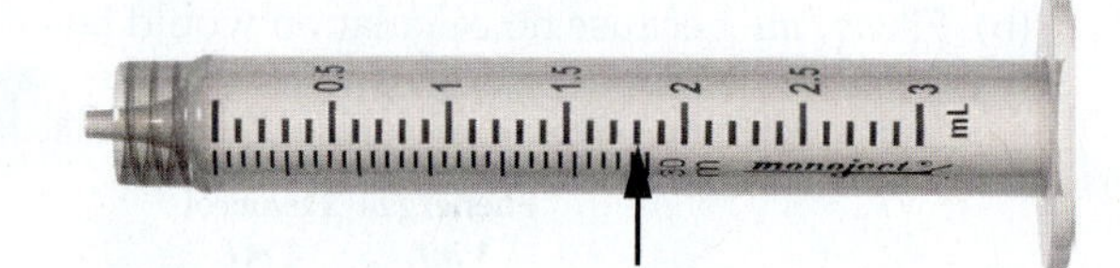

5. 35-*mL* syringe; 18 *mL*

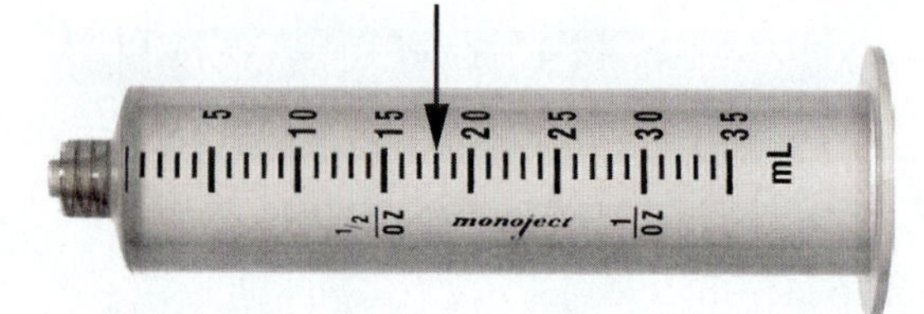

6. 12-*mL* syringe; 9.2 *mL*

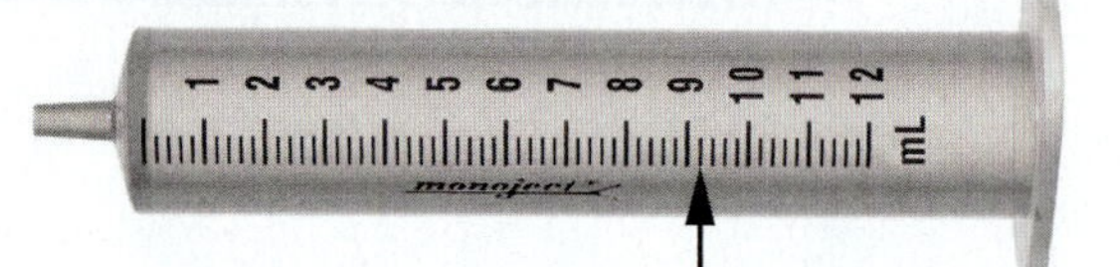

7. 50-*unit* Lo-Dose insulin syringe; 33 *units*

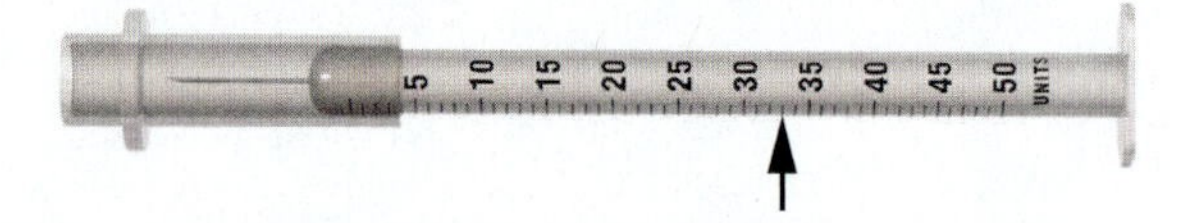

8. 100-*unit* insulin syringe; 66 *units*

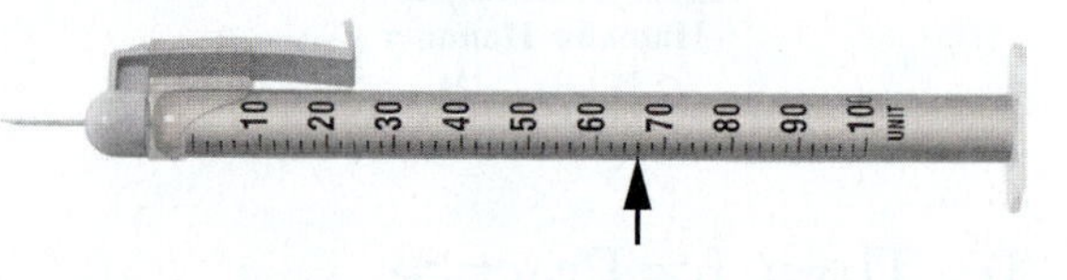

9. 0.5-*mL* syringe; 0.09 *mL*

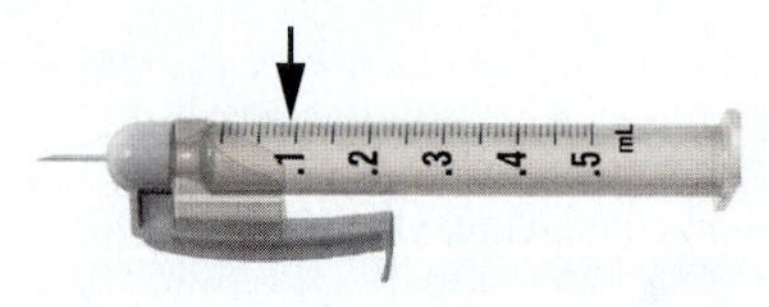

10. 100-*unit* insulin syringe; 67 *units*

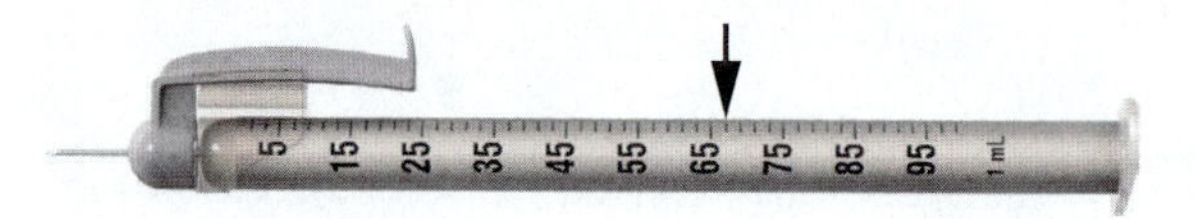

11. 12-*mL* syringe; 10.4 *mL*

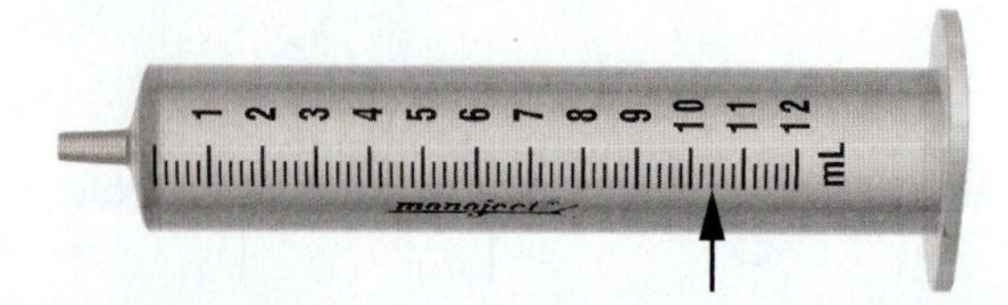

12. 1-*mL* tuberculin syringe; 0.75 *mL*

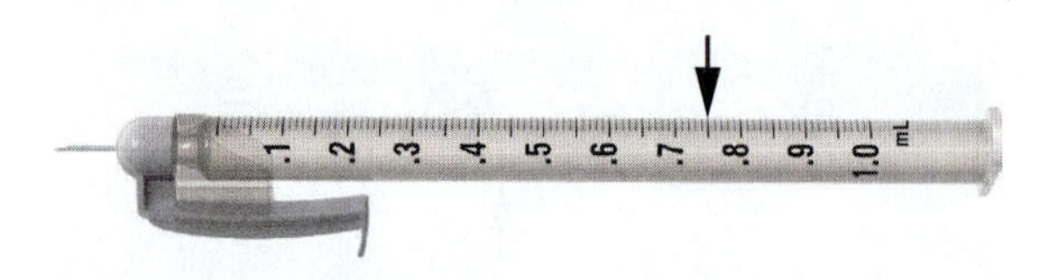

13. 12-*mL* syringe; 11.2 *mL*

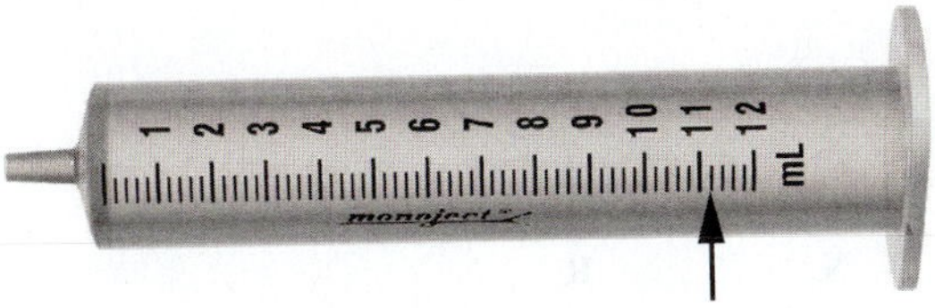

14. 35-*mL* syringe; 24 *mL*

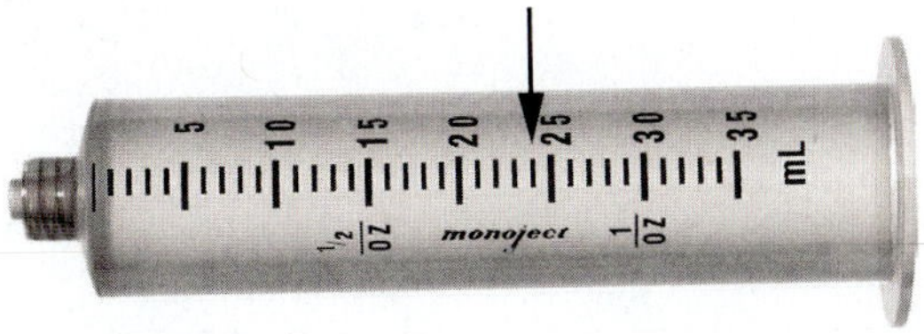

15. 2.4 *mL*

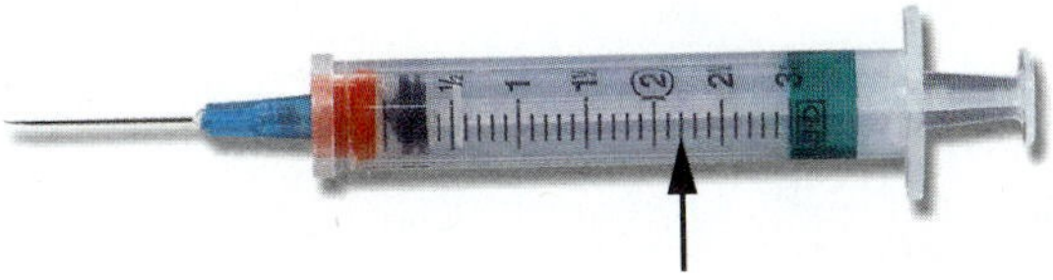

16. 22 *units*

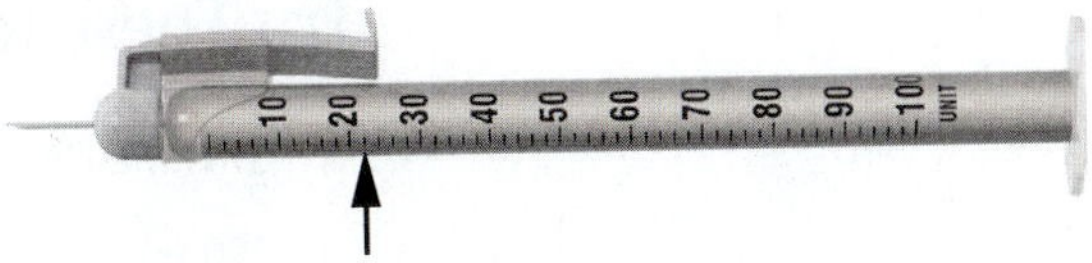

17. 1.6 *mL*

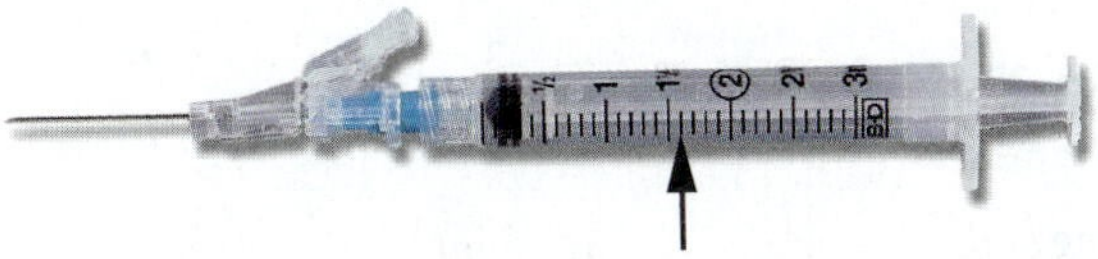

18. 0.4 *mL*

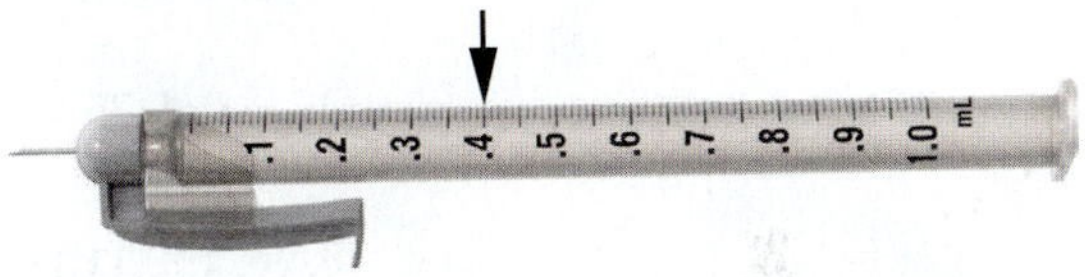

19. 4 *units*

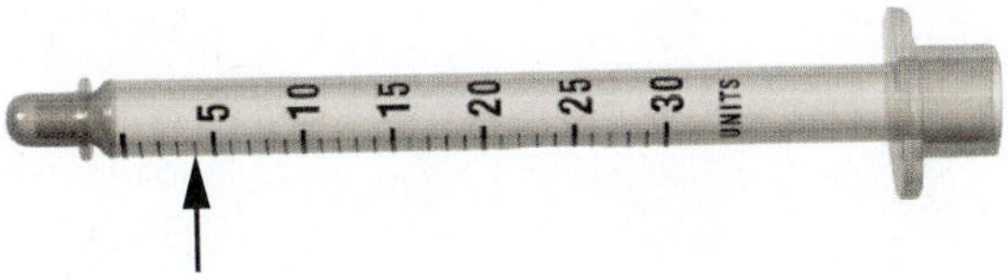

20. 1.5 *mL*

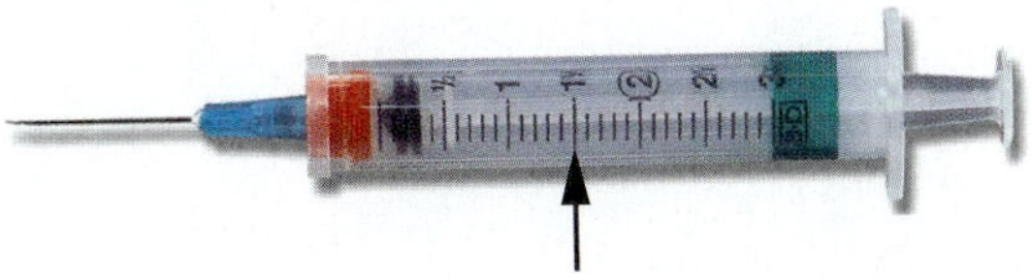

Cumulative Review Exercises

1. (a) no insulin (b) 2 *units* (c) notify MD stat
2. 4 *mL*
3. 4 *mL*
4. 2 *mL*
5. 4 *mL*
6. 2 *t*
7. 0.68 *g*
8. 90.9 *kg*
9. 3 *tab*
10. 1 *g*
11. 0.5 *mL*, 1 *mL* syringe
12. 1.98 m^2
13. 30 *unit* Lo-Dose syringe, 23 *units* in total
14. 1.5 *mL*, 3 *mL* syringe
15. 1 *mL*, 1 *mL* syringe

Chapter 8

Case Study 8.1

1. label (a) 1 *tab*
2. label (f) 1 *tab*
3. 1 *tab*
4. 2 *tab*
5. 240 *mL/d*
6. 0.5 *mL*

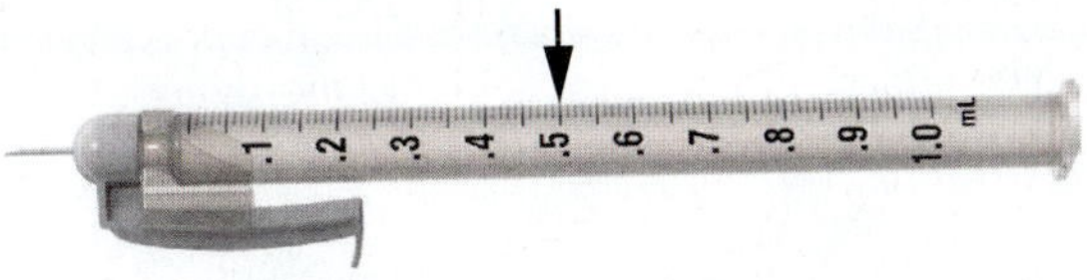

7. Withdraw 10 *units* of Humulin R insulin, then into the same syringe withdraw 34 *units* of Humulin N insulin for a total of 44 *units*.

Humulin N
Humulin R

8. 4.5 *g*

Try These for Practice

1. $\frac{1}{5}$, 1:5, 20%
2. $\frac{2}{5}$, 2:5, 40%
3. 8 *g*
4. 200 *mL*
5. 10%

Exercises

1. $\frac{1}{4}$, 1:4, 25%
2. $\frac{3}{8}$, 3:8, 37.5%
3. $\frac{3}{50}$, 3:50, 6%
4. $\frac{1}{3}$, 1:3, 33.3%
5. 40 *mg/mL*
6. 6 *mL*
7.

Ratio	Fraction	Percent
1:5	$\frac{1}{5}$	20%
1:4	$\frac{1}{4}$	25%
1:10	$\frac{1}{10}$	10%
1:200	$\frac{1}{200}$	0.5%
9:1,000	$\frac{9}{1,000}$	0.9%

8. 25 *g*
9. 2 *L*
10. $\frac{1}{4}$ strength
11. 9,000 *mg*
12. 40 *oz*
13. 800 *mL*
14. 80 *g*
15. Dissolve two 10-*g* tablets in water, then dilute with water to 200 *mL*
16. 2,250 *mg*
17. 60 *mg*
18. neither, both are the same
19. 10 *g*
20. 400 *mL*

Cumulative Review Exercises

1. 600 *mg*
2. $1\frac{1}{2}$ *oz*
3. 50 *kg*
4. 4.5 *cm*
5. 16 *oz*
6. 3.5 *lb/wk*
7. 0830 *h* Wednesday
8. 3.5 *mL*
9. 40 *mg*
10. 15 *mcg*
11. 1525 *h*
12. 42 *mL/h*
13. yes
14. 12 *mg*
15. 1.86 m^2

Chapter 9

Case Study 9.1

1. (a) 0.63 *mL*
   (b) Use a 1-*mL* syringe
2. (a) 1.5 *mL*
   (b) Use a 3-*mL* syringe
3. (a) 15.9 *mL*
   (b) Use a 20-*mL* syringe
4. 2.5 *mL*
5. (a) label (d)
   (b) 1 *tablet*
6. 1 *tab*
7. 15 *mL*
8. (a) Label i
   (b) 4 *tab*
9. $\frac{1}{2}$ *tab*
10. 60 *mg/day*

Try These for Practice

1. 1.4 *mL*
2. 1.6 *mL*
3. 4 *mL*
4. 1 *mL*
5. 0.99 *mL*

Exercises

1. 0.5 *mL*
2. 0.92 *mL*
3. 0.65 *mL*
4. 2.6 *mL*
5. 0.8 *mL*
6. (a) 0.5 *mL*
   (b) use a 1-*mL* syringe

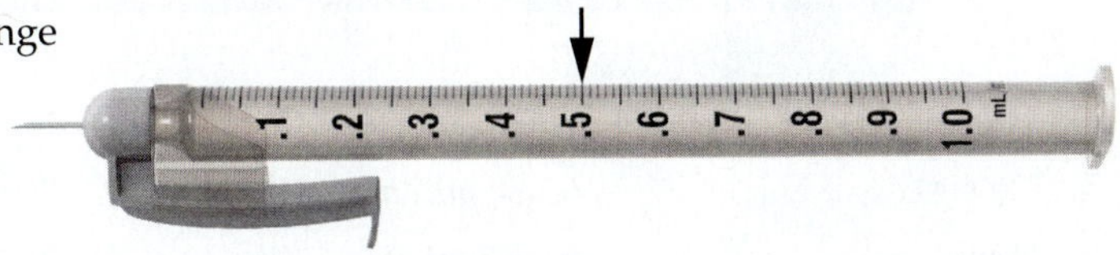

7. (a) 2.6 *mL*
   (b) use a 3-*mL* syringe

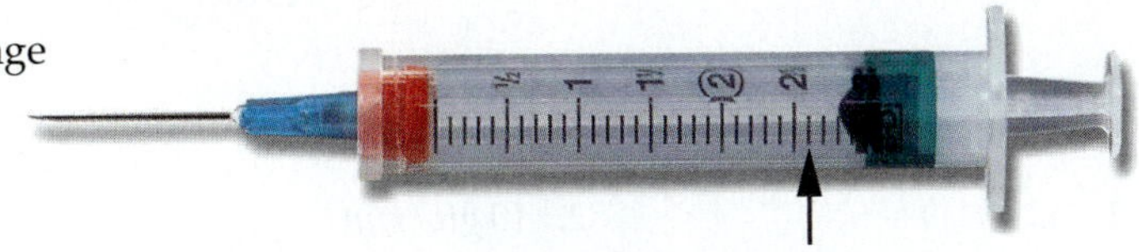

8. (a) 0.18 *mL*
   (b) 0.5 *mL*
9. (a) 0.38 *mL*
   (b) 0.5 *mL*
10. (a) 1.5 *mL*
    (b) 3 *mL*
11. (a) 2 *mL*
    (b) 3 *mL*
12. (a) 0.91 *mL*
    (b) 1 *mL*
13. (a) 2 *mL*
    (b) 16 *mL*
14. (a) 480 *mcg*/0.8 *mL* vial because 1.5 *mL* is too large a volume for a subcut
    (b) 0.76 *mL*
15. 2 *mL*
16. 1.1 *mL*
17. (a) 12 *units*;
    (b) 30 *unit* Lo-dose insulin syringe
18. 4 *units*
19. (a) minimum 1.9 *mg*;
    (b) maximum 4.8 *mg*
20. 3 *mL*

Cumulative Review Exercises

1. 150 *kg*
2. 4.5 *g*
3. No, it is an overdose.
4. 2.14 m^2
5. 0.5 *mL*
6. dexamethasone sodium phosphate
7. 4 *mg/mL*
8. IV, IM, intra-articular, soft tissue, or intralesional
9. 0.75 *mL*
10. 30 *mL*
11. 1,800 *mg*
12. 6 *mL*
13. 3 *cap*
14. (a) 2 *mL*;
    (b) 3 *mL* syringe
15. (a) 3,409 *units*;
    (b) 0.85 *mL*
    (c) 1 *mL* tuberculin syringe

Chapter 10

Case Study 10.1

1. 0.8 *mL*
2. 90 *mcgtt/min*
3. 0.21 *mL*
4.

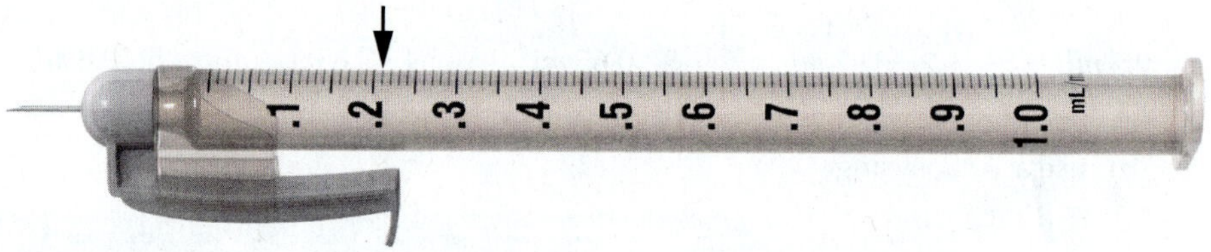

5. 126 *mg/day*
6. 80 *mL/h*
7. 2,160 *mL*
8. 24 *mL*
9. 6.7 *mL*
10. 785.5 *mL*

Try These for Practice

1. 42 *mL/h*
2. 10 *gtt/min*
3. 300 *mL*
4. 1935 *h*
5. 120 *mL*

Exercises

1. $63 \frac{mL}{h}$
2. 125 *mcgtt/min*
3. 28 *gtt/min*
4. 30 *mL/h*
5. 80 *mL*
6. 42 *mL/h*
7. 28 *gtt/min*
8. (a) 133 *mL/h*
   (b) 250 *mL/h*
   (c) no 88% increase
9. 11:32 P.M. the same day
10. 8 *h*

11. 240 *mL*
12. 480 *mL*
13. (a) 28 *gtt/min*
    (b) 33 *gtt/min*
    (c) Yes, 18% increase
14. 22.5 *mL*
15. 6 am Tuesday
16. 264 *mL*
17. 0800 *h* the same day
18. 1:38 P.M. the same day
19. (a) 17 *gtt/min*
    (b) 21 *gtt/min*
    (c) No
20. 100 *mL*

Cumulative Review Exercises

1. 165 *cm*
2. 4 *oz*
3. 85 *kg*
4. 56 *mm*
5. 1655 *h*
6. 4,500 *mg*
7. 2.5%
8. 1.91 m^2
9. 40 *mg/mL*
10. 27.3 *mg*
11. b
12. It is safe; 3 *tab*
13. 7.5 *mL*
14. 3 *mL*
15. 19 *mL/h*

Chapter 11

Case Study11.1

1. 125 *mL/h*
2. 0.75 *mL*
3. 0.25 *mL*
4. 0.71 *mL*
5. 26 *gtt/min*
6. 170 *mL/h*
7. (a) 300 *mL/h*
   (b) 25 *mL/h*
8. 3 *mL/h*
9. 90 *mU/h*
10. 0.5 *mL*

Try These for Practice

1. 100 *mL/h*, 5 *mg/min*
2. (a) 600 *mL/h*
   (b) 50 *mg/min*
3. 0825 *h* the same day
4. 33 *mL/h*
5.

	Dosage Rate	Flow Rate
initial	0.2 mg/min	30 mL/h
	0.24 mg/min	36 mL/h
	0.28 mg/min	42 mL/h
	0.32 mg/min	48 mL/h
	0.36 mg/min	54 mL/h
max	0.4 mg/min	60 mL/h

Exercises

1. 56 *gtt/min*
2. 320 *mcg/min*
3. 60 *mL/h*
4. 1 *mg/min*
5. (a) 25 *mL*
   (b) 23.9 *mL*
   (c) 448 *mL/h*
   (d) 30.3 *mg/min*
6. 33 *mg/min*

7. 17 *mcgtt/min*

8. (a) 0.4 *mL*
(b) 1 *mL/min*
(c) 0.5 *mL*
(d) 12 *sec*

9. (a) 500 *mg*
(b) 50 *mL*

10. 20 *mg/min*

11. 44 *mg/min*

12. 20 *min*

13. 12.5 *mL*

14. (a) 36 *mL/h*
(b)

Dosage Rate	Flow Rate
3 *mcg/min* (initial)	36 *mL/h*
5 *mcg/min*	60 *mL/h*
7 *mcg/min*	84 *mL/h*
9 *mcg/min*	108 *mL/h*
11 *mcg/min* (maximum)	132 *mL/h*

15. 400 *mcg/min*

16. 4 *mg/min*

17. 104 *mL/h*, 10 *mg/min*

18. (a) 15 *mL*
(b) 15 *mL*
(c) 0.83 *mg/min*

19. 36.7 *mg/mL*

20. 2.5 *mL*

Cumulative Review Exercises

1. 3.4 *mL*

2. 10 *lb* 8 *oz*

3. 0.22 *mL*

4. 2 m^2

5. No, it is not safe.

6. (a) 563 *mg*
(b) 7 *mL*
(c) 27 *mL/h*
(d) 2.3 *mg/min*

7. 4.2 *cm*

8. 15 *mL*

9. (a) 3.9 *mL*
(b) 3.8 *mL*

10. 1 *tab*

11. 50 *mg*

12. not safe; contact the prescriber

13. 500 *mcg*

14. 4.9 *mL*

15. 10 *gtt/min*

Chapter 12

Case Study 12.1

1. 1,600 *mL* DFM

2. add 18.2 *mL*, give 2.5 *mL*

3. 103 *mL/h*

4. Yes, the dose is safe.

5. 0.62 *mL* (rounded down)

6. 3 *cap* label (f)

7. 1,000 *mcg*

8. 1 *tab*

9. 9.3 *mL* (rounded down)

10. 5 *mL* label (d)

11. 176 *mcg/day*

Try These for Practice

1. Yes, it is safe; administer 50 *mg*.

2. Yes, it is safe.

3. 1 *t*

4. 5 *mL*

5. 9.1 *mL*

Exercises

1. 15 mL
2. Yes, it is safe.
3. No, it is an overdose
4. 0.08 mL
5. 450 mg/d
6. 9.8 mL
7. 56 mL/h
8. 4.3 mL
9. 11.7 mL
10. (a) 68 mg
    (b) 500 mL/h
11. 2 vials, withdraw 5 mL
12. 0.5 mL
13. 26 mL
14. 1 mL/min
15. 35 mL/h
16. 3 mL
17. (a) 318- 795 mg/day
    (b) yes
    (c) 3 mL
18. 0.52 mL, 1 mL syringe
19. 33 mL/h
20. 0.43 mL

Cumulative Review Exercises

1. 4.2 cm
2. 9 g
3. 30 gtt/min
4. 2.25 mg/min
5. 0.5 mL
6. 68 mL/h
7. 10 h
8. 0.375 mg
9. 2 mg
10. 2.24 m^2
11. 900 $units/h$
12. 125 mL/h
13. Add 6 oz of water to 18 oz of Isomil to make 24 oz of $\frac{3}{4}$ strength Isomil for the 24 h period.
14. 6.25 mL
15. 0.8 mg

Answers to the Comprehensive Self-Tests

Comprehensive Self-Test 1

1. 0.3 g of Omnicef
2. 5 mL of Kaletra
3. (a) 1 mL
   (b) 0.25 mL
4. (a) 0.67 mL
   (b) 1-mL syringe
5. 24 mg/h
6. 1 *capsule* of Depakene
7. (a) 25 mL
   (b) 0.5- or 1-mL syringe
8. 9.1 mg
9. 27.3 *units*
10. 158 mL/h
11. (a) yes
    (b) 200 mL/h
12. 50 $mcgtt/min$
13. 12.2 mL
14. 1,626 mL/d
15. 50 *doses*
16. (a) 4 mg/mL
    (b) 40 mg/h
    (c) 0.17 mg/min
17. 15.9 mL

18. (a) No, the dose is not safe; it is not enough
    (b) Do not give the medication, contact the prescriber

19. (a) 0.03 *mL*
    (b) 1 *mL*

20. (a) 4.5 *g*
    (b) 311 *mL/h*

21. (a) Yes, the dose is safe; it is between the minimum dose of 375 *mg* and the maximum dose of 750 *mg*.
    (b) 16 *mL*

22. 2 *vials*

23. 2.2 *mL*

24. (a) 0.75 *mL*
    (b) at least $1\frac{1}{2}$ *minutes*

25. 200 *units/h*

Comprehensive Self-Test 2

1. 10 *mL*

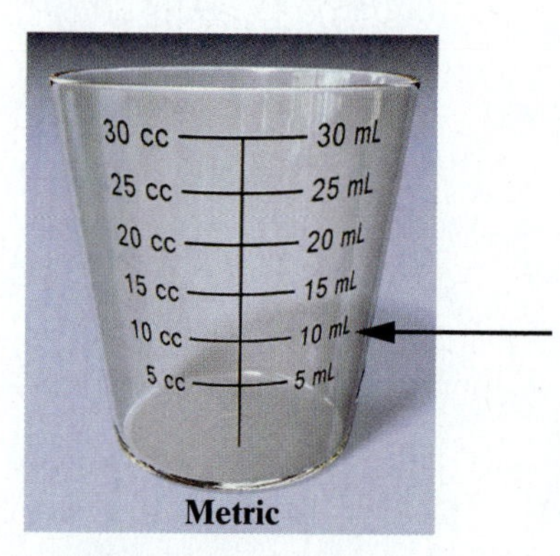

2. (a) 5 *mL*
   (b) 2.5 *mL q30 sec*

3. 7 *g* of Zovirax

4. 1 *mL* of ampicillin

5. (a) Yes, it is safe
   (b) 7.5 *mL*

6. 2 *mg*

7. 0.29 *mL*

8. (a) yes
   (b) 2.4 *mL*

9. 17 *gtt/min*

10. 28 *tab*

11. 25 *mL/h*

12. 2,500 *units/h*

13. 3 *units/h*

14. (a) 0.4 *mL*
    (b) 0.5 *mL*

15. yes

16. 1,760 *mL/d*

17. No, the dose is too low; contact the prescriber

18. 7.5 *mL/h* of dopamine

19. 1.2 *mL* of Solu-Cortef (hydrocortisone sodium succinate)

20. Yes, the prescribed dose is safe

21. 50 *mL* of Mannitol

22. 141.6 *mg* of Norvir (ritonavir)

23. 25 *gtt/min* of D5W

24. 2 *tab* of Synthroid (levothyroxine)

25. 0.8 *mL* of heparin

Comprehensive Self-Test 3

1. 650 *mcg/min*
2. 15 *mL*
3. 0.75 *mL*
4. 0.4 *mL*
5. 38 *gtt/min*
6. 50 *g*
7.
8. 4 *mL*
9. (a) 200 *mL/h*
   (b) 2 *g/d*
10. 0.25 *mL*
11. 0.3 *mL*
12. 22.5 *mL/h*
13. 18 *units/h*
14. 2 *mL*
15. 0.5 *mL*
16. (a) 436 *mg/d*
    (b) 727 *mg/d*
    (c) yes
17. 160 *mg*, 50 *mL/h*
18. 25 *gtt/min*
19. 1 m^2
20. 0.5 *mL*
21. 1.25 *mL/min*, 25 *gtt/min*, 13 *hours* 20 *minutes*
22. 2,000 *mL*
23. 30 *mL*
24. 10 *mg*, 60 *mL*
25. 21 *mL/h*

Comprehensive Self-Test 4

1. 1,500 *units/h*
2. (a) Yes, the dose is safe
   (b) 0.8 *mL*
3. (a) 6 *mg*
   (b) 6 *mL*
   (c) 1.5 *mL* every 15 *sec*
4. 1.4 *mL*
5. 0.12 *g*
6. 1100 *h* the next day
7. 8 *tab*
8. yes
9. (a) 1.2 *mL*
   (b)
10. (a) 436 *mg/d*
    (b) 872 *mg/d*
    (c) 2.75 *mL*
11. 2 *g*
12. 75 *mL/h*
13. 2,500 *mL/d*, 104 *mL/h*
14. no
15. 4.5 *mL/h*
16. 6 *mL/h*
17. 2.5 *mL*
18. 2 *cap*, 3.15 *g*
19. 30 *mL*
20. 21 *mL/h*
21. 45 *mL*, 2.75 *mL/h*
22. 0.7 *mL*
23. 3-*mL* syringe
24. Take 600 *mL* of Sustacal and dilute to 900 *mL*
25. 0400 *h* the next day

Appendix B

FDA and ISMP Lists of Look-Alike Drug Names with Recommended Tall Man Letters

Since 2008, ISMP has maintained a list of drug name pairs and trios with recommended, **bolded** tall man (uppercase) letters to help draw attention to the dissimilarities in look-alike drug names. The list includes mostly generic-generic drug name pairs, although a few brand-brand or brand-generic name pairs are included. The U.S. Food and Drug Administration (FDA) list of drug names with recommended tall man letters was initiated in 2001 with the agency's Name Differentiation Project (www.ismp.org/sc?id=520).

While numerous studies between 2000 and 2016 have demonstrated the ability of tall man letters alone or in conjunction with other text enhancements to improve the accuracy of drug name perception and reduce errors due to drug name similarity,[1-9] some studies have suggested that the strategy is ineffective.[10-12] The evidence is mixed due in large part to methodological differences and significant study limitations. Nevertheless, while gaps still exist in our full understanding of the role of tall man lettering in the clinical setting, there is sufficient evidence to suggest that this simple and straightforward technique is worth implementing as one among numerous strategies to mitigate the risk of errors due to similar drug names. To await irrefutable, scientific proof of effectiveness minimizes and undervalues the study findings and anecdotal evidence available today[13] that support this important risk-reduction strategy. As such, the use of tall man letters has been endorsed by ISMP, The Joint Commission (recommended but not required), the U.S. Food and Drug Administration (as part of its Name Differentiation Project), as well as other national and international organizations, including the World Health Organization and the International Medication Safety Network (IMSN).[14]

Table 1 provides an alphabetized list of FDA-approved established drug names with recommended tall man letters.

Table 1 FDA-Approved List of Generic Drug Names with Tall Man Letters

Drug Name with Tall Man Letters	Confused With
aceta**ZOLAMIDE**	aceto**HEXAMIDE**
aceto**HEXAMIDE**	aceta**ZOLAMIDE**
bu**PROP**ion	bus**PIR**one
bus**PIR**one	bu**PROP**ion
chlorpro**MAZINE**	chlorpro**PAMIDE**
chlorpro**PAMIDE**	chlorpro**MAZINE**

Table 1

Drug Name with Tall Man Letters	Confused With
clomi**PHENE**	clomi**PRAMINE**
clomi**PRAMINE**	clomi**PHENE**
cyclo**SERINE**	cyclo**SPORINE**
cyclo**SPORINE**	cyclo**SERINE**
DAUNOrubicin	**DOXO**rubicin
dimenhy**DRINATE**	diphenhydr**AMINE**
diphenhydr**AMINE**	dimenhy**DRINATE**
DOBUTamine	**DOP**amine
DOPamine	**DOBUT**amine
DOXOrubicin	**DAUNO**rubicin
glipi**ZIDE**	gly**BURIDE**
gly**BURIDE**	glipi**ZIDE**
hydr**ALAZINE**	hydr**OXY**zine – **HYDRO**morphone
HYDROmorphone	hydr**OXY**zine – hydr**ALAZINE**
hydr**OXY**zine	hydr**ALAZINE** – **HYDRO**morphone
medroxy**PROGESTER**one	methyl**PREDNIS**olone - methyl**TESTOSTER**one
methyl**PREDNIS**olone	medroxy**PROGESTER**one - methyl**TESTOSTER**one
methyl**TESTOSTER**one	medroxy**PROGESTER**one - methyl**PREDNIS**olone
mito**XANTRONE**	Not specified
ni**CAR**dipine	**NIFE**dipine
NIFEdipine	ni**CAR**dipine
predniso**LONE**	predni**SONE**
predni**SONE**	predniso**LONE**
risperi**DONE**	r**OPINIR**ole
r**OPINIR**ole	risperi**DONE**
sulf**ADIAZINE**	sulfi**SOXAZOLE**
sulfi**SOXAZOLE**	sulf**ADIAZINE**
TOLAZamide	**TOLBUT**amide
TOLBUTamide	**TOLAZ**amide
vin**BLAS**tine	vin**CRIS**tine
vin**CRIS**tine	vin**BLAS**tine

SOURCE: FDA and ISMP Lists of Look-Alike Drug Names with Recommended Tall Man Letters from Institute for Safe Medication Practices. Copyright © 2016 by Institute for Safe Medication Practices. Used by permission of Institute for Safe Medication Practices.

Table 2 provides an alphabetized list of additional drug names with recommendations from ISMP regarding the use and placement of tall man letters. This is not an official list approved by FDA. It is intended for voluntary use by healthcare practitioners, drug information vendors, and medication technology vendors. Any product label changes by manufacturers require FDA approval.

To promote standardization regarding which letters to present in uppercase, ISMP follows a tested methodology whenever possible called the CD3 rule.[15] The methodology suggests working from the left of the drug name first by capitalizing all the characters to the right once 2 or more dissimilar letters are encountered, and then, working from the right, returning 2 or more letters common to both words to lowercase letters. When the rule cannot be applied because there are no common letters on the right side of the name, the methodology suggests capitalizing the central part of the word only. When application of this rule fails to lead to the best tall man lettering option (e.g., makes names appear too similar, makes names hard to read based on pronunciation), an alternative option is considered.

ISMP suggests that the **bolded**, tall man lettering scheme provided by FDA and ISMP for the drug name pairs listed in **Tables 1** and **2** be followed to promote consistency.

Table 2 ISMP List of Additional Drug Names with Tall Man Letters***

Drug Name with Tall Man Letters	Confused With
ALPRAZolam	**LOR**azepam – clonaze**PAM**
a**MIL**oride	am**LODIP**ine
am**LODIP**ine	a**MIL**oride
ARIPiprazole	**RABE**prazole
AVINza*	**INV**anz*
aza**CITID**ine	aza**THIO**prine
aza**THIO**prine	aza**CITID**ine
car**BAM**azepine	**OX**carbazepine
CARBOplatin	**CIS**platin
ce**FAZ**olin	cefo**TE**tan – cef**OX**itin – cef**TAZ**idime – cef**TRIAX**one
cefo**TE**tan	ce**FAZ**olin – cef**OX**itin – cef**TAZ**idime – cef**TRIAX**one
cef**OX**itin	ce**FAZ**olin – cefo**TE**tan – cef**TAZ**idime – cef**TRIAX**one
cef**TAZ**idime	ce**FAZ**olin – cefo**TE**tan – cef**OX**itin – cef**TRIAX**one
cef**TRIAX**one	ce**FAZ**olin - cefo**TE**tan - cef**OX**itin - cef**TAZ**idime
Cele**BREX***	Cele**XA***
Cele**XA***	Cele**BREX***
chlordiaze**POXIDE**	chlorpro**MAZINE****
chlorpro**MAZINE****	chlordiaze**POXIDE**
CISplatin	**CARBO**platin
clo**BAZ**am	clonaze**PAM**
clonaze**PAM**	clo**NID**ine – clo**ZAP**ine – clo**BAZ**am – **LOR**azepam
clo**NID**ine	clonaze**PAM** - clo**ZAP**ine – Klono**PIN***
clo**ZAP**ine	clonaze**PAM** – clo**NID**ine
DACTINomycin	**DAPTO**mycin
DAPTOmycin	**DACTIN**omycin
DEPO-Medrol*	**SOLU**-Medrol*
diaze**PAM**	dil**TIAZ**em
dil**TIAZ**em	diaze**PAM**
DOCEtaxel	**PACL**itaxel
DOXOrubicin**	**IDA**rubicin
DULoxetine	**FLU**oxetine – **PAR**oxetine
e**PHED**rine	**EPINEPH**rine
EPINEPHrine	e**PHED**rine
epi**RUB**icin	eri**BUL**in
eri**BUL**in	epi**RUB**icin
fenta**NYL**	**SUF**entanil
flavox**ATE**	fluvoxa**MINE**
FLUoxetine	**DUL**oxetine – **PAR**oxetine
flu**PHENAZ**ine	fluvoxa**MINE**
fluvoxa**MINE**	flu**PHENAZ**ine - flavox**ATE**
guai**FEN**esin	guan**FACINE**
guan**FACINE**	guai**FEN**esin
Huma**LOG***	Humu**LIN***
Humu**LIN***	Huma**LOG***
hydr**ALAZINE****	hydro**CHLORO**thiazide – hydr**OXY**zine**
hydro**CHLORO**thiazide	hydr**OXY**zine** – hydr**ALAZINE****

** Brand names always start with an uppercase letter. Some brand names incorporate tall man letters in initial characters and may not be readily recognized as brand names. An asterisk follows all brand names on the ISMP list.*

*** These drug names are also on the FDA list.*

**** The ISMP list is not an official list approved by FDA. It is intended for voluntary use by healthcare practitioners and drug information and technology vendors. Any manufacturers' product label changes require FDA approval.*

Table 2

Drug Name with Tall Man Letters	Confused With
HYDROcodone	oxy**CODONE**
HYDROmorphone**	morphine – oxy**MOR**phone
HYDROXYprogesterone	medroxy**PROGESTER**one**
hydr**OXY**zine**	hydr**ALAZINE**** – hydro**CHLORO**thiazide
IDArubicin	**DOXO**rubicin** – idaru**CIZU**mab
idaru**CIZU**mab	**IDA**rubicin
in**FLIX**imab	ri**TUX**imab
INVanz*	**AVIN**za*
ISOtretinoin	tretinoin
Klono**PIN***	clo**NID**ine
La**MIC**tal*	Lam**ISIL***
Lam**ISIL***	La**MIC**tal*
lami**VUD**ine	lamo**TRI**gine
lamo**TRI**gine	lami**VUD**ine
lev**ETIRA**cetam	lev**OCARN**itine – levo**FLOX**acin
lev**OCARN**itine	lev**ETIRA**cetam
levo**FLOX**acin	lev**ETIRA**cetam
LEVOleucovorin	leucovorin
LORazepam	**ALPRAZ**olam – clonaze**PAM**
medroxy**PROGESTER**one**	**HYDROXY**progesterone
met**FORMIN**	metro**NIDAZOLE**
methazol**AMIDE**	meth**IMA**zole – met**OL**azone
meth**IMA**zole	met**OL**azone - methazol**AMIDE**
met**OL**azone	meth**IMA**zole – methazol**AMIDE**
metro**NIDAZOLE**	met**FORMIN**
metyra**PONE**	metyro**SINE**
metyro**SINE**	metyra**PONE**
mi**FEPRIS**tone	mi**SOPROS**tol
mi**SOPROS**tol	mi**FEPRIS**tone
mito**MY**cin	mito**XANTRONE****
mito**XANTRONE****	mito**MY**cin
Nex**AVAR***	Nex**IUM***
Nex**IUM***	Nex**AVAR***
ni**CAR**dipine**	ni**MOD**ipine – **NIFE**dipine**
NIFEdipine**	ni**MOD**ipine – ni**CAR**dipine**
ni**MOD**ipine	**NIFE**dipine** – ni**CAR**dipine**
Novo**LIN***	Novo**LOG***
Novo**LOG***	Novo**LIN***
OLANZapine	**QUE**tiapine
OXcarbazepine	car**BAM**azepine
oxy**CODONE**	**HYDRO**codone – Oxy**CONTIN*** – oxy**MOR**phone
Oxy**CONTIN***	oxy**CODONE** – oxy**MOR**phone
oxy**MOR**phone	**HYDRO**morphone** – oxy**CODONE** – Oxy**CONTIN***
PACLitaxel	**DOCE**taxel
PARoxetine	**FLU**oxetine – **DUL**oxetine
PAZOPanib	**PONAT**inib

** Brand names always start with an uppercase letter. Some brand names incorporate tall man letters in initial characters and may not be readily recognized as brand names. An asterisk follows all brand names on the ISMP list.*

*** These drug names are also on the FDA list.*

**** The ISMP list is not an official list approved by FDA. It is intended for voluntary use by healthcare practitioners and drug information and technology vendors. Any manufacturers' product label changes require FDA approval.*

(Continued)

Table 2 *(continued)*

Drug Name with Tall Man Letters	Confused With
PEMEtrexed	**PRALA**trexate
penicill**AMINE**	penicillin
PENTobarbital	**PHEN**obarbital
PHENobarbital	**PENT**obarbital
PONATinib	**PAZOP**anib
PRALAtrexate	**PEME**trexed
Pri**LOSEC****	**PRO**zac*
PROzac*	Pri**LOSEC***
QUEtiapine	**OLANZ**apine
qui**NID**ine	qui**NINE**
qui**NINE**	qui**NID**ine
RABEprazole	**ARIP**iprazole
ra**NITI**dine	ri**MANTA**dine
rif**AMP**in	rif**AXIM**in
rif**AXIM**in	rif**AMP**in
ri**MANTA**dine	ra**NITI**dine
Risper**DAL***	r**OPINIR**ole**
risperi**DONE****	r**OPINIR**ole**
ri**TUX**imab	in**FLIX**imab
romi**DEP**sin	romi**PLOS**tim
romi**PLOS**tim	romi**DEP**sin
r**OPINIR**ole**	Risper**DAL***– risperi**DONE****
Sand**IMMUNE***	Sando**STATIN***
Sando**STATIN***	Sand**IMMUNE***
s**AX**agliptin	**SIT**agliptin
SEROquel*	**SINE**quan*
SINEquan*	**SERO**quel*
SITagliptin	s**AX**agliptin – **SUMA**triptan
Solu-**CORTEF***	**SOLU**-Medrol*
SOLU-Medrol*	Solu-**CORTEF*** – **DEPO**-Medrol*
SORAfenib	**SUNI**tinib
SUFentanil	fenta**NYL**
sulf**ADIAZINE****	sulfa**SALA**zine
sulfa**SALA**zine	sulf**ADIAZINE****
SUMAtriptan	**SIT**agliptin – **ZOLM**itriptan
SUNItinib	**SORA**fenib
TEGretol*	**TREN**tal*
tia**GAB**ine	ti**ZAN**idine
ti**ZAN**idine	tia**GAB**ine
tra**MAD**ol	tra**ZOD**one
tra**ZOD**one	tra**MAD**ol
TRENtal*	**TEG**retol*
val**ACY**clovir	val**GAN**ciclovir
val**GAN**ciclovir	val**ACY**clovir
ZOLMitriptan	**SUMA**triptan
Zy**PREXA***	Zyr**TEC***
Zyr**TEC***	Zy**PREXA***

* *Brand names always start with an uppercase letter. Some brand names incorporate tall man letters in initial characters and may not be readily recognized as brand names. An asterisk follows all brand names on the ISMP list.*

** *These drug names are also on the FDA list.*

*** *The ISMP list is not an official list approved by FDA. It is intended for voluntary use by healthcare practitioners and drug information and technology vendors. Any manufacturers' product label changes require FDA approval.*

SOURCE: FDA and ISMP Lists of Look-Alike Drug Names with Recommended Tall Man Letters from Institute for Safe Medication Practices.

References

1) DeHenau C, Becker MW, Bello NM, Liu S, Bix L. Tallman lettering as a strategy for differentiation in look-alike, sound-alike drug names: the role of familiarity in differentiating drug doppelgangers. *Appl Ergon.* 2016;52:77–84.
2) Filik R, Purdy K, Gale A, Gerrett D. Drug name confusion: evaluating the effectiveness of capital ("tall man") letters using eye movement data. *Soc Sci Med.* 2004;59(12):2597–601.
3) Filik R, Purdy K, Gale A, Gerrett D. Labeling of medicines and patient safety: evaluating methods of reducing drug name confusion. *Hum Factors.* 2006;48(1):39–47.
4) Grasha A. Cognitive systems perspective on human performance in the pharmacy: implications for accuracy, effectiveness, and job satisfaction (Report No. 062100). Alexandria (VA): NACDS. 2000.
5) Darker IT, Gerret D, Filik R, Purdy KJ, Gale AG. The influence of 'tall man' lettering on errors of visual perception in the recognition of written drug names. *Ergonomics.* 2011;54(1):21–33.
6) Or CK, Chan AH. Effects of text enhancements on the differentiation performance of orthographically similar drug names. *Work.* 2014;48(4):521–8.
7) Or CK, Wang H. A comparison of the effects of different typographical methods on the recognizability of printed drug names. *Drug Saf.* 2014;37(5):351–9.
8) Filik R, Price J, Darker I, Gerrett D, Purdy K, Gale A. The influence of tall man lettering on drug name confusion: a laboratory-based investigation in the UK using younger and older adults and healthcare practitioners. *Drug Saf.* 2010;33(8):677–87.
9) Gabriele S. The role of typography in differentiating look-alike/sound-alike drug names. *Healthc Q.* 2006; 9(Spec No):88–95.
10) Schell KL. Using enhanced text to facilitate recognition of drug names: evidence from two experimental studies. *Appl Ergon.* 2009;40(1):82–90.
11) Irwin A, Mearns K, Watson M, Urquhart J. The effect of proximity, tall man lettering, and time pressure on accurate visual perception of drug names. *Hum Factors.* 2013;55(2):253–66.
12) Zhong W, Feinstein JA, Patel NS, Dai D, Feudtner C. Tall man lettering and potential prescription errors: a time series analysis of 42 children's hospitals in the USA over 9 years. *BMJ Qual Saf.* Published Online First: November 3, 2015.
13) Leape LL, Berwick MB, Bates DW. What practices will most improve safety? Evidence-based medicine meets patient safety. *JAMA.* 2002;288(4):501–7.
14) Position statement on improving the safety of international non-proprietary names of medicines (INNs). Horsham (PA): International Medication Safety Network; November 2011.
15) Gerrett D, Gale AG, Darker IT, Filik R, Purdy KJ. Tall man lettering. Final report of the use of tall man lettering to minimise selection errors of medicine names in computer prescribing and dispensing systems. Loughborough University Enterprises Ltd; 2009.

Appendix C
Commonly Used Abbreviations

To someone unfamiliar with prescription abbreviations, medication orders may look like a foreign language. To interpret prescriptive orders accurately and to administer drugs safely, a qualified person must have a thorough knowledge of common abbreviations. For instance, when the prescriber writes, "**hydromorphone 1.5 *mg* IM *q*4 *h* prn**," the healthcare professional knows how to interpret it as "hydromorphone, 1.5 *milligrams*, intramuscular, every 4 *hours*, whenever necessary." For measurement abbreviations, refer to Appendix D.

Abbreviation	Meaning
ā	before *(abante)*
ac	before meals *(ante cibum)*
ad lib	as desired *(ad libitum)*
A.M., am	morning
amp	ampule
b.i.d.	two times a day
BP	blood pressure
c̄	with
C	Celsius; centigrade
cap	capsule
CBC	complete blood count
cc	cubic centimeter
CVP	central venous pressure
D/W	dextrose in water
D5W or D5/W or D_5W	5% dextrose in water
daw	dispense as written
Dx	diagnosis
elix	elixir
ER	extended release
F	Fahrenheit
g	gram
gr	grain
GT	gastrostomy tube
gtt	drop
h, hr	hour
hs	hour of sleep; bedtime *(hora somni)*
IC	intracardiac
ID	intradermal
IM	intramuscular; intramuscularly
IV	intravenous; intravenously
IVP	intravenous push
IVPB	intravenous piggyback

Abbreviation	Meaning
kg	kilogram
KVO	keep vein open
L	liter
LA	long acting
lb	pound
LIB	left in bag, left in bottle
LOS	length of stay
MAR	medication administration record
mcg	microgram
mcgtt	microdrop
mEq	milliequivalent
mg	milligram
min	minute
mL	milliliter
mU	milliunit
NDC	national drug code
NGT	nasogastric tube
NKA	no known allergies
NKDA	no known drug allergies
NKFA	no known food allergies
NPO	nothing by mouth *(per ora)*
NS	normal saline
NSAID	nonsteroidal anti-inflammatory drug
OTC	over the counter
oz	ounce
PEG	percutaneous endoscopic gastrostomy tube
P	pulse
pc	after meals *(post cibum)*
PEJ	percutaneous endoscopic jejunostomy
PICC	peripherally inserted central catheter
P.M., pm	afternoon, evening
PO	by mouth *(per os)*

Abbreviation	Meaning
POST-OP	after surgery
PR	by way of the rectum
PRE-OP	before surgery
prn	when required or whenever necessary
Pt	patient
pt	pint
q	every *(quaque)*
qh	every hour *(quaque hora)*
q2h	every two hours
q3h	every three hours
q4h	every four hours
q6h	every six hours
q8h	every eight hours
q12h	every twelve hours
q.i.d.	four times a day *(quarter in die)*
R	respiration
R/O	rule out
Rx	prescription, treatment

Abbreviation	Meaning
$\bar{s}$	without *(sine)*
SIG	directions to the patient
SL	sublingual
SR	sustained release
stat	immediately *(statum)*
subcut	subcutaneous
supp	suppository
susp	suspension
T or tbs	tablespoon
t or tsp	teaspoon
T	temperature
t.i.d.	three times a day *(ter in die)*
tab	tablet
TPN	total parenteral nutrition
USP	United States Pharmacopeia
V/S	vital signs
wt	weight

Appendix D

Units of Measurement in Metric and Household Systems

Abbreviations			
Volume			
Metric		**Household**	
milliliter	*mL*	teaspoon	*t* or *tsp*
liter	*L*	tablespoon	*T* or *tbs*
cubic centimeter	*cc*	fluid ounce	*oz*
microdrop	*mcgtt*	pint	*pt*
drop	*gtt*	quart	*qt*
Weight			
Metric		**Household**	
microgram	*mcg*	ounce	*oz*
milligram	*mg*	pound	*lb*
gram	*g*		
kilogram	*kg*		
Length			
Metric		**Household**	
millimeter	*mm*	inch	*in*
centimeter	*cm*	foot	*ft*
meter	*m*		
Area			
Metric			
square meter	m^2		

Appendix E

Celsius and Fahrenheit Temperature Conversions

Reading and recording a temperature is a crucial step in assessing a patient's health. Temperatures can be measured using either the Fahrenheit (F) scale or the Celsius or centrigrade (C) scale. Celsius/Fahrenheit equivalency tables make it easy to convert Celsius to Fahrenheit, or vice versa. Still, it is useful to be able to make this conversion yourself.

You can use the following formulas to convert from one temperature scale to the other:

$$C = \frac{F - 32}{1.8} \text{ and } F = 1.8\,C + 32$$

For those unfamiliar with algebra, the following rules are equivalent to the algebraic formulas.

First rule: To convert to Celsius. Subtract 32 and then divide by 1.8.

Second rule: To convert to Fahrenheit. Multiply by 1.8 and then add 32.

NOTE

Temperatures are rounded to the nearest tenth.

Example E.1

Convert 102.5° *F* to *Celsius*.

Using the first rule, you subtract 32.

$$\begin{array}{r} 102.5 \\ -32.0 \\ \hline 70.5 \end{array}$$

Then you divide by 1.8.

$$\begin{array}{r} 39.17 \\ 1.8\overline{)70.5000} \end{array}$$

So, 102.5° *F* equals 39.2° *C*.

Example E.2

Convert 3° *C* to *Fahrenheit*.

Using the second rule, you first multiply by 1.8.

$$\begin{array}{r} 1.8 \\ \times\ 3 \\ \hline 5.4 \end{array}$$

Then you add 32.

$$\begin{array}{r} 5.4 \\ +32.0 \\ \hline 37.4 \end{array}$$

So, 3° *C* equals 37.4° *F*

For those unfamiliar with the Celsius system, the following rhyme might be useful:

Thirty is hot
Twenty is nice
Ten is chilly
Zero is ice

Appendix F
Diluting Stock Solutions

A stock solution is one in which a pure drug is already dissolved in a liquid. The strength of each stock solution is written on the label. If the order is for a stronger solution, you will need to prepare a new solution. However, if the order is for a weaker solution, you can dilute the stock solution to the prescribed strength. To find out how much stock solution to take, use the following formula.

$$\frac{\text{Amount prescribed} \times \text{Strength prescribed}}{\text{Strength of stock}} = \text{Amount of stock}$$

Example F.1

How would you prepare 1 *L* of a 25% solution from a 50% stock solution? Because this example does not indicate whether the drug in the solution is a solid or a liquid in its pure form, you may choose either *grams* or *milliliters* for the amount of the pure drug, and the choice will have no effect on the answer. *Grams* are chosen in the following solution.

Given: Amount prescribed: 1,000 *mL*

Strength prescribed: 25% or $\frac{25\ g}{100\ mL}$

Strength of stock: 50% or $\frac{50\ g}{100\ mL}$

Find: Amount of stock: ? *mL*

$$\frac{\text{Amount prescribed} \times \text{Strength prescribed}}{\text{Strength of stock}} = \text{Amount of stock}$$

Substituting the given information into the formula, you get

$$\frac{1{,}000\ mL \times \frac{25\ g}{100\ mL}}{\frac{50\ g}{100\ mL}} = ?\ mL$$

This complex fraction may be written as a division problem as follows:

$$1{,}000\ mL \times \frac{25\ g}{100\ mL} \div \frac{50\ g}{100\ mL} = ?\ mL$$

This division problem may be changed to a multiplication problem by inverting the last fraction. Now, cancel and multiply.

$$1{,}000\ mL \times \frac{25\ \cancel{g}}{\cancel{100\ mL}} \times \frac{\cancel{100\ mL}}{50\ \cancel{g}} = 500\ mL$$

So, you would take 500 *mL* of the 50% stock solution and add water to the level of 1,000 *mL*.

Example F.2

How would you prepare 2,500 *mL* of a 1:10 boric acid solution from a 40% stock solution of this antiseptic?

Given: Amount prescribed: 2,500 *mL*

Strength prescribed: 1:10 or $\frac{1\ mL}{10\ mL}$

Strength of stock: 40% or $\frac{40\ mL}{100\ mL}$

Find: Amount of stock: ? *mL*

$$\frac{2{,}500\ mL \times \frac{1\ \cancel{mL}}{10\ \cancel{mL}}}{\frac{40\ \cancel{mL}}{100\ \cancel{mL}}} = \text{Amount of stock}$$

$$2{,}500\ mL \times \frac{1}{10} \div \frac{40}{100} = ?\ mL$$

$$\overset{250}{\cancel{2{,}500}} \times \frac{1}{\underset{1}{\cancel{10}}} \times \frac{100}{40} = 625\ mL$$

So, you would take 625 *mL* of the 40% stock solution of boric acid and add water to the level of 2,500 *mL*.

Example F.3

How would you prepare 500 *mL* of a 1:25 solution from a 1:4 stock solution of the antiseptic Argyrol?

Given: Amount prescribed: 500 *mL*

Strength prescribed: 1:25 or $\frac{1\ mL}{25\ mL}$

Strength of stock: 1:4 or $\frac{1\ mL}{4\ mL}$

Find: Amount of stock: ? *mL*

$$\frac{500\ mL \times \frac{1\ \cancel{mL}}{25\ \cancel{mL}}}{\frac{1\ \cancel{mL}}{4\ \cancel{mL}}} = \text{Amount of stock}$$

$$500\ mL \times \frac{1}{25} \div \frac{1}{4} = ?\ mL$$

$$\overset{20}{\cancel{500}}\ mL \times \frac{1}{\underset{1}{\cancel{25}}} \times \frac{4}{1} = 80\ mL$$

So, you would take 80 *mL* of a 1:4 stock solution of Argyrol and add water to the level of 500 *mL*.

Exercises

1. How would you prepare 200 mL of a 5% solution from a 20% stock solution?
2. How would you prepare 500 mL of a 1:4 solution from a 1:3 stock solution?
3. How would you prepare 1 L of a 0.45% solution from a 0.9% stock solution?
4. How would you prepare 200 mL of a 25% solution from a 35% stock solution?
5. How would you prepare 2 L of a 1:5 solution from a $\frac{1}{2}$ strength stock solution?

Answers

1. Take 50 mL of the stock solution and add water to the level of 200 mL.
2. Take 375 mL of the stock solution and add water to the level of 500 mL.
3. Take 500 mL of the stock solution and add water to the level of 1 L.
4. Take 143 mL of the stock solution and add water to the level of 200 mL.
5. Take 800 mL of the stock solution and add water to the level of 2 L.

Appendix G
Apothecary System

The apothecary system is one of the oldest systems of drug measurement. Although the apothecary system was used in the past to write prescriptions, it has largely been replaced by the metric system. Apothecary units are rarely used on drug labels, but when they are, the metric equivalents are also provided.

> **NOTE**
>
> In the apothecary system, the abbreviation or symbol for the unit is placed before the quantity (as in *drams* 8). *Ounces* are used for liquid volume in both the household and apothecary systems. To avoid errors, the abbreviations *dr* and *oz* are preferred over the formerly used abbreviations ℥ and ʒ.

Liquid Volume in the Apothecary System

The equivalents for the units of measurement for liquid volume in the apothecary system are shown in Table G.1 along with their abbreviations.

Table G.1 Common Equivalents for Apothecary Liquid Volume Units

ounce (*oz*) 1 = *drams* (*dr*) 8
dram (*dr*) 1 = *minims* 60

> **NOTE**
>
> Decimal numbers are never used in the apothecary system.

Example G.1

How many *minims* would be equivalent to *dr* $\frac{1}{6}$?

$$dr\,\frac{1}{6} = minims?$$

Because *dr* 1 = *minims* 60, the unit fraction is $\frac{minims\ 60}{dr\ 1}$

$$\frac{\cancel{dr}\ 1}{6} \times \frac{minims\ 60}{\cancel{dr}\ 1} = minims\ 10$$

So, *minims* 10 are equivalent to *dr* $\frac{1}{6}$.

Example G.2

How many *ounces* would be equivalent to *dr* 4?

$$dr\ 4 = ounces\ ?$$

Because *dr* 8 = *ounce* 1, the unit fraction is $\frac{oz\ 1}{dr\ 8}$

$$\frac{\cancel{dr}\ 4}{1} \times \frac{oz\ 1}{\cancel{dr}\ 8} = ounce\frac{1}{2}$$

So, *dr* 4 is equivalent to *oz* $\frac{1}{2}$.

Weight in the Apothecary System

The *grain* (*gr*) is the only unit of weight in the apothecary system that is used in administering medications.

Roman Numerals

Dosages in the apothecary system are sometimes written using Roman numerals. Table G.2 shows Roman numerals.

Table G.2 Roman Numerals

	Roman Numerals
1	I
2	II
3	III
4	IV
5	V
6	VI
7	VII
8	VIII
9	IX
10	X
15	XV
20	XX
$\frac{1}{2}$	ss
$1\frac{1}{2}$	iss
$7\frac{1}{2}$	viiss

Equivalents of Common Units of Measurement

Tables G.3 and G.4 list some common equivalent values for weight, volume, and length in the metric, household, and apothecary systems of measurement. Although these equivalents are considered standards, many of them are approximations.

NOTE

Here are some useful equivalents:
1 *t* = 5 *mL* = *dr* 1
2 *T* = 30 *mL* = *oz* 1 = *dr* 8

Table G.3 Equivalent Values for Units of Weight

Metric		Apothecary		Household
60 *milligrams (mg)*	=	*grain (gr)* 1		
1 *gram (g)*	=	*grains (gr)* 15		
1 *kilogram (kg)*			=	2.2 *pounds (lb)*

Table G.4 Equivalent Values for Units of Volume

Metric		Apothecary		Household
1 *milliliter (mL)*	=	*minims* 15		
5 *milliliters (mL)*	=	*dram (dr)* 1	=	1 *teaspoon (t)*
15 *milliliters (mL)*	=	*ounce (oz)* $\frac{1}{2}$	=	1 *tablespoon (T)*
30 *milliliters (mL)*	=	*ounce (oz)* 1	=	2 *tablespoons (T)*
500 *milliliters*	=	*ounces (oz)* 16	=	1 *pint (pt)*
1,000 *milliliters*	=	*ounces (oz)* 32	=	1 *quart (qt)*

Metric–Apothecary Conversions

Example G.3

Convert 40 *milligrams* to *grains*.

$$40\ mg = gr\ ?$$

Because 60 *mg* = *gr* 1, the unit fraction is $\frac{gr\ 1}{60\ mg}$

$$\frac{40\ \cancel{mg}}{1} \times \frac{gr\ 1}{60\ \cancel{mg}} = gr\frac{2}{3}$$

So, 40 *milligrams* are equivalent to *grain* $\frac{2}{3}$.

Example G.4

Convert 0.12 *milligrams* to *grains*.

$$0.12\ mg = gr\ ?$$

Because 60 *m* = *gr* 1, the unit fraction is $\frac{gr\ 1}{60\ mg}$

$$\frac{0.12\ \cancel{mg}}{1} \times \frac{gr\ 1}{60\ \cancel{mg}} = \frac{gr\ 0.12}{60} \times \frac{100}{100} = \frac{gr\ 12}{6000} = gr\frac{1}{500}$$

So, 0.12 *milligrams* are equivalent to *grain* $\frac{1}{500}$.

Example G.5

Convert 1.5 *grams* to an equivalent weight in *grains*.

$$1.5\ g = gr?$$

Because $1\ g = gr\ 15$, the unit fraction is $\frac{gr\ 15}{1\ g}$

$$\frac{1.5\ \cancel{g}}{1} \times \frac{gr\ 15}{1\ \cancel{g}} = gr\ 22.5$$

A decimal number cannot be used in the apothecary system. Therefore, 22.5 must be written in fractional form as $22\frac{1}{2}$.

So, 1.5 *grams* are equivalent to *grains* $22\frac{1}{2}$.

NOTE

Grains are apothecary units and are expressed as fractions or whole numbers. Therefore, *grains* 22.5 should be expressed as *grains* $22\frac{1}{2}$.

Example G.6

Convert *grain* $\frac{1}{300}$ to *milligrams*.

$$gr\frac{1}{300} = ?\ mg$$

Because $1\ gr = 60\ mg$, the unit fraction is $\frac{60\ mg}{gr\ 1}$

$$\frac{\cancel{gr}\ 1}{300} \times \frac{60\ mg}{\cancel{gr}\ 1} = 0.2\ mg$$

So, *grain* $\frac{1}{300}$ is equivalent to 0.2 *milligrams*.

Example G.7

Convert *grains* $7\frac{1}{2}$ to *grams*.

$$gr\ 7\frac{1}{2} = ?\ g$$

Because $gr\ 15 = 1\ g$, the unit fraction is $\frac{1\ g}{gr\ 15}$

$$\frac{\cancel{gr}\ 15}{2} \times \frac{1\ g}{\cancel{gr}\ 15} = \frac{1}{2}g = 0.5\ g$$

So, *grains* $7\frac{1}{2}$ are equivalent to 0.5 *gram*.

NOTE

Grams are metric units, so they are expressed as decimals or whole numbers. Therefore, $\frac{1}{2}$ *gram* is expressed as 0.5 *gram*.

Household-Apothecary Conversions

Example G.8

Convert *ounces* 2 to *tablespoons*.

$$oz\ 2 = ?\ T$$

Because $oz\ 1 = 2\ T$, the unit fraction is $\frac{2\ T}{oz\ 1}$

$$\frac{\cancel{oz}\ 2}{1} \times \frac{2\ T}{\cancel{oz}\ 1} = 4\ T$$

So, *ounces* 2 are equivalent to 4 *tablespoons*.

Exercises

1. $oz\ 1 = dr\ ?$
2. $dr\ 1 = minims?$
3. $dr\ 12 = oz?$
4. $dr\ 1\frac{1}{2} = minims?$
5. $oz\ 64 = dr?$
6. $dr\ 1 = ?\ t = minims\ ? = ?\ mL$
7. $oz\ 1 = ?\ T = dr\ ? = ?\ mL$
8. $1\ cup = ?\ glass = oz\ ? = ?\ pt$
9. $gr\ 1 = ?\ mg$
10. $1\ g = gr\ ?$
11. $0.006\ mg = gr?$
12. $gr\ 3\frac{3}{4} = ?\ mg$

Answers

1. $dr\ 8$
2. $minims\ 60$
3. $oz\ 1\frac{1}{2}$
4. $minims\ 90$
5. $dr\ 512$
6. $dr\ 1 = 1\ t = minims\ 60 = 5\ mL$
7. $oz\ 1 = 2\ T = dr\ 8 = 30\ mL$
8. $1\ cup = 1\ glass = oz\ 8 = \frac{1}{2}pt$
9. $60\ mg$
10. $gr\ 15$
11. $gr\ \frac{1}{10{,}000}$
12. $225\ mg$

Index

E

F

M

N

O

T

U

V